Learning Surgery

Learning Surgery
The Surgery Clerkship Manual

Editor

Stephen F. Lowry, MD, FACS, FRCS Edin (Hon.)

Professor and Chair, Department of Surgery, University of Medicine
and Dentistry of New Jersey, Robert Wood Johnson Medical School,
New Brunswick, New Jersey

Associate Editors

Rocco G. Ciocca, MD
Associate Professor, Department of Surgery, Division of Vascular
Surgery, University of Medicine and Dentistry of New Jersey, Robert
Wood Johnson Medical School, New Brunswick, New Jersey

Candice S. Rettie, PhD
Adjunct Assistant Professor, Department of Surgery, Division of
Vascular Surgery, University of Medicine and Dentistry of New
Jersey, Robert Wood Johnson Medical School, New Brunswick, New
Jersey

With 96 Illustrations

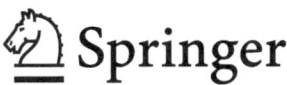

Editor:
Stephen F. Lowry, MD, FACS, FRCS Edin (Hon.)
Professor and Chair, Department of Surgery, University of Medicine and
Dentistry of New Jersey, Robert Wood Johnson Medical School, New
Brunswick, NJ 08901, USA

Associate Editors:
Rocco G. Ciocca, MD
Associate Professor, Department of Surgery, Division of Vascular Surgery,
University of Medicine and Dentistry of New Jersey, Robert Wood Johnson
Medical School, New Brunswick, NJ 08903, USA

Candice S. Rettie, PhD
Adjunct Assistant Professor, Department of Surgery, Division of Vascular
Surgery, University of Medicine and Dentistry of New Jersey, Robert Wood
Johnson Medical School, New Brunswick, NJ 08903, USA

Assistant Editor:
Micki Vodarsik
Department of Surgery, Office of the Chairman, University of Medicine and
Dentistry of New Jersey, Robert Wood Johnson Medical School, New
Brunswick, NJ 08901, USA

Library of Congress Cataloging-in-Publication Data
Learning surgery : the surgery clerkship manual / [edited by] Stephen F. Lowry,
    Rocco G. Ciocca, Candice Rettie.
        p. ; cm.
    Includes bibliographical references and index.

    1. Surgery—Handbooks,   manuals,   etc.   2. Clinical   clerkship—Handbooks,
manuals, etc.   I. Lowry, Stephen F.   II. Ciocca, Rocco G.   III. Rettie, Candice
    [DNLM: 1. Surgery—Handbooks.   2. Surgical Procedures, Operative—Hand-
books.   3. Clinical Clerkship—Handbooks. WO 39 L438 2004]
    RD37.L43 2004
    617—dc22   2004056548

Printed on acid-free paper.
ISBN-13: 978-1-4419-1978-6   e-ISBN-13: 978-0-387-28310-4

9 8 7 6 5 4 3 2 1

springeronline.com

To our students
who inspire us with their passion for learning
and
to our practicing colleagues
who share in the commitment to
providing optimal surgical care for our patients

Preface

The successful practice of surgery embraces the concept of life-long learning. Indeed, every field of surgical specialization now boasts of comprehensive textbooks which run to thousands of pages. To the newly arrived student of surgery or to the practitioner faced with the occasional surgical problem, the scope of knowledge can seem overwhelming. This book is designed to assist our colleagues endeavoring to learn the core concepts and common problems of surgical practice. We have chosen not to dwell upon the arcane aspects of surgical knowledge or technique that are the purview of the specialist. Rather, this volume is meant to provide much of the knowledge content demanded of the clerkship participant as well as the non-surgical, referring physician.

Several unique features have been utilized for this purpose. First, we have emphasized evidence-based approaches to surgical practice throughout the text. For this purpose, we have liberally (and literally) adapted evidence-based tables from the first edition of the comprehensive textbook *Surgery: Basic Science and Clinical Evidence* which I was privileged to be a coeditor with my colleagues: Drs. Jeff Norton, Randy Bollinger, Fred Chang, Sean Mulvihill, Harvey Pass, and Rob Thompson. Second, we have adapted many of the learning objectives defined by the Association for Surgical Education and outlined these at the beginning of each chapter. Many chapters are presentation focused rather than bearing the more traditional disease or organ system orientation. Each chapter is introduced by one or more brief case studies that focus upon key concepts and common presentations of the illnesses under discussion. Finally, diagnosis and management algorithms are included in most chapters to guide both the learning and doing processes.

I express my gratitude for the efforts of my colleagues in the Department of Surgery at Robert Wood Johnson Medical School who have contributed unselfishly of their knowledge in the construct of this edition. I know them personally to be master clinicians and educators in their field. There is much wisdom embedded in their contributions. I hope the reader can share in this wisdom as well as their commitment to *learning surgery*.

Stephen F. Lowry
MD, FACS, FRCS Edin (Hon.)
New Brunswick, NJ

Acknowledgments

We wish to thank Beth Campbell of Springer who helped us finish this journey and Laura Gillan who started us on the pathway. Barbara Chernow has, as always, provided us with her expert guidance and unwavering standard of excellence. The editors of *Surgery: Basic Science and Clinical Evidence* provided constant support and encouragement and the contributors to the first edition of this textbook set the standard for documenting the evidence-based practice of surgery.

Stephen F. Lowry
MD, FACS, FRCS Edin (Hon.)

Content

Part I   Introduction to Clinical Surgery in the Surgical Clerkship Setting

Contributors

Doreen M. Agnese, MD
Department of Surgical Oncology, The Arthur G. James Cancer Hospital and Richard J. Solove Research Institute, The Ohio State University, Columbus, OH, USA

Joseph G. Barone, MD
Department of Surgery/Urology, University of Medicine and Dentistry of New Jersey, Robert Wood Johnson Medical School, New Brunswick, NJ, USA

Carla Braxton, MD, MBA
Department of Surgery, University of Kansas Hospital, Kansas City, KS, USA

Gregory R. Brevetti, MD, FACS, FACC
Department of Cardiothoracic Surgery, SUNY Brooklyn, Brooklyn, NY, USA

Lucy S. Brevetti, MD
Department of Vascular Surgery, University of Medicine and Dentistry of New Jersey, Robert Wood Johnson Medical School, New Brunswick, NJ, USA

Randall S. Burd, MD, PhD
Department of Surgery, Division of Pediatric Surgery, University of Medicine and Dentistry of New Jersey, Robert Wood Johnson Medical School, New Brunswick, NJ, USA

James J. Chandler, AB, MD
Department of Surgery, University of Medicine and Dentistry of New Jersey, Robert Wood Johnson Medical School, New Brunswick, NJ, USA

Rocco G. Ciocca, MD
Division of Vascular Surgery, University of Medicine and Dentistry of New Jersey, Robert Wood Johnson Medical School, New Brunswick, NJ, USA

Siobhan A. Corbett, MD
Department of Surgery, University of Medicine and Dentistry of New Jersey, Robert Wood Johnson Medical School, New Brunswick, NJ, USA

John M. Davis, MD
University of Medicine and Dentistry of New Jersey, Robert Wood Johnson Medical School, New Brunswick, NJ *and* Department of Surgery, Jersey Shore University Medical Center, Neptune, NJ, USA

Theodore E. Eisenstat, MD
Department of Surgery, University of Medicine and Dentistry of New Jersey, Robert Wood Johnson Medical School, New Brunswick, NJ, USA

Albert Frankel, MD
Department of Surgery, University of Medicine and Dentistry of New Jersey, Robert Wood Johnson Medical School, New Brunswick, NJ, USA

Charles J. Gatt, Jr., MD
Department of Orthopaedic Surgery, University of Medicine and Dentistry of New Jersey, Robert Wood Johnson Medical School, New Brunswick, NJ, USA

Jeffrey Hammond, MD, MPH
Department of Surgery, University of Medicine and Dentistry of New Jersey, Robert Wood Johnson Medical School, New Brunswick, NJ, USA

Thomas J. Kearney, MD, FACS
Department of Surgery and the Cancer Institute of New Jersey, University of Medicine and Dentistry of New Jersey, Robert Wood Johnson Medical School, New Brunswick, NJ, USA

John E. Langenfeld, MD
Division of Cardiothoracic Surgery, University of Medicine and Dentistry of New Jersey, Robert Wood Johnson Medical School, New Brunswick, NJ, USA

David A. Laskow, MD
Department of Surgery, University of Medicine and Dentistry of New Jersey, Robert Wood Johnson Medical School, New Brunswick, NJ, USA

James W. Lim, MD
Department of Surgery, University of Medicine and Dentistry of New Jersey, Robert Wood Johnson Medical School, New Brunswick, NJ, USA

Stephen F. Lowry, MD, FACS, FRCS Edin (Hon.)
Department of Surgery, University of Medicine and Dentistry of New Jersey, Robert Wood Johnson Medical School, New Brunswick, NJ, USA

John T. Malcynski, MD, FACS, FCCP
Department of Surgery, Section of Trauma Surgery and Surgical Critical Care, University of Medicine and Dentistry of New Jersey, Robert Wood Johnson Medical School, New Brunswick, NJ, USA

Gary B. Nackman, BS, MD
Department of Surgery, University of Medicine and Dentistry of New Jersey, Robert Wood Johnson Medical School, New Brunswick, NJ, USA

J. Martin Perez, MD
Department of Surgery, University of Medicine and Dentistry of New Jersey, Robert Wood Johnson Medical School, New Brunswick, NJ, USA

Michael Perrotti, MD, FACS
Department of Surgery (Urology), Albany Medical College, Albany, NY, USA

M. Nerissa Prieto, MS, MD
Department of Surgery, University of Medicine and Dentistry of New Jersey, Robert Wood Johnson Medical School, New Brunswick, NJ, USA

Candice S. Rettie, PhD
Department of Surgery, Division of Vascular Surgery, University of Medicine and Dentistry of New Jersey, Robert Wood Johnson Medical School, New Brunswick, New Jersey

Scott R. Shepard, MD
Division of Neurosurgery, University of Medicine and Dentistry of New Jersey, Robert Wood Johnson Medical School, New Brunswick, NJ, USA

Alan J. Spotnitz, MD, MPH
Department of Surgery, University of Medicine and Dentistry of New Jersey, Robert Wood Johnson Medical School, New Brunswick, NJ, USA

John P. Sutyak, MD, EdM
Department of Surgery, Southern Illinois University School of Medicine, Springfield, IL, USA

Philip D. Wey, MD, FACS
Department of Surgery, Division of Plastic Surgery, University of Medicine and Dentistry of New Jersey, Robert Wood Johnson Medical School, New Brunswick, NJ, USA

Robert E. Weiss, MD
Department of Surgery (Urology), Department of Surgery, University of Medicine and Dentistry of New Jersey, Robert Wood Johnson Medical School, New Brunswick, NJ, USA

Susannah S. Wise, MD
Division of General Surgery, University of Medicine and Dentistry of New Jersey, Robert Wood Johnson Medical School, New Brunswick, NJ, USA

I

Introduction to Clinical Surgery in the Surgical Clerkship Setting

Perioperative Care of the Surgery Patient

Rocco G. Ciocca

Objectives

1. To describe features of a patient's clinical history that influence surgical decision making. Consider known diseases, risk factors, urgency of operation, medications, etc.
2. To discuss tools that may assist in preoperative risk assessment. Consider laboratory studies, imaging studies, etc. Include the following:
   - Pulmonary (example: exercise tolerance, pulmonary function testing)
   - Cardiovascular (ASA classification, Goldman criteria, echocardiography, thallium studies, Doppler)
   - Renal (blood urea nitrogen, creatinine dialysis history)
   - Metabolic (nutritional assessment, thyroid function).

Case

An 87-year-old man is seen in the emergency room. He is complaining of vague abdominal pain over the past few months. He has had a markedly diminished appetite with associated weight loss. During a rather cursory initial physical examination, the emergency room physician palpates a firm, slightly tender mass in the patient's right upper quadrant. A surgical consult is requested.

Introduction

One might wonder what is unique in the surgical assessment of a patient that differentiates it from any other medical evaluation. The answer is nothing and everything.

A good medical evaluation and a good surgical evaluation really should contain many of the same components. A **surgical evaluation should include a thorough history and physical exam**. Close attention to the patient's underlying medical conditions is critical and comes into play when the surgeon is trying to assess the risks for a given patient of a particular operation. This is particularly pertinent when evaluating the 87-year-old patient in the case presented here.

The **main differences between the two types of evaluations are acuity and the need to frequently make a difficult decision with limited data in the surgical scenario**. The decisions made by a surgeon frequently involve subjecting patients to a procedure that may either save their life or hasten their demise. (These decisions are not unique to surgeons but also are often experienced by interventionalists.) The question is: How can one maximize the former while minimizing the latter?

A great deal can be said for experience and time, and few would argue that the more experience one has the better one's judgment becomes. Education begets experience to some degree, and therefore it is incumbent on the budding physician to read and absorb as much material as possible. (Later chapters in this text will help you do that.) It is extremely important to correlate the material that one has read to clinical cases. Therefore, the art of medicine is a constant learning and rereading of given topics.

Since patients' presentations can be confusing, **it is necessary for the physician to develop a systematic evaluation of a patient**. This systematic organized approach, in fact, forms the essence of the surgical approach. The organization of preoperative preparation forms the basis of this chapter. What does it take to safely and properly prepare a patient for an operation?

As a surgical resident frequently called to the emergency room or clinic to evaluate a patient with a "surgical" problem, always approach the patient with the following questions in mind: **(1) Does the patient need to be operated on?** If the answer is no, then the problem is not surgical and appropriate medical therapy or consultation can be set up. If the answer is yes, then the question is: When? Emergently, urgently, or can the operation be done electively? This leads to the next question: **(2) Does the patient need to be admitted to the hospital?** If the answer is yes, then the appropriate therapy needs to be started (intravenous fluid, antibiotics, standard preoperative testing) (See **Algorithm 1.1.**).

History and Physical Examination

The foundation of both medicine and surgery begins with a thorough history and physical examination. Often, they are the only necessary diagnostic evaluations prior to surgery. We have become dependent on myriad diagnostic studies that, while at times helpful, are sometimes unnecessary, expensive, overutilized, time-consuming, and, occasionally, dangerous. A well-performed history and a physical exam have none of these disadvantages.

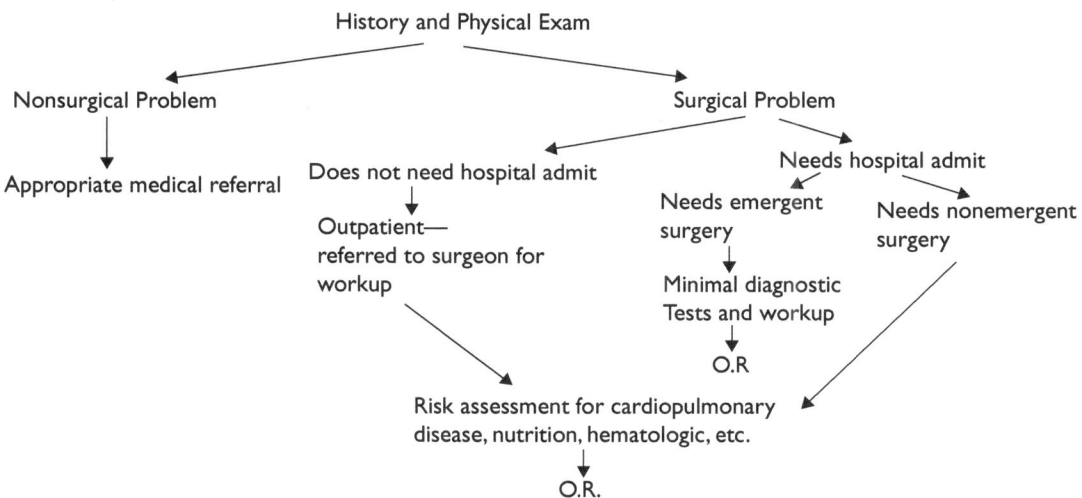

Algorithm 1.1. Patient presents with complaint.

While specifics of the history and physical exam differ depending on the specific complaint of the patient and are discussed in greater detail in the ensuing chapters, there are a few constants to keep in mind. **The first constant is to take some time to listen to the patient.** As simple and as seemingly easy as this is to do, it is something that all physicians, on occasion, fail to do. It can be time-consuming, since patients do not always clearly and concisely articulate their problem. It is important, however, to let patients explain their problem. Based on the chief complaint or complaints, the physician then can ask more directed questions to illuminate the problem further. Very often, the physician needs to act like a good newspaper reporter, concisely obtaining the What, Where, When, and How of a problem: What is the problem? Where does it hurt? When did it start? How does it make you feel? How bad is it? How did it happen? The answers to these questions are important and frequently diagnostic.

Another critically important component of the patients' history includes a **listing of their past medical history**, usually starting with whether or not they have ever experienced earlier episodes of their current problem. If they have, then a description of the type and success of the therapy may be helpful. One should inquire, in a systematic manner, about any history of major medical illnesses. Particular attention to any history of previous surgery is of obvious import. The patient's past medical history in the case presented at the beginning of this chapter is critically important.

Family history may be important and pertinent to patients' presentation. The patients' **social history** also may provide insight into their problem. This certainly will give the examiner a clearer understanding of what the patient does and what sort of familial or social support the patient may have. Always inquire, in as nonjudgmental manner as possible, about social habits such as smoking, alcohol intake, illegal drug use, and sexual practices. As delicate and uncomfortable as these questions may be to both the patient and examiner, the answers are clinically and at times critically important.

Patients sometimes lack insight regarding their health. **A thorough listing, including dosages, of medications** is necessary and frequently provides insight into the patient's underlying medical conditions. Inclusion of any adverse reactions or allergies to medications is of obvious import.

The physical exam should begin with an overall observation of the patient. Does he/she appear robust and healthy or frail and chronically ill? This so-called "eyeball" test, while difficult to scientifically validate, can be helpful, particularly when the patient's presenting problem requires urgent or emergent surgical intervention. The exam should be thorough and systematic. **It is helpful to examine the patient in a head-to-toe manner.** This makes intuitive sense, and, if one performs the examination in the same order each time, the likelihood of missing an important physical finding decreases. Avoid the tendency to examine first, and sometimes only, the body area for which the patient has a complaint. The specifics of the physical exam will be dealt with more thoroughly in later chapters.

Risk Assessment

Cardiac

It is estimated that more than 3 million patients with coronary artery disease undergo surgery every year in the United States. Of these patients, approximately 50,000 patients sustain a perioperative myocardial infarction (MI). The mortality of a perioperative MI is high, roughly 40%. **The challenge is proper assessment of an individual for coronary artery disease and whether preoperative intervention actually improves the patient's final outcome or merely shifts morbidity and mortality to another procedure or healthcare professional.** This is one area where evidence-based medicine has made an attempt to provide healthcare professionals/surgeons with guidelines (**Tables 1.1, 1.2, 1.3,** and **1.4**).

The above-cited data and tables are helpful. **Elective surgery should be avoided or postponed in patients who have suffered a recent MI or who have unstable angina.** These patients are at greatest risk of having an MI perioperatively within the first 30 days of their initial MI (27%). This risk decreases over the ensuing weeks and drops to about 5% after 6 months. Shorter delays may be acceptable for patients who must be operated upon sooner than 6 months after an MI. For these patients, full hemodynamic monitoring may be beneficial.

One cannot emphasize enough the need to optimize the patient's underlying cardiac conditions prior to surgery. Congestive heart failure should be controlled, blood pressure optimized, cardiac rhythm stabilized, and medications fine-tuned. Frequently, the surgeon must handle these issues, but a cardiologist or primary care physician can be extremely helpful in achieving these goals.

Table 1.1. Risk stratification parameters and criteria for cardiac events following noncardiac surgery.

Parameter	Low risk	Intermediate risk	High risk
Clinical characteristic	Advanced age	Mild angina	Myocardial infarction within previous 7–30 days
	Abnormal ECG (LVH, LBBB, ST-T abnormalities)	Prior myocardial infarction	Unstable or severe angina
	Atrial fibrillation or other nonsinus rhythm	Previous or compensated congestive heart failure	
	Low functional capacity (climb <1 flight stairs with bag of groceries)	Diabetes mellitus	
	Hypertension		
	History of stroke		
Type of operation (partial list) Low: <1% cardiac risk; High: >5% cardiac risk.	Endoscopic procedures	Carotid endarterectomy	Emergent major surgery
	Skin or skin structure operation (i.e., groin hernia, breast procedure)	Head and neck procedure	Aortic and other major vascular procedures, including peripheral procedures
	Cataract excision	Intraabdominal procedures	Long procedures/major fluid shifts or blood loss
		Intrathoracic procedures	
		Orthopedic surgery	
		Prostate surgery	
Characteristics of ECG stress test (i.e., treadmill)	No ischemia	Ischemia at moderate-level exercise (heart rate 100–130)	Ischemia at low-level exercise (heart rate <100)
	Ischemia only at high-level exercise (heart rate >130)	ST depression >0.1 mV	ST depression >0.1 mV
	ST depression >0.1 mV	Typical angina	Typical angina
	Typical angina	Three or four abnormal leads	Five or more abnormal leads
	One or two abnormal leads	Persistent ischemia 1–3 min after exercise	Persistent ischemia >3 min after exercise

Source: Reprinted from Barie PS. Perioperative management. In: Norton JA, Bollinger RR, Chang AE, et al, eds. Surgery: Basic Science and Clinical Evidence. New York: Springer-Verlag, 2001, with permission.

Table 1.2. Cardiac risk index system (CRIS).

Factors	Points
History	
Age >70 years	5
Myocardial infarction <6 months ago	10
Aortic stenosis	3
Physical examination	
S_3 gallop, jugular venous distention, or congestive heart failure	11
Bedridden	3
Laboratory	
PO_2 <60 mm Hg	3
PCO_2 >50 mm Hg	3
Potassium <3 mEq/dL	3
Blood urine nitrogen >50 mg/dL	3
Creatinine >3 mg/dL	3
Operation	
Emergency	4
Inrathoracic	3
Intraabdominal	3
Aortic	3

Approximate cardiac risk (percent incidence of major complications):

	Class[a]				
	Baseline	I	II	III	IV
Minor surgery	1	0.3	1	3	19
Major noncardiac surgery, age >40 years	4	1	4	12	48
Abdominal aortic surgery, or age >40 with other characteristics	10	3	10	30	75

[a] CRIS class I, 0–5 points; class II, 6–12 points; class III, 13–25 points; class IV, ≥26 points.
Source: Adapted from Goldman L, Caldera DL, Nussbaum SR, et al. Multifactorial index of cardiac risk in noncardiac surgical procedures. N Engl J Med 1977;297:845–850. Reprinted from Barie PS. Perioperative management. In: Norton JA, Bollinger RR, Chang AE, et al, eds. Surgery: Basic Science and Clinical Evidence. New York: Springer-Verlag, 2001, with permission.

The amount of testing that goes on in the name of cardiac risk assessment is staggering. The American College of Cardiology/American Heart Association Guideline Algorithm for Perioperative Cardiovascular Evaluation of Noncardiac Surgery provides useful and reasonable recommendations, which, if followed, may avoid unnecessary and expensive studies.

Pulmonary

In patients with a history of pulmonary disease or for those who will require lung resection surgery, preoperative assessment of pulmonary function is of value. Postoperative respiratory complications are leading causes of postoperative morbidity and mortality, ranking second only to cardiac complications as immediate causes of death.

History and physical exam can be helpful in assessing a patient's risk of pulmonary problems, and, frequently, these are all that are necessary. Routine chest x-rays are of little value in a patient with a normal physical exam and at low risk based on history. Certainly, a chest x-ray (posteroanterior and lateral) may be helpful in a patient with a history of chronic obstructive pulmonary disease (COPD), shortness of breath (SOB), and physical findings consistent with congestive heart failure (CHF) or upper respiratory infections or as screening for metastatic disease.

Preoperative laboratory testing is generally not predictive of perioperative pulmonary problems. Studies often confirm what a careful physician already has deciphered from a history and physical exam.

Table 1.3. Evaluation steps corresponding to American College of Cardiology/American Heart Association (ACC/AHA) guideline algorithms for perioperative cardiovascular evaluation of noncardiac surgery.

Step 1.	What is the urgency of the proposed surgery? If emergent, detailed risk assessment must be deferred to the postoperative period.
Step 2.	Has the patient had myocardial revascularization within the past 5 years? If so, further testing is generally unnecessary if the patient is stable/asymptomatic.
Step 3.	Has the patient had a cardiologic evaluation within the past 2 years? If so, further testing is generally unnecessary if the patient is stable/asymptomatic.
Step 4.	Does the patient have unstable symptoms or a major predictor of risk? Unstable chest pain, decompensated congestive heart failure, symptomatic arrhythmias, and severe valvular heart disease require evaluation and treatment before elective surgery.
Step 5.	Does the patient have intermediate clinical predictors of risk, such as prior myocardial infarction, angina pectoris, prior or compensated heart failure, or diabetes? Consideration of the patient's capacity to function and the level of risk inherent in the proposed surgery can help identify patients who will benefit most from perioperative noninvasive testing.
Step 6.	Patients with intermediate risk and good-to-excellent functional capacity can undergo intermediate-risk surgery with very little risk. Consider additional testing for patients with multiple predictors about to undergo higher-risk surgery.
Step 7.	Further testing can be performed on patients with poor functional capacity in the absence of clinical predictors of risk, especially if vascular surgery is being planned.
Step 8.	For high-risk patients about to go to high-risk surgery, coronary angiography or even cardiac surgery may be less than the noncardiac operation. Clinical, surgery-specific, and functional parameters are taken into account to make the decision. Indications for coronary revascularization are identical whether or not considered in preparation for noncardiac surgery.

Source: Adapted from Eagle KA, Brundage BH, Chaitman BR, et al. ACC/AHA guidelines for perioperative cardiovascular evaluation for noncardiac surgery. Report of the American College of Cardiology/American Heart Association Task Force on Practice Guidelines (Committee on Perioperative Cardiovascular Evaluation for Noncardiac Surgery). J Am Coll Cardiol 1996;27:910–948. Copyright 1996 The American College of Cardiology Foundation and American Heart Association Inc. Permission for one time use. Further reproduction is not permitted without the permission of the ACC/AHA. Reprinted from Barie PS. Perioperative management. In: Norton JA, Bollinger RR, Chang AE, et al, eds. Surgery: Basic Science and Clinical Evidence. New York: Springer-Verlag, 2001, with permission.

Table 1.4. Guidelines to perioperative cardiovascular evaluation of noncardiac surgery.

Indications for assessment of left ventricular function at rest (radionuclide angiography, echocardiography, contrast ventriculography)

Level I: (helpful)	Patients with current or poorly controlled congestive heart failure
Level II: (possibly helpful)	Patients with prior congestive heart failure or dyspnea of unknown etiology
Level III: (not helpful)	Routine testing of ventricular function in patients without prior congestive heart failure

Indications for cardiac catheterization

Level I:	High-risk results during noninvasive testing
	Unstable chest pain syndrome
	Nondiagnostic or equivocal noninvasive testing result in high-risk patient before high-risk procedure
Level II:	Intermediate results from noninvasive testing
	Nondiagnostic or equivocal noninvasive testing result in low-risk patient before high-risk procedure
	Urgent noncardiac surgery after a recent acute myocardial infarction
	Perioperative myocardial infarction
Level III:	Low-risk noninvasive testing result in patient with known coronary artery disease, before a low-risk procedure
	Screening before a noninvasive test
	Asymptomatic patient with normal exercise tolerance after coronary revascularization
	Normal coronary angiography in previous 5 years
	Revascularization impossible, contraindicated, or refused a priori

Source: Adapted from Eagle KA, Brundage BH, Chaitman BR, et al. ACC/AHA guidelines for perioperative cardiovascular evaluation for noncardiac surgery. Report of the American College of Cardiology/American Heart Association Task Force on Practice Guidelines (Committee on Perioperative Cardiovascular Evaluation for Noncardiac Surgery). J Am Coll Cardiol 1996;27:910–948. Copyright 1996 The American College of Cardiology Foundation and American Heart Association Inc. Permission for one time use. Further reproduction is not permitted without permission of the ACC/AHA. Reprinted from Barie PS. Perioperative Management. In: Norton JA, Bollinger RR, Chang AE, et al, eds. Surgery: Basic Science and Clinical Evidence. New York: Springer-Verlag, 2001, with permission.
Summary of evidence-based recommendations for supplemental evaluation of the American College of Cardiology/American Heart Association Task Force on Practice Guidelines, Committee on Perioperative Cardiovascular Evaluation for Noncardiac Surgery, 1996.

An elevated serum bicarbonate concentration suggests chronic respiratory acidosis, while polycythemia may suggest chronic hypoxemia. A room air blood gas may provide useful baseline information so that one is not surprised that the postoperative arterial blood gas findings are so abnormal. A room air arterial oxygen tension (Pao_2) less than 60 mm Hg correlates with pulmonary hypertension, whereas a $Paco_2$ greater than 45 mm Hg is associated with increased perioperative morbidity. Spirometry before and after bronchodilators is simple and easy to obtain. Analysis of forced expiratory volume in 1 second (FEV_1) and forced vital capacity (FVC) usually provides enough information for clinical decision making. Dyspnea is assumed to occur when FEV_1 is less than 2 L, whereas an FEV_1 less than 50% of the predicted value correlates with exertional dyspnea. In patients with COPD, the FVC decreases less than the FEV_1, resulting in an FEV_1/FVC ratio less than 0.8. Spirometry correlates with the development of postoperative atelectasis and pneumonia, particularly if FEV_1 is less than 1.2 L or less than 70% of predicted, or FEV_1/FVC is less than 0.65. If spirometric parameters improve by 15% or more after bronchodilator therapy, such therapy should be continued. If pulmonary resection is planned, then split-lung function can be obtained. An FEV_1 of approximately 800 mL from the contralateral lung is required to proceed with pneumonectomy. For abdominal surgery, there is no indication for evaluation beyond spirometry and arterial blood gas analysis.

Patients may be well served by a preoperative discussion with their surgeon or respiratory therapist regarding the role of postoperative incentive spirometry and pulmonary toilet procedures. The patients need to be informed of the need for their active involvement postoperatively if they are to avoid pulmonary complications such as atelectasis and pneumonia. They also should be reassured that, while they will have some postoperative discomfort, measures will be taken to assure that they will have adequate pain relief.

Perhaps the most useful intervention is for the smoking patient to cease smoking prior to surgery. Cessation of cigarette smoking is very important for those who smoke more than 10 cigarettes per day. Short-term abstinence (48 hours) decreases the carboxyhemoglobin to that of a nonsmoker, abolishes the effects of nicotine on the cardiovascular system, and improves mucosal ciliary function. Sputum volume decreases after 1 to 2 weeks of abstinence, and spirometry improves after about 6 weeks of abstinence.

Prophylaxis for venous thromboembolism is covered in Chapter 29.

Nutritional

There is a strong inverse correlation between the body's protein status and postoperative complications in populations of patients undergoing elective major gastrointestinal surgery and, to a lesser extent, other forms of surgery. With this in mind, it would seem useful to assess the nutritional status of a patient prior to surgery and possibly intervene preoperatively if a deficit is unmasked. While this makes intuitive sense, there in not much evidence to support improved clinical outcome via aggressive nutritional supportive measures.

While there are many clinical and laboratory measures that can help assess a patient's nutritional status, there is no "gold standard." Parameters such as weight loss, albumin, prealbumin, and immune competence (measured by delayed cutaneous hypersensitivity or total lymphocyte count) have been used to classify patients into states of mild, moderate, and severe malnutrition, but, by themselves, individual markers may not accurately represent the nutritional status of the patient. Preoperative weight loss is an important historical factor to obtain, if possible. In general, a weight loss of 5% to 10% over a month or 10% to 20% over 6 months is associated with increased complications from an operation. A more thorough history of weight loss in the patient in the case presented at the beginning of this chapter will be important.

While no one marker is predictive of surgical outcome, combinations of measurements have been used to quantify the risk for subsequent complications. The prognostic nutrition index (PNI) correlates with poor outcome in the following equation:

$$PNI\,(\%) = 158 - 16.6\,(ALB) - 0.78\,(TSF) - 0.20\,(TFN) - 5.8\,(DH)$$

where PNI is the risk of complication occurring in an individual patient, ALB is the serum albumin (g/dL), TSF is the triceps skin fold thickness (mm), TFN is serum transferring (mg/dL), and DH is delayed hypersensitivity reaction to one of three recall antigens (0, nonreactive; 1, <5-mm indurations; 2, >5-mm indurations). Because delayed hypersensitivity is uncommon in clinical practice, the equation has been simplified by substituting the lymphocyte score, using a scale of 0 to 2, where 0 is less than 1000 total lymphocytes/mm^3, 1 is 1000 to 2000 total lymphocytes/mm^3, and a score of 2 is more than 2000 total lymphocytes/mm^3. The higher the score using either of these equations, the greater the risk of postoperative complications.

Nutritional issues are discussed in greater detail in Chapter 3. **It is important to take the patient's nutritional state into consideration after surgery. In the majority of well-nourished patients, little needs to be done other than to ensure that they resume a normal diet as soon as possible after surgery, preferably within 5 to 10 days. In patients who are severely malnourished, aggressive nutritional support may be of some benefit, with most of the benefit occurring in the early postoperative period.**

Hematologic

An obvious concern for a surgeon who is about to induce iatrogenic injury to a patient is that of bleeding and the patient's inherent ability to form clots. The patient's ability to form clots is always a double-edged concern. On the one hand, the surgeon depends on it so that the patient does not exsanguinate from the intervention (fortunately, an exceedingly rare event). Conversely, a patient in a hypercoaguable state may suffer from a thromboemblic event that could be life threatening. In addition, a growing number of patients requiring surgical intervention are chronically anticoagulated for a number of reasons, e.g., Afib, previous valve replacement, history of hypercoaguablity, etc., and the surgeon needs to have a strategy to deal with these patients.

The best test for clotting problems is a thorough history and physical. Historical information of importance includes whether the patient or a family member has had a prior episode of bleeding or a thromboembolic event, and whether the patient has a history of prior transfusions, prior surgery, heavy menstrual bleeding, easy bruising, frequent nosebleeds, or gum bleeding after brushing teeth. Information on the coexistence of kidney or liver disease, poor dietary habits, excessive ingestion of alcohol, and use of aspirin, other nonsteroidal antiinflammatory drugs (NSAIDs), lipid lowering drugs, or anticoagulants must be ascertained. If the history is negative and the patient has not had a previous significant hemostatic challenge, then the likelihood of a bleeding or thrombotic event is exceedingly rare and the value of preoperative coagulation testing is low.

The standard "coags" routinely ordered as screening test—the prothrombin time (PT), activated partial thromboplastin time (aPTT), and platelet count—identify abnormalities of importance in only 0.2% of patients. This underscores the importance of adopting a reasonable strategy of ordering only those diagnostic tests indicated by the patient's history. If a clinically important coagulopathy is identified, therapeutic strategies for management of various coagulation disorders in preparation for surgery are listed in Table 1.5.

Caring for patients who are taking anticoagulants requires careful planning. A good deal of the planning hinges upon how urgently the surgery needs to be performed and the indication for the anticoagulation. Most patients who take warfarin and who are to undergo ambulatory or same-day admission elective surgery can be managed simply by having them discontinue their warfarin for several days prior to surgery. If there is concern that the patient should not be without anticoagulation, the patient can be systemically anticoagulated with unfractionated intravenous heparin. The heparin infusion is discontinued approximately 4 hours prior to surgery (the half-life of heparin is about 90 minutes), and surgery proceeds with good hemostasis. There is growing interest in the use of low molecular weight heparin (LMWH) as a bridge for surgery, and it is an attractive option, yet data are currently insufficient to provide a definitive recommendation for its use.

Antibiotic Prophylaxis

This topic is discussed in greater detail in future chapters. Suffice it to say that surgery is an insult to the body's immune system and infection is frequently an unwanted side affect. Antibiotic therapy may help decrease the incidence of postoperative infection. Antibiotic therapy must be used judiciously so as to avoid overuse and selection of resistant strains of bacteria. Table 1.6 summarizes the evidence-based guidelines for prevention of surgical site infections.

Lab Studies

The studies that are generally performed include a complete blood count, serum electrolytes, PT, and aPTT. A type and screen or type and crossmatch should be requested for operations where blood transfusions are likely (Table 1.7).

Table 1.5. Preoperative management of selected coagulation disorders.

Diagnosis	Treatment
Factor deficiencies	
Hemophilia A: Mild, factor VIII >10%	Desmopressin, 0.3 mg/kg i.v. q 12–24 h × 5–7 days for minor surgery.
Severe	Factor VIII concentrate (level 50–75% for mild–moderate injury, 75–100% for severe insults).
	Dose: 1 U will increase F VIII level by 2% in a 70-kg patient; give one-half i.v. q 12 h or 1/24 dose i.v. q 1 h by infusion after the initial bolus.
	Levels should be maintained for 5–7 (moderate injury) or 7–14 days (severe injury), as delayed bleeding is typical. Levels of 25–30% are adequate for a minor operation.
Hemophilia B: Mild	Desmopressin, 0.3 mg/kg i.v. q 12–24 h.
Severe	Factor IX concentrate (level 50–75% for mild–moderate injury, 75–100% for severe insults).
	Dose: 1 U will increase F IX level by 2% in a 70-kg patient; give one-half i.v. q 18–24 h after the initial bolus. Levels should be maintained for 5–7 (moderate injury) or 7–14 days (severe injury), as delayed bleeding is typical. Levels of 10–25% are adequate for a minor operation.
von Willebrand's disease: Type 1	Desmopressin, 0.3 mg/kg i.v. q 12–24 h × 5–7 days. Tachyphylaxis can be restored by a 24-h drug holiday to allow repletion of endothelial stores. Keep VIII: vWF 60% for 24–72 h for minor surgery 80% for 5–7 days for major surgery.
Type 2	Trial of desmopressin (unpredictable effect).
	Cryoprecipitate (contains 80–100 units vWF/10 units).
Liver disease (multifactorial)	Based on specific defect. Fresh-frozen plasma to keep PT/aPTT <1.3 × control (difficult to correct factor VII deficiency).
	Vitamin K, 10 mg i.m., if vitamin K deficiency suspected.
	Platelet count >50,000–100,000.
	Cryoprecipitate if low fibrinogen (<100–150 mg/dL), factor VIII.
	Warfarin (vitamin K deficiency, factor II, VII, IX, X).
	Fresh frozen plasma to keep PT <1.3 × control. Vitamin K, 10 mg i.m., if the patient does not require immediate correction (<12–48 h) or short-term anticoagulation.
Platelet abnormalities	
Thrombocytopenia	Transfuse platelets <50,000 if bleeding or invasive procedure is anticipated; <20,000 otherwise.
Idiopathic thrombocytopenic purpura	Intravenous immunoglobulin, 2 g/kg over 2–4 days (VERY expensive).
	Platelet infusion after ligation of the splenic artery during splenectomy if the response to immune globulin is poor.
Drug-induced	Discontinue all noncritical medications.
	Transfuse platelets only if surgery cannot be delayed to allow spontaneous recovery.
Uremia	Aggressive hemodialysis?
	Transfuse to hematocrit ~30% to allow improved adhesion?
	Desmopressin, 0.3 mg/kg i.v. q 12–24 h (rapid effect of short duration).
	Cryoprecipitate, 10 units (rapid effect but short duration).
	Conjugated estrogens, 25 mg i.v./day for 3 days (slow onset of action but effective for up to 2 weeks).

Source: Reprinted from Kudsk KA, Jacobs DO. Nutrition. In: Norton JA, Bollinger RR, Chang AE, et al, eds. Surgery: Basic Science and Clinical Evidence. New York: Springer-Verlag, 2001, with permission.

Table 1.6. Summary of evidence-based guidelines for the prevention of surgical site infection (wound infection).[a]

Preparation of the patient
Level I: Identify and treat all infections remote to the surgical site before elective operations. Postpone elective operations until the infection has resolved.
Do not remove hair preoperatively unless hair at or near the incision site will interfere with surgery. If hair is removed, it should be removed immediately beforehand, preferably with electric clippers.
Level II: Control the blood glucose concentration in all diabetic patients.
Encourage abstinence from tobacco for a minimum of 30 days before surgery.
Indicated blood transfusions should not be withheld as a means to prevent surgical site infection.
Patients should shower or bathe with an antiseptic agent at least the night before surgery.
Wash and clean the incision site before antiseptic skin preparation.

Hand/forearm antisepsis
Level II: Keep nails short.
Scrub the hands and forearms up to the elbows for at least 2–5 min with an appropriate antiseptic.

Antimicrobial prophylaxis
Level I: Administer antibiotic prophylaxis only when indicated.
Administer the initial dose intravenously, timed such that a bactericidal concentration of the drug is established in serum and tissues when the incision is made. Maintain therapeutic levels of the agent in serum and tissues for the duration of the operation. Levels should be maintained only until, at most, a few hours after the incision is closed.
Before elective colon operations, additionally prepare the colon mechanically with enemas or cathartic agents. Administer nonabsorbable oral antimicrobial agents in divided doses on the day before surgery.
For high-risk cesarean section, administer the prophylactic antibiotic agent immediately after the umbilical cord is clamped.
Level II: Do not use vancomycin routinely for surgical prophylaxis.

Surgical attire and drapes
Level II: A surgical mask should be worn to cover fully the mouth and nose for the duration of the operation, or while sterile instruments are exposed.
A cap or hood should be worn to cover fully hair on the head and face.
Wear sterile gloves after donning a sterile gown.
Do not wear shoe covers for the prevention of surgical site infection.
Use surgical gowns and drapes that are effective barriers when wet.
Change scrub suits that are visibly soiled or contaminated by blood or other potentially infectious materials.

Asepsis and surgical technique
Level I: Adhere to principles of asepsis when placing intravascular devices or when dispensing or administering intravenous drugs.
Level II: Handle tissue gently, maintain hemostasis, minimize devitalized or charred tissue and foreign bodies, and eradicate dead space at the surgical site.
Use delayed primary skin closure or allow incisions to heal by secondary intention if the surgical site is contaminated or dirty.
Use closed suction drains when drainage is necessary, placing the drain through a separate incision distant from the operative incision. Remove drains as soon as possible.

Postoperative incision care
Level II: A sterile dressing should be kept for 24–48 h postoperatively on an incision closed primarily. No recommendation is made regarding keeping a dressing on the wound beyond 48 h.
Wash hands before and after dressing changes and any contact with the surgical site.
Use sterile technique to change dressings.
Educate the patient about surgical site infections, relevant symptoms and signs, and the need to report them if noted.

[a] Centers for Disease Control and Prevention, 1999; level III guidelines excluded.
Source: Adapted from Mangram AJ, Horan TC, Pearson ML, et al. Guideline for prevention of surgical site infection, 1999, with permission. Hospital Infection Control Practices Advisory Committee. Infect Control Hosp Epidemiol 1999;20:250–278. Reprinted from Barie PS. Perioperative management. In: Norton JA, Bollinger, RR, Chang AE, et al, eds. Surgery: Basic Science and Clinical Evidence. New York: Springer-Verlag, 2001, with permission.

Table 1.7. Selected surgical procedures and likelihood of blood transfusion.

Low (<15%) risk: no likely benefit from preoperative autologous donation
Childbirth
Cesarean section
Cholecystectomy
Transurethral prostatectomy
Vaginal delivery
Vaginal hysterectomy
High (>50%) risk: likely benefit from preoperative autologous donation
Abdominal hysterectomy
Cardiac surgery
Colorectal surgery
Craniotomy
Mastectomy
Radical prostatectomy
Spinal surgery
Total joint replacement
Vascular graft surgery

Source: Reprinted from Barie PS. Perioperative management. In: Norton JA, Bollinger RR, Chang AE, et al, eds. Surgery: Basic Science and Clinical Evidence. New York: Springer-Verlag, 2001, with permission.

Additional studies that are frequently ordered include a urinalysis, urine pregnancy test, and, when indicated, liver function studies. **While the list of additional studies could go on and on, the important principle to understand is that few of these studies are helpful when routinely ordered. Selective laboratory evaluation, coupled with a thorough history and physical exam, will prove to be both safer and more cost-effective.**

Imaging Studies

The disease process being treated should dictate the imaging studies ordered. In general, physicians order too many rather than too few. Most patients can be brought to the operating room safely based on the performance of good history and physical exam. **Diagnostic imaging studies should be ordered to fine-tune the history and physical and so that appropriate surgical planning decisions can be made.**

A frequently asked question is: Who needs a chest x-ray prior to surgery? Routine chest x-rays are of very little value. This routine order is somewhat historical, carrying over from the days of prevalent tuberculosis. Healthy young patients with no evidence of pulmonary disease benefit little from a chest x-ray. It is rare in a patient who has a normal pulmonary exam that the chest x-ray significantly alters the operation for which it was ordered. It is more reasonable to obtain a chest x-ray in an elderly patient, and, at times, this results in interesting findings, such as a lesion requiring further workup.

Informed Consent

Informed consent should be viewed as an opportunity for the surgeon to take some time to explain to the patient why an operation is necessary, what the operation entails, what sort of recovery to expect, and what complications might be incurred. The discussion should be **frank and honest while sensitive to obvious anxieties of the preoperative patient.** It is also helpful, when possible, to have this discussion **in the presence of a concerned spouse or family member.** Time should be given for all involved to ask questions. With this in mind, the discussion may best be done sometime well in advance of the operation. This understandably is not always possible. The discussion, when possible, also should include nonoperative therapies for the given disease process.

Case Evaluation

When considering the approach to the surgical patient as it applies to the case cited at the beginning of this chapter, there are several important considerations. First, the patient most likely does have a surgical problem and most likely requires an operation. He most likely does not require an emergency operation, and therefore the physicians attending to the patient have some time to fully evaluate the problem with an appropriate series of laboratory tests and diagnostic studies. A thorough and honest assessment of the patient's comorbid conditions and risks for major surgery is necessary prior to proceeding with a significant operation.

Summary

The successful approach to the surgical patient requires the physician to understand the anatomic and physiologic problems with which the patient presents, listen to the patient, collect a detailed history, and then perform a complete physical exam. Based on the history and physical, a diagnosis, or at least a working differential diagnosis, is derived. Appropriate laboratory, screening, and diagnostic studies are ordered. A discussion of the findings and treatment alternatives takes place. Although the aforementioned steps are not unique to surgery, the difference lies in the fact that a surgeon undertakes the aforementioned steps en route to an intervention. The intervention may be minor and expose the patient to minimal risk or it may be very significant and may permanently alter the patient's life. Patients place their well-being in the surgeon's hands. To earn that trust, surgeons must be well trained, exhibit good judgment, understand the limitations of their patients based on their comorbidities, and understand the limitations of their own ability.

Selected Readings

Arozullah AM, Khuri SF, Henderson WG, et al. Development and validation of a multifactorial risk index for predicting postoperative pneumonia after major noncardiac surgery. Ann Intern Med 2001;135(10):847–857.

Barie PS. Perioperative management. In: Norton JA, Bollinger RR, Chang AE, et al, eds. Surgery: Basic Science and Clinical Evidence. New York: Springer-Verlag, 2001.

Eagle KA, Brundage BH, Chaitman BR, et al. Guidelines for perioperative cardiovascular evaluation for noncardiac surgery. Report of the American College of Cardiology/American Heart Association Task Force on Practice Guidelines (Committee on Perioperative Cardiovascular Evaluation for Noncardiac Surgery). J Am Coll Cardiol 1996;27:910–948.

Goldman L. Cardiac risk for vascular surgery. J Am Coll Cardiol 1996;27:799–802.

Goldman L, Caldera DL, Nussbaum SR, et al. Multifactorial index of cardiac risk in noncardiac surgical procedures. N Engl J Med 1977;297:845–850.

Hathaway WE, Goodnight SH Jr. Disorders of Hemostasis and Thrombosis. A Clinical Guide. New York: McGraw-Hill, 1993.

Heyland DK, MacDonald S, Keefe L, Drover JW. Total parental nutrition in the critically ill patient: a meta-analysis. JAMA 1998;280:2013–2019.

King MS. Preoperative evaluation. Am Fam Physician 2000;62(2):308–311.

Kudsk KA, Jacobs DO. Nutrition. In: Norton JA, Bollinger RR, Chang AE, et al, eds. Surgery: Basic Science and Clinical Evidence. New York: Springer-Verlag, 2001.

Mangram AJ, Horan TC, Pearson ML, et al. Guideline for prevention of surgical site infection, 1999. Hospital Infection Control Practice Advisory Committee. Infect Control Hosp Epidemiol 1999;20:250–278.

Marshall JC. Risk prediction and outcome description in critical surgical illness. In: Norton JA, Bollinger RR, Chang AE, et al, eds. Surgery: Basic Science and Clinical Evidence: New York: Springer-Verlag, 2001.

Wall RT. Anesthesia. In: Norton JA, Bollinger RR, Chang AE, et al, eds. Surgery: Basic Science and Clinical Evidence. New York: Springer-Verlag, 2001.

Practicing Evidence-Based Surgery

Candice S. Rettie and Gary B. Nackman

Objectives

1. To know the definition of evidence-based medicine (EBM).
2. To appreciate the role that EBM plays in contributing to the provision of quality patient care.
3. To apply EBM concepts to the delivery of patient care:
   - To articulate meaningful clinical questions.
   - To understand the basic concepts that facilitate effective literature searches.
   - To acquire the basic skills necessary to evaluate the quality and relevance of the search results.
   - To acquire the basic skills necessary to integrate EBM into the practice of medicine.

Case

Patient: Mr. Edwards is a 45-year-old white man.

Presenting problem: Pain and dragging sensation in left groin.

History of present illness: Three days ago, when lifting a very large pine tree that blew over in a recent windstorm, the patient felt a sudden pain in his left groin. The acute pain resolved, but he continues to feel a "dragging" sensation in same area. He has not noticed any bulge in his groin.

Past medical history: Negative: No prior episodes; no chronic illnesses.

Past surgical history: Cholecystectomy 3 years ago.

Review of systems: Noncontributory:
- Gastrointestinal: Denies change in bowel habits; no history of constipation; no hematochezia; no nausea and vomiting.
- Genitourinary: Denies difficulty or pain with urination or night-time urgency/frequency.

Pertinent social/family history: Non–union worker who loads and unloads delivery trucks.

Physical examination:

- Vitals: BP: 120/75; Temp: 37.5°C; HR: 72; Resp: 12.
- Abdomen: flat, soft, nontender, no masses. Upon standing, a bulge observed in left inguinal region: no erythema, nontender, easily reduced.
- Rectal exam: prostate within normal limits.

The Relevance of Evidence-Based Medicine

Many of the issues involved in the care of patients include "age-old" traditions that may be based on empiricism. The first cholecystectomy was performed in 1882. Until several decades ago, drainage of the gallbladder bed following cholecystectomy was the standard of care and was based on the belief that drainage of the affected area would promote healing and reduce postoperative complications. Through the 1970s, students and residents heard from their instructors and supervisors: "This is how my mentor taught me to drain the gallbladder bed, so you should do it this way, too." With advances in surgical science, the study of the efficacy of drainage following cholecystectomy clearly indicated that drainage of the gallbladder bed did not improve clinical outcomes. Even though the traditional dogma had been rebuked by demonstrating no need for routine drainage, the clinical practice took decades to change.

A significant challenge in medicine is to maintain the learning process throughout one's career, to keep current with the most recent evidence and practice guidelines, to understand the science behind the evidence and the guidelines, and thereby to continue providing optimal patient care. Even seasoned clinicians, when faced with the need to make a complex clinical decision, ask: "What are the practice guidelines for treating patients with this disease?" Implementing the practice guidelines in a routine manner is not sufficient. It is important to understand the studies that resulted in the practice guidelines and the implications of these findings for your specific patient. Remaining current with important developments and thoughtfully integrating new information into your patient's care are essential elements of the practice of surgery, whether one is a student, resident, or an experienced attending physician. **Evidence-based medicine is the purposeful integration of the most recent, best evidence into the daily practice of medicine** (See **Algorithm 2.1.**).

Evidence-Based Medicine (EBM), as a formal approach to the practice of medicine, was defined in the 1980s by David Sackett and his colleagues as

the conscientious, explicit, and judicious use of current best evidence in making decisions about the care of individual patients. The practice of evidence-based medicine means integrating individual clinical expertise with the best available clinical evidence from systematic research. In short, evidence-based med-

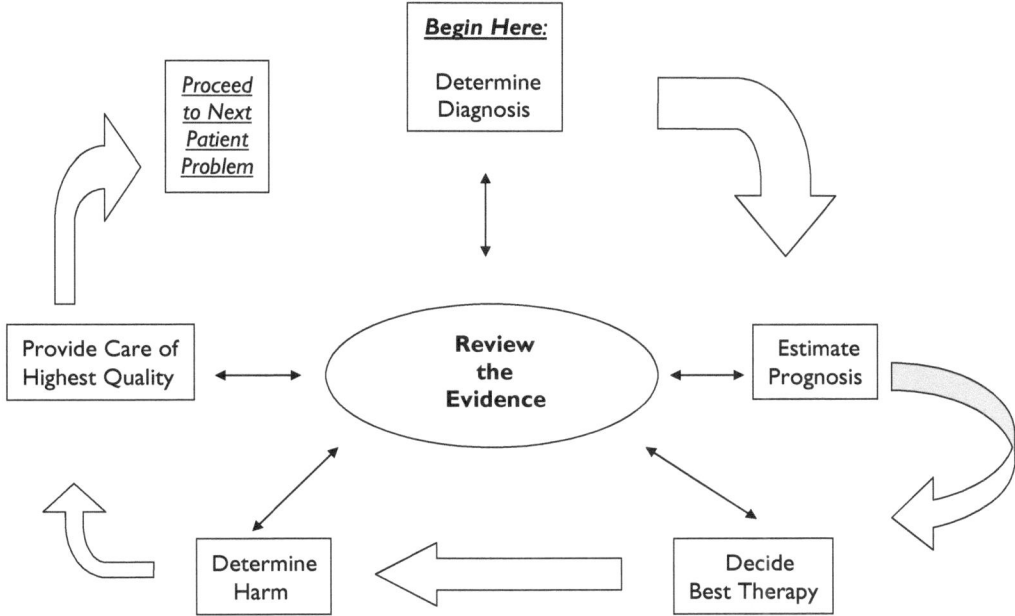

Algorithm 2.1. The practice of evidence-based patient care.

icine means systematically searching for the best evidence rather than relying on expert opinion or anecdotal experience.[1]

EBM is never a substitute for clinical expertise. In providing patient care, **EBM should be integrated with clinical acumen, in the context of the patient's preferences and values:**

Good doctors use both individual clinical expertise and the best available external evidence and neither alone is enough. Without clinical expertise, practice risks becoming tyrannized by external evidence, for even excellent external evidence may be inapplicable to or inappropriate for an individual patient. Without current best external evidence, practice risks becoming rapidly out of date, to the detriment of the patients.[2]

Implicit in this definition of EBM is the premise that an individual patient's case must drive the search for, and the application of, relevant and high-quality evidence. Further, "best evidence" refers to the data and the conclusions derived from systematic research, such as information provided through the Cochrane Library (http://www.update-software.com/cochrane/). The Cochrane Library is the gold standard for EBM databases. Expert opinion and anecdotal experience are not systematic research. However, current best evidence must be integrated with clinical acumen (derived from experience, expert opinion, and anecdotal evidence) and with the preferences and values of the patient.

---

[1] Sackett DL, Richardson WS, Rosenberg W, Haynes RB. Evidence-Based Medicine: How to Practice and Teach EBM. New York: Churchill Livingstone, 1997.
[2] Ibid.

Patients with a similar disease process may vary in their presentation and in their response to treatment. Therefore, it is essential to realize that, even with the best evidence, the application of that evidence must be considered in the context of the unique attributes of each patient. Further, patient autonomy, as expressed in differences in expectations and preferences, must be considered when developing a patient management plan.

If you still have doubts about the importance of practicing EBM in the practice of surgery, there are three compelling reasons to support the use of EBM in your practice. First, a common characteristic of physicians is their desire and obligation to provide optimal care for their patients and, as much as is possible, to facilitate the patients' return to their previous state of health. Since optimal medical care for patients changes over time with progress in technology and improved understanding of patient outcomes, it is necessary *to have the tools that ensure your ability to remain current*. Evidence-based medicine provides a framework to allow the physician lifelong learning opportunities.

Second, today's patients are better educated and often seek a collaborative relationship with their physician. They may have read the latest findings from National Institutes of Health (NIH) trials and often participate in patient advocacy groups. Current knowledge and critical appraisal of the professional literature is a vital component of your skill set as a physician. Through critical appraisal of the literature, you can provide the appropriate context for the information obtained by patients. Your clinical acumen, combined with your knowledge of the scientific method and levels of evidence, allows you to respond professionally and meaningfully to your patient's questions about his or her care.

Third, physicians must play an increasingly high-profile role in the development of public policy. The best evidence and an understanding of why it is the best are necessary if medicine, as a profession, is going to be the final arbiter of its practice.

The Practice of Evidence-Based Surgery

The practice of evidence-based surgery integrates the art of surgery (well-honed clinical acumen, "good hands," and interpersonal awareness) with use of the best information provided by contemporary science. The five central precepts of evidence-based surgery are as follows.

1. **The clinical problem, not the physician's habits or institutional protocols, should determine the type of evidence to be sought.** It has been recognized that "clinical pathways" or "optimaps" aid in the care of patients, streamlining cost-effective care. The correct application of the evidence-based approach to patient care demands that, in following clinical protocols, one always must be mindful that the quality of the evidence being used to develop a treatment plan meets the specific needs of the individual patient.

2. **Clinical decision making should be based on the clinical data obtained by the practitioner and application of the best available scientific evidence.** Data obtained from conducting a history and physical examination provide the foundation for clinical decision making. These data then are evaluated in the context of the current best evidence. Clinical decision making is the result of applying the best that science and clinical acumen have to offer in the unique context of the individual patient.

3. **It frequently has been stated that the literature is complex and often contradictory. The challenge is for the physician to be able to judge the validity of a study and the applicability of the findings for guiding the care of the specific patient. Identifying the best evidence refers to reading the literature critically with a basic understanding of epidemiologic and biostatistical methods.** Without an understanding of the basic concepts of research design and statistics, one is unable to critically review the relevance and validity of a study.

4. **Conclusions derived from identifying and critically appraising evidence are useful only if they are put into the context of the individual patient's needs and then put into action in managing patients or making healthcare decisions.** Physicians need to be able to obtain meaningful information in real time to improve clinical decision making.

5. **Performance should be evaluated constantly.** It is important to monitor the outcome of your care and communicate with colleagues the success and failures of treatment, as demonstrated in the classic morbidity and mortality conference. Understanding the relationship between care and outcomes has been the hallmark of surgical care since the days of Billroth in the 19th century. Being accountable for one's actions and taking action to eliminate untoward outcomes are hallmarks of the excellent surgeon.

The practice of evidence-based surgery begins with gathering data to understand what brings the patient to the surgeon's office. As with the traditional practice of surgery, it is necessary to ask meaningful questions about the patient's problem. The answers to the questions are obtained from a focused history and physical examination of the patient. The information that is obtained is organized into a differential diagnosis list. The process of asking questions then shifts from posing questions designed to elicit accurate data about the patient to posing questions about the available evidence regarding how to best care for the patient. **This additional step of systematically obtaining relevant, current, scientific evidence to guide clinical decision making is what differentiates evidence-based practice from traditional practice.**

How to Use the Current Best Evidence

The most effective way of using evidence to provide clinical care is with a "bottom-up" "approach." Clinical reasoning is based on acquiring information to answer questions. The clinician's task is to understand the nature of the patient's problem. **Clinical expertise drives the** posing of relevant questions and the obtaining of useful information to better characterize the patient's problem. The questions posed in the process of clinical decision making are answered by using the best evidence available. For example, a properly randomized controlled trial is rated as more scientific and, therefore, as more reliable and valid than clinical wisdom and acumen or published expert opinion. Finally, the question is put into context by integrating the best external evidence with individual clinical expertise and patient choice.

A common question is how or where to get the current best evidence. Your reference librarian will be an invaluable resource. There are several on-line databases and resources that are useful, including the Cochrane Library, EBM journals such as *Evidence Based Medicine*, the National Institutes of Health databases, and other Web databases:

http://cebm.jr2.ox.ac.uk/
http://www.cebm.utoronto.ca/
http://www.guidelines.gov/index.asp
http://www.nlm.nih.gov/medlineplus.

The content of these databases is described briefly in **Appendix 2.A.**

How Do You Appraise the Evidence?

There are several types of evidence. **The most desirable evidence is provided by randomized, controlled trials. Study designs also include less rigorous experimental designs and quasi-experimental designs, such as case series, case-control studies, and cohort studies. Quasi-experimental methods, meta-analyses, outcome studies, and practice guidelines provide an overall assessment of a topic by analyzing multiple studies that used various research designs.** The study designs and the elements of randomized controlled trials are summarized in **Tables 2.1** and **2.2.**

The **levels of evidence** refer to a grading system for assessing medical studies by classifying them according to the scientific rigor or the quality of the evidence (outcomes). The levels of evidence are ordered to give the best rating to studies in which the risk of bias is reduced, as reflected by the a priori design of the study (its scientific rigor) and the actual quality of the study. Studies of evidence are clas-

Table 2.1. Hierarchy of study designs.

	Control group	Prospective follow-up	Random allocation of subjects
Case series	No	No	No
Case-control study	Yes	No	No
Cohort study	Yes	Yes	No
Randomized controlled trial	Yes	Yes	Yes

Source: Reprinted from McLeod RS. Evidence-based surgery. In: Norton JA, Bollinger RR, Chang AE, et al, eds. Surgery: Basic Science and Clinical Evidence. New York: Springer-Verlag, 2001, with permission.

Table 2.2. Elements of a randomized controlled trial.
1. **Stating the research question**
2. **Selecting the subjects**
3. **Allocating the subjects**
4. **Describing the maneuver**
   a. **The interventions**
   b. **Minimizing potential biases**
   c. **Baseline and follow-up maneuvers**
5. **Measuring outcome**
   a. **Assessing treatment effectiveness**
   b. **Assessing side effects and toxicity**
6. **Analyzing the data**
7. **Estimating the sample size**
8. **Ethical considerations**
9. **Administrative issues**
   a. **Feasibility of the trial**
   b. **Administration of the trial**
   c. **Data management**
   d. **Funding issues**

Source: Reprinted from McLeod RS. Evidence-based surgery. In: Norton JA, Bollinger RR, Chang AE, et al, eds. Surgery: Basic Science and Clinical Evidence. New York: Springer-Verlag, 2001, with permission.

sified into three levels, determined by the scientific rigor of the study's design. See **Table 2.3**.

In addition to reviewing the outcomes of specific, randomized, clinical trials, systematic reviews, meta-analyses, and practice guidelines can be extremely useful in dealing with specific patient problems or in updating of knowledge. **Systematic reviews** follow a defined protocol for the purpose of integrating the results of multiple studies when methodologic differences preclude conducting a meta-analysis. Guidelines for evaluating the quality of systematic reviews are presented in **Table 2.4**.

Table 2.3. Levels of evidence.

I	**Evidence obtained from at least one properly randomized controlled trial**
II-1	**Evidence obtained from well-designed controlled trials without randomization**
II-2	**Evidence obtained from well-designed cohort or case-control analytic studies, preferably from more than one center or research group**
II-3	**Evidence obtained from comparisons between times or places with or without the intervention; dramatic results in uncontrolled experiments (such as the results of treatment with penicillin in the 1940s) could also be included in this category**
III	**Opinions of respected authorities, based on clinical experience, descriptive studies, or reports of expert committees**

Source: Reprinted from McLeod RS. Evidence-based surgery. In: Norton JA, Bollinger RR, Chang AE, et al, eds. Surgery: Basic Science and Clinical Evidence. New York: Springer-Verlag, 2001, with permission.

A review conducted using the **meta-analysis** process differs from the typical techniques used in the creation of a review article. The meta-analysis includes the development of specific criteria to be applied to the existing literature for the purpose of determining which studies are suitable for further evaluation. After inclusion criteria are met, the meta-analysis can combine the results of several studies to increase the "statistical power" of the data set, a vital step in determining the adequacy of the sample size. One of the difficulties inherent in meta-analytic reviews is the variable quality of the articles cited. While there are statistical methods to control for the variability, it is important to understand how quality is defined. The quality of an article is assessed by determining the reliability (replicability and consistency of the findings) and the validity (meaningfulness) of the findings. The important issue is how to evaluate the studies.

The **standards for reviewing an article** are as follows:

- Were there **clearly defined groups of patients** who shared essential characteristics of interest in the study?
- Were the **measurements** of treatment exposure and clinical outcome **reliable (consistent or replicable) and valid (meaningful)**?
- Was the **follow-up adequate** in duration and depth?
- Do the results satisfy some **"diagnostic test for causation"**?

Validity refers to how well a technique (or measure) measures what it is supposed to measure. There are three kinds of validity: content, criterion, and construct validity. **Content validity** refers to the degree to which a measure (e.g., a lab study) actually represents (is specific for) the entity (e.g., a disease) being measured. For example, creatinine clearance is indicative of renal function; therefore, creatinine clearance has content validity when it is used to measure renal function. **Criterion validity** is related to how well the measurement (e.g., a lab study) predicts another characteristic (e.g., sign or symptom) associated with the entity (e.g., disease). For example, creatinine clearance does not

Table 2.4. Guidelines for using a review.

1. Did the overview address a focused clinical question?
2. Were the criteria used to select articles for inclusion appropriate?
3. Is it unlikely that important, relevant studies were missed?
4. Was the validity of the included studies appraised?
5. Were the assessments of the studies reproducible?
6. Were the results similar from study to study?
7. What are the overall results of the review?
8. How precise were the results?
9. Can the results be applied to my patient care?
10. Were all the clinically important outcomes considered?
11. Are the benefits worth the harms and costs?

Source: Adapted from Oxman AD, Cook DJ, Guyatt GH. Users' guides to the medical literature. VI. How to use an overview. Evidence-Based Medicine Working Group. JAMA 1994;272:1367–1371. Copyright © 1994 American Medical Association. All Rights Reserved. Reprinted from McLeod RS. Evidence-based surgery. In: Norton JA, Bollinger RR, Chang AE, et al, eds. Surgery: Basic Science and Clinical Evidence. New York: Springer-Verlag, 2001, with permission.

Table 2.5. Are the results of this diagnostic study valid?

1. Was there an independent, blind comparison with a reference ("gold") standard of diagnosis?
2. Was the diagnostic test evaluated in an appropriate spectrum of patients (like those in whom it would be used in practice)?
3. Was the reference standard applied regardless of the diagnostic test result?

Source: Reprinted from Sackett DL, Richardson WS, Rosenberg W, Haynes RB. Evidence-Based Medicine: How to Practice and Teach EBM. New York: Churchill Livingstone Inc., 1997. Copyright © 1997 Elsevier Ltd. With permission from Elsevier.

clearly predict the presence of lower extremity claudication with ambulation; therefore, in a study of renal function, use of creatinine clearance as an indicator of lower extremity ischemia would not be recommended, since creatinine clearance does not have criterion validity for predicting claudication upon ambulation. Construct validity is more nebulous. **Construct validity** refers to a specific pattern of relationships among similar variables that are characteristic of an entity, such that two or more of the characteristics are more strongly related to each other than to a third characteristic. Usually, the outcome is measured by several independent measures, and the similarity of the measures is assessed. For example, in children there is a strong positive correlation between age and height, shoe size, and the total score on a test of general knowledge. Whereas height and shoe size generally have a strong positive correlation to each other, total score on the knowledge test has a weaker correlation to age and shoe size.

Validity of the data can be determined by reviewing the data that are presented in the article. Sample sizes should be specified, and descriptive statistics of the samples should be provided. The baseline measures of the groups should be specified so that the reader can determine whether or not the groups were similar in their initial baseline measures. See **Tables 2.5**, **2.6**, and **2.7** for descriptions of how to determine validity in different types of studies.

Reliability refers to the replicability of the findings. Generally, replicating the measures and evaluating the degree of agreement assesses reliability. Were the methods specified? Were the techniques used in the study consistently applied?

Clinical **practice guidelines** are user-friendly statements that integrate best evidence and other knowledge to guide clinical decision

Table 2.6. Is this evidence about prognosis valid?

1. Was a defined, representative sample of patients assembled at a common (usually early) point in the course of their disease?
2. Was patient follow-up sufficiently long and complete?
3. Were objective outcome criteria applied in a "blind" fashion?
4. If subgroups with different prognoses are identified:
   • Was there adjustment for important prognostic factors?
   • Was there validation in an independent group of "test-set" patients?

Source: Reprinted from Sackett DL, Richardson WS, Rosenberg W, Haynes RB. Evidence-Based Medicine: How to Practice and Teach EBM. New York: Churchill Livingstone Inc., 1997. Copyright © 1997 Elsevier Ltd. With permission from Elsevier.

Table 2.7. Are the results of this systematic review valid?

1. Is it an overview of randomized trials of the treatment you're interested in?
2. Does it include a methods section that describes:
   a. Finding and including all the relevant trials?
   b. Assessing their individual validity?
3. Were the results consistent from study to study?

Source: Reprinted from Sackett DL, Richardson WS, Rosenberg W, Haynes RB. Evidence-Based Medicine: How to Practice and Teach EBM. New York: Churchill Livingstone Inc., 1997. Copyright © 1997 Elsevier Ltd. With permission from Elsevier.

making. As with any evidence, one must review carefully the "review" to determine the quality of the conclusions. **Practice guidelines are systematically developed protocols (not rules) about appropriate health care for specific clinical circumstances.** The guidelines usually are **flexible** so that the individual patient characteristics, common local practice, and individual practitioner preferences can be accommodated. The most rigorously developed guidelines are **evidence based**, preferably based on the findings of level I and II studies. A recent review of over 275 current, published, peer-reviewed clinical practice guidelines identified areas of concern in the development of the guidelines. Analysis of the methods used to identify, summarize, and evaluate evidence in the development of peer-reviewed clinical guidelines found dismal levels of methodologic rigor, especially in the identification and summary of evidence. The specifications of the patient population, the interventions, and the outcomes of interest frequently were inadequate. A strength of most guidelines is that they do specify recommendations for clinical practice and for how to individualize patient care. Guidelines for assessing practice guidelines are presented in **Table 2.8**.

Table 2.8. Guideline for assessing practice guidelines.

1. Were all important options and outcomes clearly specified?
2. Was an explicit and sensible process used to identify, select, and combine evidence?
3. Was an explicit and sensible process used to consider the relative value of different outcomes?
4. Is the guideline likely to account for important recent developments?
5. Has the guideline been subject to peer review and testing?
6. Are practical, clinically important, recommendations made?
7. How strong are the recommendations?
8. What is the impact of uncertainty associated with the evidence and values used in guidelines?
9. Is the primary objective of the guideline consistent with your objective?
10. Are the recommendations applicable to your patients?

Source: Adapted from Hayward RSA, Wilson MC, Tunis SR, Bass EB, Guyatt GH, for the Evidence Based Medicine Working Group. User's guide to the medical literature. VIII. How to use clinical practice guidelines. Are recommendations valid? JAMA 1995;274:570–574. Copyright © 1995 American Medical Association. All rights reserved. Reprinted from McLeod RS. Evidence-based surgery. In: Norton JA, Bollinger RR, Chang AE, et al, eds. Surgery: Basic Science and Clinical Evidence. New York: Springer-Verlag, 2001, with permission.

Table 2.9. Different ways of finding out whether a treatment sometimes causes harm.

		Adverse outcome		
		Present (case)	Absent (control)	Totals
Exposed to the treatment	Yes (cohort)	a	b	a + b
	No (cohort)	c	d	c + d
	Totals	a + c	b + d	a + b + c + d

Source: Reprinted from Sackett DL, Richardson WS, Rosenberg W, Haynes RB. Evidence-Based Medicine: How to Practice and Teach EBM. New York: Churchill Livingstone Inc., 1997. Copyright © 1997 Elsevier Ltd. With permission from Elsevier.

The validity of recommendations from clinical guidelines can be evaluated by considering the following issues:

- Specify **important decisions and related patient outcomes: Were all the critical decision points and the associated patient outcomes clearly identified?**
- Use the **evidence relevant to each decision option: Was it identified, validated, and combined in a sensible and explicit way?**
- Identify the **relative preferences of the key stakeholders: Are the** outcomes of decisions (including benefits, risks, and costs) identified and explicitly considered?
- Robustness of the **clinical guideline: Does it maintain its structure, while providing the flexibility necessary to accommodate clinically sensible variations in practice?**

Finally, it is essential to be familiar with basic epidemiology and biostatistics so that the clinical relevance of the evidence that you obtained from your search can be determined. In general, it is helpful to be able to calculate two types of statistics:

1. Odds ratios, likelihood ratios
2. Sensitivity/specificity

Examples of epidemiologic and biostatistical tests are provided in **Tables 2.9, 2.10,** and **2.11.**

Essential Elements of an EBM Question

The EBM process begins with asking questions that arise as a care plan is developed for the patient. The first step is to know how to ask the question(s). Questions need to focus on the meaningful clinical components of caring for the patient. Sackett[3] specifies **four essential elements** to an EBM question:

---

[3] Ibid.

Table 2.10. A teaching byte for introducing likelihood ratios.

Objective: To provide a quick example of diagnostic test results for explaining and illustrating likelihood ratios at the bedside.

Key information to remember: 10, 30, 50, 9, 1 (you may find it easier to remember them as single digits 1, 3, 5, 9, 1 and then add zeros to the first three of them; or remember that the first three ascend as odd digits beginning with 1 and the final two descend; or whatever works for you!)

Put them in a table:

		Target disorder		Likelihood ratio	
		Present	Absent		
Diagnostic test result	Most abnormal	10%	1%	10%/1% = 10	SpPin
		30%	9%	30%/9% = 3.3	Up a bit
	Mid-zone	50%	50%	50%/50% = 1	No use
		9%	30%	9%/30% = 0.3	Down a bit
	Most normal	1%	10%	1%/10% = 0.1	SnNout
	Totals	100%	100%		

(Alternatively, you could enter them as counts and convert them to % or decimal fractions)

(Simply the same numbers as the previous column, but in the reverse order)

Using the nomogram or hand calculations, you can take clinically sensible pretest probabilities and see how different test results take you to posttest probabilities.

For example, for a pretest of 50%,* the posttest probabilities are (from top to bottom):

- 10/11[†]= 91% (in most situations, you've ruled in the diagnosis; analogous to a SpPin[‡])
- 3.3/4.3 = 77% (the diagnosis is more likely, but not decisively so)
- 1/2 = 50% (right back where you started from, because the test result's LR of 1 means that pretest probability is unchanged by the test)

Source: Reprinted from Sackett DL, Richardson WS, Rosenberg W, Haynes RB. Evidence-Based Medicine: How to Practice and Teach EBM. New York: Churchill Livingstone Inc., 1997. Copyright © 1997 Elsevier Ltd. With permission from Elsevier.

Table 2.11. Types of statistical tests.

Data type	Statistical test (with no adjustment for prognostic factors)	Procedure test (with adjustment for prognostic factors)
Binary (dichotomous)	Fisher exact test or chi-square	Logistic regression (Mantel–Haenszel)
Ordered discrete	Mann-Whitney U-test	
Continuous (normal distribution)	Student's *t*-test	Analysis of covariance (ANCOVA) (multiple regression)
Time to event (censored data)	Log-rank Wilcoxon test	Log-rank (Cox's proportional hazards)

Source: Reprinted from McLeod RS. Evidence-based surgery. In: Norton JA, Bollinger RR, Chang AE, et al, eds. Surgery: Basic Science and Clinical Evidence. New York: Springer-Verlag, 2001, with permission.

1. *Patient or problem* being addressed
2. *Intervention*, whether by nature or by clinical design (a cause, a prognostic factor, or treatment, etc.), being considered
3. *Comparison intervention*, when relevant
4. *Outcome* or outcomes of clinical interest

The acronym **PICO** is useful in remembering the elements. See **Table 2.12** for a description of the elements and ways to frame your question.

Clinical Application

This section focuses on the application of the EBM algorithm (**Algorithm 2.1**) to the clinical case presented at the beginning of this chapter and the process for asking questions in the development of a treatment plan.

How Do You Use Your Questions?

Determine the answer to the following queries:

- Which question is most important to the patient's well-being?
- Which question is most feasible to answer within the time you have available?
- Which question is most interesting to you?
- Which question are you most likely to encounter repeatedly in your practice?

Once you have selected your question(s), the next step is to gather and review the evidence.

The evidence-based practice algorithm (**Algorithm 2.1**) that is presented at the beginning of this chapter provides a structure for developing questions that focus on each step in the process of clinical decision making. **The steps in clinical decision making as presented in the algorithm are: achieving a diagnosis, estimating prognosis, deciding on the best therapy, determining harm, and providing care of the highest quality.** To apply the algorithm, a patient problem is selected. The case of Mr. Edwards (see case at beginning of the chapter) serves as an example. Mr. Edwards has made an appointment with his physician because of a dragging sensation in his groin that has persisted for 3 days after he felt a sharp pain while lifting a heavy object. Mr. Edwards wants to find out if anything can, or should, be done about it.

For Mr. Edwards' physician, however, the clinical question becomes more complicated. Using the algorithm, five questions are generated that will guide the clinical decision making:

- What is the most likely diagnosis for an acute pain in the groin that has evolved into a persistent dragging sensation in the same area?
- What is the prognosis if the condition is not treated?
- What is the best therapy to treat the condition?
- What harm is likely to come to the patient as a result of the recommended therapy?

Table 2.12. The four elements of well-built clinical questions.

	1. Patient or problem	2. Intervention (a cause, a prognostic factor, a treatment, etc.)	3. Comparison intervention (if necessary)	4. Outcome(s)
Tips for building	Starting with your patient, ask, "How would I describe a group of patients similar to mine?" Balance precision with brevity	Ask, "Which main intervention am I considering?" Be specific	Ask, "What is the main alternative to compare with the intervention?" Again, be specific	Ask, "What can I hope to accomplish?" or "What could this exposure really affect?" Again, be specific
Example	"In patients with heart failure from dilated cardiomyopathy who are in sinus rhythm . . ."	". . . would adding anticoagulation with warfarin to standard heart failure therapy . . ."	". . . when compared with standard therapy alone . . ."	". . . lead to lower mortality or morbidity from thromboembolism. Is this enough to be worth the increased risk of bleeding?"

Source: Reprinted from Sackett DL, Richardson WS, Rosenberg W, Haynes RB. Evidence-Based Medicine: How to Practice and Teach EBM. New York: Churchill Livingstone Inc, 1997. Copyright © 1997 Elsevier Ltd. With permission from Elsevier.

Table 2.13. Differential diagnosis of groin masses.

Inguinal hernia	Hydrocele
Femoral hernia	Testicular mass
Lipoma	Testicular torsion
Lymphadenitis	Epididymitis
Lymphadenopathy	Ectopic testicle
Abscess	Femoral aneurysm or pseudoaneurysm
Hematoma	Cyst
Varicocele	Seroma

Source: Reprinted from Scott DJ, Jones DB. Hernias and abdominal wall defects. In: Norton JA, Bollinger RR, Chang AE, et al, eds. Surgery: Basic Science and Clinical Evidence. New York: Springer-Verlag, 2001, with permission.

- What is the optimal care for the patient (that is grounded in the patient's preferences and life situation, evaluating the literature, understanding local resources, and the clinician's experience)?

Step 1: Achieving a Diagnosis

The clinical process for determining a diagnosis is to obtain a history, conduct a physical examination, generate differential diagnoses, and order relevant labs and studies. The essential information from the history and physical examination is consistent with a diagnosis of left inguinal hernia. In creating the differential, however, it is important to ensure that other reasonable explanations of an abdominal mass are considered. **Table 2.13** lists alternative diagnoses that can be considered.

Achieving a diagnosis, the first step of the EBM algorithm, has the same related elements as every other step:

- *Patient's primary complaint or the problem of interest* (pain in the groin)
- *Intervention or action* (history and physical exam)
- *Comparison of alternative interventions* (identify labs/studies to be ordered)
- *Outcome of clinical interest* (diagnostic accuracy/cost-effectiveness of each lab/study)

The process for generating a question to guide clinical decision making regarding achieving a diagnosis is summarized in **Table 2.14**.

The question can be phrased as follows: **What role do labs and clinical studies have in diagnosing the reason for a sudden onset of**

Table 2.14. Step 1: Achieving a diagnosis.

	Creating an evidence-based medicine question			
Element:	Patient problem	Intervention	Comparison intervention	Outcome of clinical interest
Question components:	Male patient with pain in L groin	H/PE to determine diagnosis (DX)	H/PE *and* labs/studies to determine DX	Diagnostic accuracy, cost-effectiveness

pain in the groin that occurred during heavy lifting and was followed by several days' duration of dragging sensation? To evaluate the relevance of the studies for diagnostic utility with regard to a patient's condition, apply the following criteria: look for "gold standard" evaluations; check to see if the diagnostic test was used in an appropriate spectrum of patients; and, finally, determine whether or not the reference standard was applied to the study results, regardless of the diagnostic test result. By following these steps, the quality of the study and its relevance to the patient can be determined so that the physician can make a decision about whether or not to incorporate the findings into the patient's care plan.

With regard to Mr. Edwards, the literature is reviewed and confirms that the gold standard for diagnosing hernia is a thorough history and physical examination. Based on the data obtained through the history and physical examination, an initial list of differential diagnoses is developed. Based on epidemiologic data, it is fairly certain that Mr. Edwards has an inguinal hernia. Approximately 680,000 inguinal hernia repairs are performed annually in the United States, and more than 90% are performed on males. However, it is important to exclude alternative diagnoses. Other diagnoses that could present with persistent groin pain are placed on the differential list. After confirming the adequacy of the list, it is clear that the most likely diagnosis is a hernia. The next step is to classify the type of hernia, since this will help to determine the preferred course of treatment (Table 2.15).

Step 2: Estimating a Prognosis

Continuing through the algorithm, perform step 2: estimating a prognosis. To estimate a prognosis, you must be confident of the accuracy of your diagnosis. It is clear that the hernia is neither incarcerated nor strangulated. However, the natural course of the condition indicates that there is a significant probability that either of these two events

Table 2.15. Nyhus classification of groin hernias.

Type 1. Indirect inguinal hernia—normal internal inguinal ring
Type 2. Indirect inguinal hernia—enlarged internal inguinal ring but intact inguinal canal floor

Type 3. Posterior wall defect
  A. Direct inguinal hernia
  B. Indirect inguinal hernia—enlarged internal inguinal ring with destruction of adjacent inguinal canal floor, e.g., massive scrotal, sliding, or pantaloon hernias
  C. Femoral hernias

Type 4. Recurrent hernia
  A. Direct
  B. Indirect
  C. Femoral
  D. Combined

Source: Reprinted from Scott DJ, Jones DB. Hernias and abdominal wall defects. In: Norton JA, Bollinger RR, Chang AE, et al, eds. Surgery: Basic Science and Clinical Evidence. New York: Springer-Verlag, 2001, with permission.

Table 2.16. Step 2: Estimating a prognosis.

	Creating an evidence-based medicine question			
Element	Patient problem	Intervention	Comparison intervention	Outcome of clinical interest
Question component	Male, acute onset L groin pain	Observation	Operative intervention	Likelihood of incarceration/ strangulation

could occur. **Table 2.16** specifies how to create a question to guide clinical decision making at this point.

The question becomes: **For a patient with a left inguinal hernia, what treatment should you recommend (observation or surgery) to reduce the likelihood of incarceration or strangulation of the hernia?** One must be able to define what the natural history of a condition is before a risk-benefit analysis may be completed.

The literature is searched to determine the probability of an adverse outcome related to the medical condition, in this case incarceration and strangulation. To evaluate the studies for validity with regard to estimating Mr. Edwards' prognosis, apply the following four criteria:

- Determine the **characteristics of the patients in the study** (defined, representative sample assembled at a common point in the course of their disease).
- Determine **the adequacy of the follow-up** (sufficient duration and comprehensiveness).
- Was the **objective outcome criteria applied in a blinded manner** (the evaluators were unaware of the patient's specific treatment)?
- For studies divided into subgroups with different prognoses, were appropriate **adjustments made for important prognostic factors**? Was there **a control group of "test-set" patients**?

Step 3: Deciding on the Best Therapy

Step 3 in the algorithm is **deciding on the best therapy for your patient**. The essential element in framing the question about best therapy focuses on what interventions (cause/prognostic factor/ treatment/etc.) should be considered. This process is critical to the development of a treatment recommendation that is individualized for each patient.

For Mr. Edwards, surgery will become necessary; the natural history of a hernia is that it becomes larger with the passage of time, does not resolve spontaneously, and can result in intestinal obstruction or strangulation. In this specific example, it is difficult to identify published studies in which patients with inguinal hernia were randomized prospectively to operative versus nonoperative therapy. Historically, however, prior to the common practice of elective repair, hernias were known as the most common cause of intestinal obstruction. Therefore, prophylactic hernia repair became the the standard of care. Prophylactic hernia repair is considered to be the optimal intervention, based on the best available data (level III: historical observation, the wisdom of

Table 2.17. Step 3: Deciding on the best therapy.

Creating an evidence-based medicine question				
Element	Patient problem	Intervention	Comparison intervention	Outcome of clinical interest
Question component	Male, L inguinal hernia	Open operative procedure	Laparoscopic procedure	Optimal operative procedure for reducing inguinal hernia

experts). Unless a patient is so debilitated that his life expectancy is very short or his comorbid conditions are so severe that operative risks are considered to be unacceptable, one should consider prophylactic repair. Hernia surgery poses an acceptable level of risk when compared to the high likelihood of intestinal obstruction or strangulation without elective preventive surgery. A literature search also reveals that the risk of hernia strangulation is thought to be greatest in the period soon after initial presentation.[4]

Based on the prognosis determined from talking with experts and reviewing the literature, it is clear that the optimal treatment is surgery. The literature identifies three treatment options: observation with reevaluation in 2 weeks, immediate surgery, and elective surgery 6 months hence. Reducing the risk of the potential complications of hernias (incarceration and strangulation) is best achieved through minimizing the time until surgery.

Mr. Edwards' treatment plan develops as follows:

- Preferred treatment is elective surgery, scheduled as soon as possible, with biweekly follow-up by the primary care physician during the interim and patient education related to the signs and symptoms of an incarcerated or strangulated hernia.
- The less preferable treatment is indefinite observation with a follow-up visit to the surgeon in 6 months.

The next EBM question that guides the development of a plan for Mr. Edwards is: What type of operative procedure is best? The essential element is specifying comparison "interventions," for example, comparing open and laparoscopic techniques. **Table 2.17** specifies the components of your clinical decision-making question regarding best therapy.

The evidence-based question about estimating best therapy becomes: For a male patient with a simple left inguinal hernia, is a laparoscopic or open procedure the preferred approach? (The question can be answered by checking Chapter 35, "Hernias and Abdominal Wall Defects," by D.J. Scott and D.B. Jones, in Surgery: Basic Science and Clinical Evidence, cited above, for the techniques to repair primary inguinal hernias.)

---

[4] Gallegos NC, Dawson J, et al. Risk of strangulation in groin hernias. Br J Surg 1991;78(10):1171–1173. Rai S, Chandra SS, et al. A study of the risk of strangulation and obstruction in groin hernias. Aust N Z J Surg 1998;68(9):630–634.

Table 2.18. Step 4: Determining harm.

	Creating an evidence-based medicine question			
Element	Patient problem	Intervention	Comparison intervention	Outcome of clinical interest
Question component	Male with L inguinal hernia	Laparoscopic	Open	Adverse effects, time to recovery

In reviewing the studies for treatment, there are two major questions to be answered: Was there **randomized assignment of patients to experimental conditions** and were they analyzed in the groups to which they were assigned? Was the **attrition rate reported** and were all patients who entered the study accounted for at the conclusion of the study?

In a quick search of Cochrane's database, you find two prospective, nonrandomized trials describing the outcomes of using an open approach (the Lichtenstein approach) to repair primary inguinal hernias: one by Kark et al[5] reporting a series of 3175 and one by Lichtenstein's group[6] reporting 4000 repairs. With the use of the open Lichtenstein approach, the rate of recurrence varied from 0.5% to 0.1%, with minimal complications, and patients usually returned to work within 2 weeks. A search for prospective studies of laparoscopic techniques yields Phillips et al's[7] multicenter study of 3229 transabdominal preperitoneal (TAPP) repairs and Felix et al's[8] retrospective, multicenter study of 10,053 TAPP repairs. The recurrence rate was 0.4% to 0.6%. It is apparent that the two approaches yield comparable results.

Step 4: Determining Harm

In reviewing studies of negative outcome, two basic questions must be answered:

1. Does the intervention cause an **adverse effect** in *some patients*?
2. And, if so, was the particular intervention responsible for the **negative outcome** in the *specific patient*?

Answering the two questions above will frame the next set of EBM questions that are needed to develop the plan for Mr. Edwards. In framing this iteration of EBM questions, the essential element that must be considered is **specifying the clinical outcome of interest**. See **Table 2.18** for an example of the components of the next EBM question that will guide the process of clinical decision making for Mr. Edwards.

---

[5] Kark AE, Kurzer MN, Belsham PA. 3175 primary inguinal hernia repairs: advantages of ambulatory open mesh repair using local anesthesia. J Am Coll Surg 1998;186:447–455.
[6] Amid PK, Shulman AG, Lichtenstein IL. Open "tension-free" repair of inguinal hernias: the Lichtenstein technique. Eur J Surg 1996;162:447–453.
[7] Phillips EH, Arregui M, Carrol BJ, et al. Incidence of complications following laparoscopic hernioplasty. Surg Enosc 1995;9:1621.
[8] Felix EL, Michas CA, Gonzalez MH. Laparoscopic hernioplast: TAPP vs TEP. Surg Endosc 1995;9:984–989.

Table 2.19. Step 5: Providing care of the highest quality.

	Creating an Evidence-Based Medicine Question			
Element:	Patient problem	Intervention	Comparison intervention	Outcome of clinical interest
Question component:	Male with L inguinal hernia, no acute distress, primary wage earner for family—hourly worker with no paid time off; wife has excellent insurance	Open approach	Laparoscopic approach	Minimal time away from work

Source: Reprinted from Scott DJ, Jones DB. Hernias and abdominal wall defects. In: Norton JA, Bollinger RR, Chang AE, et al, eds. Surgery: Basic Science and Clinical Evidence. New York: Springer-Verlag, 2001.

The EBM question becomes: For a 45-year-old man with a simple left inguinal hernia, which procedure is most likely to have the maximum likelihood of immediate success and also is most likely to prevent recurrence? The focus of the question is obtaining data about the adverse outcomes associated with the use of open versus laparoscopic operative techniques.[9] There are several level I studies that explicitly compare the Lichtenstein (open) and TAPP (laparoscopic) procedures.[10] Other studies have compared TEP and other open. After reviewing the information, you conclude that the major difference between the two laparoscopic procedures versus the open Lichtenstein procedure is that, although laparoscopic procedures cost significantly more, laparoscopic procedures appear to allow patients to return to work more quickly. Operative time and complication rates are not notably different.

Step 5: Providing Care of the Highest Quality

In the final step in the algorithm, **the element that is emphasized is assuring that the clinical decision making of the physician optimized the outcome** for Mr. Edwards. **Table 2.19** specifies the relevant components of the clinical decision-making question. The evidence is summa-

---

[9] Liem MSL, Van Der Graff Y, Van Steensel CJ, et al. Comparison of conventional anterior surgery and laparoscopic surgery for inguinal-hernia repair. N Engl J Med 1997;336:1541–1547. Champault G, Rizk N, Cathleine JM, et al. Inguinal hernia repair: totally pre-peritoneal laparoscopic approach versus Stoppa operation, randomized trial: 100 cases. Hernia 1997;1:31–36. Wright DM, Kennedy A, Baxter JN, et al. Early outcome after open versus extraperitoneal endoscopic tension-free hernioplasty: a randomized clinical trial. Surgery (St. Louis) 1996;119:552–557.

[10] Paganini AM, Lezoches E, Carle F, et al. A randomized, controlled, clinical study of laparoscopic vs open tension-free inguinal hernia repair. Sur Endosc 1998;12:979–986. Payne JH, Grininger LM, Izawa MT, et al. Laparoscopic or open inguinal herniorrhaphy? A randomized prospective trial. Arch Surg 1994;129:973–981.

rized and explained to Mr. Edwards so that he can be a participant in his care and give informed consent to the treatment of his choice. It turns out that he is an hourly worker, without paid time off. His wife's health insurance will cover any reasonable and customary costs. *The patient's most important concern is that he is able to return to work in the shortest time possible.* Given the information about the risks and benefits inherent to each procedure, he elects to have the laparoscopic hernia repair.

Summary

Evidence-based medicine provides a systematic approach to ensuring the delivery of the highest quality of care possible to patients. It draws on the best evidence available to inform the practice of skilled and experienced clinicians. The quality of the evidence ranges from useful but potentially biased single-case studies to randomized clinical trials that meet the strictest standards of scientific rigor. Additional useful evidence can be obtained from meta-analyses, outcome studies, and practice guidelines.

Evidence-based medicine has five core tenets for practicing medicine:

- Clinical decision making should be based on the best available scientific evidence.
- The clinical problem, rather than the habits or protocols, should determine the type of evidence to be sought.
- Identifying the best evidence means thinking informed by epidemiologic and biostatistical methods.
- Conclusions derived from identifying and critically appraising evidence are useful only if put into action in managing patients or making healthcare decisions.
- Performance should be constantly evaluated.

The evidence-based medicine algorithm for delivering quality patient care contains five clinical objectives:

1. Achieving a diagnosis
2. Estimating the prognosis
3. Deciding on the best therapy
4. Determining harm
5. Providing care of the highest quality

Application of the five core tenets of evidence-based medicine to the five clinical objectives promotes the optimal practice of surgery. The acronym for developing an effective question to guide the application of evidence to the practice of surgery is PICO: patient problem, intervention, comparison intervention, and outcome of clinical interest.

Three "pearls" to keep in mind:

- Clinical wisdom is invaluable but never above question.
- The best evidence is only as good as the clinician who applies the information to deliver patient care.
- Clinical acumen and experience form the essential base on which the practice of evidence-based medicine rests.

Selected Readings

Dawson-Saunders B, Trapp RG. Basic and Clinical Biostatistics, 2nd ed. Norwalk, CT: Appleton & Lange, 1994.

Glasziou P, Irwig L, Bain C, Colditz G. Systematic Reviews in Health Care: A Practical Guide. New York: Cambridge University Press, 2001.

McLeod RS. Evidence-based surgery. In: Norton JA, et al, eds. Surgery: Basic Science and Clinical Evidence. New York: Springer-Verlag, 2001.

Reeves S, Koppel I, Barr H, Freeth D, Hammick M. Twelve tips for undertaking a systematic review. Medical Teacher 2002;24:358–363.

Sackett DL, Richardson WS, Rosenberg W, Haynes RB. Evidence-Based Medicine: How to Practice and Teach EBM. New York: Churchill Livingstone, 1997.

Sackett DL, Rosenberg MC, Muir Gray JA, et al. Evidence-Based Medicine: How to Practice and Teach EBM, 2nd ed. London: Churchill Livingstone, 2000.

Appendix 2.A: Useful Evidence-Based Web Sites

http://cebmjr2.ox.ac.uk/

The National Health Service of Great Britain, Division of Research and Development, Centre for Evidence-Based Medicine sponsors this Web site. The contents include the following resources:

- Evidence-based on call: current, reviewed, evidence-based information for clinicians
- EBM toolbox: clinical tools for practitioners
- Levels of evidence: descriptions of several taxonomies for categorizing levels of evidence
- Glossary
- Downloads of various applications

http://www.cebm.utoronto.ca/

The University of Toronto's Centre for Evidence-Based Medicine sponsors this Web site for the purpose of disseminating and evaluating resources for the practice of evidence-based medicine. The contents include the following resources:

- Instructional module on asking evidence-based questions
- PDA downloads
- Glossary
- Gateway to resources on the Internet, including journals, CDs, textbooks, and other Web sites.

http://www.guidelines.gov/

The Agency of Healthcare Research and Quality, in partnership with the American Medical Association (AMA) and the American Association of Health Plans, sponsors the National Guideline Clearinghouse (NGC) Web site. The contents include the following:

- Browser for current practice guidelines
- A site to compare guidelines
- Practice resources

http://nlm.nih.gov/medlineplus/

The National Library of Medicine and the National Institutes of Health sponsor this Web site. The contents include the following:

- Health topics—information on conditions, diseases, and wellness, and a medical encyclopedia
- Drug information
- Dictionaries
- Other resources:
  - Link to Clintrials.gov, a Web site that provides information about clinical research studies

3

Nutrition Support in the Surgery Patient

Stephen F. Lowry

Objectives

1. To understand the decision-making process for initiating, maintaining, and terminating Specialized Nutritional Support (SNS) in surgical patients.
2. To understand the decision-making process for calculating nutritional requirements, gaining access for SNS, and monitoring for complications during SNS.

Cases

Case 1

A 67-year-old man with obstructing esophageal cancer presents for consideration of surgical therapy. He has lost 25 pounds (15% of normal body weight) over the past 4 months, is unable to swallow anything except liquids, and has near-complete loss of appetite. He has no other past history of significance and takes medications only for hypertension. His appearance is gaunt with obvious loss of body fat and muscle wasting. There is mild peripheral edema. The remainder of the physical exam is unremarkable. Workup suggests that he is a candidate for esophageal resection. His albumin is $2.7\,g/L$ and his hemoglobin is $9\,g/L$ with microcytic indices. All other determinations are normal.

Case 2

A previously healthy 27-year-old woman is the restrained driver in a head-on collision. She is diagnosed with intraabdominal injuries and undergoes emergency laparotomy. At operation, a crush injury to the pancreas and duodenum is repaired as is a mesenteric tear and grade II liver laceration. Appropriate external drainage of the injury sites is undertaken. She has lost approximately 1000 mL of blood and has received 4000 mL of crystalloid solutions intraoperatively. She will be transferred to the intensive care unit (ICU) for initial postoperative care. No other major injuries are noted.

Implications of Nutritional Support for Clinical Outcomes

Many of the illnesses and injuries subject to surgical intervention and care promote alterations of metabolism that place patients at some risk of malnutrition-specific morbidities. It widely is assumed that mal-nutrition, especially within the context of hypermetabolism, increases the risk of infection, leads to wound-healing failure, prolongs rehabil-itation, and diminishes responses to adjunctive therapies. Active intervention, in the form of specialized nutrition support (SNS) tech-nologies, provides the potential to attenuate these consequences and, at least partially, to restore adequate nutritional status.

Consideration of SNS in surgical patients requires an under-standing of the therapeutic risks and benefits as well as the timing of intervention, and an analysis of the effectiveness of therapy. Algo-rithm 3.1 provides a logical approach to these issues. These consider-ations are undertaken repeatedly during the course of surgical care and may be modulated by changes in patient status and prognosis. **It is axiomatic that it is always preferable to provide nutrients via the intestinal tract, but the capacity to effectively and efficiently do so may be altered by changes in clinical condition.**

Assessing Nutritional Status

When considering SNS intervention, there are several issues that must be addressed at the outset. The most pressing issue is whether the patient already has manifestations of "malnutrition." There is a **strong inverse correlation between body protein status and the incidence of postoperative complications** in patients undergoing major elective (gastrointestinal) surgery. Unfortunately, the consensus regarding the most appropriate manner used to assess protein status is lacking, and the clinician often faces the dilemma of a continuum of nutritional situations ranging from seemingly normal to that of severe cachexia and wasting. Readily obtainable parameters, such as weight loss (especially in relation to normal or ideal body weight), circulating protein levels (such as albumin), surrogate markers of immune func-tion (such as lymphocyte count), as well as physical examination for evidence of muscle wasting (loss of temporal or other skeletal muscle mass), should be sought in all patients was done in **Case 1**. How such parameters translate into nutritional risk is a matter of some conjecture.

There is clearly no "gold standard" for determining nutritional status because the influence of disease and injury independently may

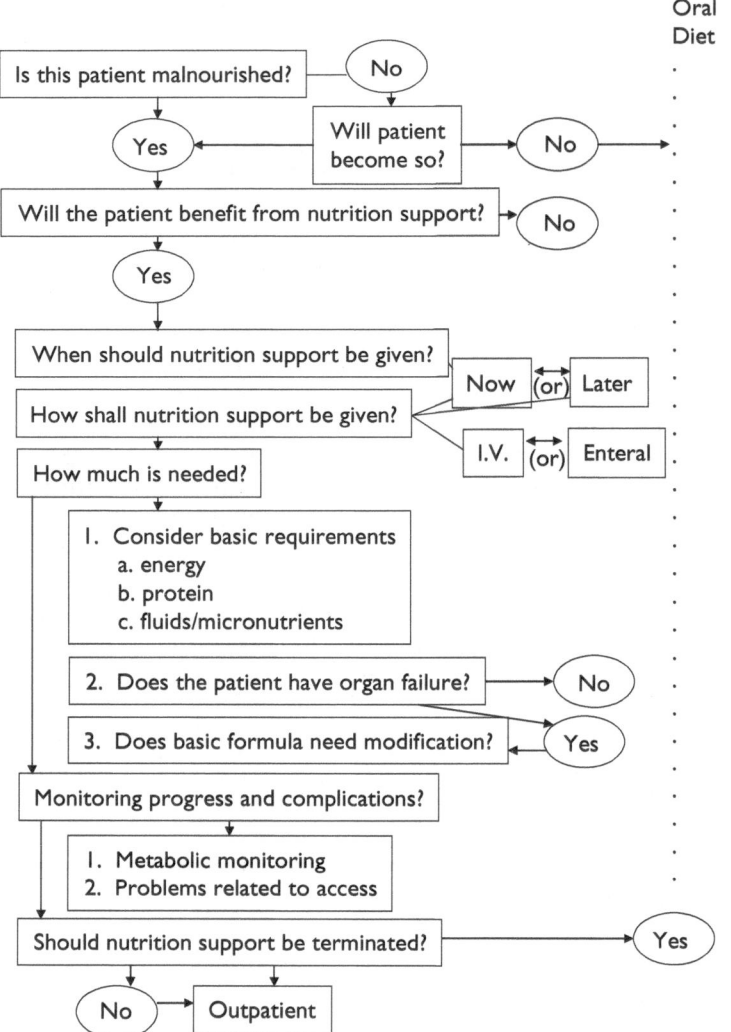

Algorithm 3.1. Algorithm for decision analysis for nutritional support.

influence most biochemical or anthropometric parameters. Malnutrition appears to be a continuum that is influenced by altered intake and the degree of antecedent/concurrent metabolic stress. At a minimum, **accurate documentation of weight loss** over prior weeks and months is an indicator of the potential degree of malnutrition. Decisions regarding the immediacy or need for SNS can be undertaken with an evidence-based approach when considered in conjunction with the magnitude and duration of future metabolic stresses imposed by injury or major surgery. In summary, there are several general categories that define the **current indications for SNS**. They include (1) patients who are **overtly malnourished** and require restoration of protein and energy stores in preparation for or in conjunction with other therapies;

(2) patients who are **unable or unwilling to eat** and who will become malnourished without SNS intervention; (3) patients in whom **use of the digestive tract is inadequate or unsafe**; and (4) patients in whom the **magnitude and duration of hypermetabolism likely will lead to malnutrition** without SNS.

Defining the Benefits and Timing of Nutritional Support

Although the effect of SNS in patients with modest malnutrition is unclear, there are significant class I data describing the impact of SNS in nontrauma/noncritically ill well-nourished and severely malnourished surgical patients. As noted in **Table 3.1**, SNS, either enteral or parenteral, generally demonstrated little or no impact on postoperative patient outcome and, in some series, was associated with increased complications. By contrast, patients with severe malnutrition (weight loss >10–12%) **(Case 1)** did benefit from preoperative or perioperative SNS. At present, it is unclear in these patients whether the benefit of SNS was derived from the pre- and/or postoperative phase of SNS.

The above results raise the issue of whether patients with elective surgery should undergo a period of preoperative SNS. At present, resource constraints likely will preclude any efforts unless the patient already is receiving SNS for the underlying illness. It is prudent, however, to be attentive to preoperative nutrient intake and urge supplemental oral feedings, where possible.

In the absence of antecedent malnutrition, indications instituting postoperative or injury SNS involves a more complex decision process **(Case 2)**. The clinician is required to **consider the complexity of the surgical/injury process, the magnitude and duration of hypermetabolism, and the prospects for early return to oral feeding. Absent a favorable response to each of the above parameters, the immediate or early (within 5 days) institution of SNS at least must be considered.**

In some patients, such as those with extensive burns or severe, complex injuries **(Case 2)** or patients expected to require additional surgery or cytotoxic therapies, the decision for early initiation of SNS is straightforward. Despite a general lack of class I evidence to support this decision, few would argue with such a decision. Indeed, SNS should be considered during the operative planning or intraoperatively so that an access route can be provided (such as a jejunostomy tube or central venous catheter).

The majority of patients do not require postoperative SNS. But the nutritional status should be reassessed throughout the hospital stay. Should clinical conditions change and/or complications develop, it may be prudent to initiate SNS at a subsequent point. As a general rule, **SNS should be considered in any patient who does not return to nearly adequate or normal oral intake status within 5 to 7 days of admission.** As a general rule, SNS is not of benefit unless provided for 7 days or more.

Table 3.1. Perioperative and early feeding studies with substantial number of well-nourished or moderately malnourished patients.

Author	Year	Class of evidence	Conclusions
Veterans Affairs Total Parenteral Nutrition Cooperative Study Group[a]	1991	I	Of 395 malnourished patients requiring laparotomy or noncardiac thoracotomy randomized to 7–15 days preoperative nutrition ($n = 192$) or no perioperative nutrition support ($n = 203$) and monitored for 90 days following surgery, the rates of major complications were similar in patients with mild or moderate degrees of malnutrition with more infectious complications in the TPN group ($p = .01$) but more noninfectious complications in the control group ($p = .02$); 90-day mortality rates were also similar. Only in severely malnourished patients did TPN significantly reduce noninfectious complications (5% vs. 43%, $p = .03$) with no increase in infectious complications.
Fan[b]	1994	I	A randomized prospective study of 124 patients undergoing resection of hepatocellular carcinoma randomized to perioperative intravenous nutrition with 35% branched-chain amino acids, dextrose, and lipid (50% medium-chain triglycerides) for 14 days in addition to oral diet or control group (oral diet alone). Postoperative morbidity rate reduced in perioperative fed group (34% vs. 55%) because of fewer septic complications (17% vs. 37%) and less deterioration of liver function as measured by indocyanine green. There were no significant differences in deaths although most of the benefit occurred in cirrhotic patients undergoing major hepatectomy.
Brennan[c]	1994	I	A prospective, randomized trial of 117 moderately malnourished patients randomized to postoperative parenteral nutrition ($n = 60$, albumin = 3.1, 5.8% preoperative body weight loss) or standard i.v. fluids ($n = 57$, albumin = 3.3, 6.8% preoperative body weight loss). Complications were significantly greater in TPN-fed patients with a significant increase in intraabdominal abscess and major complications.
Heslin[d]	1997	I	Of 195 well-nourished patients undergoing esophageal, gastric, pancreatic, or gastric resection randomized to jejunal feedings ($n = 97$; albumin 4.08 ± 0.04 g/dL) or i.v. feedings ($n = 98$; albumin = 4.1 ± 0.06 g/dL), no significant differences found in the number of major, minor, or infectious wound complications between groups and no difference in hospital mortality or length of stay. There was one small-bowel necrosis in the enterally fed group.
Doglietto[e]	1996	I	Their 678 patients with normal or mild malnutrition undergoing major elective abdominal surgery randomized to protein-sparing therapy or no specialized nutrition had similar operative mortality rates and postoperative complication rate.
Watters[f]	1997	I	Patients undergoing esophagectomy or pancreatoduodenectomy were randomized to postoperative early jejunal feedings ($n = 13$; albumin = 4.08 ± 5 g/dL) or no enteral feeding ($n = 15$; 4.1 ± 4 g/dL) during the first 6 postoperative days. Postoperative vital capacity and fractional expired volume were lower in the fed group and postoperative mobility was lower in the fed group in this well-nourished group of patients at low risk of nutrition-related complications. This study was confounded by increased epidural anesthesia in the enterally fed group.

Table 3.1. *Continued*

Author	Year	Class of evidence	Conclusions
Daly[g]	1992	I	Studied 85 patients randomized to standard (n = 44; albumin = 3.0 ± 1.2 g/dL) vs. supplemented (n = 41; albumin = 3.3 g/dL) enteral diets with 77 eligible patients. Infectious and wound complications (p = .02) and length of stay (p = .01) significantly shorter for supplemented group. Diets were not isonitrogenous.
Daly[h]	1995	I	Studied 60 patients with upper gastrointestinal lesions requiring resection randomized to standard enteral diet (n = 30) or diet supplemented with arginine, omega-3 fatty acids, and nucleotides (n = 30). Patients were moderately malnourished with albumins less than 3.4. Length of stay and infectious/wound complications significantly reduced (p < .05 for both) in supplemented group. Patients also randomized to jejunal feedings during radiation chemotherapy tolerated chemotherapy significantly better.

TPN, total parenteral nutrition.

[a] The Veteran Affairs Total Parenteral Nutrition Cooperative Study Group. Perioperative total parenteral nutrition in surgical patients. N Engl Med 1991;325:525–532.

[b] Fan ST, Lo CM, Lai EC, et al. Perioperative nutritional support in patients undergoing hepatectomy for hepatocellular carcinoma. N Engl J Med 1994;331:1547–1552.

[c] Brennan MF, Pisters PWT, Posner M, et al. A prospective, randomized trial of total parenteral nutrition after major pancreatic resection for malignancy. Ann Surg 1994;220:436–444.

[d] Heslin MJ, Latkany L, Leung D, et al. A prospective, randomized trial of early enteral feeding after resection of upper gastrointestinal malignancy. Ann Surg 1997;226:567–577.

[e] Doglietto GB, Gallitelli L, Pacelli F, et al. Protein-sparing therapy after major abdominal surgery: lack of clinical effects. Ann Surg 1996;223:357–362.

[f] Watters JM, Kirkpatrick SM, Norris SB, et al. Immediate postoperative enteral feeding results in impaired respiratory mechanics and decreased mobility. Ann Surg 1997;226:368–377.

[g] Daly JM, Lieberman MD, Goldfine J, et al. Enteral nutrition with supplemental arginine, RNA, and omega-3 fatty acids in patients after operation: immunologic, metabolic, and clinical outcome. Surgery (St. Louis) 1992;112:56–67.

[h] Daly JM, Weintraub FN, Shou J, et al. Enteral nutrition during multimodality therapy in upper gastrointestinal cancer patients. Ann Surg 1995;221:327–338.

Source: Reprinted from Kudsk KA, Jacobs DO. Nutrition. In: Norton JA, Bollinger RR, Chang AE, et al, eds. Surgery: Basic Science and Clinical Evidence. New York: Springer-Verlag, 2001, with permission.

Defining the Route of Nutritional Support

Specialized nutritional support may be provided intravenously, enterally, or by some combination of both. Although parenteral and enteral nutrition likely promote similar metabolic efficacy, current class I data strongly suggest that enteral feeding is associated with a lower overall rate of complications. No data exist currently to suggest that mortality is influenced adversely by the choice of feeding route.

The clinician always should consider feeding options during the decision-making process. While it is clearly preferable to establish an enteral feeding conduit, some conditions may preclude full use of this route for a variable period of time. Some patients tolerate limited enteral feedings despite cautionary clinical conditions (e.g., peritonitis). Given the objective to provide adequate SNS, extended (days) efforts to establish full SNS via the intestinal tract are unwarranted in the face of severe malnutrition and/or hypermetabolism. Providing at least some intravenous SNS should be considered if a significant caloric and protein deficit will be incurred.

Establishing Access for Nutritional Support

Whether done pre-, intra-, or postoperatively, care must be taken to **establish a secure and safe portal for delivery of SNS. The portal should be dedicated solely to the purposes of SNS,** as there is evidence to suggest that violating the condition increases complications. Once established and maintained by the above criteria, these portals need not be changed routinely unless there is clinical or laboratory evidence of dysfunction or infection.

Access for Parenteral Nutrition

The preferred method for obtaining access for intravenous SNS is with a subclavian vein catheter. This usually provides a secure site that can be maintained in a sterile fashion. In some circumstances, a multiple-lumen catheter is inserted to provide for other monitoring options, but one lumen must be dedicated to SNS administration. Barring a subclavian insertion site, other options include jugular vein as well as peripheral catheter insertion sites. Such sites are more prone to complications of infection, dislodgment, and venous thrombosis and should be replaced with a more secure or permanent catheter at the earliest opportunity. Protocols for changing dressings and intravenous tubings for SNS central vein catheters should be maintained.

Access for Enteral Nutrition

Although some patients tolerate direct intragastric tube feedings, this practice is discouraged in patients who are prone to aspiration (critically ill, unconscious, etc.). Most patients with severe injury or after laparotomy have gastroparesis, and hence cannot tolerate gastric feedings. **It is judicious to assume that any patient requiring prolonged enteral SNS will require feedings distal to the stomach.** Numerous options for such feeding conduits are available. Some can be placed at the bedside using flexible small-bore tubes, while others require intra-operative, radiographically guided, or endoscopically assisted placement. Consideration of these options should begin as soon as practical after admission. (See Chapter 7, "Nutrition," by Kenneth A. Kudsk and Danny O. Jacobs, cited above for further details and illustrations.)

Combined Enteral and Parenteral Nutrition

Although it is unknown what proportion of nutrients need to be provided enterally to achieve optimal results, a combination of both enteral and intravenous feeding may promote early, adequate nutrition. This is accomplished more readily if the parenteral SNS is given via a central vein catheter, although small-bore peripheral access may be used for a limited time. Such catheters are prone to vein thrombosis if the dextrose concentration exceeds 10%, and thus this route is more limiting in duration and patient comfort.

Defining the Nutritional Prescription

The initial approach to defining nutritional requirements in surgical patients assumes no difference either between the routes of feeding or among patients on the basis of antecedent nutritional status. While there are differences between commonly prescribed intravenous SNS formulas and available enteral formulas, for purposes of defining individual patient requirements, initial considerations revolve around **estimates of energy and protein needs**. For these initial calculations, it is important to have **a measure or a reasonable estimate of preinjury body weight**. For subsequent refinements in the prescription, **knowledge of current fluid and electrolyte status and of organ function** is necessary. (For more details, see Chapter 4.)

Basic Requirements

Energy
Although there are several proposed methods for estimating energy needs, the most widely used are the Harris-Benedict equations, which define basal energy expenditure (BEE) (**Table 3.2**). These equations account for gender, age, height, and weight and provide a rough estimate of the basal (nonstressed) energy expenditure. This calculation therefore can be used once these simple parameters are ascertained. In the absence of these parameters, one may utilize the estimates provided in **Table 3.3**. While there are other, and perhaps more precise, methods of energy needs assessment, all involve obtaining more detailed biochemical or calorimetric data. As a first approximation, the Harris-Benedict formulas usually are sufficient.

Once this calculation has been performed, one next needs to estimate the degree of hypermetabolism arising from the underlying condition. For instance, an elective operation with minimal blood loss and complexity increases the energy expenditure by 10% to 20% above the BEE. Hence, the prescription for energy needs should encompass this stress factor and be targeted at 1.10 to 1.20 times the Harris-Benedict calcu-

Table 3.2. Calculating resting metabolic expenditure.

Resting metabolic expenditure (RME) in kilocalories per day, can be estimated by using the Harris-Benedict equations:

For men
$66.47 + 13.75 (W) + 5 (H) - 6.76 (A)$

For women
$65.51 + 9.56 (W) + 2.86 (H) - 4.68 (A)$

W, weight in kilograms; H, height in centimeters; A, age in years.
Source: Reprinted from Kudsk KA, Jacobs DO. Nutrition. In: Norton JA, Bollinger RR, Chang AE, et al, eds. Surgery: Basic Science and Clinical Evidence. New York: Springer-Verlag, 2001, with permission.

Table 3.3. Energy and protein needs for surgical patients.

Condition	Kcal/kg/day	Protein/kg/day	NPC:N
Normal to moderate malnutrition	(low stress) 25–30	1.0	150:1
Moderate stress	25–30	1.5	120:1
Hypermetabolic, stressed	30–35	1.5–2.0	90–120:1
Burns	35–40	2.0–2.5	90–120:1

Source: Reprinted from Kudsk KA, Jacobs DO. Nutrition. In: Norton JA, Bollinger RR, Chang AE, et al, eds. Surgery: Basic Science and Clinical Evidence. New York: Springer-Verlag, 2001, with permission.

lation. As shown in **Table 3.3**, other surgical conditions increase this stress factor proportionally.

Sources of Nonprotein Calories for SNS

Glucose. The limit of glucose oxidation is approximately 5 to 7 mg/kg/min. Consequently, there is an upper limit of the amount of parenteral or enteral glucose that should be administered. Therefore, patients should not receive more than 500 to 600 g of glucose/day in an effort to keep their respiratory quotient near 1.0. Providing a majority of nonprotein calories as glucose, however, promotes retention of nitrogen. Excess levels of glucose promote fat deposition and may be associated with impairment of respiratory function and hyperglycemia.

Lipids. Alternative sources of nonprotein calories include various forms of lipid. While enteral formulas contain various medium- and long-chain lipid moieties, those available for parenteral administration are primarily omega-6-polyunsaturated long-chain fatty acids derived from vegetable oils. While such formulations are tolerated well by most patients, attention to lipid clearance and lipid sensitive diseases requires vigilance. The maximum recommended dose of lipid administration is 2.0 to 2.5 g/kg/day, and rates of administration in excess of this seldom are indicated. At a minimum, lipids must be provided at >5% of total calories to prevent essential fatty acid deficiency.

Protein
While the normal intake of protein in healthy, well-nourished adults is approximately 0.8 g/kg/day, these requirements are increased in stressed patients. In the absence of measured nitrogen (protein) losses, it is recommended that such patients receive 1.5 to 2.0 g/kg/day of protein (note: divide by 6.25 to obtain nitrogen equivalent).

Some patients with anticipated excessive losses (e.g., burns or open wounds) may require higher levels of nitrogen intake for maximum benefit. Other patients with severely contracted lean body mass may require less than 1.5 g/kg/day, as do patients with renal impairment and the inability to clear a normal or increased nitrogen load.

Although there is much discussion about the appropriate composition of protein or parenteral amino acid formulas, little data currently exist to suggest that these more expensive mixtures significantly improve outcome. To date, "designer formulas" for enhancing immune function have been documented to benefit only trauma patients. (See Chapter 7, "Nutrition," by Kenneth A. Kudsk and Danny O. Jacobs, cited above, for more discussion.)

Fluid and Micronutrients

Once the determination of energy and protein needs has been established, attention turns to defining the concentration of electrolytes, trace minerals, and other micronutrients that must be administered. Documenting fluid status (as discussed in Chapter 4) also requires careful physical examination and a review of intake/output records and changes in body weight to assess this condition.

It is essential to evaluate recent laboratory determinations for the presence of preexisting micronutrient imbalances. Efforts to correct any severe abnormalities should begin before instituting SNS. Barring the existence of such electrolyte or acid–base disorders, a standard range of micronutrient administration may be initiated at the onset of SNS (**Table 3.4**). These recommendations for micronutrient administration have been established from common clinical practice, but each **patient must be evaluated individually at the outset of SNS therapy and at regular intervals throughout the course of treatment**. Dramatic and life-threatening changes in electrolyte concentration as well as other serious metabolic abnormalities may evolve rapidly in patients with serious illness. (For more details, see Monitoring Progress and Complications, below.)

Modifications for Organ Dysfunction

Patients with organ failures require adjustments to both protein and micronutrient prescriptions. Patients with heart failure may require limitations of both fluid (reduced volume) and electrolyte (sodium) administration. Similarly, patients with renal insufficiency require attention to both volume and several electrolyte levels. Such patients

Table 3.4. Electrolyte concentrations in parenteral nutrition (PN).

Electrolyte	Recommended central PN doses	Recommended peripheral PN doses	Usual range of doses
Potassium (mEq/L)	30	30	0–120 (CVL) 0–80 (PV)
Sodium (mEq/L)	30	30	0–150
Phosphate (mmol/L)	15	5	0–20
Magnesium (mEq/L)	5	5	0–16
Calcium (mEq/L) (as gluconate)	4.7	4.7	0–10
Chloride (mEq/L)	50	50	0–150
Acetate (mEq/L)	40	40	0–100

CVL, central venous line; PV, peripheral vein.
Source: Reprinted from Kudsk KA, Jacobs DO. Nutrition. In: Norton JA, Bollinger RR, Chang AE, et al, eds. Surgery: Basic Science and Clinical Evidence. New York: Springer-Verlag, 2001, with permission.

should continue to receive adequate calories, with adjustments in the glucose load depending on the level of tolerance. Patients with liver disease may need reductions in the protein content as well as fluid and electrolyte levels of SNS formulas. Specialized amino acid formulas for hepatic failure may be used judiciously in selected patients.

Basic Formulations for Nutritional Support

Although there are numerous options for providing both enteral and parenteral formulations, the basic requirements are outlined below and in the referenced tables. The reader is referred to more detailed descriptions of these prescriptions elsewhere. (See Chapter 7 "Nutrition," by Kenneth A. Kudsk and Danny O. Jacobs, cited above.) The standard provisions outlined herein may be modified by the clinical considerations outlined above. In addition, the provider must be aware of the varying content of electrolytes in these formulations as well as of other micronutrients and vitamins (such as vitamin K). The latter, for instance, may not be appropriate for patients requiring anticoagulation therapy. **The clinicians should familiarize themselves with the content and concentrations of any SNS formulation before it is initiated.** An extensive listing of currently available enteral and parenteral nutrition formulations is provided in **Tables 3.5, 3.6, 3.7,** and **3.8**. An outline for standard orders for nutritional support is shown in **Table 3.9**. This is intended as a template for the initial prescription and should be modified according to clinical conditions.

Enteral Formulas
There are several basic categories of enteral formulas:

Standard, isotonic formulas contain an appropriate balance of carbohydrate, protein, and fat and usually are tolerated well because of low osmolarity (approximately 300 mOsm/L) and caloric density (1.0 kcal/mL). These are considered low-residue diets in that they do not contain fiber and are used in stable patients with significant hypermetabolism.

Standard, fiber-containing formulas are similar to the isotonic products and usually contain both a higher protein content as well as soluble and insoluble fiber. These often are fed to critically ill patients via jejunostomy tubes and appear to reduce the incidence of diarrhea.

High-density formulas provide a caloric density of 1.5 to 2.0 kcal/ml and may be appropriate for patients requiring volume restriction. Osmolarity is higher than standard formulas and the propensity for diarrhea is increased. These formulas are tolerated better by intragastric feeding.

Elemental/peptide-based formulas contain predigested proteins that may promote absorption in patients with malabsorption. Their higher osmolarity and lower fat content require a slower infusion rate initially.

Special formulas for organ dysfunction have been designed specifically for patients with established or evolving organ failure. Formu-

Table 3.5. Some enteral feeding formulas.

Product, supplier	kcal/mL	Total calorie/ nitrogen	Liters to provide 100% RDA vitamins and minerals	mOSm	Protein	Carbohydrate	Fat	Na	K	Features
Precision LR, Sandoz	1.1	239	1.7	530	26	248	1.6	30	2.3	P, F
Travasorb STD, Baxter	1	184	2	560	30	190	14	40	30	P, U, MCT
Reabilan, O'Brien	1	175	3	350	32	131	39	30	32	L, U, MCT
Travasorb, Baxter	1	154	1.9	450	35	136	35	30	31	L, E, MCT
Ensure, Ross	1	153	1.9	450	37	145	37	37	40	L, F
Resource Crystals, Sandoz	1	154	1.9	450	37	145	37	37	40	F
Resource Power, Sandoz	1	178	1.9	450	37	145	37	37	40	P, F
Enrich, Ross	1	148	1.4	480	40	162	37	37	40	L, E, High residue
Compleat, Reg, Sandoz	1	131	1.5	405	43	128	43	57	36	L, U
Ensure HN, Ross	1	125	1.3	470	44	141	35	40	40	L, F
Precision HN, Sandoz	1	125	2.8	525	44	216	1.3	43	23	P, F
Reabilan HN, O'Brien	1.3	125	2.9	490	58	158	52	43	43	L, U, MCT
Meritene, Doyle	1	104	1.2	550	58	110	32	38	41	L, F
Sustacal, Mead Johnson	1	79	1	625	61	140	23	41	53	L, F
Meritene Powder, Doyle	1	104	1.2	690	66	113	32	44	68	P, F
Sustacal Powder, M.J.	1.3	80	0.8	899	77	180	34	54	87	Mixed w/whole milk
Isotonic:										
Precision isotonic, Sandoz	1	183	1.6	300	29	144	30	20	25	P, F
Isocal, Mead Johnson	1	167	1.9	300	34	133	44	23	34	L, U, MCT
Entrition, Biosearch	1	154	2	300	35	136	35	31	31	L, U
Osmolite, Ross	1	153	1.9	300	37	145	39	24	26	L, U, MCT
Compleat Modified, Sandoz	1	131	1.5	300	4.3	141	37	29	36	L, U
Peptamen, Clintec Nutrition	1	131	2	260	40	127	39	22	16	L, U, MCT
Osmolite HN, Ross	1	125	1.3	310	44	141	37	40	40	L, U, MCT
Isotein HN, Sandoz	1.2	86	1.8	300	68	156	34	27	27	P, F, MCT
For impaired gastrointestinal tract and other special situations:										
Tolerex, Eaton	1	284	1.8	550	21	226	1.5	20	30	P, U
Vivonex T.E.N., Eaton	1	149	2	630	38	206	2.8	20	20	P, U, BCAA
Surgical liquid, Diet Ross	0.7	117	1.2	545	38	136	0	36	21	P, F
Criticare HN, Mead Johnson	1	148	2	650	38	222	3.4	28	34	L, U

Continued

Table 3.5. *Continued*

Product, supplier	kcal/mL	Total calorie/nitrogen	Liters to provide 100% RDA vitamins and minerals	mOSm	Protein	Carbohydrate	Fat	Na	K	Features
Vital HN, Ross	1	125	1.5	460	42	185	11	20	34	P, F, MCT
Trauma-aid HBC, McGaw	1	132	3	640	56	166	7	23	30	P, F, MCT, BCAA
Stresstein, Sandoz	1.2	97	2	910	70	173	27	29	29	P, U, MCT, BCAA
Travasorb MCT, Baxter	1.5	100	1.3	450	74	185	49	23	26	L, F, MCT
Impact, Novartis	1	91	1.5	375	56	130	28	48	36	L, U, MCT, fish oil
Perative, Ross	1.3	122	1.2	425	67	177	37	45	44	L, U, MCT, arginine
Alitraq, Ross	1	120	1.5	480	53	165	16	44	31	F, F, glutamine
Subdue, Mead Johnson	1	120	1.2	330	50	127	34	48	41	L, F, MCT
Immun-aid, McGaw	1	77	2	460	80	120	22	25	27	P, MCT, BCAA, arginine
For specific pathologic entities:										
Aminiaid, McGaw	1.9	362	Packets of 112 g, 467 cal, 470 mOsm/L	1095	23	384	25	14	<5	For renal failure
Travasorb renal, Baxter										For renal failure
Hepatic aid IL, McGaw	1.1	174	Packets of 96 g, 378 cal, 480 mOsm/L	460	44	158	34	<5	<6	For liver failure
Travasorb hepatic, Baxter										For liver failure
Pulmocare, Ross	1.5	150	1	490	63	106	92	57	49	To decrease CO$_2$ production
High calorie density:										
Ensure Plus, Ross	1.5	146	1.6	600	55	200	53	50	54	L, F
Sustacal HC, Mead Johnson	1.5	134	1.2	650	61	190	57	37	38	L, F
Ensure Plus HN, Ross	1.5	125	0.9	650	62	200	50	51	47	L, F
Magnacal, Sherwood	2	154	1	590	70	250	80	44	32	L, F
Isocal HCN, Mead Johnson	2	145	1.5	690	75	224	91	35	36	L, F, MCT
Twocal HN, Ross	2	126	0.9	700	84	217	90	46	59	L, F, MCT

P, powder; L, liquid; F, flavored; U, Unflavored; BCAA, Branched-chain amino acids; MCT, medium-chain triglycerides.

Protein, carbohydrate, and fat are expressed as gram per liter (g/L) standard dilution, Na and K are expressed as milliequivalents per liter (mEq) standard dilution.

Source: Reprinted from Kudsk KA, Jacobs DO. Nutrition. In: Norton JA, Bollinger RR, Chang AE, et al, eds. Surgery: Basic Science and Clinical Evidence. New York: Springer-Verlag, 2001, with permission.

Table 3.6. Some parenteral amino acid solutions.

	Novamine 15%	Travasol 10%	TrophAmine 6%
Protein equivalent (g/100 mL)	15	10	6
Total nitrogen (g/100 mL)	2.3	1.6	0.93
Osmolarity (mOsm/L)	1300	998	525
pH	5.6	6	5.5
Essential amino acids (mg/100 mL)			
Isoleucine	749	600	490
Leucine	1040	730	840
Lysine	1180	580	490
Methionine	749	400	200
Phenylalanine	1040	560	290
Threonine	349	420	260
Tryptophan	250	180	120
Valine	960	580	470
Nonessential amino acids (mg/100 mL)			
Cysteine			<14
Arginine	1470	1150	730
Alanine	2170	2070	320
Proline	894	680	410
Glycine	1040	1030	220
Serine	592	500	230
Tyrosine			15

Source: Reprinted from Kudsk KA, Jacobs DO. Nutrition. In: Norton JA, Bollinger RR, Chang AE, et al, eds. Surgery: Basic Science and Clinical Evidence. New York: Springer-Verlag, 2001, with permission.

Table 3.7. Fatty acid content of intravenous lipid preparations.

	Intralipid	Liposyn II	Liposyn III
Manufacturer	Clintec Nutrition	Abbott	Abbott
concentration (%)	10	10	10
	20	20	20
Oil (%)			
Safflower		5	
		10	
Soybean	10	5	10
	20	10	20
Fatty acid content (%)			
Linoleic	50	65.8	54.5
	50	65.8	54.5
Oleic	26	17.7	22.4
	26	17.7	22.4
Palmitic	10	8.8	10.5
	10	8.8	10.5
Linoleic	9	4.2	8.3
	9	4.2	8.3
Stearic	3.5	3.4	4.2
	3.5	3.4	4.2
Osmolarity (mOsm/L)	260	276	284
	260	258	292

Source: Reprinted from Kudsk KA, Jacobs DO. Nutrition. In: Norton JA, Bollinger RR, Chang AE, et al, eds. Surgery: Basic Science and Clinical Evidence. New York: Springer-Verlag, 2001, with permission.

Table 3.8. Central parenteral nutrition.

	Central	Peripheral
Daily calories	2000–3000	1000–1500
Protein	Variable	56–87 g
Volume of fluid required	1000–3000 mL	2000–3500 mL
Duration of therapy	≥7 days	5–7 days
Route of administration	Dedicated central venous catheter	Peripheral vein or multiuse central catheter
Substrate profile	55–60% carbohydrate 15–20% protein 25% fat	30% carbohydrate 20% protein 50% fat
Osmolarity	~2000 mOsm/l	~600–900 mOsm/l

Source: Reprinted from Kudsk KA, Jacobs DO. Nutrition. In: Norton JA, Bollinger RR, Chang AE, et al, eds. Surgery: Basic Science and Clinical Evidence. New York: Springer-Verlag, 2001, with permission.

Table 3.9. Standard orders for nutritional support.

1. Confirm correct feeding tube or intravenous device placement.
2. Prescribe the formula composition.
3. Prescribe the rate of advancement and target rate of the nutrient.
4. Add vitamin K.
5. Intake and output should be recorded each shift.
6. Order laboratory tests to monitor complications and efficacy of nutritional therapy.
   Initial: Chemistry profile, serum magnesium, complete blood count (CBC), PT/PTT
   Start-up: SMA-6 daily for 3 days, Mg, PO_4
   Maintenance:
     SMA-20 every Monday and Thursday
     Magnesium, CBC every Monday
7. Monitor blood glucose every 6 hours during start-up; continue every 12 hours for CPN (or more often as clinically indicated).
   Add vitamin K.
8. Enteral-specific orders
   a. Gastric feedings: elevate head of bed 45 degrees.
   b. Gastric feedings: Check gastric residuals every 4 hours. Hold feedings for 4 hours if the residual is greater than the hourly rate, and notify physician if two consecutive measurements are excessive.
   c. Irrigate feeding tubes with 20 mL of tap water after each intermittent feeding or t.i.d., when tube is disconnected, or before and after medications are administered via tube.
   d. For obstructed tubes not cleared with simple pressure, instill 10 mL of a solution of 1 tablet Viokase, one tablet $NaHCO_3$, and 30 mL of warm tap water; repeat once.
   e. For jejunal feedings, do *not* interrupt for diagnostic tests or NPO status.

PT, prothrombin time; PTT, partial thromboplastin time; SMA-6, Sequential Mutliple Analysis—six different serum tests.
Source: Reprinted from Borzotta AP. Physiologic aspects of surgical disease. In: Polk HC Jr., Gardner B, Stone HH, eds. Basic Surgery, 5th ed. St. Louis: Quality Medical Publishing, Inc., 1995.

las for renal and hepatic failure as well as newly promoted "immune enhancing" products are available. These formulas may prove useful in managing the complications associated with specific conditions, although evidence that they prolong life is limited.

Complications of Enteral Feeding: The most common complications of enteral feeding include diarrhea, aspiration, vomiting, distention, metabolic abnormalities, and tube dislodgment. Aspiration is reduced by avoiding intragastric feeding in patients with reflux or in those who must be recumbent. Gastric residual volumes should be checked regularly, and prokinetic agents may benefit some patients. Diarrhea may represent a more complex diagnostic dilemma, and patients should be evaluated for *Clostridium difficile* infection and other medications as an etiology. Fiber containing feedings may reduce this problem. Attention always must be given to the new onset of pain or distention in patients with intestinal feeding tubes. Small-bowel intussusception, necrosis, perforation, and pneumatosis intestinalis have been reported in such patients. Other causes of abdominal pathology, including (a)calculous cholecystitis, are not infrequent in patients who require SNS.

Parenteral Formulas

The basic content and prescription of parenteral nutrition formulations are shown in **Table 3.8**. *Central parenteral* formulas are often standardized by hospital pharmacies and usually include a hypertonic (>10%) dextrose source combined with amino acids. Intravenous fat emulsions may be mixed with this solution or provided as a separate infusion. Electrolytes and trace minerals are added to these solutions before infusion, and virtually all such solutions are given via volume controlled pumps. Additional additives, such as insulin, may be included in the solutions or provided by other means, as needed.

Peripheral parenteral contains lower concentrations of dextrose (<10%) in combination with amino acids. Additives similar to those used in central vein feedings may be used. Peripheral vein nutrition is a less optimal form of feeding in that adequate caloric support cannot be achieved except in unusual circumstances. Consequently, it is seldom used except where there are no other options or during the transition phase to full enteral feeding status.

Complications of Parenteral Feeding: Tolerance to parenteral feedings should be evaluated throughout the course. In that acute parenteral nutrition is most common in patients who are critically ill, consideration always must be given to fluid status as well as glucose intolerance and electrolyte abnormalities. An acute shift toward anabolism may unmask preexisting body electrolyte deficiencies (see Monitoring Progress and Complications, below.) Control of blood glucose is important as well as an awareness that acute discontinuation of feedings may result in hypoglycemia. Abnormalities of acid–base balance also occur more frequently in such patients, and alterations in electrolyte composition (such as acetate salts) of solutions may be indicated. As always, patients with indwelling catheters must be monitored carefully for infection. An abrupt change in glucose tolerance may indicate infection related to the catheter or another source.

Monitoring Progress and Complications

Defining a plan for monitoring the results of SNS is an integral part of the prescription and, like all therapies, **an awareness that changes in formulations and that life-threatening complications can arise is essential**. In general, all patients should be metabolically and hemodynamically stable before the initiation of SNS. This may require a modest delay before such therapy begins, but it allows a determination of any associated morbidities that might influence the progress of treatment or, in some cases, the preclusion of SNS from terminally ill patients. **Emergencies related to SNS begin after efforts to initiate therapy have begun.**

Problems Related to Access

These problems can be life-threatening and include misadventures related to placement of enteral or parenteral feeding portals. Acute pneumothorax, inadvertent arterial puncture, air embolism, and perforation of the vena cava or heart can accompany attempts at central venous access. These must be dealt with expeditiously and definitively. Insertion of catheters by experienced personnel serves to minimize these complications.

More frequently, however, it is the initial misplacement of the catheter or latent events such as insertion-site infection or vessel thrombosis that provide troubling morbidities to patients. Current practice dictates that the **proper placement of any feeding catheter must be confirmed before SNS is begun**. These complications are monitored by a rigorous adherence to sterility guidelines and protocols and by regular physical examination of the patient. A constant awareness of the potential for these events promotes early intervention and treatment.

Problems related to placement of enteral feeding portals arise with similar, if not greater, frequency. Although it is increasingly popular to return to intragastric feeding, proper tube placement and function also must be assured. The ability to frequently monitor gastric residual volumes is helpful. Problems of aspiration, especially in patients prone to reflux, may preclude this route of enteral nutrient provision. Under such circumstances, the placement of small-bore feeding catheters either transgastrically or transcutaneously requires experienced personnel. Careful attention to maintenance of tube patency is important. Ideally, only nutrient solutions should be provided by these tubes. As noted above, enteral feeding tubes may cause abdominal distention or symptoms that must be investigated.

Metabolic Monitoring

It is essential that all patients have adequate biochemical screening before and after the initiation of SNS. While it is unclear how frequent these parameters should be determined, as a general rule, critically ill patients should have determinations performed at least two to three times per week or during the initiation of SNS, while more stable patients may be evaluated one to two times per week. **Careful, daily physical examination is an essential component of the monitoring regimen. Problems related to access portals as well as organ dysfunction and fluid imbalance may be detected initially, or solely, on this basis.**

Problems of Deficiency

The initial prescription, as outlined above, includes provisions for routine electrolytes as well as for those that may be dramatically altered during SNS (magnesium, phosphate). Routine monitoring for trace minerals (zinc, copper, etc.) is not done unless there is suspicion of a deficiency. A determination of red blood cell indices may help to define iron deficiency (not routinely provided in intravenous nutrition). Evaluation of basic bleeding parameters is undertaken to detect the presence of vitamin K deficiency, which also may develop in parenterally fed patients. Liver biochemical tests may detect changes in hepatic function. Although these parameters may increase during SNS by 1.5 to 2.0 times above normal even in the absence of significant pathology, further increases may indicate the need for additional evaluation.

As noted above, relatively rare deficiencies may become manifest during the course of SNS. Thiamine deficiency may occur in patients receiving large carbohydrate loads. Megaloblastic anemia also may occur secondary to folate deficiency. Trace mineral deficiencies may be a latent problem, especially in patients with preexisting malnutrition and prolonged inflammatory conditions. Attention should be given to patients with previous compromise of intestinal absorption.

Problems of Excess

Significant changes in overall clinical status as well as specific organs may provoke a state of excess provision. The most overt of these is glucose intolerance, which may occur for many reasons. Stress diabetes is a common event in severely injured patients. At least daily evaluation of glucose tolerance, by blood or urine sampling, is indicated in all patients. More frequent determinations are warranted during initiation of SNS in critically ill patients. **An abrupt increase in glucose levels in an otherwise stable patient must suggest infection until proven otherwise.**

Glucose excess also may precipitate or aggravate pulmonary problems in some patients. If the rate of endogenous glucose oxidation is exceeded, carbon dioxide retention may result in respiratory distress or weaning problems in ventilated patients. Glucose excess also may cause liver dysfunction in some patients.

Other evidence of nutrient excess occurs during conditions of evolving organ dysfunction. While a modest rise in blood urea nitrogen frequently may accompany SNS, any increase above twice normal or in association with increases in creatinine warrants consideration of protein or amino acid intolerance. A reduction in volume and nitrogen load as well as evaluation of electrolyte tolerance may be indicated. Protein intolerance also may occur in patients with underlying liver dysfunction. Under such circumstances, a reduction in nitrogen load or alteration in amino acid formulation may be indicated.

Terminating Nutritional Support

The decision to **terminate SNS** rests upon several factors, including **the ability of the patient to tolerate oral feedings, the achievement of initial therapeutic goals, and the expectation of additional therapies that will improve quality of life and prolong outcome.** Once SNS has been initiated, the decision to terminate therapy must rely on sound clinical judgment, but the clinician should be able to address each of the above issues in the affirmative. The vast majority will be able to be weaned from SNS before hospital discharge. It is preferable to assure that the patient is capable of taking oral intake before complete termination of SNS. This may be done by reducing the amount of SNS by one half while assessing swallowing and digestion of oral diet. There is no evidence to suggest that this level of SNS suppresses appetite. Some patients may require liquid diets as a transition to solid food, but this does not necessitate an interruption of the tapering schedule. Once the oral diet is tolerated, SNS may be discontinued. In patients who have been receiving supplemental insulin, peripheral low-dose dextrose infusions minimize the chances of hypoglycemia.

A limited number of patients may require continuation of SNS after discharge from the hospital. This decision requires input from several sources, including family and home healthcare agencies as well as social work and nursing professionals. Efforts to identify at the earliest possible time patients in need of outpatient SNS are warranted. This provides time to arrange for this more complex therapy.

For some patients none of the weaning indications are reasonable expectations. In such cases, the judgment as to continuation of SNS requires a mutual decision among patient and family, the provider, and other interested parties.

Summary

Specialized nutritional support (SNS) is a necessary adjunctive therapy in some portion of hospitalized surgical patients. An understanding of the indications, techniques, and complications of SNS is necessary to practice modern surgical care. While most surgical patients do not require SNS, the continued monitoring of patients and appropriate initiation of SNS may reduce the incidence of complication and promote the early restoration of functional status.

Examples of the judicious use of SNS can be derived from the presented cases. In **Case 1**, where the patient has established cachexia, the initiation of SNS *before* operation might serve to diminish postoperative complications. In **Case 2**, SNS should be instituted at an early juncture, particularly if the patient does not steadily recover from her injuries.

Selected Readings

Brennan MF, Pisters PWT, Posner M, et al. A prospective, randomized trial of total parenteral nutrition after major pancreatic resection for malignancy. Ann Surg 1994;220:436–444.

Daly JM, Lieberman MD, Goldfine J, et al. Enteral nutrition with supplemental arginine, RNA, and omega-3 fatty acids in patients after operation: immunologic, metabolic, and clinical outcome. Surgery (St. Louis) 1992; 112:56–67.

Daly JM, Weintraub FN, Shou J, et al. Enteral nutrition during multimodality therapy in upper gastrointestinal cancer patients. Ann Surg 1995;221: 327–338.

Doglietto GB, Gallitelli L, Pacelli F, et al. Protein-sparing therapy after major abdominal surgery: lack of clinical effects. Ann Surg 1996;223:357–362.

Fan ST, Lo CM, Lai EC, et al. Perioperative nutritional support in patients undergoing hepatectomy for hepatocellular carcinoma. N Engl J Med 1994;331:1547–1552.

Heslin MJ, Latkany L, Leung D, et al. A prospective, randomized trial of early enteral feeding after resection of upper gastrointestinal malignancy. Ann Surg 1997;226:567–577.

Kudsk KA, Jacobs DO, Nutrition. In: Norton JA, Bollinger RR, Chang AE, et al, eds. Surgery: Basic Science and Clinical Evidence. New York: Springer-Verlag, 2001.

Mueller JM, Brenner U, Pichlmaier H. Preoperative parenteral feeding in patients with gastrointestinal carcinoma. Lancet 1982;1:68.

The Veteran Affairs Total Parenteral Nutrition Cooperative Study Group. Perioperative total parenteral nutrition in surgical patients. N Engl J Med 1991;325:525–532.

Watters JM, Kirkpatrick SM, Norris SB, et al. Immediate postoperative enteral feeding results in impared respiratory mechanics and decreased mobility. Ann Surg 1997;226:369–377.

4

Fluid, Electrolyte, and Acid–Base Disorders in the Surgery Patient

Stephen F. Lowry

Objectives

1. To understand the normal electrolyte composition of body fluids and how they are modified by injury and surgical disease.
2. To understand the importance of evaluating fluid status.
3. To recognize the clinical manifestation of common electrolyte abnormalities and methods for their correction.
4. To understand the common manifestation of acid–base abnormalities.

Cases

Case 1

A 72-year-old man undergoes subtotal colectomy for massive lower GI bleeding. He receives five units of blood during and following operation and is NPO for 6 days while receiving dextrose 5% in water (D5/W) at a rate of 125 mL/hour. Urine output remains normal with specific gravity of 1.012. On the sixth postoperative day, he is disoriented and combative. Among the results of workup are serum sodium = 119 mEq/L, potassium = 3.6 mEq/L, chloride = 85 mEq/L, glucose = 120 mg/dL, blood urea nitrogen (BUN) = 24.

Case 2

A 40-year-old woman presents with a 1 week history of persistent upper abdominal pain in association with nausea and vomiting. She tolerates only small amounts of clear fluids by mouth. No diarrhea is present. Physical examination is unrevealing except for loss of skin turgor and reduced breath sounds over the right chest. Lab results include sodium = 138 mEq/L, potassium = 2.6 mEq/L, HCO_3 =

43 mEq/L. A blood gas is obtained, revealing pH = 7.57, Pao_2 = 98 mm Hg, $Paco_2$ = 52 mm Hg, base excess = 10.

Case 3

A 58-year-old woman presents with a 1-week history of confusion, lethargy, and persistent nausea. She has new complaints of back and hip pain. Past history includes a mastectomy for breast cancer 5 years previously. Laboratory values obtained during evaluation include hematocrit (Hct) = 41, white blood count (WBC) = 9000, platelets = 110,000, sodium = 137 mEq/L, potassium = 3.8 mEq/L, BUN = 25 mg/dL, albumin = 3.4 g/dL, bilirubin = 1.5 g/dL, alkaline phosphatase = 350 IU/L, calcium = 14.2 mg/dL.

Introduction

An understanding of changes in fluid, electrolyte, and acid–base concepts is fundamental to the care of surgical patients. These changes can range from mild, readily correctable deviations to life-threatening abnormalities that demand immediate attention. This chapter outlines some of the physiologic mechanisms that initiate such imbalances and methods to systematically evaluate the diverse clinical and biochemical data that lead to decisions regarding therapy. **The information and data presented below are intended for application in adult patients**, although the principles espoused also are germane to pediatric patients.

Basic Concepts

The Stress Response

The normal **physiologic response to injury or operation produces a neuroendocrine response that preserves cellular function and promotes maintenance of circulating volume. This is readily demonstrable in terms of retention of water and sodium and the excretion of potassium.** Many stimuli can produce this response, including many associated with trauma or operation. Activation of several endocrine response pathways increases the levels of antidiuretic hormone (ADH), aldosterone, angiotensin II, cortisol, and catecholamines. Hyperosmolarity and hypovolemia are the principal stimulants for ADH release, which increases renal water resorption from the collecting ducts and raises urine osmolarity. Aldosterone, the principal stimulus for renal potassium excretion, also is increased by angiotensin II, which can increase both renal sodium and water retention. Aldosterone also is increased by elevated levels of potassium, a common consequence of tissue injury. Hydrocortisone and catecholamine release also contribute to the excretion of potassium.

Body Fluid Compartments

Total body water (TBW) approximates 60% of body weight (BW) and is divided among the intracellular volume (ICV) as 40% of BW and an extracellular volume (ECV) representing 20% of BW. The ECV is divided further into an interstitial fluid volume (IFV) pool, which is roughly 15% of BW, and the intravascular or plasma volume (PV), which approximates 5% of BW. The TBW is the solvent for most of the solutes in the body, and it is assumed that water moves freely between the ECV and ICV in an effort to equalize the concentration of solutes within each space. However, the solute and colloid concentrations of the ICV and ECV differ markedly. The ECV contains most of the body sodium, while the predominant ICV cation is potassium. Albumin represents the dominant osmotically active colloid within the ECV and virtually is excluded from the ICV. The exogenous administration of electrolytes results in the distribution of that ion to the usual fluid compartment of highest preferential concentration.

Electrolytes

When an electrolyte dissolves in water, it releases positive and negative ions. Although, as noted above, their concentrations vary between fluid compartments, the distribution of water across fluid compartments seeks to equalize the concentration of total solutes and other osmotically active particles. When considering electrolyte problems, it is useful to use the milliequivalent (mEq) measure of their chemical combining capacity. In some cases, this must be converted from the weight expression milligram (mg) expressed on the laboratory report. **Table 4.1** assists in this conversion.

A millimole (mM) is the atomic weight of a substance expressed in milligrams. A milliosmole (mOsm) is a measure of the number of osmotically active particles in solution. Since mOsm does not depend on valence, the mM dissolved in solution will be the same as mOsm. **The osmolarity of a solution depends on the number of active particles per unit of volume (mOsm/L).** The normal osmolarity of serum is $290 \pm 10\,\text{mOsm/L}$. The effective osmolarity (tonicity) involves the mea-

Table 4.1. Data for serum electrolytes.

Electrolyte	Normal	
	mg/dL	mEq/L
Sodium	322	140
Potassium	17.5	4.5
Calcium	10	5
Magnesium	2.4	2
Chloride	35.7	102
Phosphorus	3.4	2.0

Source: Reprinted from Pemberton LB, Pemberton DK. Treatment of Water, Electrolyte, and Acid-Base Disorders in the Surgical Patient. New York: McGraw Hill, 1994. With permission of The McGraw-Hill Companies.

surement of two solutes, sodium and glucose, that represent nearly 90% of ECV osmolarity. This can be modified by addition of urea concentration, especially in conditions of uremia. The formula for calculating approximate osmolarity is:

$$POSM = 2 \times plasma\ [Na^+] + [glucose]/20 + [BUN]/3$$

Because water moves freely between fluid compartments, ECV osmolarity (or tonicity) is equivalent to that in the ICV.

Maintenance Requirements

There are several principles that underlie the prescription for replacing fluid and electrolytes in surgical patients. This includes a knowledge of normal maintenance requirements as well as replacement for losses.

Water

The normal losses of water include sensible (measurable) losses from urine (500–1500 mL/day) and feces (100–200 mL/day), as well as insensible (unmeasurable) loses from sweat and respiration (8–12 mL/kg/day). Cutaneous insensible losses increase by approximately 10% for each degree C above normal. A method to roughly calculate daily normal water requirements is shown in **Figure 4.1**. The water of biologic oxidation (catabolism) contributes up to 300 mL/day and can be subtracted from these calculations. For healthy adults, an estimated daily maintenance fluid requirement approximates 30 to 35 mL/kg/day.

Sodium

Sodium losses in urine can vary widely but, in general, approximate daily intake. The normal kidney can conserve sodium to a minimum level of 5 to 10 mEq/L. A figure of 70 to 100 mEq Na/day is a reasonable estimate of maintenance level.

Potassium

The normal excretion of potassium approximates 40 to 60 mEq/day. Since the renal conservation of potassium is not as efficient as for sodium, this is the minimum level of daily replacement in healthy adults (0.5–1.0 mEq/kg/day).

Summary of Normal Maintenance Fluids for Surgical Patients

In the absence of other comorbidities or prolonged injury/operation induced stress, the NPO surgical patient is adequately maintained by infusion of variable combinations of dextrose (D5) and saline (up to 0.5 N) containing solutions, with approximately 15 to 20 mEq/L of potassium added. The rate of infusion should be adjusted to achieve water replacement as outlined above. Such parenteral solutions, when

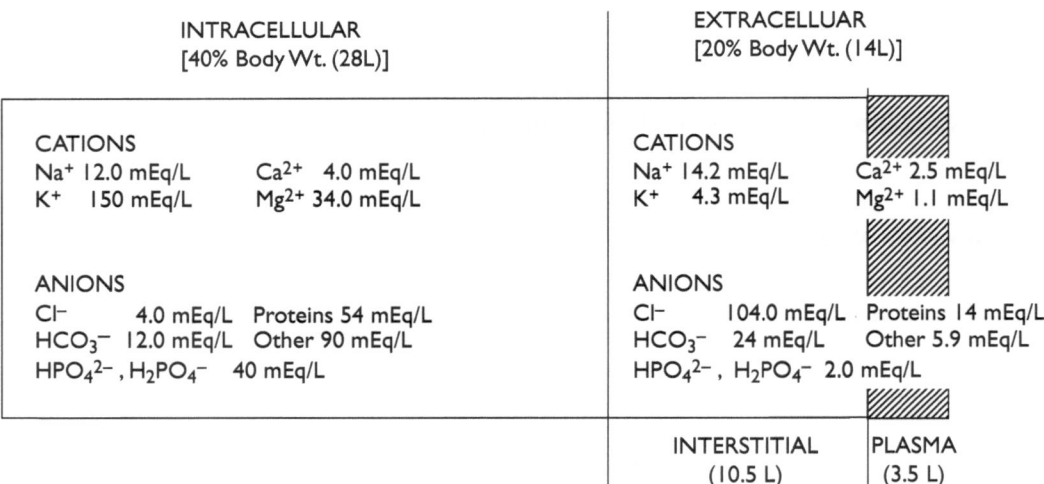

Total Body Water
[60% Body Wt. (42L)]

Figure 4.1. Distribution of body water and electrolytes in a healthy 70-kg male. (Adapted from Narins RG, Krishna GC. Disorders of water balance. In: Stein JH, ed. Internal Medicine, 2nd ed. Philadelphia: Lippincott Williams & Wilkins. Reprinted from Nathens AB, Maier RV. Perioperative Fluids and Electrolytes. In: Norton JA, Bollinger RR, Chang AE, et al, eds. Surgery: Basic Science and Clinical Evidence. New York: Springer-Verlag, 2001, with permission.)

given at an appropriate rate of infusion, suffice to manage the majority of postoperative patients.

Perioperative Fluid and Electrolyte Requirements

The management of fluid and electrolytes in the stressed surgical patient requires a systematic approach to the changing dynamics and demands of the patient. Consideration of existing maintenance requirements, deficits or excesses, and ongoing losses requires regular monitoring and flexibility in prescribing. While the majority of patients require only minor, if any, adjustments in parenteral fluid intake, some present challenging and life-threatening situations.

Fluid Sequestration

Following injury or operation, the **extravasation of intravascular fluid into the interstitium leads to tissue edema ("third space").** Estimates of this volume for general surgery patients range from 4 to 8 mL/kg/h and this volume may persist for up to 24 hours or longer. **This loss of functional ECV must be considered as an additional ongoing loss in the early postoperative or injury period.**

Gastrointestinal Losses

Additional ongoing losses from intestinal drains, stomas, tubes, and fistulas also must be documented and replaced. The fluid volume and electrolyte concentration of such losses vary by site and should be recorded carefully. Replacement of such losses should approximate the known, or measured, concentration of electrolytes (**Table 4.2**).

Intraoperative Losses

Careful attention to the operative record for replacement of fluids during surgery always is warranted. Usually, additional fluids for prolonged operations and for operations upon open cavities is warranted. Surgeons must know what fluids and medications were given during the procedure so that they can write appropriate postoperative fluid orders. Orders for intravenous fluids may need to be rewritten frequently to maintain normal heart rate, urine output (0.5–1.0 mL/kg/h), and blood pressure.

Defining Problems of Fluid and Electrolyte Imbalance

Fluid balance and electrolyte disorders can be classified into disturbances of (1) extracellular fluid volume; (2) sodium concentration; and (3) composition (acid–base balance and other electrolytes). When confronted with an existing problem of fluid or electrolyte derangement, it is helpful initially to analyze the issues of fluid (water) and electrolyte imbalance separately.

Fluid Status

The initial issue is whether a deficit or excess of water exists. A deficiency of extracellular volume can be diagnosed clinically (**Table 4.3**). Acutely, there may be no changes in serum sodium, whereas repeated studies may demonstrate changes in sodium as well as in BUN.

Table 4.2. Volume and composition of gastrointestinal fluid losses.

Source	Volume (mL)	Na^+ (mEq/L)	Cl^- (mEq/L)	K^+ (mEq/L)	HCO_3^- (mEq/L)	H^+ (mEq/L)
Stomach	1000–4200	20–120	130	10–15	—	30–100
Duodenum	100–2000	110	115	15	10	—
Ileum	1000–3000	80–150	60–100	10	30–50	—
Colon (diarrhea)	500–1700	120	90	25	45	—
Bile	500–1000	140	100	5	25	—
Pancreas	500–1000	140	30	5	115	—

Source: Reprinted from Nathens AB, Maier RV. Perioperative fluids and electrolytes. In: Norton JA, Bollinger RR, Chang AE, et al, eds. Surgery: Basic Science and Clinical Evidence. New York: Springer-Verlag, 2001, with permission.

Table 4.3. Extracellular fluid volume.

Type of Sign	Symptoms of deficit		Symptoms of excess	
	Moderate	Severe	Moderate	Severe
Central nervous system	Sleepiness Apathy Slow responses Anorexia Cessation of usual activity	Decreased tension reflexes Anesthesia of distal extremities Stupor Coma	None	None
Gastrointestinal	Progressive decrease in food consumption	Nausea, vomiting Refusal to eat Silent ileus and distention	At operation: Edema of stomach, colon, lesser and greater omenta, and small bowel mesentery	
Cardiovascular	Orthostatic hypotension Tachycardia Collapsed veins Collapsing pulse	Cutaneous lividity Hypotension Distant heart sounds Cold extremities Absent peripheral pulses	Elevated venous pressure Distention of peripheral veins Increased cardiac output Loud heart sounds Functional murmurs Bounding pulse High pulse pressure Increased pulmonary second sound Gallop	Pulmonary edema
Tissue	Soft small tongue with longitudinal wrinkling Decreased skin turgor	Atonic muscles Sunken eyes	Subcutaneous pitting edema Basilar rales	Anasarca Moist rales Vomiting Diarrhea
Metabolic	Mild decrease in temperature (97°–99°R)	Marked decrease in temperature (95°–98°R)	None	None

Source: Reprinted from Shires GT, Shires GT III, Lowry S. Fluid, electrolyte and nutritional management of the surgical patient. In: Schwartz SI, ed. Principles of Surgery, 6th ed. New York: McGraw-Hill, 1994. With permission of The McGraw-Hill Companies.
R = rectal.

Under chronic conditions, an assessment of ECV also may be determined from serum sodium level and osmolarity. A high serum sodium (>145 mEq/L) indicates a water deficit, whereas low serum sodium (<135 mEq/L) confirms water excess. **The sodium level provides no information about the body sodium content**, merely the relative amounts of free water and sodium. If serum osmolarity is high, it is important to consider the influence of other osmotically active particles, including glucose. Elevated glucose should be treated and will restore, at least partially, serum osmolarity.

Water Excess

Although water excess may coexist with either sodium excess or deficit, the most common postoperative variant, hypo-osmolar hyponatremia, may develop slowly with minimal symptoms. Rapid development results in neurologic symptoms that may eventuate in convulsions and coma if not properly addressed as discussed in **Case 1**. **A serum sodium less than 125 mEq/L demands immediate attention.** Other causes of hyponatremia are listed in **Table 4.4**. (See **Algorithm 4.1** for treatment.)

The treatment of water excess involves removing the excess water, adding sodium, or using both approaches to increase serum osmolarity. Restriction of water intake often suffices in that continued sensible and insensible losses will assure free water loss. (The amount of excess water may be estimated by: BW in kg × 0.04 = L of water excess.) In cases in which sodium administration is necessary (i.e., symptomatic

Table 4.4. Causes of hyponatremia.

Pseudohyponatremia (normal plasma osmolarity)
Hyperlipidemia, hyperproteinemia
Dilutional hyponatremia (increased plasma osmolarity)
Hyperglycemia, mannitol
True hyponatremia (reduced plasma osmolarity)
Reduction in ECF volume
Plasma, GI, skin, or renal losses (diuretics)
Expanded ECF volume
Congestive heart failure
Hypoproteinemic states (cirrhosis, nephrotic syndrome, malnutrition)
Normal ECF volume
SIADH
Pulmonary or CNS lesions
Endocrine disorders (hypothyroidism, hypoadrenalism)
Drugs (e.g., morphine, tricyclic antidepressants, clofibrate, antineoplastic agents, chlorpropamide, aminophylline, indomethacin)
Miscellaneous (pain, nausea)

SIADH, syndrome of inappropriate antidiuretic hormone secretion.
Source: Reprinted from Nathens AB, Maier RV. Perioperative fluids and electrolytes. In: Norton JA, Bollinger RR, Chang AE, et al, eds. Surgery: Basic Science and Clinical Evidence. New York: Springer-Verlag, 2001, with permission.

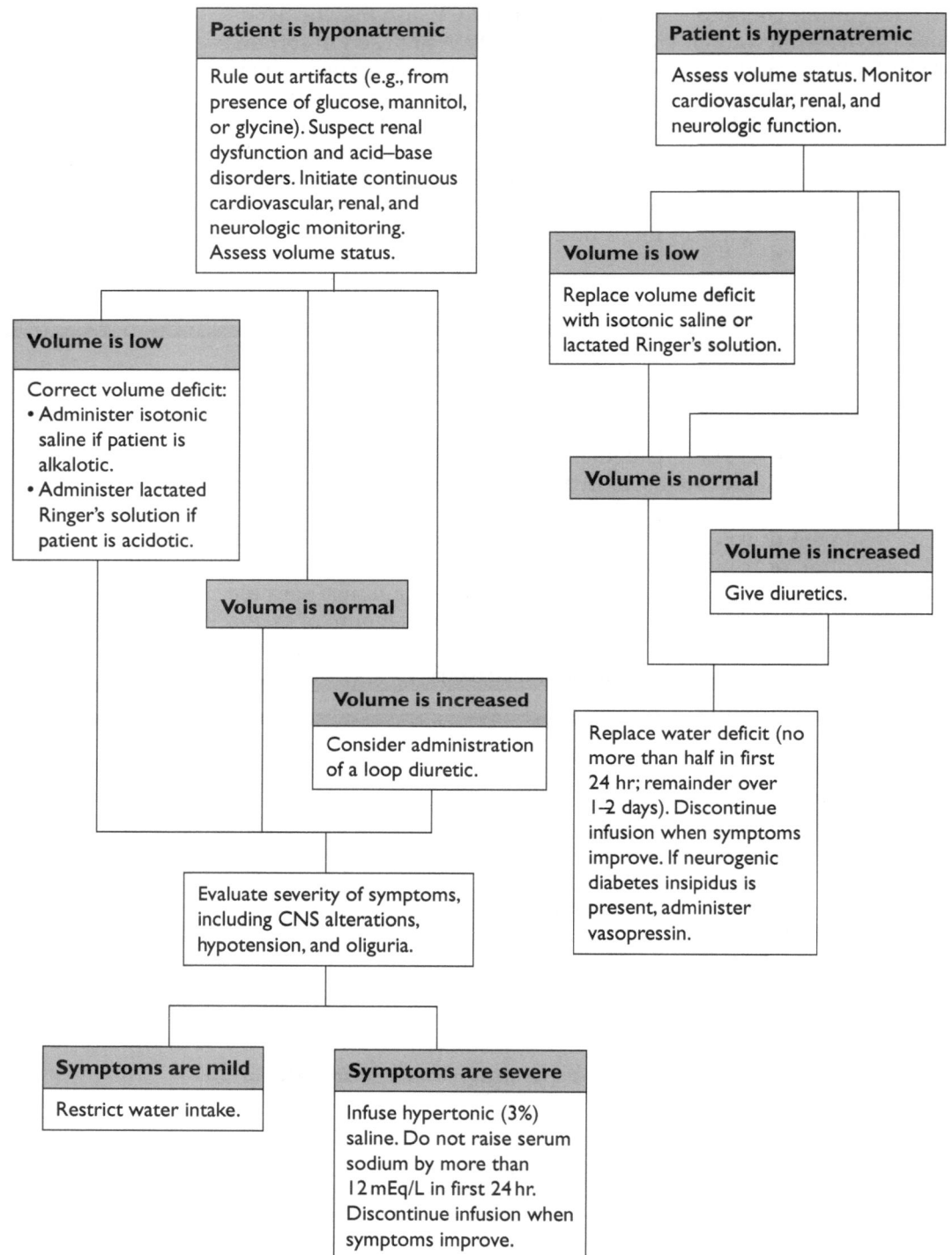

Algorithm 4.1. Initial assessment of patient with fluid and electrolyte imbalance. (Reprinted from Van Zee KJ, Lowry SF. Life-threatening electrolyte abnormalities. In: Wilmore DW, Cheung LY, Harken AH, et al, eds. ACS Surgery: Principles and Practice (Section 1: Resuscitation). New York: WebMD Corporation, 1997.)

hyponatremia), a rise in serum sodium may be achieved by administration of the desired increase of sodium (in mEq/L) = 0.6 (% of BW as TBW) × BW (in kg). An uncommon but devastating complication of raising serum sodium too rapidly is central pontine demyelinating syndrome. This may occur if sodium is increased at a rate >0.5 mEq/L per hour. To prevent this complication, it is generally recommended that symptomatic patients receive one half of the calculated sodium dose (using hypertonic sodium solutions, such as 3% saline) over 8 hours to bring serum sodium into an acceptable range (120–125 mEq/L), as would be appropriate in **Case 1**. The remaining dose then may be infused over the next 16 hours. Do not use hypotonic saline solutions until the serum sodium is in an acceptable range. Medications that antagonize ADH effect, such as demeclocycline (300–600 mg b.i.d.), also may be used cautiously, especially in patients with renal failure.

Water Excess Caused by SIADH

The **syndrome of inappropriate ADH** (SIADH) results from increased ADH secretion in the face of hypo-osmolarity and normal blood volume. **The criteria for this diagnosis also include a reduced aldosterone level with urine sodium >20 mEq/L, serum< urine osmolarity, and the absence of renal failure, hypotension, or edema.** The syndrome of inappropriate ADH results from several diseases, including malignant tumors, central nervous system (CNS) diseases, pulmonary disorders, medications, and severe stress. The primary treatments for SIADH are management of the underlying condition and water restriction (<1000 mL/day). Administration of hypotonic fluids should be avoided.

Water Deficit

A deficit of ECV is the most frequently encountered derangement of fluid balance in surgical patients. It may occur from shed blood, loss of gastrointestinal fluids, diarrhea, fistulous drainage, or inadequate replacement of insensible losses. More subtle are "third-space" losses (e.g., peritonitis) or sequestration of fluids intraluminally and intramurally (e.g., bowel obstruction). Similar to changes in conditions of water excess, a severe or rapidly developing deficit of water may cause several symptoms (**Table 4.3**). Lab tests for serum sodium (>145 mEq/L) and osmolarity (>300 mOsm/L) establish the diagnosis. Water deficit results from loss of hypotonic body fluids without adequate replacement or intake of hypertonic fluids without adequate sodium excretion. Patients with decreased mental status or those unable to regulate their water intake are prone to this problem. Patients who are NPO, cannot swallow, or are receiving water-restricted (hypertonic) nutritional regimens also develop this disorder. Excess water loss may result from insensible sources (lungs, sweat) or from excessive gastrointestinal (GI) or renal losses. Large renal losses of hypotonic urine are referred to as diabetes insipidus (DI), which may be of central origin (lack of ADH secretion) or renal (reduces concentrating ability). The most common cause of central DI is trauma. This form often is reversible. Other causes include infections and tumors of the pituitary region. Nephrogenic DI refers to a renal inability to concentrate urine and can be caused by hypercalcemia, hypokalemia, as well as drugs such as lithium. Once a diagnosis of water deficit is entertained, evaluation of urine concentrations can be useful.

While water deficit may be associated with either sodium excess or deficit (see **Algorithm 4.1**), the specific treatment of water deficit must include the administration of free water as a dextrose solution (D5W). Treatment must be done urgently for serum sodium levels >160 mEq/L. Up to 1 L of D5W may be given over 2 to 4 hours to correct the hypernatremia.

Sodium Concentration Changes

As noted earlier, the sodium cation is responsible primarily for maintaining the osmotic integrity of ECV. The signs and symptoms of hyponatremia and hypernatremia can be detected clinically (**Table 4.5**), especially if changes occur rapidly. More commonly, these changes occur over several days, as noted above. Under such circumstances, mixed volume and concentration abnormalities often occur. Consequently, it is important that volume status is assessed initially before any conclusion as to changes in concentration or composition is ascribed.

Sodium Excess

In surgical patients, this condition is **caused primarily by excess sodium intake (as may occur with infusion of isotonic saline)** and renal retention. The proximal signal for these events is a stress response to injury or operation. Chronic sodium excess usually results in edema and weight gain. Classic vascular signs of expanded ECV or frank heart failure may occur, especially in patients with diseases prone to causing edema [congestive heart failure (CHF), cirrhosis, nephrotic syndrome]. **Treatment of sodium excess includes eliminating or reducing sodium intake, mobilization of edema fluid for renal excretion (such as osmotic diuretics for fluid and solute diuretics for sodium), and treatment of any underlying disease that enhances sodium retention.** An algorithm for assessment of fluid status and acute sodium changes is shown in **Algorithm 4.1**.

Sodium Deficit

In the surgical patient, this condition usually occurs via loss of sodium without adequate saline replacement. Several additional sources of sodium loss should be considered, including gastrointestinal fluids and skin. Third-space losses of sodium (and water) also can be extensive after major injury or operation. The symptoms and signs of sodium deficit arise from hypovolemia and reduced tissue perfusion. Under such circumstances, urine sodium is low (<15 mEq/L) and osmolarity is increased (>450 mOsm/L). Prerenal azotemia may be evident (serum BUN/creatinine ratio >20:1). Loss of skin turgor also may occur. Treatment of sodium deficit is directed toward correction of the sodium and water contraction of the ECV. If hypotension is present, this must be treated with normal saline or lactated Ringer's

Table 4.5. Consequences of abnormal sodium concentration.

Type of sign	Hyponatremia (water intoxication)	Hypernatremia (water deficit)
Central nervous system	**Moderate:** Muscle twitching Hyperactive tendon reflexes Increased intracranial pressure (compensated phase) **Severe:** Convulsions Loss of reflexes Increased intracranial pressure (decompensated phase)	**Moderate:** Restlessness Weakness **Severe:** Delirium Maniacal behavior
Cardiovascular	Changes in blood pressure and pulse secondary to increased intracranial pressure Tachycardia Hypotension (if severe)	
Tissue	Salivation, lacrimation, watery diarrhea "Fingerprinting" of skin (sign of intracellular volume excess) Decreased saliva and tears Dry and sticky mucous membranes Red, swollen tongue Flushed skin	
Renal	Oliguria that progresses to anuria Oliguria	
Metabolic	None Fever	

Source: Reprinted from Shires GT, Shires GT III, Lowry S. Fluid, electrolyte and nutritional management of the surgical patient. In: Schwartz SI, ed. Principles of Surgery, 6th ed. New York: McGraw-Hill, 1994. With permission of The McGraw-Hill Companies.

Table 4.6. Composition of parenteral fluids (Electrolyte Content, mEq/L).

Solutions	Cations				Anions		Osmolality (mOsm)
	Na	K	Ca	Mg	Cl	HCO$_3$	
Extracellular fluid	142	4	5	3	103	27	280–310
Ringer's lactate	130	4	3	—	109	28*	273
0.9% sodium chloride	154	—	—	—	154	—	308
D$_5$ 45% sodium chloride	77	—	—	—	77	—	407
D$_5$ W	—	—	—	—	—	—	253
M/6 sodium lactate	167	—	−1	—	—	167*	334
3% sodium chloride	513	—	—	—	513	—	1026

Source: Reprinted from Borzotta AP. Nutritional support. In: Polk HC Jr, Gardner B, Stone HH, eds. Basic Surgery, 5th ed. St. Louis: Quality Medical Publishing Inc., 1995.

solution. A mild sodium deficit without symptoms may be treated over several days if the losses of sodium have been reduced.

Administration of fluids for water and sodium requires knowledge of the current fluid and electrolyte status of the patient, understanding of the level of stress, and appreciation for actual or potential sources of ongoing fluid and electrolyte losses. Having estimated the fluid and sodium status of the patient, administration of appropriate volumes of water and sodium usually is done by the intravenous route. Standard solutions of known contents nearly always are used, and the prescribing physician must be familiar with these basic formulas (**Table 4.6**). Abnormalities of other electrolytes (K, Ca, P, Mg: see Abnormalities of Electrolytes, below) usually require specific fluid solutions or addition of these ions to standard solutions. Changes in acid–base balance also may require special alkalotic or acidotic solutions to correct these abnormalities (**Tables 4.7** and **4.8**).

Table 4.7. Alkalinizing solutions.*

Solution	Tonicity	% Solution	Volume	Electrolytes total mEq	
				Na	HCO$_3$
NaHCO$_3$	Isotonic	1.5	1 L	180	180
NaHCO$_3$	Hypertonic	7.5	50 mL	45	45
NaHCO$_3$	Hypertonic	8.3	50 mL	50	50
Na lactate 1/6 molar	Isotonic	1.9	1 L	167	167
NaHCO$_3$	Hypertonic	5.0	500 mL	300	300

* Some IV alkalinizing solutions are provided with their tonicity, concentration, volume, and mEq of Na and HCO$_3$. The liver converts each mEq of Na lactate of 1 mEq of NaHCO$_3$. 3.75 g of NaHCO$_3$ contains 45 mEq of NA and 45 mEq of HCO$_3$. Solution 1 is made by taking 800 mL of 5% D/W and adding four ampules of 50 mL (200 mL) of 7.5% NaHCO$_3$. Also, one or more 50-mL ampules of 7.5 NaHCO$_3$ (No. 2) can be added to 1 L of 5% D/W or $^1/_2$N saline and will provide 1 amp. = 45, 2 amps. = 90, and 3 amps. = 135 mEq of Na and HCO$_3$ to the IV solution.

Source: Reprinted from Pemberton LB, Pemberton DK. Treatment of Water, Electrolyte, and Acid-Base Disorders in the Surgical Patient. New York: McGraw-Hill, 1994. With permission of The McGraw-Hill Companies.

TABLE 4.8. Acidifying solutions.*

Solution	Tonicity	Percent	Volume	Electrolytes total mEq	
				NH$_4$	C1
NH$_4$ C1	Hypertonic	26.75	20 mL	100	100
NH$_4$ C1	Hypertonic	2.14	1 L	400	400
HC1	Isotonic	0.1 N	1 L	100	100

* Acidifying solutions that can be used to treat metabolic alkalosis. These solutions would be used only if KC1 and NaC1 IV solutions were unable to correct the alkalosis. *Source:* Reprinted from Pemberton LB, Pemberton DK. Treatment of Water, Electrolyte, and Acid-Base Disorders in the Surgical Patient. New York: McGraw-Hill, 1994. With permission of The McGraw-Hill Companies.

Disorders of Composition

By definition, composition changes include alterations in acid–base balance plus changes in concentration of potassium, calcium, magnesium, and phosphate.

Acid–Base Balance

There are four major buffers in the body: proteins, hemoglobin, phosphate, and bicarbonate. All serve to maintain the hydrogen ion concentration within a physiologic range. Bicarbonate is by far the largest of these buffer pools and follows the equation:

$$H^+ + HCO_3 \leftrightarrow H_2CO_3 \leftrightarrow H_2O + CO_2$$

This buffer system involves regulation of CO_2 by the lungs and HCO_3 by the kidneys. Changes in CO_2 are reflected as $Paco_2$ in arterial blood gases. Respiratory acid–base abnormalities are identified readily by determination of $Paco_2$. By contrast, **there are no definitive means to identify a "metabolic" acid–base abnormality**. Two approaches have been used. The first is the concept of **anion gap**, which is used to identify a nonvolatile or fixed acid–base abnormality. Given that many blood anions are not measured routinely, the difference between the measured cations and anions is called the "anion gap" [Anion gap = Na – (HCO$_3$ + Cl)]. The normal value is 12. Metabolic acidosis is the most common reason for increases with accumulation of anions such as lactate, acetoacetate, sulfates, and phosphates. (Note: hyperchloremic acidosis may occur without an anion gap.)

The second approach involves measurements of base excess and base deficit. **Base excess** measures the amount of nonvolatile acid loss or extra base that has increased the total buffer base. **Base deficit** measures the amount of lost base or extra acid that has decreased the buffer base. The normal value is 0 ± 2.5 mEq/L. Base excess (>2.5 mEq/L) represents metabolic alkalosis, whereas base deficit (<–2.5 mEq/L) represents metabolic acidosis. The four types of acid–base abnormalities are shown in **Table 4.9**.

- **Respiratory acidosis** results from hypoventilation with retention of CO_2. This frequently occurs in postoperative patients who have received heavy sedation or have been extubated prematurely.

Table 4.9. Commonly encountered acid-base disorders.

Type of acid–base disorder	Defect	Common causes	$\dfrac{BHCO_3}{H_2CO_3} = \dfrac{20}{1}$	Compensation
Respiratory acidosis	Retention of CO_2 (decreased alveolar ventilation)	Depression of respiratory center: morphine, CNS injury	↑ Denominator ratio <20:1	Renal Retention of bicarbonate Excretion of acid salts, increased ammonia formation Chloride shift into red cells
Respiratory alkalosis	Excessive loss of CO_2 (increased alveolar ventilation)	Hyperventilation: Emotional distress, severe pain, assisted ventilation, encephalitis	↓ Denominator ratio >20:1	Renal Excretion of bicarbonate, retention of acid salts, decreased ammonia formation
Metabolic acidosis	Retention of fixed acids *or* loss of base bicarbonate	Diabetes, azotemia, lactic acid accumulation, starvation Diarrhea, small bowel fistulas	↓ Numerator ratio <20:1	Pulmonary (rapid) Increased rate and depth of breathing Renal (slow) as in respiratory acidosis
Metabolic alkalosis	Loss of fixed acids Gain of base bicarbonate Potassium depletion	Vomiting or gastric suction with pyloric obstruction Excessive intake of bicarbonate Diuretics	↑ Numerator ratio >20:1	Pulmonary (rapid) Increased rate and depth of breathing Renal (slow) as in respiratory alkalosis

CNS, central nervous system.

Source: Reprinted from Shires GT, Shires GT III, Lowry S. Fluid, electrolyte and nutritional management of the surgical patient. In: Schwartz SI, ed. Principles of Surgery, 6th ed. New York: McGraw-Hill, 1994. With permission of The McGraw-Hill Companies.

- **Respiratory alkalosis** results from hyperventilation leading to depressed arterial levels of CO_2. It may occur in patients experiencing pain or those undergoing excessive mechanical ventilation. Alkalosis causes a shift in the oxyhemoglobin-dissociation curve that can lead to tissue hypoxia. Respiratory alkalosis also can lead to reduced levels of potassium and calcium.
- **Metabolic acidosis** results from the overproduction of acid (lactate, ketoacidosis) and also may result from excessive loss of bicarbonate from diarrhea or bowel fistulas.
- **Metabolic alkalosis** is caused by loss of fixed acid or bicarbonate retention. As discussed in **Case 2**, a classic example is loss of acid-rich gastric juice via nasogastric tubes. Usually, there is an associated ECV depletion. Total body potassium and magnesium deficits mandate judicious replacement. Occasionally, 0.1 N hydrochloric acid infusions are needed to reverse the alkalosis.

Regardless of whether the initial acid–base disorder is metabolic or respiratory, a secondary compensatory response occurs within the other system. The changes associated with acute and compensated acid–base disorders are shown in **Table 4.10**. This opposes the pH abnormality and seeks to restore balance. The adequacy of that compensatory response may be impaired by a variety of associated conditions or medications. If the pH value is in the same direction as the respiratory diagnosis (low pH and elevated $Paco_2$), then the respiratory problem is primary. Opposing changes in pH and $Paco_2$ suggest a primary metabolic diagnosis.

Abnormalities of Electrolytes

Potassium: Only about 2% of total body potassium is located in the ECV. Nevertheless, slight alterations in plasma potassium may dramatically alter muscle and nerve function. As a consequence, **abnormalities of potassium concentration require expeditious treatment**.

Table 4.10. Respiratory and metabolic components of acid–base disorders.

Type of acid–base disorder	Acute (Uncompensated)			Chronic (partially compensated)		
	pH	PCO₂ (respiratory component)	Plasma HCO₃⁻* (metabolic component)	pH	PCO₂ (respiratory component)	Plasma HCO₃⁻* (metabolic component)
Respiratory acidosis	↓↓	↑↑	N	↓	↑↑	↑
Respiratory alkalosis	↑↑	↓↓	N	↑	↓↓	↓
Metabolic acidosis	↓↓	N	↓↓	↓	↓	↓
Metabolic alkalosis	↑↑	N	↑↑	↑	↑?	↑

* Measured as levels of standard bicarbonate, whole blood buffer base, CO_2 content, or CO_2 combining power. The *base excess value* is positive when the standard bicarbonate level is above normal and negative when the standard bicarbonate level is below normal.

Source: Reprinted from Shires GT, Shires GT III, Lowry S. Fluid, electrolyte and nutritional management of the surgical patient. In: Schwartz SI, ed. Principles of Surgery, 6th ed. New York: McGraw-Hill, 1994. With permission of The McGraw-Hill Companies.

Hyperkalemia (>6mEq/L) requires immediate intervention to prevent refractory cardiac arrhythmias. Sudden increases in potassium level usually are caused by infusion or increased transcellular flux resulting from tissue injury or acidosis. More chronic elevations of potassium suggest an impairment of renal excretion. **Algorithm 4.2** addresses treatment of hyperkalemia.

Hypokalemia in the surgical patient usually results from unreplaced losses of gastrointestinal fluids (diarrhea, massive emesis) (**see Table 4.2** for composition of gastrointestinal fluids). Hypokalemia also may exist or be exaggerated by renal tubular disorders, diuretic use, metabolic alkalosis, some medications, and hormonal disorders (primary aldosteronism, Cushing's syndrome). **The treatment of hypokalemia is directed toward rapid restoration of extracellular potassium concentration followed by slower replenishment of total body deficits.** This approach would be appropriate for **Case 2**. This can be accomplished by infusion of 20 to 40 mEq of potassium/hour and must be accompanied by continuous electrocardiogram (ECG) monitoring at higher rates. Restoration of other abnormalities, such as alkalosis, also should be addressed.

Calcium: Nearly 99% of body calcium is located in bone. Calcium located in body fluid circulates as free (40%) or bound to albumin (50%) or other anions. Only the free component is biologically active. **Acid–base abnormalities alter the binding of calcium to albumin. (Alkalosis leads to a reduction in ionized calcium, whereas acidosis increases ionized calcium levels.)** Most of the ingested calcium is excreted in stool. Replacement of calcium usually is not necessary for routine, uncomplicated surgical patients. However, attention to replacement may be required in patients with large fluid shifts, immobilization, and especially in patients with surgical thyroid or parathyroid disorders.

Hypercalcemia most often results from hyperparathyroidism and malignancy. Symptoms of hypercalcemia may include confusion, lethargy, weakness, anorexia, vomiting, constipation, and pancreatitis. Nephrogenic diabetes insipidus also may result. Serum calcium concentrations above 14mg/dL or any level associated with ECG abnormalities requires urgent treatment. Virtually all such patients, such as the one described in **Case 3**, are dehydrated and require hydration with saline. Additional treatments may include diuretics as well as diphosphanates, calcitonin, or mithramycin. Steroids may be useful in some patients.

Hypocalcemia results from several mechanisms, including low parathormone activity, low vitamin D activity, and conditions referred to as pseudohypocalcemia (low albumin, hyperventilation). Acute conditions such as pancreatitis, massive soft tissue infections, high-output gastrointestinal fistulas, and massive transfusion of citrated blood also may lead to acute hypocalcemia. The early symptoms of hypocalcemia include numbness or tingling of the circumoral region or fingertips. Tetany and seizure may occur at very low calcium levels. Replacement of calcium requires an appreciation of the causes and symptoms. For

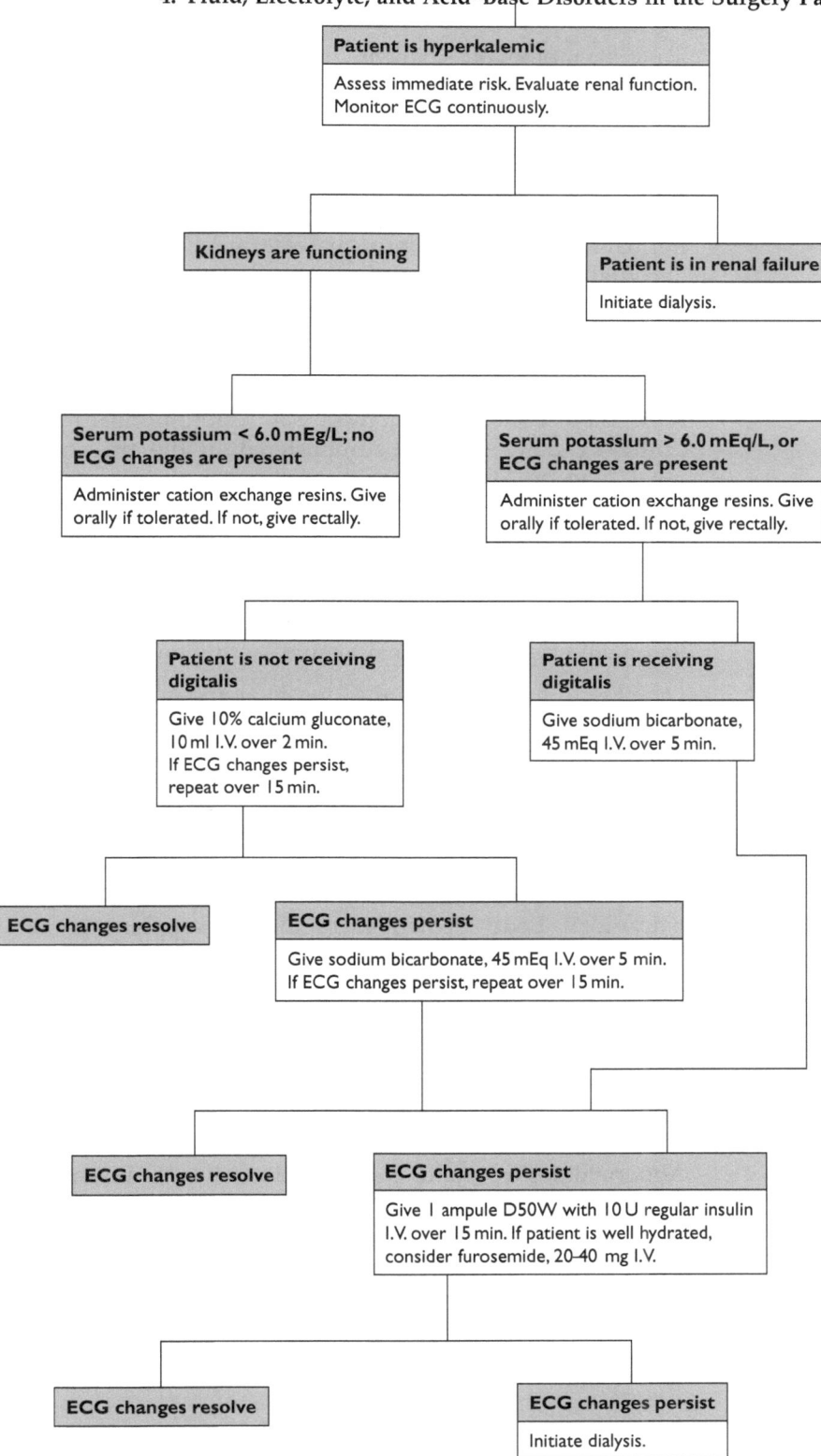

Algorithm 4.2. Assessment and treatment of hyperkalemia. (Reprinted from Van Zee KJ, Lowry SF. Life-threatening electrolyte abnormalities. In: Wilmore DW, Cheung LY, Harken AH, et al, eds. ACS Surgery: Principles and Practice (Section 1: Resuscitation). New York: WebMD Corporation, 1997, with permission.)

acute symptomatic patients, intravenous replacement may be necessary.

Magnesium: Approximately 50% of body magnesium is located in bone and is not readily exchangeable. Like potassium, magnesium is an intracellular cation that tends to become depleted during alkalotic conditions. Magnesium absorption occurs in the small intestine, and the normal dietary intake approximates 20 mEq/day.

Hypomagnesemia may occur secondary to malabsorption, diarrhea, hypoparathyroidism, pancreatitis, intestinal fistulas, cirrhosis, and hypoaldosteronism. It also may occur during periods of refeeding after catabolism or starvation. Low magnesium levels also often accompany hypocalcemic states, and the symptoms of deficiency are similar. Often, repletion of both ions is necessary to restore normal function. Up to 2 mEg/kg daily may be administered in the presence of normal renal function. Attention to restoration of any fluid deficits also is mandatory.

Hypermagnesemia most frequently occurs in the presence of renal failure. Acidosis exacerbates this condition. Use of magnesium-containing antacids also may lead to elevated serum levels. Emergency treatment of symptomatic hypermagnesemia requires calcium salts, and definitive treatment may require hydration and renal dialysis.

Phosphate: Phosphate is the most abundant intracellular anion, whereas only 0.1% of body phosphate is in the circulation. Consequently, blood levels do not reflect total body stores.

Hypophosphatemia may result from reduced intestinal absorption, increased renal excretion, hyperparathyroidism, massive liver resection, or inadequate repletion during recovery from starvation or catabolism. Tissue oxygen delivery may be impaired due to reduced 2,3-diphosphoglycerate levels. Muscle weakness and malaise accompany total body depletion. Prolonged supplementation may be necessary in severely depleted patients.

Hyperphosphatemia often occurs in the presence of impaired renal function and may be associated with hypocalcemia. Hypoparathyroidism also reduces renal phosphate excretion.

Summary

Abnormalities of fluid balance, electrolyte imbalance, and acid–base status are very common in surgical patients. While one must address acute, life-threatening abnormalities expeditiously, a systematic approach to evaluating each patient should be a routine component of surgical care. Addressing fluid, electrolyte, and acid–base status is part of the care plan for every patient. The surgeon should anticipate clinical conditions that can present with or eventuate in such abnormalities.

Selected Readings

Goldborger E. Primer of Water, Electrolyte and Acid–Base Syndromes, 7th ed. Philadelphia: Lea & Febiger, 1986.

Nathens AB, Maier RV. In: Norton JA, Bollinger RR, Chang AE. et al, eds. Surgery: Basic Science and Clinical Evidence. New York: Springer-Verlag, 2001.

Pemberton LB, Pemberton PG. Treatment of Water, Electrolyte, and Acid–Base Disorders in the Surgical Patient. New York: McGraw-Hill, 1994.

Polk HC, Gardner B, Stone HH. Basic Surgery, 5th ed. St. Louis: Quality Medical Publishing, 1995.

Shires GT, Shires GT III, Lowry S. Fluid electrolyte and nutritional management of the surgical patient. In: Schwartz SI, ed. Principles of Surgery, 6th ed. New York: McGraw-Hill, 1994.

5

Surgical Critical Care

John T. Malcynski

Objectives

To describe the priorities in evaluating and treating a critically ill surgical patient:

- to identify immediate life-threatening situations and treat them accordingly.
- to discuss the systems approach to organ dysfunction in the evaluation and treatment of the critically ill surgical patient.

Cases

Case 1

A 28-year-old male unrestrained driver was involved in a head-on motor vehicle crash and found to have a grade III liver laceration that the trauma surgeon wants to manage nonoperatively. In addition, the patient is intubated due to a severe pulmonary contusion that has resulted in a significant hypoxemia. As the patient is brought into the intensive care unit (ICU) for you to manage, you note his skin is cool, pale, and mottled. As the nurse obtains initial vital signs, she tells you that his heart rate is 120 beats per minute and his blood pressure is 90/50 mm Hg.

Case 2

A 69-year-old woman has just arrived from the operating room after undergoing a sigmoid colectomy with Hartmann's pouch and an end colostomy. As the surgeon drops off the patient in your care, he comments that there was a large amount of stool contamination in the abdomen that seemed to be present for several days. Due to a large amount of intraoperative fluids, the anesthesiologist decided to keep the patient intubated. You note that her heart rate is in the 100s and her blood pressure is 80/45. Her skin is not noticeably cool to the touch.

Introduction

It is not uncommon for a medical condition or illness to involve multiple organ systems. In addition to the primary anatomic insult and the problems that result, a cascade of physiologic derangements may occur that involve multiple, seemingly unrelated, organ systems. This usually is the case in the surgical critical care patient, where an initiating event, such as major trauma, burns, or infection, along with any premorbid conditions, results in a life-threatening situation that requires an understanding of complex physiologic interactions. **The clinical condition characterized by severe dysfunction of multiple organ systems is termed multiple organ dysfunction system (MODS).** The exact mechanisms of MODS have yet to be determined, but we do know that it is mediated by a series of complex interactions between intracellular components, such as cytokines, the neuroendocrine system, and extrinsic products, such as endotoxin. The resultant condition is that of capillary leak, myocardial depression, and massive fluid balance changes. It is the task of the surgical intensivist, along with the facilities of the multidisciplinary ICU, to understand the interactions between the affected organ systems, dictate a course of support, and aid in the recovery of the patient.

As with any discipline, a **thorough history and physical examination** are imperative in beginning to understand the process or processes at hand. This includes any premorbid conditions, such as heart or lung disease, as well as details of the latest insult that initiated the process at hand. Elements, such as injuries from a traumatic event, details of a surgical procedure, or the likely focus of infection, are helpful in determining what steps need to be taken to provide appropriate support to the patient.

In addition, conditions that are immediately life threatening are addressed and treated in a systematic approach. As in other algorithms, such as Advanced Cardiac Life Support (ACLS) and Advanced Trauma Life Support (ATLS), following the **ABC principle by conducting a primary survey (Table 5.1)** ensures that the clinician addresses the most critical conditions in the order of their potential to cause death.

Algorithm 5.1 provides a basic framework for the methodical approach to the care of a patient in the ICU.

History and Physical Examination

History

As stated earlier, knowing the patient's history (**Table 5.2**) is essential for adequately treating a critically ill patient with multiple organ dysfunction. **Premorbid conditions,** such as a history of congestive heart failure (CHF) or renal insufficiency, **greatly affects the magnitude to which a patient may respond to the illness and the therapies instituted to treat it.** As in the trauma patient in **Case 1**, identification of all injuries is crucial in helping avoid potentially hazardous therapeutic

Table 5.1. Elements of the primary survey.

1. Airway
Evaluation
Ensure airway is patent

Problem
Obstruction from foreign body
Anatomic obstruction (tongue)
Physiologic obstruction (vomitus, secretions)

Therapy
Endotracheal/orotracheal intubation
Surgical airway (cricothyrotomy/tracheostomy)

2. Breathing
Evaluation
Ensure air is moving equally between both lungs

Problem
Tension pneumothorax
Hemothorax
Lung or lobar collapse

Therapy
Needle thoracostomy
Tube thoracostomy

3. Circulation
Evaluation
Ensure adequate cardiovascular state

Problem
Bleeding (GI hemorrhage, external bleeding source)
Shock—inadequate circulation for maintenance of cellular function
    (hemorrhagic, cardiogenic, septic, neurogenic)

Therapy
Adequate intravenous access (large-bore peripheral venous access,
    large-bore central venous access)
Fluid/blood product administration
Invasive circulatory monitoring
Pharmacologic support (vasopressors/inotropes)
Control of primary source of blood loss

measures, such as anticoagulation in a patient with a liver laceration
or closed head injury. A list of preillness medications helps avoid possible drug interactions from medications given in the ICU.

Physical Examination

In this technologic age of invasive monitoring and other advanced
diagnostic modalities, it is easy to overlook the physical examination
in the evaluation of the critically ill patient. By merely touching a
patient and noting the temperature of the skin, one can diagnose that
a patient is in shock and even determine the type of shock, such as in
the patient with mottled, cool skin who is in hypovolemic shock. This
is the situation in **Case 1**, where the cool, pale, mottled skin should alert
the clinician that a derangement in the patient's hemodynamics exists.

The loss of breath sounds over a lung field in a mechanically ventilated patient who experiences a sudden drop in blood pressure can reveal a tension pneumothorax. In this situation, waiting for further diagnostic tests may prove to be detrimental and may result in the patient's death.

A systematic approach to the physical exam, especially when conducted the same way for each patient, ensures that no elements of the exam are neglected or missed. Depending on the examiner's preference, this usually is carried out anatomically from "head to toe" or using a systemic approach, such as commencing with the neurologic system and ending with the musculoskeletal system (**Table 5.3**).

Diagnostics and Management

Because critically ill patients frequently have dysfunction involving multiple organ systems, **diagnostic measures and subsequent therapies are directed at the system involved. Not uncommonly, the treatment of one system has an effect on other organ systems.** For example, improving cardiac performance also may improve renal function. This complex nature of the interactions between organ systems adds an extra challenge to the intensivist. To provide a basic approach

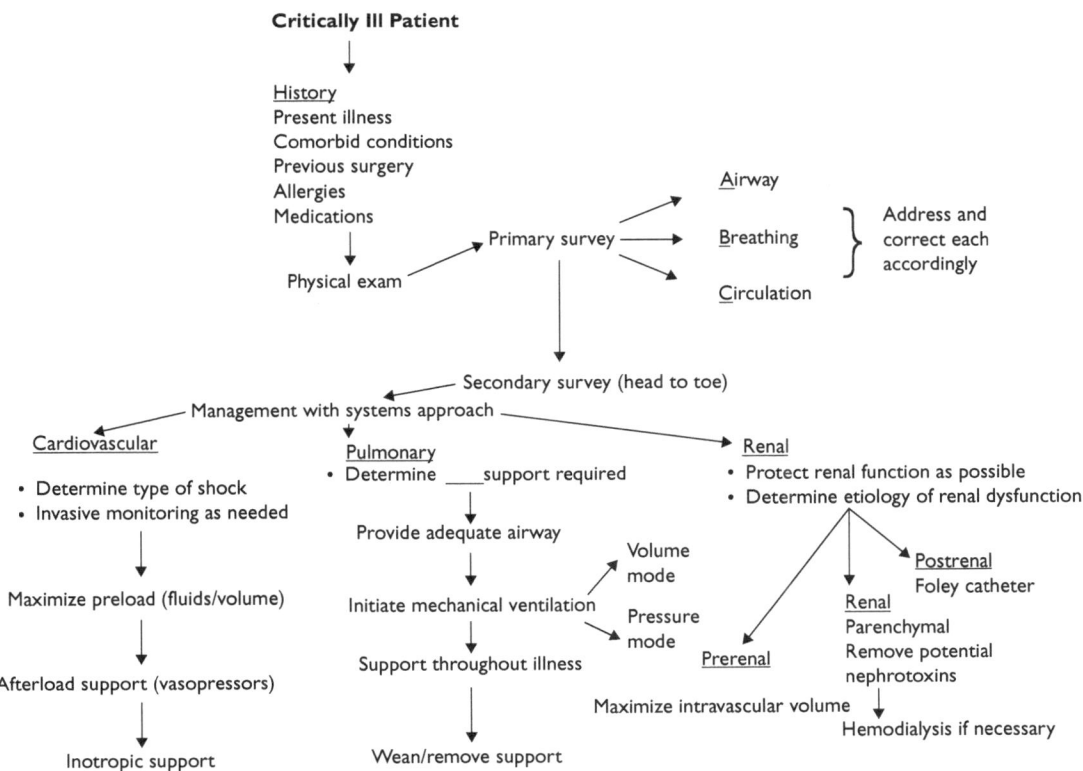

Algorithm 5.1. Evaluation and management of the critically ill patient.

Table 5.2. Important elements to be considered in the history.

Initiating insult
Blood loss and transfusions
Foci of infection
Medical conditions
Cardiac disease
Pulmonary dysfunction/chronic obstructive pulmonary disease
Hepatic disease/cirrhosis
Renal insufficiency
Bleeding disorders
Peptic ulcer disease
Surgical history
Coronary artery bypass graft
Gastrointestinal procedures
Medications
Allergies
History of cancer

to such problems encountered in the surgical critical care patient, this chapter discusses individual organ systems, focusing on pathophysiologic changes, diagnosis, and treatment. Although virtually all organ systems, from the endocrine to the immunologic, are affected in some manner, those that are treated most commonly by the intensivist are the **cardiovascular, pulmonary, and renal systems**. Since this chapter is designed to provide a general overview of surgical critical care, these three organ systems are the primary focus of discussion.

Table 5.3. A few of the elements of the physical exam that should be evaluated and documented.

General	*Abdomen*
Level of alertness	Bowel sounds
Glasgow coma score	Diarrhea
Movement of extremities	Distention
Head, ears, eyes, nose, and throat	Blood (upper or lower)
Scleral icterus	*Skin*
Mucous membranes	Turgor
Jugular venous distention	Temperature
Heart	Peripheral edema
Rhythm	Capillary refill
Rate	Pulses
Murmurs	
Lungs	
Character of breath sounds	
Coarse	
Rales	
Diminished	
Secretions	

Cardiovascular Dysfunction

Shock is defined as the body's inability to maintain adequate perfusion at the cellular level. Despite the etiology of the shock state, it is the failure of the cardiovascular system to provide this perfusion. This state presents with hypotension, either by a systolic blood pressure (SBP) less than 90 mm Hg or a mean arterial pressure (MAP) less than 60 mm Hg. MAP can easily be calculated by the following formula:

$$MAP = \frac{1}{3}[(SBP - DBP)/DBP]$$

where DBP is the diastolic blood pressure.

Details on the types of shock—hypovolemic/hemorrhagic, cardiogenic, septic, neurogenic, spinal, anaphylactic—are described in Chapter 7. **Determination of the type of shock is very important because treatment strategies may differ depending on the etiology.** Each of the case presentations represents a patient in shock; however, the cause of each is different. The patient in **Case 1** clearly is in **hemorrhagic/hypovolemic shock** due to blood loss from his liver laceration. The patient in **Case 2** most likely is in **septic shock** from fecal peritonitis. Physical examination may give clues to the process at hand, but often this is not a reliable means by which to institute a therapy. It is in this situation that the technology of the ICU comes into play, and **invasive hemodynamic monitoring can be very helpful**.

As the term implies, **invasive monitoring** involves the placement of devices, such as catheters, into the body, whether it be a central vein, peripheral artery, or the heart itself. **By using such devices, circulatory information, such as preload, afterload, and inotropy, as well as cardiac performance indicators, such as cardiac output, can be determined.**

Preload

Preload refers to the load or tension on the myocardium when it begins to contract. Preload is determined by the quantity or volume of blood in the ventricle at the end of diastole, just before systole is to occur. When initiating cardiovascular support, preload should be maximized prior to the initiation of vasopressors. This usually is facilitated by the use of invasive monitoring.

Central venous pressure (CVP) measures right-side cardiac pressures by way of a catheter placed into the superior vena cava (SVC), with the actual pressure obtained at the junction of the SVC and the right atrium (RA). The CVP measurements are accurate in determining preload provided certain conditions, such as right-sided heart failure, pericardial tamponade, or high positive end-expiratory pressures (PEEP) requirements while on mechanical ventilation, are not present. If the CVP is low, one almost always can be assured that preload is not optimal.

Measurement of the **pulmonary artery occlusion pressure (PAOP)** is a more invasive monitoring technique that estimates the volume of the left ventricle. A catheter is inserted into the central venous system and passed into the right atrium, through the tricuspid valve, and into the right ventricle. From the right ventricle, the catheter is directed by the natural flow of blood into a dependent branch of the pulmonary artery (PA) until a balloon at the tip of the catheter eventually occludes flow from that artery. This also is known as wedging the balloon into the PA, thus the term **wedge pressure**. With the balloon occluding further flow in the PA branch, a stagnant column of blood results from the distal tip of the pressure transducer. Since no flow exists in this column of blood, one can assume that the pressure measured at the column is the same all along the column, which traverses the pulmonary capillary bed to the pulmonary veins into the left atrium (LA). Provided that there is no mitral valvular disease, such as mitral regurgitation, this pressure also should be accurate for the pressure of the left ventricle (LV). This point of measurement is obtained at end diastole, just before the LV contracts when the mitral valve is open. It then is possible to correlate this pressure with the volume of the LV. This correlation, however, only is possible provided that the compliance—the ability of the ventricle to stretch adequately given the volume of blood it receives—of the LV is not impaired, as in the case of diastolic dysfunction, when the diseased ventricle is too stiff to adequately expand. In this case, high filling pressures may be seen by a small volume of blood in the ventricle. **Case 1** and **Case 2** both describe a patient with an inadequate preload. However, the etiology of each is quite different. The patient in **Case 1** suffers from hypovolemia as a result of a massive hemorrhage, whereas the patient in **Case 2** represents hypovolemia as a result of systemic inflammatory response syndrome (SIRS) with resultant intravascular fluid extravasation. It is imperative that preload is maximized in each case, despite the different etiologies.

Afterload

Afterload is the pressure against which the ventricle must pump. It typically is thought of as the resistance or tone that the arterial vasculature exhibits against the flow of blood as it travels through the vessel, where resistance is related to flow and pressure in the following equation:

$$Resistance = Pressure/Flow.$$

The resistance of the arterial vasculature, otherwise known as **systemic vascular resistance (SVR)**, can be determined by the following formula:

$$SVR = MAP - CVP/CO$$

where CO is the cardiac output. Once preload is optimized, afterload is addressed by the administration of agents that either increase or decrease the vascular tone, depending on the type of shock present (**Table 5.4**). In cases in which vascular tone is decreased, such as septic shock, α-adrenergic receptor agonists, such as norepinephrine, epinephrine, phenylepherine, or dopamine, commonly are used. This is the situation with the patient in **Case 2**, who is exhibiting signs of septic shock secondary to the fecal contamination within her abdomen. Hypovolemia is compounded with a loss of vascular tone, which

Table 5.4. Vasoactive drugs and receptor activities for the treatment of shock.

Class and drug	Blood pressure	Systemic vascular resistance	Cardiac output	Heart rate	Isotrope		Renal blood flow	Coronary blood flow	MvO₂
					Low-dose	High-dose			
Alpha only									
Phenylephrine	↑↑↑	↑↑↑	↓↓↓	↓↓↓	±	±	↓↓↓↓	±↑↑	↑
Alpha and beta									
Norepinephrine	↑↑	↑↑↑	↓↓↑↑	↓↓±	↑	↑	↓↓↓	↑↑↑	↑↑
Epinephrine	↑±	↑±	↑↑↑↑	↑↑↑	↑↑	↑↑↑	↓±	↑↑↑	↑↑↑
Dopamine	↑↑	↑↑	↑↑	↑	±	↑↑	↑↑↑	↑↑	↑↑
Beta only									
Isoproterenol	↑±	↓↓	↑↑↑↑	↑↑↑↑	↑↑↑	↑↑↑↑	±	↑↑↑	↑↑↑↑
Dobutamine	↓↓	↓↓↓	↑↑↑	↑↑	↑↑↑	↑↑↑	±	↑↑↑	↑↑↑
Beta-blocker									
Propranolol	±↓↓	±→	↓↓↓	↓↓↓↓	↓↓	↓↓↓	→	↓↓↓	↓↓↓
Metoprolol	↓↓↓	±↑	↓↓	↓↓↓	↓↓	↓↓↓	±	↓↓	↓↓
Other									
Nitroglycerine	±↓	↓↓	±↑	±↑	±	±	±↑	→→→	↓↓↓
Hydralazine	↓↓↓	↓↓↓	±↑	±↑↑	±	±	±↑	→	↓↓↓
Prazosin	↓↓↓	↓↓	±↑	±	±	±	±↑	→	↓↓↓
Nitroprusside	↓↓	↓↓↓	↑↑↑	±↑↑	±	±	±↑↑	±	↓↓↓

Source: Reprinted from Pettitt TW, Cobb JP. Critical care. In: Doherty GM, Bauman DS, Creswell LL, Goss JA, Lairmore TC, eds. The Washington Manual of Surgery. Philadelphia: Lippincott Williams & Wilkins, 1996. With permission from Lippincott Williams & Wilkins.

ultimately will require vasoactive support. It should be stated again that it is vital to ensure that adequate intravascular volume or preload is attained prior to the initiation of vasopressors, since these agents can result in end-organ hypoxia and injury due to their vasoconstrictive properties. Organs particularly at risk are the kidneys and the gastrointestinal tract.

Inotropy

Inotropy is the contractility of the myocardium and the force at which it occurs. According to Starling's law, the contractility of the heart increases up to a critical point as the force against the myocardial fibers increases. A further increase of force causes a decrease of the contractility. This force generated against the myocardial fibers is a result of blood entering the ventricle and causing it to expand. If, after preload is maximized, cardiac indices are less than desirable, manifested by a low stroke volume or cardiac output, inotropic agents may be administered to help improve cardiac performance. Dobutamine, a beta agonist, or the phosphodiesterase inhibitors amrinone and milrinone all increase cardiac contractility and thus cardiac output. It should be noted that as these agents increase the contractility of the myocardium, the oxygen requirement of the heart also increases and may worsen an already ischemic heart.

Pulmonary Dysfunction

The inability of a patient's lungs to provide the body with adequate oxygen amounts in order to maintain cellular function (oxygenation) or the inability to adequately expel carbon dioxide (ventilation) is what is known as pulmonary dysfunction. When noninvasive means of support, such as supplemental oxygen administration, is adequate in compensating for this dysfunction, the term **pulmonary insufficiency** is used. When more aggressive and invasive means of support are required, such as mechanical ventilation, the term **pulmonary failure** is used.

Etiology

There are many causes for pulmonary insufficiency and failure that involve all aspects of the respiratory system (**Table 5.5**). It is important to determine the etiology of the failure and look for potentially reversible causes, although support of the respiratory system is accomplished essentially in the same way.

A major cause of pulmonary dysfunction in the surgical ICU is the **acute respiratory distress syndrome (ARDS)**. This condition commonly is seen in patients who have experienced severe trauma, are septic, or have undergone a major operative procedure possibly requiring a massive transfusion. This condition is the result of a systemic state of inflammation known as SIRS, cited above, in which numerous cellular components, such as cytokines and interleukins, along with extrinsic mediators, such as bacterial lipopolysaccharide (LPS), act on endothelial cells, causing an alteration in their permeability, which results in a "leak" of intravascular components (both proteinaceous

Table 5.5. Some common categories and causes of pulmonary dysfunction.

Neuromuscular
   Brainstem injury/stroke
   Spinal cord injury
   Polio
   Amyotrophic lateral sclerosis

Mechanical
   Airway obstruction (foreign body, trauma)
   Flail chest
   Pneumothorax
   Diaphragmatic injury

Parenchymal
   Pneumonia
   Pulmonary contusion
   Acute respiratory distress syndrome
   Congestive heart failure

Miscellaneous
   Drug overdose
   Anaphylaxis

and serous) into nonvascular spaces. This manifestation on the lung causes the alveoli to flood with water and protein to the extent that the alveoli are hindered markedly in their ability to transport oxygen into the blood. Although the lungs are affected and altered by SIRS, the disease process at hand usually is not a result of a primary lung problem, but it is merely an organ system where SIRS manifests.

Three criteria must be present to accurately define a condition as being ARDS (**Table 5.6**). The Po_2/Fio_2 ratio of less than 200 denotes a severe hypoxia. A healthy individual breathing room air ($Fio_2 = 0.21$) should have a Po_2 of approximately 100 mm Hg, making the P/F ratio 476. A pulmonary artery wedge pressure less than 18 is necessary to rule out a cardiogenic etiology for the pulmonary edema. Pulmonary edema in the face of an elevated pulmonary capillary wedge pressure (PCWP) usually is a result of CHF and must be differentiated from ARDS. Finally, bilateral infiltrates on the chest x-ray (CXR) ensure that a pattern of pulmonary edema is present and that pneumonia is not all that is responsible for the hypoxia.

Treatment

Two separate processes, **oxygenation** and **ventilation**, must be considered when planning to support the respiratory system. Each compo-

Table 5.6. Three criteria that must be present to accurately diagnose acute respiratory distress syndrome.

1. Po_2/Fio_2 ratio <200
2. Pulmonary capillary wedge pressure <18
3. Bilateral patchy infiltrates on chest x-ray

nent is relatively independent of the other but equally as important. Oxygenation is the process in which atmospheric oxygenation is transported to red blood cells via lung alveoli. Oxygen acts as the end receptor in the mitochondrial electron transport chain that is involved in cellular respiration. Ventilation is the process in which the lung releases carbon dioxide, a waste product from substrate metabolism, from the blood into the atmosphere.

The first decision to make in pulmonary management is whether to initiate support by way of mechanical ventilation. Typically, the parameters used in determining the need for such support are the following:

1. respiratory rate >30 breaths per minute
2. Pao_2 <60 mm Hg
3. $Paco_2$ >60 mm Hg

Severe tachypnea may cause excessive fatigue and exhaustion, while hypoxemia and hypercapnea reflect the inability to oxygenate or ventilate accordingly. Not all parameters need to be met in order to initiate mechanical ventilatory support.

The initial step in providing mechanical ventilation is securing an airway. This usually is accomplished by inserting a balloon-cuffed tube into the trachea by way of a nasotracheal or orotracheal route. This tube is then attached to connection tubing that is then connected to the ventilator.

Next, the ventilator is adjusted to the desired settings. The intensivist has several different ventilatory modes he may employ in meeting his objective. These modes primarily describe the means by which a breath is delivered from the machine to the patient, either by volume or by pressure. When a breath is delivered by volume, a designated volume is set on the ventilator, and the ventilator delivers that set amount of gas. A pressure mode delivers an amount of gas into the lungs up to a given pressure that is set on the ventilator. The volume of gas administered is determined by how compliant the lungs are and how much they can stretch with a given force of air. Compliance is calculated as the change in volume divided by the change in pressure:

$$dV/dP$$

where normal is 100 mL/cm H_2O. A lung that is very sick may have a low compliance (<20) and therefore be very stiff. A pressure limit of 35 cm water may generate only a tidal volume of 200 cc, whereas the same pressure limit of 35 cm would generate 800 cc in a healthy lung. The advantage of a pressure control is that, by limiting the pressure to which the lung will be subjected, there is less of a chance of causing injury to the lung, known as barotrauma, from excessive airway pressures that sometimes may result when using a volume mode.

The next decision to make is determining whether mandatory breaths are to be administered or whether only supported breaths are required. It is possible even to have a combination of each. **Mandatory breaths,** as the term implies, involves setting a given number of breaths that the patient will receive. This number may be the only breaths the patient receives or may be in addition to breaths that the patient contributes, with or without additional support from the ventilator. Supported breaths are initiated by the patient, usually with a determined level of support supplied or assisted by the ventilator.

When a suitable ventilatory mode is determined according to the patient's clinical status, the goal is to achieve appropriate minute ventilation—the volume of gas exhaled in 1 minute—in order to maintain a eucapnic state. This is accomplished by setting the desired tidal volume and respiratory rate. Tidal volume usually is calculated to be 10 to 12 mm per Kilogram of body weight. A recent exception is in the case of a patient with ARDS, where prospective studies have shown that 6 to 8 mm Hg/g body wt. may have a protective effect on the lung and reduce overall mortality. Next, a respiratory rate is determined to achieve a minute ventilation of 8 to 12 L/min. An arterial blood gas is drawn 30 minutes after support has been initiated, and the Pco_2 is evaluated. The tidal volume or respiratory rate is adjusted accordingly to bring the Pco_2 to a desirable level. The more common ventilatory modes and their comparisons are listed in **Table 5.7.**

After the desired ventilatory mode and parameters are chosen, **the priority of oxygenating the patient is addressed**. This is accomplished by selecting a level for both the fractional inspired oxygen (Fio_2) and PEEP. The Fio_2 is the percentage of oxygen mixed with nitrogen that is to be delivered to the patient. The ranges are from atmospheric oxygen concentration of 21% or 0.21 to supplying 100% or 1.0 oxygen. Typically, the Fio_2 is started at 1.0 and then titrated to a level to maintain oxygen saturation between 92% and 95%.

A person with a minimal alveolar-arterial (A-a) gradient usually will end up with an Fio_2 set at 0.4; PEEP, which is the residual pressure in the alveoli at the end of expiration, is added to help prevent atelectasis. With a minimal A-a gradient, PEEP usually is set at 5 cm H_2O, which also is known as **physiologic PEEP**. Higher levels of PEEP can be added to facilitate oxygenating the patient, especially when a large diffusion gradient exists, as in ARDS. It is thought that PEEP helps to improve the functional residual capacity (FRC) of the lung and aids in recruiting unused alveoli. In addition, PEEP may play a role in thinning out the thick proteinaceous fluid layer in the alveoli, thus promoting oxygen diffusion across the basement membrane of the alveoli. Disadvantages of PEEP, especially at higher levels in the 20- to 30-cm H_2O range, include barotrauma to the airways, resulting in a tension pneumothorax and a decline in cardiac output as a result of decreased cardiac filling from compression of the pulmonary veins from such high intrathoracic pressures. In cases of severe life-threatening hypoxia, other ventilator strategies can be employed, such as reversing the inspiratory to expiratory (I:E) ratio, thus allowing a longer time for oxygen to diffuse across diseased basement membrane. This strategy, however, involves an unnatural breathing pattern and usually requires that a patient be sedated heavily or even chemically paralyzed in order to allow this ventilatory mode to be effective.

Ventilatory support is continued throughout the patient's acute illness. As the patient resolves the illness at hand, the intensivist is

Table 5.7. Conventional ventilator modes.

Mode	Description	Advantages	Disadvantages	Uses
A. Volume-limited	Set tidal volume; peak inspiratory pressure varies	Ensures adequate tidal volume	Barotrauma in those with very poor lung compliance	
1. Assist/control (A/C)	Both spontaneous (patient-initiated, "assisted") and ("controlled") breaths have same tidal volume	Minimal work of breathing	Easy for patient to hyperventilate. Makes assessment of ventilatory muscle strength difficult to evaluate	Weak, heavily sedated, or paralyzed
2. Intermittent mandatory ventilation (IMV)	Tidal volume of machine-initiated ("mandatory") breaths set; no ventilator support for spontaneous breaths	Allows gradual decrease of support by decreasing rate of mandatory breaths	No support for spontaneous breaths	Often used in combination with PSV for weaning
B. Pressure-limited	Set peak inspiratory pressure; tidal volume varies	Decreased risk of barotrauma	Does not ensure tidal volume	
1. Pressure control ventilation (PCV)	Inspiratory pressure and rate set	Inverse ratio ventilation (IRV); increased alveolar "recruitment"	Requires heavy sedation and/or paralytics	Patients with very poor lung compliance
2. Pressure support ventilation (PSV)	Inspiratory pressure set; no rate	Most comfortable of the conventional modes	Increased risk of hypoventilation	Awake patients; often used in combination with IMV for weaning

Source: Reprinted from Cobb JP. Critical care: a system-oriented approach. In: Norton JA, Bollinger RR, Chang AE, et al, eds. Surgery: Basic Science and Clinical Evidence. New York: Springer-Verlag, 2001, with permission.

able to decrease the amount of work that is being accomplished by the ventilator as well as the amount of oxygen required.

Discontinuation of Mechanical Ventilation

There are as many strategies employed to wean a patient off the ventilator as there are ventilatory modes. The most common involves the **gradual decrease in the minute ventilation supported by the machine, allowing the patient to supply the difference**. This is done either by gradually decreasing the number of mandatory breaths given to the patient or decreasing the amount of pressure supplied to the patient during the supported breaths. Several prospective studies have evaluated these popular strategies and can be reviewed in **Table 5.8**.

Once it is decided that a patient has a good chance of discontinued ventilatory support, that is, is on minimal assisted settings with a low FiO_2 while maintaining an acceptable minute ventilation without being fatigued from tachypnea, consideration is made regarding removing the breathing tube or extubating the patient. Traditional parameters use such indices as the spontaneous tidal volume and the vital capacity a patient can generate as well as the degree of negative pressure or negative inspiratory force (NIF) a patient can generate. Recently, an index has been used to predict the success of keeping a patient off the ventilator once extubated. This index is known as the Rapid Shallow Breathing Index (RSBI) and is determined by the number of breaths in 1 minute divided by the tidal volume of each breath (f/Vt). Patients with an RSBI less than 100 have a high rate of success (in the order of 80%+) in remaining extubated.

Table 5.8. Prospective, randomized, controlled clinical trials comparing strategies to wean mechanical ventilation (level I evidence).

Authors and reference	No. of patients	Comparisons	Duration of ventilation before randomization	Duration of ventilation after randomization	Conclusion
Brochard et al.[a]	109	IMV vs. PSV vs. T-piece	17 vs. 11 vs. 14 days	9.9 vs. 5.7 vs. 8.5 days	PSV best
Esteban et al.[b]	130	IMV vs. PSV vs. T-piece	6.5 vs. 10.8 vs. 11.5 days	5 vs. 4 vs. 3 days	T-piece best
Ely et al.[c]	300	Routine vs. daily T-piece	3 vs. 2.5 days	3 vs. 2 days	Daily T-piece better
Kollef et al.[d]	357	Routine vs. protocol	2.4 vs. 1.7 days	1.5 vs. 1.2 days	Protocol better

[a] Brochard L, Rauss A, Benito S, et al. Comparison of three methods of gradual withdrawal from ventilatory support during weaning from mechanical ventilation [see comments]. Am J Respir Crit Care Med 1994;150(4):896–903.
[b] Esteban A, Frutos F, Tobin MJ, et al. A comparison of four methods of weaning patients from mechanical ventilation. Spanish Lung Failure Collaborative Group [see comments]. N Engl J Med 1995;332(6):345–350.
[c] Ely EW, Baker AM, Dunagan DP, et al. Effect on the duration of mechanical ventilation of identifying patients capable of breathing spontaneously [see comments]. N Engl J Med 1996;335(25):1864–1869.
[d] Kollef MH, Shapiro SD, Silver P, et al. A randomized, controlled trial of protocol-directed versus physician-directed weaning from mechanical ventilation [see comments]. Crit Care Med 1997;25(4):567–574.
Source: Reprinted from Cobb JP. Critical care: a system-oriented approach. In: Norton JA, Bollinger RR, Chang AE, et al, eds. Surgery: Basic Science and Clinical Evidence. New York: Springer-Verlag, 2001, with permission.

Renal Dysfunction

Renal dysfunction is not a rare occurrence in the surgical ICU. Associated many times with SIRS and multisystem organ failure (MSOF), renal dysfunction, which may lead to renal failure, carries a substantial mortality rate in ICU patients, approaching 50% in some investigations. It is this fact that encourages the surgical intensivist to attempt to "protect" the kidneys as much as possible during a critical illness. This usually is accomplished by maximizing renal perfusion while simultaneously minimizing any potential nephrotoxins.

Early signs of renal dysfunction are characterized by a prolonged decrease in urine output and a rise in the blood urea nitrogen (BUN) and serum creatinine. Late signs of frank renal failure include fluid overload, hyperkalemia, platelet dysfunction, acidosis, and even pericardial effusion. When renal dysfunction is first suspected, all etiologies should be sought out and corrected, if possible. This usually is thought out anatomically by addressing the three components of renal function, namely, **prerenal, renal (parenchymal),** and **postrenal.**

The **prerenal** component regards the perfusion to the kidneys. Inadequate renal perfusion results in renal hypoxia and can lead to acute tubular necrosis (ATN). Prolonged hypotension and hypovolemia are the primary causes for a prerenal etiology of renal failure. Tests that may help determine a prerenal cause include measurement of the urine sodium or calculation of the **fractional excretion of sodium** (FE Na). A urine sodium less than 10 mEq/L sodium implies sodium conservation, with functional renal tubules that can reabsorb salt, and points to a prerenal picture, while a urine sodium greater than 20 mEq/L usually represents the inability of injured renal tubules to conserve sodium, thus wasting salt. The fractional excretion of sodium tends to be a more reliable test and is determined by obtaining urine and serum levels of sodium and creatinine and using the following formula:

$$(Urine\ Na \times Serum\ Cr/Serum\ Na \times Urine\ Cr) \times 100$$

A value less than 1 implies prerenal syndrome, while a value greater than 1 implies a parenchymal etiology.

Prerenal failure is treated by maximizing filling pressures and intravascular volume, ensuring that renal perfusion is optimum. Judicious use of vasopressors is warranted, however, because, while they can increase blood pressure, they can cause a profound constriction of the renal arteries and actually decrease the perfusion to the kidneys. Drugs such as dopamine and furosamide do increase urine output, but there is no scientific proof that these agents prevent or improve renal function, nor have they been shown to improve overall survival when used in such situations. It is clear that nonoliguric renal failure (>500 cc urine/day) carries a more favorable prognosis with respect to return of renal function and overall survival than does oliguric renal failure (<500 cc urine/day), but conversion of oliguric renal failure to nonoliguric renal failure using dopamine or furosamide has no effect on either renal function or survival.

Renal parenchymal failure involves the kidney and the actual renal tubules. This usually is referred to as ATN, which entails actual cellular death of the nephrons and loss of viable kidney tissue. See **Table 5.9** for the common causes of ATN.

Treatment for this type of renal failure consists of maximizing renal perfusion and removing any potential nephrotoxins. The natural history of ATN occurs over a period of 10 to 14 days. This is noted by a serial increase in the BUN and serum creatinine. Resolution of ATN is characterized by an eventual plateau of the serum creatinine until the level begins to fall. If by day 14 the creatinine level does not plateau, the chances of renal function returning are very slim. Finally, a postrenal etiology for renal dysfunction should be ruled out. Postrenal causes are a result of an obstruction of urine at the level of the ureters or below that results in an oliguric or anuric state. An increase of BUN and serum creatinine also may be discovered.

Although less common than the previous two types of renal dysfunction, on occasion **postrenal dysfunction** may be the only explanation for the problem. Bilateral ureteral obstruction or bladder outlet obstruction from a clogged urethral catheter are the more common etiologies. Simply changing the urethral catheter may be all that is required to resolve the issue. An abdominal ultrasound may be helpful in determining if hydroureters or hydronephroses are present.

The patients in both **Case 1 and Case 2** are susceptible to the development of renal failure, despite the difference in their physiologic state. Each has the potential for renal hypoperfusion that can lead to ATN. It is crucial for the clinician to make every effort to maintain renal perfusion while avoiding potential nephrotoxins, if possible.

Occasionally in the ICU, a patient requires hemodialysis as a result of the manifestations of the renal failure. These manifestations usually are life threatening and require immediate attention. Here is a list of the emergency indications requiring hemodialysis in the ICU:

Volume overload/CHF
Severe acidosis
Hyperkalemia
Uremia/platelet dysfunction/bleeding

Continuous veno-veno hemofiltration and dialysis (CVVHD) is a form of hemodialysis performed in some tertiary centers. As the term implies, this technique involves the continuous circulation of blood

Table 5.9. Common causes of acute tubular necrosis.

Prolonged hypotension and ischemia
IV x-ray contrast
Nephrotoxic drugs (aminoglycosides, furosemide)
Rhabdomyolysis/myoglobin
Transfusion reaction
Hemolytic-uremic syndrome
Hepatorenal syndrome

through a specially designed hemodialysis machine that removes a smaller amount of fluid from the patient on an hourly basis. It also is equipped with a membrane that can address the metabolic consequences of ATN. The advantage of CVVHD is that smaller amounts of fluid can be removed over a longer period of time, resulting in less drastic fluid shifts for the patient. Disadvantages include systemic anticoagulation, which keeps the venous lines from clotting, and the need for specialized personnel.

Summary

The critically ill surgical patient often has multiple organ system dysfunction, which requires the surgical intensivist to use a methodical approach in treating such patients. A thorough history and a thorough physical examination are essential initial steps in the management scheme. Frequently, invasive monitoring techniques are required to supply additional information about the patient's status and to help guide therapeutic maneuvers. It is important to realize that, despite using the systems approach for the management of the critically ill, treatment of one system has an effect on the others, resulting in both positive and negative repercussions.

Selected Readings

Bernard GR, Artigas A, Brigham KL, et al. Report of the American-European consensus conference on ARDS: definitions, mechanisms, relevant outcomes and clinical trial coordination. The Consensus Committee. Intensive Care Med 1994;20:225–232.

Bone RC, Balk RA, Cerra FB, et al. Definitions for sepsis and organ failure and guidelines for the use of innovative therapies in sepsis. The ACCP/SCCM Consensus Conference Committee. American College of Chest Physicians/Society of Critical Care Medicine. Chest 1992;101:1644–1655.

Cobb JP. Critical care: a system-oriented approach. In: Norton JA, Bollinger RR, Chang AE, et al., eds. Surgery: Basic Science and Clinical Evidence. New York: Springer-Verlag, 2001:277–290.

Fink MP. Monitoring techniques and complications in critical care. In: Norton JA, Bollinger RR, Chang AE, et al., eds. Surgery: Basic Science and Clinical Evidence. New York: Springer-Verlag, 2001:291–303.

Kollef MH, Schuster DP. The acute respiratory distress syndrome. N Engl J Med 1995;332:27–37.

Marshall JC. Risk prediction and outcome description in critical surgical illness. In: Norton JA, Bollinger RR, Chang AE, et al., eds. Surgery: Basic Science and Clinical Evidence. New York: Springer-Verlag, 2001:305–320.

Moore FA, Moore EE. Evolving concepts in the pathogenesis of postinjury multiple organ failure. Surg Clin North Am 1995;75:257–277.

Principles of Infection: Prevention and Treatment

John M. Davis

Objectives

1. To learn which operative procedures require prophylactic antibiotics.
2. To learn the proper timing and duration of prophylactic antibiotics.
3. To learn the proper conduct in the Operating Room (OR) and the scientific basis for the procedures done in the OR to prevent infections.
4. To learn the diagnosis and management of soft tissue infections.
5. To learn the diagnosis and management of intraabdominal infections.

Cases

Case 1

A 69-year-old woman is admitted with right upper quadrant pain and tenderness and known gallstones found incidentally during an ultrasound for uterine fibroids. Subsequent to the diagnosis, she had an attack of biliary colic requiring an outpatient visit to her local emergency room. Her blood work in the emergency room included a fasting blood glucose level that was elevated at a level of 240 mg/dL. Outpatient blood testing prior to her surgery revealed a direct bilirubin level of 3.5 mg/dL.

Case 2

You are a third-year medical student beginning your third-year clerkship with surgery. You are instructed by the course director to have the chief resident orient you to your duties. The chief resident tells you to come to the operating room quickly to help on an emergency operation. When you arrive at the operating room, you are given a scrub suit and are faced with a variety of head covers and shoe covers. Some surgeons are putting on shoe covers while others are putting on dirty, old running shoes and not using shoe covers. The head nurse tells you that you are in violation of hospital code by not wearing a head cover in the hallways outside the operating room. When you reach the operating room, the surgeon and the chief resident already are at the operating table, having washed their hands for less than 2 minutes. You are left to scrub by yourself. What soap should you use? For how long should you scrub?

Case 3

An obese 55-year-old man had an emergency colectomy for perforated diverticulitis. At surgery, a large segment of sigmoid colon was involved with the infectious process. The colon was thickened by chronic inflammation, surrounded by a watery exudate, with omentum and small bowel adherent to the sigmoid colon. An end colostomy was constructed after the segment of diseased colon was removed. The distal end of the colon was closed with a stapler. The patient had no significant medical history, but on admission he had significant hypertension and a blood sugar of 340mg/dL. The wound was closed, including the skin, and the patient was transferred to the intensive care unit. Now, on postoperative day three, he is febrile with a peak temperature of 39°C (102.2°F), and has a heart rate of 105bpm. The wound is erythematous, swollen, and tender.

Introduction

Control of infection in the surgical patient should be considered in three components as indicated in **Algorithm 6.1**. The preoperative (prehospital) component consists of whatever **medical conditions** the patient brings to the hospital. Evaluation of this component dictates a careful review of the patient's general health, so that appropriate antibiotics, when necessary, may be administered in a timely fashion. Other health conditions, such as smoking, should be stopped so that they have minimum effect during the surgical procedure. The second component is the **operative environment**. Care of the patient during this phase involves following appropriate conduct in the OR in order to minimize contamination and taking full advantage of the modern concepts regarding surgical infection. In this component, the timing of antibiotics and possible re-dosing of antibiotics need to be considered. The third component is **microbial factors**. Here, the local hospital bacterial flora is important. The transmission of resistance organisms or the particular infestation of a highly virulent organism is the factor that determines whether a patient develops an infection. For this component, the surgeon needs to consider the antibiotic sensitivities so that proper antibiotics are given.

An **infection manifests itself when local or systemic host factors, environmental factors, and the microbes overwhelm the host.** When this occurs in the postoperative period, the patient needs to be evalu-

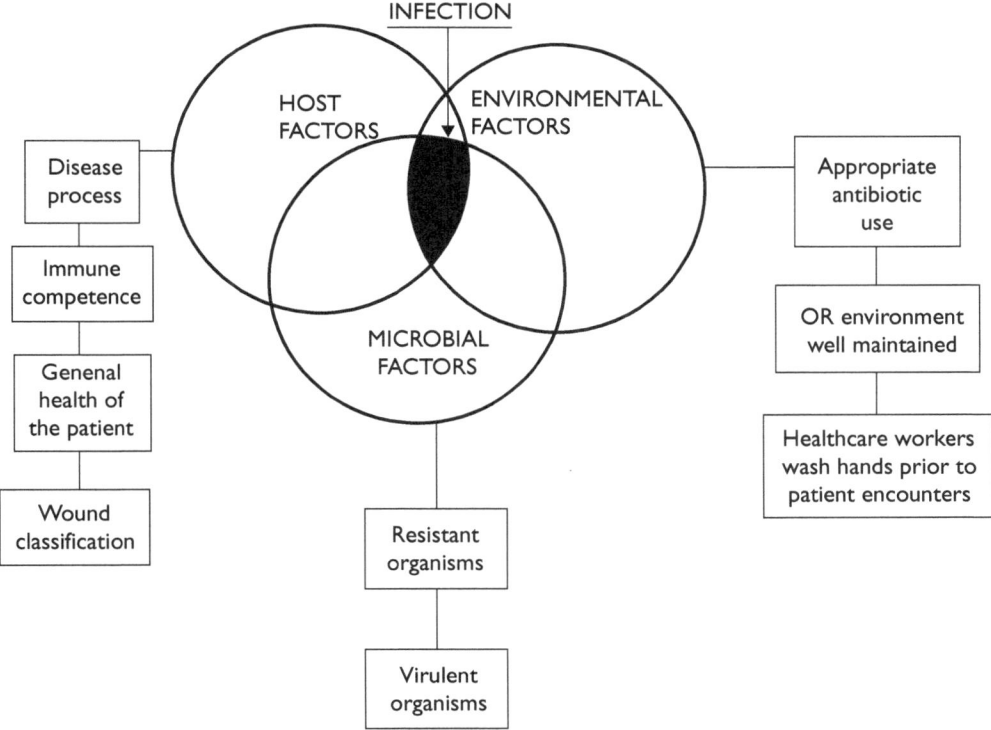

Algorithm 6.1. The risk factors for developing a wound infection: the susceptibility of the host, the virulence of the invasive bacteria, and the environmental conditions in which the wound is made.

ated carefully. The wound needs to be assessed with respect to the **post-operative signs of sepsis, specifically, fever, elevated white blood count, wound erythema, and wound tenderness.** An early diagnosis of a postoperative infection can minimize its impact on the speed of recuperation. Delay in the diagnosis and management of an infection can result in devastating, if not life-threatening, complications.

Preoperative Antibiotics

The second half of the 20th century ushered in the "antibiotics era." Since the introduction of antibiotics, **it increasingly has become evident that most operative infections are caused by bacteria from the patient's own body that reach the wound at the time of the surgery. Consequently, for antibiotics to work effectively, they have to be "on board" at the time of this inoculation in order to prevent the infection.** The risk that any postoperative wound will get infected is based on the complexity and duration of the operation. Since clean operations do not violate bacterial-bearing organs, the infection rate is very low. A wound classification system was devised in the 1970s that identifies the infection risk following surgery. **Table 6.1** shows the

Table 6.1. Choice of antibiotics by wound classification.

Wound classification	Approximate infection rate	Indications	Drug of choice
Clean	1%	Foreign-body implantation Coronary bypass Peripheral vascular	Cefazolin 1–2 g IV

Clean-contaminated	5–8%	Gastroduodenal
		  Perforated
		  Obstructed
		  Bleeding
			Cefazolin 1–2 g IV

		Biliary tract
		  >70 years old
		  Acute cholecystitis
		  Obstructive jaundice
		  Common duct stones
		  Nonfunctioning
		    gallbladder
			Cefazolin 1–2 g IV

		Colorectal	Neo/erythro (PO) or cefotetan 1–2 g IV
		Genitourinary	Ciprofloxacin 400 mg IV
		Ob-Gyn	Cefotetan 1–2 g IV
Contaminated	15%	Penetrating abdominal trauma Accidental spillage during elective surgery	Cefotetan 1–2 g IV
Dirty	50%	Drainage of an abscess	Dependent on site and likely etiology of infection

wound classification, specific indications for antibiotic therapy, and the recommended drug of choice.

Clean Cases

Prophylactic antibiotics generally are not recommended for those patients having clean operative procedures, since the minimal benefit that might result is equivalent to the risk of a side effect from the antibiotic. The routine use of antibiotics in operative procedures in which there is no identifiable benefit, such as breast biopsies, is not advised. Antibiotics are given only in operations that require the implantation of a foreign body, such as an orthopedic device, prosthetic mesh, or a vascular graft. Therefore, antibiotics are not recommended routinely in clean cases.

Several factors affect on the patient's **risks for postoperative surgical infection.** Many of the following factors are based on a wound surveillance protocol that was initiated by Peter Cruse in the early 1970s[1]: **age of the patient, nutritional status, diabetes, smoking, obesity,**

---

[1] Cruse, PJ, Foord R. A five-year prospective study of 23,649 surgical wounds. Arch Surg 1973;107:206–210.

existing infections, colonization of the wound of the skin with microorganisms, length of preoperative stay of the patient, and altered immune status. In **Case 1**, the patient has an elevated white blood count (WBC) and serum bilirubin indications that the gallbladder contains an active bacterial infection. These factors have been identified by multivariant or univariant analysis as increasing the risk of a wound infection. However, these risk factors are not necessarily independent predictors of a wound infection, which means that, by definition, a longer operative time involves more dissection, more blood loss, more dead space, and, therefore, a number of other factors that may increase the risk of a wound infection. Recent prospective studies indicate that the use of blood transfusions increases the risk of a wound sepsis by severalfold. Diabetes frequently is seen in patients who are overweight and elderly. Therefore, all three factors (age, obesity, and diabetes) may be dependent on one another. **Table 6.2** summarizes the evidence-based guidelines for the prevention of surgical site infection.

The emergence of vancomycin-resistant enterococcus (VRE) in the early 1990s has led to national guidelines recommending the restricted use of this antimicrobial agent in an attempt to minimize the emergence of resistant strains. In patients undergoing open-heart surgery, vancomycin should be used only when the incidence of methicillin-resistant *Staphylococcus aureus* (MRSA) as a cause of postoperative wound infections is in the range of 15% to 20%. With this exception, and in penicillin-allergic patients, vancomycin should not be used for antibiotic prophylaxis.

Clean-Contaminated Cases

Since clean-contaminated surgery, which is defined as an operation in which a hollow viscus is opened in planned surgery, has a higher infection risk than clean surgery, prophylactic antibiotics are advised in most situations. As with antibiotic prophylaxis in clean operations, the critical features for antibiotic use in clean-contaminated surgery are short duration, correct dosing-time interval, narrow spectrum of activity with equivalent safety, and a good safety profile. While studies consistently show that clinical practice patterns favor the use of postoperative antibiotics, no scientific data have shown an advantage to prolonged therapy of prophylactic antibiotics after surgery. A second dose of antibiotics may be given in surgery when the operation lasts over 4 hours or when significant blood loss has occurred.

Examples of clean-contaminated operations include surgery of the stomach, gallbladder, small intestine, colon, and uncomplicated appendicitis. In each situation, preoperative preparation of the patient and consideration of their condition might entail a different approach. For example, when performing a cholecystectomy on a patient with known gallstones who has had a single attack in the several weeks prior to surgery, the surgeon does not need to administer prophylactic antibiotics, especially since this operation is amenable to a laparoscopic procedure. The wounds are small and are unlikely to become contaminated and result in a wound infection. However, for patients who have

Table 6.2. Summary of evidence-based guidelines for the prevention of surgical site infection (wound infection).[a]

Preparation of the patient

Level I:
  Identify and treat all infections remote to the surgical site before elective operations. Postpone elective operations until the infection has resolved.
  Do not remove hair preoperatively unless hair at or near the incision site will interfere with surgery. If hair is removed, it should be removed immediately beforehand, preferably with electric clippers.

Level II:
  Control the blood glucose concentration in all diabetic patients.
  Encourage abstinence from tobacco for a minimum of 30 days before surgery.
  Indicated blood transfusions should not be withheld as a means to prevent surgical site infection.
  Patients should shower or bathe with an antiseptic agent at least the night before surgery.
  Wash and clean the incision site before antiseptic skin preparation.

Hand/forearm antisepsis

Level II:
  Keep nails short.
  Scrub the hands and forearms up to the elbows for at least 2–5 min with an appropriate antiseptic.

Antimicrobial prophylaxis

Level I:
  Administer antibiotic prophylaxis only when indicated.
  Administer the initial dose intravenously, timed such that a bactericidal concentration of the drug is established in serum and tissues when the incision is made. Maintain therapeutic levels of the agent in serum and tissues for the duration of the operation. Levels should be maintained only until, at most, a few hours after the incision is closed.
  Before elective colon operations, additionally prepare the colon mechanically with enemas or cathartic agents. Administer nonabsorbable oral antimicrobial agents in divided doses on the day before surgery.
  For high-risk cesarean section, administer the prophylactic antibiotic agent immediately after the umbilical cord is clamped.

Level II:
  Do not use vancomycin routinely for surgical prophylaxis.

Surgical attire and drapes

Level II:
  A surgical mask should be worn to cover fully the mouth and nose for the duration of the operation, or while sterile instruments are exposed.
  A cap or hood should be worn to cover fully hair on the head and face.
  Wear sterile gloves after donning a sterile gown.
  Do not wear shoe covers for the prevention of surgical site infection.
  Use surgical gowns and drapes that are effective barriers when wet.
  Change scrub suits that are visibly soiled or contaminated by blood or other potentially infectious materials.

Asepsis and surgical technique

Level I:
  Adhere to principles of asepsis when placing intravascular devices or when dispensing or administering intravenous drugs.

Level II:
  Handle tissue gently, maintain hemostasis, minimize devitalized or charred tissue and foreign bodies, and eradicate dead space at the surgical site.
  Use delayed primary skin closure or allow incisions to heal by secondary intention if the surgical site is contaminated or dirty.
  Use closed suction drains when drainage is necessary, placing the drain through a separate incision distant from the operative incision. Remove drains as soon as possible.

Postoperative incision care

Level II:
  A sterile dressing should be kept for 24–48 h postoperatively on an incision closed primarily. No recommendation is made regarding keeping a dressing on the wound beyond 48 h.
  Wash hands before and after dressing changes and any contact with the surgical site. Use sterile technique to change dressings.
  Educate the patient about surgical site infections, relevant symptoms and signs, and the need to report them if noted.

* Centers for Disease Control and Prevention, 1999; level III guidelines excluded.
Source: Adapted from Mangram AJ, Horan TC, Pearson ML, et al. Guideline for prevention of surgical site infection, 1999, with permission. Hospital Infection Control Practices Advisory Committee. Infect Control Hosp Epidemiol 1999;20:250–278. Reprinted from Barie PS. Perioperative management. In: Norton JA, Bollinger RR, Chang AE, et al, eds. Surgery: Basic Science and Clinical Evidence. New York: Springer-Verlag, 2001, with permission.

had a recent attack of cholecystitis, suspected cholangitis, or common duct stones, are elderly (>70 years of age), or have diabetes, prophylactic antibiotics are used. The patient presented in **Case 1** would benefit from prophylactic antibiotics based not only on the suspicion of common duct stones as evidenced by the elevated bilirubin, but also on the fact of the current attack of pain.

In the case of colon surgery, the bowel needs to be cleansed mechanically, and appropriate antibiotics need to be given either orally or intravenously (IV). It is controversial whether both intravenous and oral antibiotics should be given. Some evidence suggests that there is a slightly lower infection rate when antibiotics are given by both routes.

In urologic surgery, prophylactic antibiotics should be given when a urinary catheter is in place or if the urine is culture-positive. The drug of choice is ciprofloxacin, since it is well concentrated in the urine and covers the enteric gram-negative bacilli, which are the common pathogens. Culture results should direct appropriate prophylaxis if resistant organisms are identified. When performing a transrectal prostate biopsy, prophylaxis with antianaerobic coverage needs to be given. Similarly, head and neck surgery generally does not require prophylactic antibiotics unless the sinuses, nasal, oral, pharynx, or hypopharynx is entered.

In patients undergoing gastric surgery for an obstructive stomach, a bleeding ulcer, or gastric cancer, prophylactic antibiotics need to be considered carefully. Since gastric cancer is known to spread to contiguous organs, the possibility of a colon resection needs to be considered. Patients should have a mechanical bowel preparation with appropriate antibiotics prior to surgery. In addition, a patient with an obstructing gastric cancer would require antibiotic coverage of anaerobic and aerobic colonization of the stomach. When surgery is confined to the upper gastrointestinal tract for benign peptic ulcer disease, the patient would need antibiotics covering only the aerobic flora. It should be remembered that the stomach poses as a barrier to bacterial colonization of the small intestine, so that when gastric pH increases as a result of antacid therapy, bacterial overgrowth occurs. A single dose of prophylactic antibiotics to cover gram-negative and gram-positive flora is considered appropriate.

For surgery of the small intestine, such as for Crohn's disease or primary tumors of the small bowel, a single dose of an antibiotic to cover the gram-negative aerobes is appropriate. When the stomach or small intestine is obstructed, the flora changes dramatically so that 1 mL of small bowel contents contains the same density of aerobic and anaerobic bacteria as 1 mL of feces. Antibiotics, therefore, need to be altered appropriately to include coverage against anaerobes.

Contaminated Cases

The difference in the management of patients with contaminated abdominal wounds compared to patients with dirty wounds is that in contaminated wounds there is bacterial soilage even though there is no active infection. Because there is no established pathogen in the

wound, a short course of antibiotics is appropriate. For example, in a patient with a penetrating abdominal wound with injured bowel, a short course of antibiotics (two to three doses) is as effective as longer therapy. Evidence indicates that shortened administration of perioperative antibiotics reduces the infection rate without increasing the emergence of resistant organisms. In addition, a short course of antibiotics reduces the incidence of side effects from the antibiotics.

Dirty Cases

When pus is encountered during an intraabdominal operative procedure, prolonged antibiotic therapy is advised in order to contain the cellulitic component of the infectious process. Standard drug regimens are recommended for uncomplicated infections that arise outside of the hospital setting. Second-generation cephalosporins, cefoxitin, cefotetan, and ticarcillin-clavulinic acid are safe single-agent drugs that are extremely effective against most community-acquired infections. These agents all are derived from penicillin, and therefore carry the risk of an allergic reaction in patients who are allergic to penicillin.

If the patient has a history of a serious penicillin allergy or an immediate anaphylactic reaction, a combination of antibiotics may be used (**Table 6.3**). The disadvantage of some of these combinations is increased toxicity. The aminoglycosides are associated with renal and ototoxicity. Perhaps, more importantly, it has been recognized that this gentamicin has an altered volume of distribution and an altered half-life in the septic patient. This results in the likelihood of providing an inadequate dose of antibiotic to a septic patient, but still exposing the patient to the risk of a toxic side effect. One way to minimize these risks is to give the patient a single daily dose of gentamicin rather than three divided doses. The drug continues to be effective because of the phenomenon called the postantibiotic effect. The postantibiotic effect of a drug is realized when a drug continues to kill microbes even when measurable tissue levels are not present. If gentamicin is given once a

Table 6.3. Therapeutic antibiotics for abdominal sepsis.

Single agents
Cefoxitin
Cefotetan
Ticarcillin-clavulinic acid
Combinations
Ciprofloxicillan + metranidazole/(clindamycin)
Aztreonam + metranidazole/(clindamycin)
Gentamicin[a] + metronidazole/(clindamycin)

[a] May also use amikacin or tobramycin.
Source: Adapted from Bohnen JMA, Solomkin JS, Dellinger EP, Bjornson HS, Page CP. Guidelines for clinical care: anti-infective agents for intraabdominal infections. Arch Surg 1992;127:83. Copyright © 1992, American Medical Association. All rights reserved.

day, then the renal function of the patient must be normal (normal creatinine). The combination of ciprofloxacin with flagyl, an antianaerobe, also is a combination therapy for penicillin-allergic patients and has the advantage of efficacy with low toxicity. Aztreonam plus flagyl is another recommended combination for penicillin-allergic patients. Aztreonam has a cross-reactivity with penicillin because it is derived from the penicillin molecule, and therefore it should not be prescribed for someone with an anaphylactic reaction to penicillin.

The decision to terminate antibiotics is a critical one. Antibiotic therapy should not be ordered for a prescribed period of time, such as 7, 10, or 14 days. Two separate studies showed that the return of gastrointestinal function, the defervescence of fever, and the return of a white count to normal value all were deemed good evidence for the termination of antibiotics. When these criteria are not met, the risk of recurrent infection was 40%, while the infection rates were less than 3% if these criteria were met.

The use of antibiotic cultures in the face of intraabdominal pus recently has been questioned. Evidence indicates that surgeons are not inclined to adjust antibiotic therapy based on culture reports, especially if the patient is doing well. However, the intraperitoneal culture report is invaluable when an unusual pathogen is encountered, such as *Pseudomonas aeruginosa*, requiring specific antibiotic therapy.

Conduct in the Operating Room

Shoe Covers, Caps, Masks, Gowns, and Gloves

Operating room (OR) conduct combines procedures that are ritualistic, with no scientific basis, and activities that have been studied extensively and are of paramount importance in preventing transmission of infection in the operating field (Case 2). The use of shoe covers is a ritual from the era of flammable anesthetic gases. Because a spark from static electricity potentially could cause an explosion, specially designed nonconductive shoes that did not conduct an electric current were made for operating room personnel. For the visitor without special nonconductive shoes, shoe covers were available. Ether and cyclopropane especially were inflammable. Occasional explosions in the operating room were devastating events. By the mid-1970s, while explosive anesthetic agents were a thing of the past, shoe covers remained part of the accoutrements of the surgeon, along with caps and masks. However, current evidence suggests that the use of shoe covers actually may enhance the transmission of bacteria from the soles of one's shoes to the surgical wound. This is likely to occur especially if one does not wash one's hands after putting on the shoe covers.

With respect to barrier precaution, the use of cap, gown, mask, and OR gloves by the operating staff in the operating room to cover areas of their body that harbor a high density of potentially pathogenic bacteria is of paramount importance. However, data indicating the degree to which these barriers fail, resulting in infection, are seriously lacking. For example, the failure of gloves in the OR has been documented; however, their failure has never been coordinated with the risk of postoperative infection, even though it has been estimated that a glove failure results in inoculation of 10^5 organisms per glove failure. This may have to do with the relative differences of bacterial density in different parts of the body. The scalp hair and face, especially around the nares, are areas of high bacterial density; bacteria easily can contaminate the wound, resulting in a wound infection. Adequate coverage of these areas is imperative to prevent infection in the surgical environment.

Preoperative Shower

Over the past 20 years, there has been a revolution in the access of patients to the surgical environment. In 1980, 90% of surgical patients came to the hospital the day before surgery. Currently, 80% to 90% of patients stay at home the night prior to surgery. The preoperative management of these patients with respect to bathing, out of necessity, has been reevaluated. **While a routine preoperative shower was standard in the 1970s, there is little evidence to indicate that this makes a difference in a patient's risk of wound infection postoperatively.**

Remote-Site Infection and Shaving

The presence of a remote-site infection, whether it is a pustule, an upper respiratory infection, or urinary tract infection, needs to be identified and treated prior to any surgical intervention. Similarly, the routine shave of the operating field done either in the OR immediately prior to surgery or the night before is not recommended. A patient whose surgical site has been shaved has an infection rate two to three times higher than patients who are not shaved. The reason for this increased risk of postoperative infection is based on numerous prospective trials, as well as on scanning electron microscopy showing small injuries to the skin of experimental animal models. These injuries show heavy bacterial colonization and inflammatory cells. The need for shaving a surgical site should be considered not for sanitary reasons but only for the convenience of the patient's wound care.

Hand Washing

With respect to the surgeon's handwashing, 30 years ago a 10-minute wash was considered the standard. However, **increasingly shorter washes have been recommended by both the American College of Surgeons and the Centers for Disease Control. An initial wash of 5 minutes before the first surgery of the day is considered the standard, with subsequent preps of 2 minutes or less.** One of the reasons for these decreasing skin prep times is the recognition that the soaps are harmful to the surgeon's skin; a surgeon with a chronic skin condition can be a greater risk to the patient with respect to postoperative infection than the duration of the skin prep. Three types of soaps currently are used: an iodophor-based soap, one with chlorhexidine and one with hexachlorophene (**Table 6.4**). Alcohol-based skin preps, which are

Table 6.4. Mechanism of action of the agents effective against both
G+ and G– organisms.

Agent	Mode of action	Antifungal activity	Comments
Chlorhexidine	Cell wall distruction	Fair	Poor against tuberculosis/toxicity (eye/ear)
Iodine/iodophor	Oxidation	Good	Broad spectrum/I absorption skin irritation
Alcohols	Denaturation of protein	Good	Rapid action/short duration/flammable

being used in Europe and have just been introduced in the U.S., offer
the advantage that they require only topical application to clean skin,
resulting in shorter skin prep times and less toxicity than soaps. In all
of these considerations, **it is important to recognize that the greater
source of infection and contamination is the nail beds of the surgeon
and the grossly evident contamination on the skin and arms.**

Core Body Temperature

A recent, carefully controlled series of experiments clearly showed that
**the presence of the cold environment in the operating room reduces
the patient's core body temperature. This reduction in the patient's
core temperature significantly increases the risk of postoperative
infection.** This requires meticulous attention to keeping the patient
warm while in the operating room and not allowing the patient to come
into the OR and remain there for long periods of time prior to the initiation of surgery.

Postoperative Care

Causes of Postoperative Fever

**Postoperative fever is an important parameter to monitor after
surgery since it can indicate that the patient has a serious postoperative infection.** A temperature is abnormal if it is one degree
Fahrenheit or one half of a degree centigrade above the normal core
temperature. Depending on the patient population studied, the incidence of a postoperative fever in surgical patients may range from 15%
to 75%. The decision of whether or not to evaluate a patient with expensive blood and radiographic tests needs to be made in the context of
whether or not these tests are likely to yield helpful results. Since half
of postoperative fevers do not have an infectious etiology, the timing,
duration, and clinical setting of a fever are important clues in indicating whether or not further tests are necessary.

 **A postoperative fever occurring in the first 2 days after surgery is
very unlikely to have an infectious cause.** After general anesthesia,

pulmonary atelectasis causes activation of the pulmonary alveolar macrophage, resulting in endogenous pyrogen release. Early postoperative fever is believed to be due to this cytokine release. **If, however, a fever occurs after postoperative day 3 or persists for more than 5 days, there is a high likelihood that an underlying infection is the cause.** In this setting, before subjecting the patient to a battery of expensive laboratory tests, a careful clinical evaluation needs to be done to look for a wound infection. The most common nosocomial infections are urinary tract infections (UTIs), wound infections, and pneumonia. The clinical setting is important, since most nosocomial UTIs follow instrumentation of the urinary tract. Similarly, nosocomial pneumonias frequently follow prolonged endotracheal intubation.

Surgical Wound Management and Surgical Wound Infection Care

What is the **correct definition of a surgical wound infection?** The rigid **criterion of pus from a wound is only one sign of wound sepsis.** The Centers for Disease Control and Prevention (CDC) expanded the definition in 1992 to include **additional criteria.**[2] **Organisms isolated aseptically from a wound, pain and tenderness, localized swelling, and redness in a wound that is deliberately opened by a surgeon all meet the criteria of a surgical site infection (Case 3). In addition, the diagnosis of a superficial wound infection by the surgeon or attending physician meets the CDC criteria for a surgical site infection. Consequently, the intention to treat a wound with antibiotics meets the criteria of a wound infection.**

Postoperative management of a wound is dictated by the wound classification. A dirty wound, in which pus was encountered at the time of surgery, is left open to prevent a wound infection. While there is no prospective randomized trial to support this approach, the incidence of a wound infection is at least 50%. By leaving the wound open and letting it heal by secondary intent (allowing it to granulate in) or by delayed primary closure (pulling the wound closed with sutures placed but not tied in the operating room or by Steri-Strips), the risk of a wound infection significantly is reduced. Since a wound closed by delayed primary closure still has a risk of becoming infected, diligent wound surveillance is required by the surgeon. This approach is not applied universally to all surgical patients. In the pediatric population, wound approximation by delayed primary closure or by secondary intent generally is not done because of the very minimal amount of subcutaneous tissue and because the mechanics of local wound care are difficult in the pediatric age group. In this case, a loosely closed wound or a wound closed over a drain may help reduce a postoperative wound infection.

---

[2] Horan TC, Gaynes RP, Martore WJ, Jarvis WR, Emori G. CDC definitions of nosocomial surgical site infections, 1992: a modification of CDC definition of surgical wound infections. Infect Control Hosp Epidemiol 1992;13:606.

If the wound results from a clean or clean-contaminated surgery, a sterile dressing is applied for the first 24 to 48 hours. After this time period, once the wound has sealed, the risk of bacterial invasion from the external environment is eliminated, and the use of a dressing is optional. When the **postoperative signs of sepsis (fever, elevated white blood count, tachycardia)** occur in the presence of a swollen and tender wound, the possibility of a wound infection needs to be considered. If the wound is only erythematous in the early postoperative period, then a trial of antibiotics is reasonable until the erythema subsides. A clinical response should be seen within 24 to 48 hours. If the patient fails to respond, the wound must be explored. Some of the stitches should be removed at the site of the most erythematous area of the wound, and, if pus is encountered, the wound should be opened further and packed with gauze.

While a postoperative infection is a nuisance and, in the past, has been associated with high costs if treated in the hospital, the more serious consequence of postoperative wound sepsis is a necrotizing soft tissue infection. Finding gas on a roentgenogram in the soft tissues or crepitance on physical exam is a sign of necrotizing infection. **Necrotizing fasciitis and clostridial myonecrosis are two terms for life-threatening infections that frequently result from neglected wounds.** While these infections are rare and not subject to extensive clinical or laboratory study, it is believed that these infections are part of a continuum of a septic wound. It is clear that a clostridial infection requires an inoculum of a clostridia species, an anaerobic environment, and muscle necrosis. The term **necrotizing fasciitis** is defined more poorly, but similarly requires an anaerobic environment. Whether tissue necrosis occurs depends on the extent of the infection and the host's ability to resist. Mortality has been related to several medical risk factors, including diabetes mellitus, hypertension, and peripheral vascular disease.

Necrotizing soft tissue infections can arise outside of the hospital setting. Trivial infections in a partially compromised host may result in a serious infection. Retrospective reviews indicate that in up to half of patients with these infections, there is no identifiable cause. In some cases, a chronic wound suddenly becomes the source of a devastating infection. Illicit drug use with infected needles has been a frequent cause in hospitals located in high drug abuse areas. Fournier's gangrene is an infection initially described in the male perineum in the 1890s. The cause initially was due to a perineal soft tissue infection originating from chronic gonococcal urethritis. Since gonorrhea has become an infrequent infection with the advent of antibiotics, other causes more commonly trigger this infection. Neglected perirectal abscess or neglected hydradenitis suppurativa are currently the more common causes and can occur in women as well as men.

Aggressive surgical debridement is the mainstay of therapy in patients with necrotizing infections, with antibiotics serving as an important adjunct to therapy. Because the wounds are anaerobic, opening them to the air and removing necrotic tissue destroys the bacteria's ability to proliferate. The use of hyperbaric oxygen has been advocated, with some evidence indicating its efficacy. The risk of middle ear damage and decompression sickness make its practical use ineffective.

Drains

Drains are a very controversial issue with regard to infection. A recent study evaluating their effectiveness in draining elective colon resections shows no increased risk of infection or other complications with a drain as opposed to without one. Additionally, however, there is no clear advantage to placing a drain as opposed to not placing it. Routine use of drainage after axillary dissection has been subjected to prospective randomized trial. Again, no distinct advantage with respect to infection could be seen with the presence or absence of drains. The presence of drains resulted in fewer postoperative visits and a greater subjective evaluation of postoperative pain. In general, the use of drains should be restricted to those situations in which there is a specific indication, and the duration of drainage should be determined and limited as much as possible.

Antibiotic Therapy

Prior to the 1940s, the only antibiotic agents available were the **sulfonamide drugs**. These antibiotics are the prototype antimetabolite; their mechanism of action is inhibiting the production of microbial folic acid. The fact that they were not microbicidal and they were not effective against common gram-positive species led to the need for the development of more potent antibiotics with a broader spectrum.

Penicillin initially was administered to a British policeman, and, subsequently, in the United States, it was given to a deathly ill woman with postpartum puerperal sepsis. The miraculous survival of these patients as a result of this natural antibiotic derived from *Penicillium notatum* and discovered accidentally by Sir Alexander Fleming, gave rise to an entire class of **B-lactam** antibiotics (**Table 6.5**). These antibacterial agents are related to penicillin by the presence of the active chemical component, the B-lactam ring. This structure kills the bacteria by the competitive binding of the enzymes, known as penicillin binding proteins, responsible for the transpeptidation and transglycosylation process during cell wall polymerization. This step is critical to the integrity of the cell wall.

Bacterial resistance to penicillin began to be reported in the 1950s, necessitating the development of chemically altered derivatives of the original molecule. Methicillin was developed in an effort to effect therapy for bacteria resistant to penicillin. This antibiotic subsequently has become known for identifying a class of bacteria that is resistant to methicillin, methicillin-resistant *Staphylococcus aureus* (MRSA).

Major side chains added to certain B-lactam–derived antibiotics altered the effectiveness and spectrum of activity of the penicillin molecule. By adding the side chains, such as clavulanate, sulbactam, or tazobactam, B-lactamase, an enzyme secreted by bacteria resistant to the penicillin molecule, may be inhibited.

The **cephalosporins** are related to the penicillin molecule by the presence of the B-lactam ring, but they were derived from a naturally occurring fungus that, like penicillin, was discovered accidentally. This molecule has given rise to a large group of drugs that have been subclassified as first-generation, second-generation, or third-generation cephalosporin. These agents, as they increase in their evolution from the first generation, lose their gram-positive efficacy and increase their effectiveness against gram-negative agents, so that cefazolin, a first-generation agent, has good gram-positive coverage, cefoxitin, a second-generation cephalosporin, has good gram-negative coverage and moderate gram-positive coverage, and ceftriaxone, a third-generation cephalosporin, has excellent gram-negative coverage but very poor gram-positive effectiveness.

The major antibiotic in the **glycopeptide** group is **vancomycin**, an antibiotic that, like the B-lactam agents, inhibits cell wall synthesis. Vancomycin disrupts cell wall synthesis through a different mechanism from the B-lactam antibiotics. The recent emergence of resistant strains of MRSA to vancomycin has led to the development of a new glycopeptide, **teicoplanin**, an agent with less renal toxicity and longer dosing intervals than vancomycin.

Quinupristine-dalfopristine is a new drug in the **streptogramin** class of agents that works by inhibiting protein synthesis. Similar to the glycopeptides, it is active against gram-positive organisms and was developed to treat resistant strains of staphylococcal species.

The **macrolide antibiotics**, such as erythromycin, inhibit protein synthesis by reversible binding to the 50S ribosomal subunit. Azithromycin and clarithromycin are broader spectrum agents with anaerobic efficacy especially good for penicillin-allergic patients. Clindamycin and chloramphenicol are unrelated structurally but have a similar mechanism of action as the macrolides. Because the mechanism of action involves reversible binding, these agents are not bactericidal but bacteriostatic.

The **aminoglycosides**, similar to the macrolide antibiotics, bind to the ribosomal subunit, but, unlike macrolide antibiotics, this binding is not reversible. Consequently, these agents are bactericidal. While the aminoglycosides were the only effective antibiotic for the Enterobacteriaceae in the 1970s, their renal and ototoxicity, combined with estimating appropriate dosing regimen, have made them unacceptable as a first-line agent for gram-negative infections.

Quinolones target the DNA synthesis by binding to one of the bacteria's DNA synthetase enzymes. They are effective primarily against gram-negative aerobes, but they also are effective against gram-positive organisms. Their usefulness is enhanced because therapeutic drug tissue levels may be achieved with oral administration as well as with the intravenous route.

Metronidazole, like the quinolones, impairs microbial growth by blocking DNA synthesis. Although its spectrum of activity is limited to the gram-negative anaerobes, it is highly effective against this group of microbes. It is well absorbed orally so that parenterally and enterally administered drugs both result in therapeutic levels in the serum.

Table 6.5. Activity of selected antimicrobial agents.[a]

	Streptococcus pyrogenes	Staphylococcus aureus	Staphylococcus epidermidis
β-Lactam agents			
Penicillins			
Penicillin G	+++++	+	+
Methicillin	+++++	++	+
Ticarcillin	+++	++	+
Ampicillin	++	+	+
Penicillin agent + β-lactamase inhibitors			
Piperacillin	+	+	—
Ampicillin-sulbactam	++	++	+
Ticarcillin-clavulanate	+++	++	+
Piperacillin-tazobactam	+	+	—
First-generation cephalosporins	+++	++++	++
Second-generation cephalosporins[b]	++	++	++
Cefoxitin	++	++	++
Cefaperazone	++	++	++
Third-generation cephalosporins[b]	±	±	—
Cefotaxime	+	±	—
Cefotetan	+	+	—
Ceftazadime	+	+	—
Ceftriaxone	+	+	—
Fourth-generation cephalosporin			
Cefapime	±	±	—
Aztreonam			
Carabapenems	++	+	+
Vancomycin	+++++	+++++	+++++
Quinupristine-dalfopristine	++++	++++	++++
Erythromycin	++++	++	++
Aminoglycosides	+	+	+
Quinolones[b]	V	V	V
Naladixic acid	—	—	—
Norfloxacin	—	—	—
Ciprofloxacin	+	—	—
Moxifloxacin	+	+	+
Trimethoprim-sulfamethoxazole	—	—	—
Clindamycin	+++	++	+
Metronidazole	—	—	—

[a] +++++ indicates maximal activity; — indicates none.
[b] V indicates variability within the group, as denoted by the difference in activity among specific agents for certain types of organisms. *Source*: from Dunn DL. Diagnosis and Treatment of Infection. In: Norton JA, Bollinger RR, Chang AE, et al, eds. Surgery: Basic Science and Clinical Evidence. New York: Springer-Verlag, 2001, with permission.

Summary

Prevention of a surgical infection requires a thorough understanding of the three component parts (factors) that may contribute to a post-operative infection: the host, the environment, and the bacteria (see **Algorithm 6.1**). The severity and likelihood of an infection are dependent on the relative balance of these three factors. Since most infections come from the patient's own body, knowing the infectious risk of an operation, using the appropriate antibiotics, and conducting a timely and efficient surgery are the most significant factors in preventing a postoperative infection. The success of treating an established infection

Table 6.5. *Continued*

Enterococcus fecalis	Enterococcus fecium	Escherichia coli	Pseudomonas aeruginosa	Anaerobes
+	+	—	—	—
+	+	—	—	—
++	++	++	++	—
+++	+++	+	—	—
+++	+++	+++	++++	+
+++	+++	++	++	++++
++	++	++	++	++++
+++	+++	++++	++++	++++
—	—	—	—	—
—	—	+++	++	V
—	—	+++	++	+++
—	—	+++	++	—
—	—	+++++	V	V
—	—	+++++	++	—
—	—	++++	+	+++
—	—	+++++	+++++	—
—	—	+++++	++	++++
—	—	+++++	++++	—
+	+	+++++	++++	++++
++++	++++	—	—	—
—	++++	—	—	—
+	+	—	—	++
++	+	+++++	++++	—
V	V	V	V	V
—	—	++	+	—
—	—	+++	++	—
++	++	++++	++++	—
++	++	++++	++++	+++
—	—	++++	++	—
++	++	—	—	++++
—	—	—	—	+++++

Source: Reprinted from Dunn DL. Diagnosis and treatment of infection. In: Norton JA, Bollinger RR, Chang AE, et al, eds. Surgery: Basic Science and Clinical Evidence. New York: Springer-Verlag, 2001, with permission.

requires an understanding of both the microbes involved and the spectrum of antibiotics to treat these microbes. Finally, the operating room environment may compromise the patient's ability to resist infection in a variety of ways. The patient's internal milieu is exposed to bacteria where the natural host defense mechanism is not effective. Keeping the patient's core body temperature in a normal range is a significant factor in preventing infection. Finally, understanding the nature and types of resistant organisms present in the specific hospital, how they are spread, and what antibiotics are recommended to treat these organisms are important both for preventing the dissemination of these organisms and for curing the patient.

Selected Readings

Aly R, Maibach HI. Comparative antibacterial efficacy of a 2-minute surgical scrub with chlorhexidine gluconate, povidone-iodine, and chloroxylenol sponge-brushes. Am J Infect Control 1988;16:173–177.

Ayliffe GA. Role of the environment of the operating suite in surgical wound infection. Rev Infect Dis 1991;13(suppl 10):S800–804.

Ayliffe GA, Noy MF, Babb JR, Davies JG, Jackson J. A comparison of preoperative bathing with chlorhexidine-detergent and non-medicated soap in the prevention of wound infection. J Hosp Infect 1983;4:237–244.

Barie PS. Perioperative management. In: Norton JA, Bollinger RR, Chang AE, et al., eds. Surgery: Basic Science and Clinical Evidence. New York: Springer-Verlag, 2001.

Bohnen JMA, Solomkin JS, Dellinger EP, Bjornson HS, Page CP. Guidelines for clinical care: antiinfective agents for intraabdominal infections. Arch Surg 1992;127:83.

Centers for Disease Control and Prevention. National Nosocomial Infections Surveillance (NNIS) report, data summary from October 1986–April 1997, issued May 1997. Am J Infect Control 1997;25:477–487.

Condon RE, Bartlett JG, Greenlee H, et al. Efficacy of oral and systemic antibiotic prophylaxis in colorectal operations. Arch Surg 1983;118:496–502.

Cruse PJ, Foord R. A five-year prospective study of 23,649 surgical wounds. Arch Surg 1973;107:206–210.

Deshmukh N, Kramer JW, Kjellberg SI. A comparison of 5-minute povidone-iodine scrub and 1-minute povidone-iodine scrub followed by alcohol foam. Milit Med 1998;163:145–147.

Dineen P, Drusin L. Epidemics of postoperative wound infections associated with hair carriers. Lancet 1973;2(7839):1157–1159.

Dougherty SH, Simmons RL. The biology and practice of surgical drains. Part 11. Curr Prob Surg 1992;29(9):635–730.

Dunn DL. Diagnosis and treatment of infection. In Norton JA, Bollinger RR, Chang AE, et al., eds. Surgery: Basic Science and Clinical Evidence. New York: Springer-Verlag, 2001.

Ford CR, Peterson DE, Mitchell CR. An appraisal of the role of surgical face masks. Am J Surg 1967;113:787–790.

Hambraeus A. Aerobiology in the operating room—a review. J Hosp Infect 1988;11(suppl A):68–76.

Horan TC, Gaynes RP, Martone WJ, Jarvis WR, Emori G. CDC definitions of nosocomial surgical site infections, 1992: a modification of CDC definition of surgical wound infections. Infect Control Hosp Epidemiol 1992;13:606.

Humphreys H, Marshall RJ, Ricketts VE, Russell AJ, Reeves DS. Theatre over-shoes do not reduce operating theatre floor bacterial counts. J Hosp Infect 1991;17:117–23.

Jensen LS, Kissmeyer-Nielsen P, Wolff B, Qvist N. Randomized comparison of leucocyte-depleted versus buffy-coat-poor blood transfusion and complications after colorectal surgery. Lancet 1996;348:841–845.

Jonsson K, Hunt TK, Mathes SJ. Oxygen as an isolated variable influences resistance to infection. Ann Surg 1988;208: 783–787.

Kaiser AB, Kernodle DS, Barg NL, Petracek MR. Influence of preoperative showers on staphylococcal skin colonization: a comparative trial of antiseptic skin cleansers. Ann Thorac Surg 1988;45:35–38.

Krizek TJ, Robson MC. Evolution of quantitative bacteriology in wound management. Am J Surg 1975;130:579–584.

Lennard ES, Hargiss CO, Schoenknecht FD. Postoperative wound infection surveillance by use of bacterial contamination categories. Am J Infect Control 1985;13:147–153.

Mangram AJ, Horan TC, Pearson ML, et al. Guideline for prevention of surgical site infection, 1999. Hospital Infection Control Prectices Advisory Committee. Infect Control Hosp Epidemiol 1999;20:250–278. Reprinted from Barie PS. Perioperative Management. In Norton JA, Bollinger RR, Chang AE, et al., eds. Surgery: Basic Science and Clinical Evidence. New York: Springer-Verlag, 2001.

Nichols RL, Smith JW, Robertson GD, et al. Prospective alterations in therapy for penetrating abdominal trauma. Arch Surg 1993;128:55–64.

Page CP, Bohnen JM, Fletcher JR, McManus AT, Solomkin JS, Wittmann DH. Antimicrobial prophylaxis for surgical wounds. Guidelines for clinical care. Arch Surg 1993;128(l):79–88.

Pitt HA, Postier RG, MacGowan AW, et al. Prophylactic antibiotics in vascular surgery. Topical, systemic, or both? Ann Surg 1980;192:356–364.

Rotter ML, Larsen SO, Cooke EM, et al. A comparison of the effects of preoperative whole-body bathing with detergent alone and with detergent containing chlorhexidine gluconate on the frequency of wound infections after clean surgery. The European Working Party on Control of Hospital Infections. J Hosp Infect 1988;11:310–320.

Seropian R, Reynolds BM. Wound infections after preoperative depilatory versus razor preparation. Am J Surg 1971;121:251–254.

Sessler DI, McGuire J, Hynson J, Moayeri A, Heier T. Thermoregulatory vasoconstriction during isoflurane anesthesia minimally decreases cutaneous heat loss. Anesthesiology 1992;76:670–675.

Sharma LK, Sharma PK. Postoperative wound infection in a pediatric surgical service. J Pediatr Surg 1986;21:889–891.

Vamvakas EC, Carven JH, Hibberd PL. Blood transfusion and infection after colorectal cancer surgery. Transfusion 1996;36:1000–1008.

7

Shock

Carla Braxton and J. Martin Perez

Objectives

1. **To define shock and differentiate the signs, symptoms, and hemodynamic features of hemorrhagic, cardiogenic, neurogenic, and septic shock.**
2. **To discuss priorities and specific points of resuscitation for each form of shock.**

Cases

Case 1

A 70-year-old male unrestrained driver in a single-car crash presents to the emergency department via paramedics. The paramedics report that the steering column was broken. The patient complains of head, neck, shoulder, and back pain with some chest discomfort. On physical exam, a moderate-sized bruise is noted over his sternum. His oxygen saturation is 89% on room air; his blood pressure is 110/60; his heart rate is 100. In the emergency department, the nurse notes that his blood pressure has decreased to 80/40 mm Hg, that his heart rate has increased to 120, and that he appears pale and anxious.

Case 2

A 24-year-old man arrives in the emergency department complaining of abdominal pain. He had noted the pain approximately 1 week ago, but he was not evaluated because the discomfort had been suppressed with over-the-counter analgesics he was taking for a toothache. On exam, he has a palpable, tender right lower quadrant mass. His temperature is 103°F; his heart rate is 115; his blood pressure is 100/60. His white blood cell count is 25,000 with 17% bands. After computed tomography (CT)-guided drainage of his appendiceal abscess, he improves until postoperative day 5, when he is noted to have a blood pressure of 80/50, a heart rate of 130, oliguria, increased respiratory rate to 35, and a change in mental status. Despite 3 L of 0.9% normal saline intravenous fluid (IVF) resuscitation, hypotension and tachycardia persist.

Introduction

Shock, by definition, is a clinical syndrome that develops due to inadequate tissue perfusion. Hypoperfusion results in insufficient delivery of oxygen and nutrients for metabolism, leading to severe vital organ dysfunction. **Organ dysfunction, combined with the body's sympathetic and neuroendocrine response to oxygen and nutrient deficiency, characterizes the shock state.** Several classification profiles have been proposed to categorize shock syndromes. **It should be emphasized that these categories of shock are not absolute, and significant overlap may be observed.** Traumatic shock, for example, may include components of each of the other primary categories. Septic shock often demonstrates hypovolemia, myocardial depression, and distributive abnormalities.

This chapter discusses the various types of shock: definitions, the diagnostic workups, and management.

Types of Shock

Hypovolemic Shock (see Algorithm 7.1)

Hypovolemia is the most common cause of shock, and hemorrhage is the most common cause of hypovolemic shock. Table 7.1 presents the physical findings in hemorrhagic shock by class of hemorrhage. Class I hemorrhage represents a loss of 10% to 15% of the blood volume and results in a minimal change in the patient's vital signs. A patient with class II hemorrhage (15–30% blood volume loss) manifests tachycardia, a decreased pulse pressure, and delayed capillary refill. The patient may be mildly anxious and have decreased urine output. Larger volume losses result in the classic presentation of hemorrhagic shock. Class III (30–40% blood volume loss) hemorrhage presents with hypotension, tachycardia, tachypnea, and mental confusion progressing to lethargy. Greater than 40% blood volume loss (>2000 mL in a 70-kg patient, class IV) presents with obtundation, profound hypotension, and anuria. Compensated hemorrhagic shock (class I and II) may progress rapidly to class IV (**Case 1**), especially in the pediatric population. In **Case 1**, the initial vital signs are normal at the scene of the accident. However, rapid transition to class IV shock is evident upon arrival at the emergency department. Recognition of the early stages of shock and appropriate early intervention are the keys to management.

Other important etiologies of hypovolemic shock are losses via the gastrointestinal or urinary tracts and extravascular fluid sequestration or "third space" fluid loss. Ongoing fluid losses through these routes may not be diagnosed as readily as is hemorrhage, and, therefore they require a higher index of suspicion. For example, severely

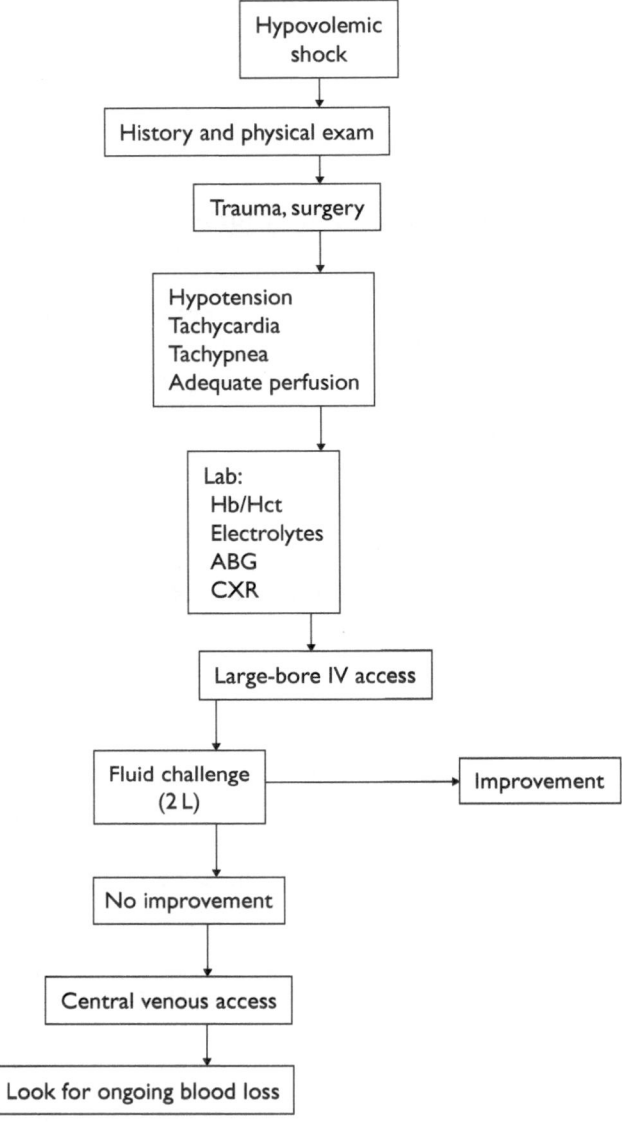

Algorithm 7.1. Algorithm for treating hypovolemic shock. ABG, arterial blood gas; CXR, chest x-ray.

burned patients require large-volume fluid replacement due to extravascular sequestration or "third space" fluid loss. Subsequent burn wound infections in such a patient could result in septic shock, adding to the complexity of management in these patients. Furthermore, a component of inhalation injury likely would add to further resuscitative fluid requirements. Processes such as peritonitis commonly lead to large-volume retroperitoneal or intraabdominal fluid sequestration. In **Case 2**, peritonitis secondary to perforated appendicitis with abscess formation leads to intraabdominal fluid sequestration, and, despite aggressive fluid resuscitation, shock persists. Septic shock, a form of severe sepsis, is evident when an infectious source is confirmed or suspected, coupled with hypoperfusion despite adequate volume resuscitation. The treatment of septic shock involves adequate fluid resuscitation, point source control of the infectious source (such as drainage of appendicial abscess in **Case 2**), and other supportive measures, such as nutritional support, ventilation, and renal replacement.

Shock following traumatic injury frequently combines aspects of several shock categories. Hypovolemia due to hemorrhage combined with tissue injury and/or bone fractures evokes a potentially more destructive proinflammatory response than hypovolemia alone. Neurogenic shock may compound a spinal cord injury. Cardiogenic shock may accompany traumatic cardiac injury, tension pneumothorax, pericardial tamponade, or myocardial contusion. **There are multiple contributors to the systemic inflammatory reaction stimulated by tissue injury. Devitalized tissue, bacterial contamination, ischemia-reperfusion injury, and hemorrhage act together to place the traumatized patient at risk for hypermetabolism, multiorgan dysfunction, and death. Therefore, the treatment of traumatic shock is aimed at quickly diagnosing the areas of injury, controlling hemorrhage, restoring circulating intravascular volume, preventing hypoxia, and limiting the extent of secondary damage introduced by inflammation and infection.** In **Case 1**, the progression to class IV shock may be due to several etiologies, including direct hemorrhagic sources, such as a ruptured spleen or liver with intraabdominal blood loss. **Exclusion of intraabdominal sources of hemorrhage must be done expeditiously because such injuries require immediate surgical treatment in the operating room.** Further sources of hemorrhage include aortic injury with hemorrhage into the chest cavity. A

Table 7.1. Physical findings in hemorrhagic shock.[a]

	Class I	Class II	Class III	Class IV
Blood loss (mL)	<750	750–1500	1500–2000	>2000
Blood loss	Up to 15%	15–30%	30–40%	>40%
Pulse rate	<100	>100	>120	>140
Blood pressure	Normal	Normal	Decreased	Decreased
Pulse pressure (mm Hg)	Normal	Decreased	Decreased	Decreased
Respiratory rate	14–20	20–30	30–40	>35
Urine output (mL/h)	>30	20–30	5–15	Negligible
CNS/mental status	Slightly anxious	Mildly anxious	Anxious, confused	Confused, lethargic

[a] Alcohol or drugs (e.g., β-blockers) may alter physical signs.
Source: Adapted from American College of Surgeons. Shock. In: Advanced Trauma Life Support Manual. Chicago: American College of Surgeons, 1997:87–107, with permission. Reprinted from Nathens AB, Maier RV. Shock and resuscitation. In: Norton JA, Bollinger RR, Chang AE, et al, eds. Surgery: Basic Science and Clinical Evidence. New York: Springer-Verlag, 2001, with permission.

nonhemorrhagic source in this patient could be a myocardial contusion with subsequent impairment of cardiac output resulting in cardiogenic shock. This may be diagnosed by echocardiography and treated with supportive measures such as inotropes.

Treatment of hypovolemic shock, regardless of the etiology, involves restoration of circulating blood volume and control of ongoing volume loss. In patients with clear evidence of shock, aggressive fluid resuscitation is of great importance. For hemorrhagic shock especially, caregivers should follow a systematic approach to resuscitation, including the airway, breathing, circulation, and disability assessment as outlined in the Advanced Trauma Life Support course. This approach may be both diagnostic and therapeutic and increases the likelihood of recognizing sources of hemorrhage.

Fluid resuscitation should be initiated with two large-bore (16 gauge or larger) catheters in the antecubital fossae and connected to the widest administration tubing available to allow for rapid volume infusion. The choice of route for vascular access (peripheral vs. central) is determined by the skill level of the practitioner and the availability of catheters required. Patient assessment for placement of intravenous catheters should take into consideration the location of fractures, open wounds, burns, and areas of potential vascular disruption. These areas should be avoided.

The choice of fluid for resuscitation begins with the most efficacious and cost effective. Rapid infusion (less than 15 minutes) of 2L of isotonic saline or a balanced salt solution should restore adequate intravascular volume. If blood pressure and heart rate do not improve following this intervention, suspect hemorrhage in excess of 1500 cc or ongoing blood loss. Blood transfusion should follow, using O-positive or O-negative blood in the most critical circumstance or type-specific or fully crossmatched blood if time allows. As a general caveat, **no time should be wasted with crossmatching if the patient has a clear source of continuing hemorrhage and remains severely unstable despite crystalloid administration.**

As a conventional approach to fluid resuscitation, crystalloid and blood product infusions are standard for patients with hemorrhagic or hypovolemic shock. There are alternate solutions, however, that include hypertonic saline, several colloid formulations, and blood substitutes (**Fig. 7.1**). Hypertonic saline (7.5% NaCl) has been studied extensively in animal models and humans with hemorrhagic shock. The hypertonic component draws water out of the intracellular space into the extracellular space in a type of "autotransfusion." This may result in significant improvement in blood pressure and cardiac output. Some formulations add 6% dextran to hypertonic saline in order to increase intravascular oncotic pressure. The beneficial effects of hypertonic saline in improving survival have not been clearly apparent in human clinical trials, with the exception of the subset of patients in shock with traumatic brain injury. (For further discussion, see Chapter 15, "Shock and Resuscitation," by A. B. Nathens and R. V. Maier, in Surgery: Basic Science and Clinical Evidence, edited by J. A. Norton et al, published by Springer-Verlag, 2001.)

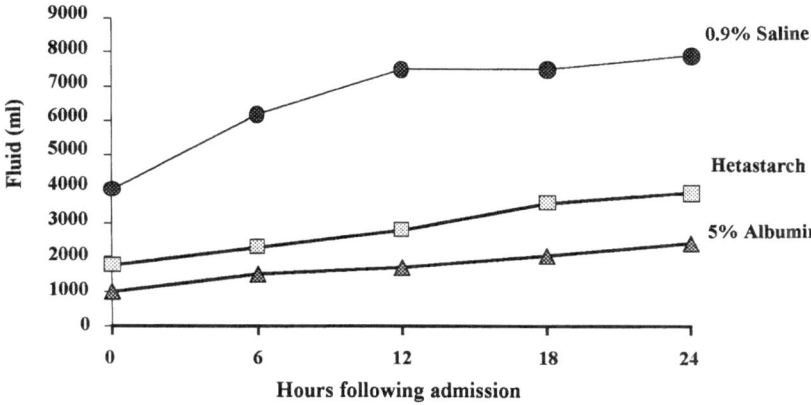

Figure 7.1. Total fluid requirements in patients with hypovolemic shock receiving either a synthetic colloid (hetastarch), 5% albumin, or 0.9% saline. Synthetic colloids have a far greater volume-expanding effect than crystalloid solutions, roughly equal to that of 5% albumin. LVEDP, left ventricular end-diastolic pressure. (Adapted from Rackow EC, Falk JL, Fein IA, et al. Fluid resuscitation in circulatory shock: a comparison of albumin, hetastarch and saline solutions in patients with hypovolemic and septic shock. Crit Care Med 1983;11:839–850. With the permission of Lippincott Williams & Wilkins. Reprinted from Nathens AB, Maier RV. Shock and resuscitation. In: Norton JA, Bollinger RR, Chang AE, et al, eds. Surgery: Basic Science and Clinical Evidence. New York: Springer-Verlag, 2001, with permission.)

The colloid versus crystalloid debate in fluid resuscitation recently has been addressed in two meta-analyses.[1] Although no single study clearly showed survival benefit in hypovolemic patients receiving crystalloid versus colloid, the meta-analyses concluded that patients resuscitated with colloid products (albumin, plasma protein products, synthetic colloids) have increased mortality. The mechanism by which albumin resuscitation leads to worse outcome has not been clarified. However, there is evidence to suggest that exogenous albumin may decrease sodium and water excretion, worsen renal failure, and impair pulmonary gas exchange.

Synthetic colloids, such as hetastarch (6% hydroxyethyl starch solution) and pentastarch, possess significant volume expansion capability. Hetastarch has a high average molecular weight and tends to remain within the intravascular space, where it can exert an oncotic effect that lasts up to 24 hours. Pentastarch has a lower average molecular weight than hetastarch, is more easily cleared in the plasma and excreted in the urine, and may cause fewer anaphylactic reactions than hetastarch. In addition, the oncotic effects of pentastarch last for approximately 12 hours and may require smaller volume infusions for similar effects on plasma expansion.

[1] Reviewers CIGA. Human albumin administration in critically ill patient: systemic review of randomized controlled trials. Br Med J 1998;317:235–240.

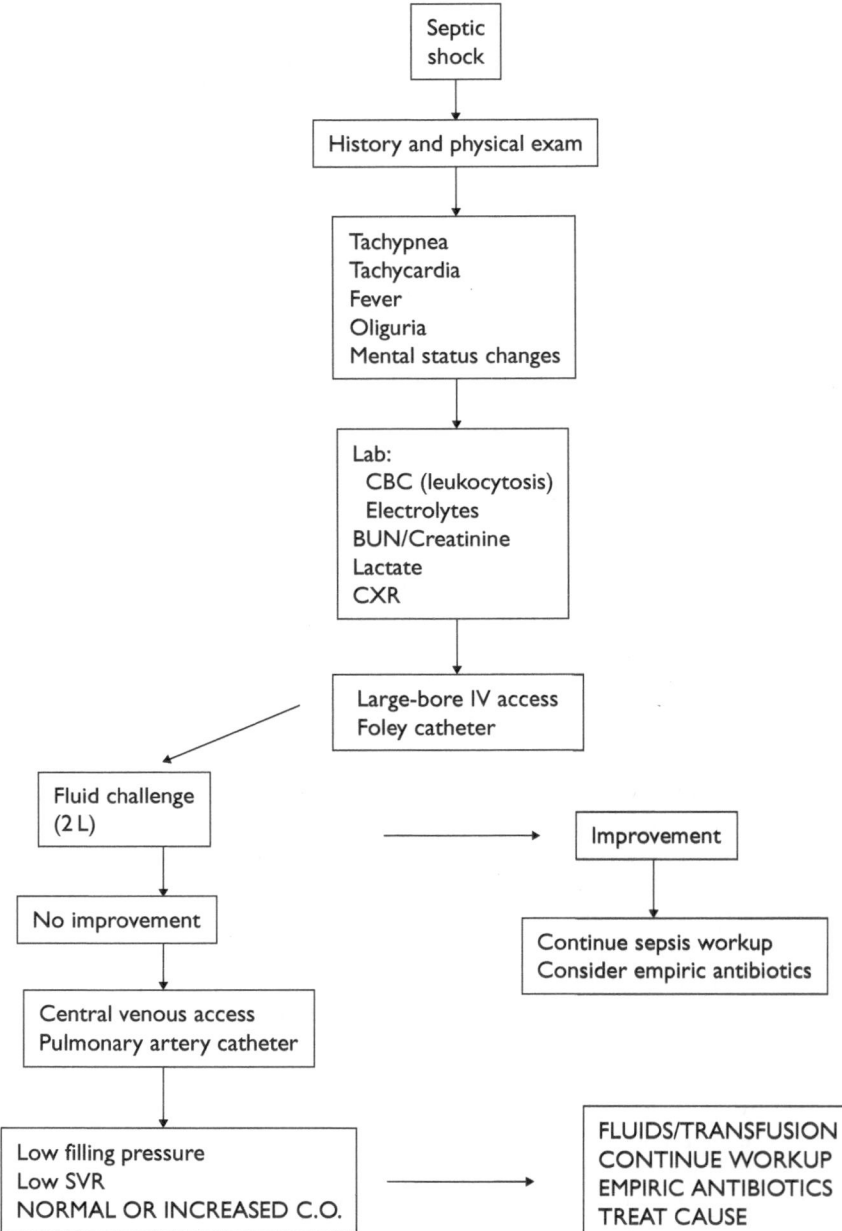

Algorithm 7.2. Algorithm for treating septic shock. SVR, systemic vascular resistance.

Septic Shock (see Algorithm 7.2)

Septic shock is the culmination of uncompensated local and systemic responses to microorganisms and their products. The resulting hypotension, hypoperfusion, and inflammation may lead to multi-system organ failure and death. Mortality rates for severe sepsis are between 20% and 50%, despite significant advances in diagnosis, antibiotic regimens, and critical care management. Bacteremia occurs in 40% to 60% of septic patients, and patients may be bacteremic without display of sepsis. Gram-positive, viral, fungal, and protozoal organisms may induce a septic response that previously was attributed only to gram-negative organisms. Bacterial products stimulate the release of proinflammatory cytokines from endothelial cells and macrophages. These mediators also contribute to the myocardial depression, vascular dilatation, hypercoagulability, impared fibrinolysis, and decreased oxygen utilization observed in severe sepsis. In **Case 2**, despite 3 L of IVF resuscitation, the patient remains hypotensive, tachycardic, and with evidence of impaired end-organ perfusion (oliguria and mental status changes). Persistent hypotension despite resuscitation could represent myocardial depression seen in sepsis, vasomotor dilatation due to inflammatory mediators, or the need for further fluid resuscitation if intravascular volume deficits were underestimated.

The symptoms of sepsis may present with varying degrees of severity. **Tachypnea, tachycardia, oliguria, and mental status changes are common clinical findings in early sepsis, often preceding fever and leukocytosis (Case 2). Laboratory findings of hyperbilirubinemia, lactic acidosis, coagulopathy, and increased serum creatinine signal hypoperfusion and end-organ ischemia. Septic decompensation is signaled by leukopenia, hypothermia, acute respiratory distress syndrome, and shock. Patients often require large-volume fluid resuscitation for hypotension due to systemic vasodilatation and increased microvascular permeability.** Vasopressor support is frequently necessary as an adjunct to volume infusion, but pressors should not be used in the place of fluid. The risk of organ damage secondary to the infusion of pressors without fluid outweighs the potential benefit of minimizing pulmonary edema by limiting volume resuscitation. For patients with renal or cardiac disease and for patients not responding to initial efforts at resuscitation, a pulmonary artery catheter may be useful to guide management.

Treatment of septic shock depends on eradication of the infectious focus as early as possible. Blood, urine, and sputum specimens should be sent for culture, along with fluid from any catheter drainage sites. Indwelling catheter sites should be examined, and catheters should be either removed or changed, as necessary. All surgical or traumatic wounds should be examined; all devitalized or infected tissue should be cultured and aggressively debrided. Computed tomography is an indispensable diagnostic tool if intraabdominal or intrathoracic infections are suspected. Abscess cavities should be percutaneously or surgically drained, whichever is appropriate. Surgical control of any ongoing contamination is mandatory. Empirical treatment with broad-spectrum antibiotics is required if the organism or site is unknown. Strong emphasis should be placed on the correct choice of antibiotic, as this has been shown to have a clinically significant impact on mortality reduction.[2] In **Case 2**, the patient has symptoms of sepsis. Given

---

[2] Leibovici L, Drucker M, et al. Septic shock in bacteremic patients: risk factors, features, and prognosis. Scand J Infect Dis 1997;29:71–75.

the prior history of appendiceal abscess drainage, recurrent intra-abdominal infection (recurrent abscess) is likely. However, blood-, urine-, sputum-, wound-, and catheter-related infection should be considered. A repeat CT scan of the abdomen would be the diagnostic modality to exclude recurrent intraabdominal abcess. Broad-spectrum antibiotics should be initiated pending the results of the diagnostic workup.

Cardiogenic Shock (see Algorithm 7.3)

Cardiogenic shock may be difficult, at least initially, to distinguish from hypovolemic shock. Both forms of shock are associated with decreased cardiac output and compensatory upregulation of the sympathetic response. Both entities also respond initially to fluid resuscitation. **The syndrome of cardiogenic shock is defined as the inability of the heart to deliver sufficient blood flow to meet metabolic demands. The etiology of cardiogenic shock may be intrinsic or extrinsic.** In **Case 1**, the development of class IV shock may be due to hemorrhage, such as an aortic injury, or may be cardiogenic, such as a myocardial contusion from blunt injury to the chest. Echocardiography would evaluate the possibility of intrinsic (infarction/contusion) or extrinsic (cardiac tamponade) myocardial dysfunction.

Intrinsic causes of cardiogenic shock include myocardial infarction, valvular disease, contusion from thoracic trauma, and arrhythmias. For patients with myocardial infarction, cardiogenic shock is associated with loss of greater than 40% of left ventricular myocardium. The normal physiologic compensation for cardiogenic shock actually results in progressively greater myocardial energy demand that, without intervention, results in the death of the patient (**Fig. 7.2**). A decrease in blood pressure activates an adrenergic response that leads to increased sympathetic tone, stimulates renin-angiotensin-aldosterone feedback, and potentiates antidiuretic hormone secretion. These mechanisms serve to increase vasomotor tone and retain salt and water. The resultant increase in systemic vascular resistance and in left ventricular end-diastolic pressure leads to increased myocardial oxygen demand in the face of decreased oxygen delivery. This, in turn, results in worsening left ventricular function, a perceived reduction in circulating blood volume, and repetition of the cycle.

Compressive cardiogenic shock occurs due to extrinsic pressure on the heart, which reduces diastolic filling, thereby impairing cardiac output. Pericardial tamponade, tension pneumothorax, diaphragmatic hernia, mediastinal hematoma, and excessive intraabdominal compartment pressure can lead to compressive (obstructive) cardiogenic shock. **Pericardial tamponade is signaled by jugular venous distention, muffled heart tones, and hypotension—Beck's triad.** Pulsus paradoxus, an inspiratory drop in systolic BP of, at least 10 mm Hg, may not be observed in patients on mechanical ventilation. Similarly, equalization of diastolic pressures may not be apparent when the right atrium is being compressed by clot. Both these scenarios complicate the diagnosis of tamponade in the post–cardiopulmonary bypass period.

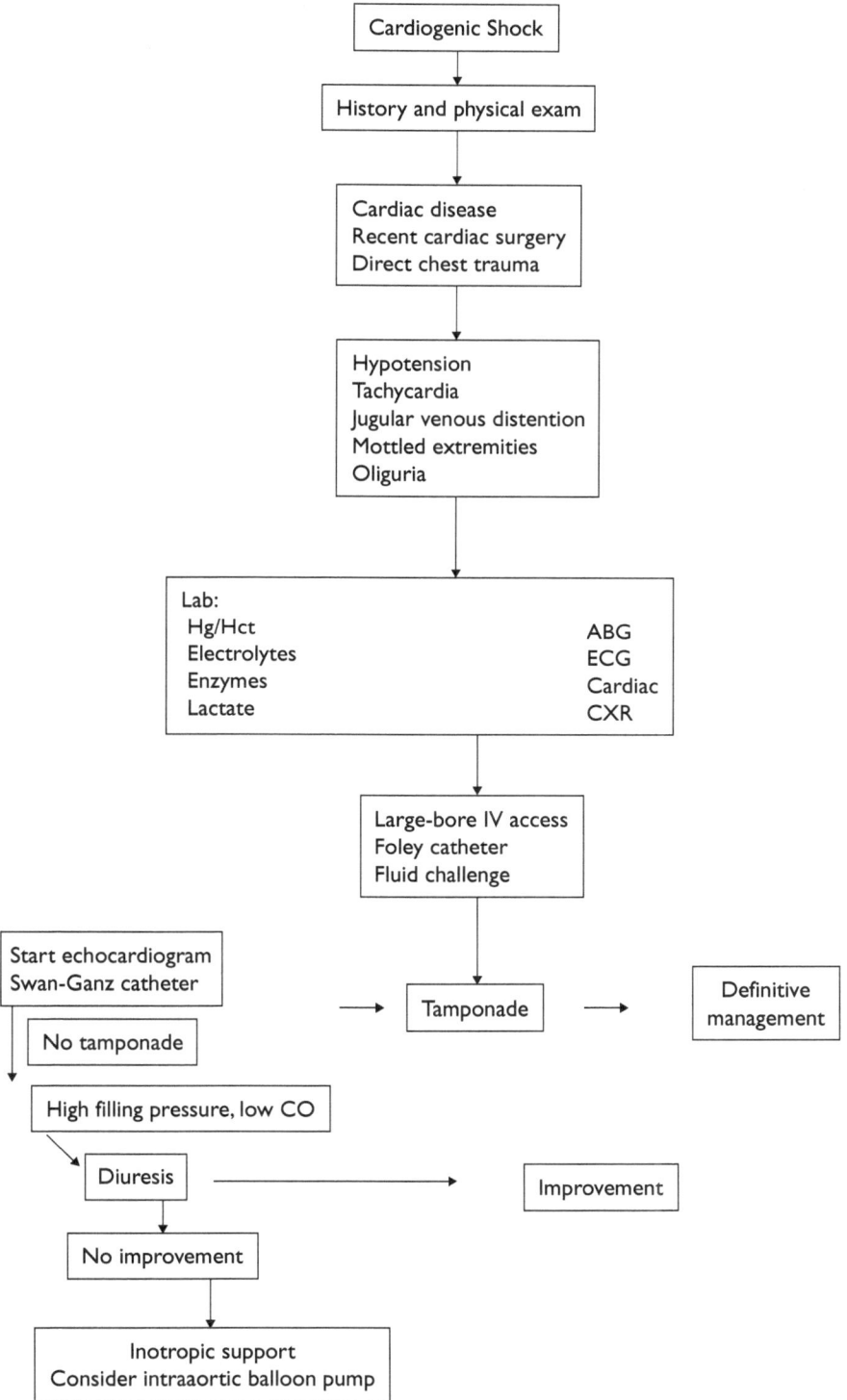

Algorithm 7.3. Algorithm for treating cardiogenic shock.

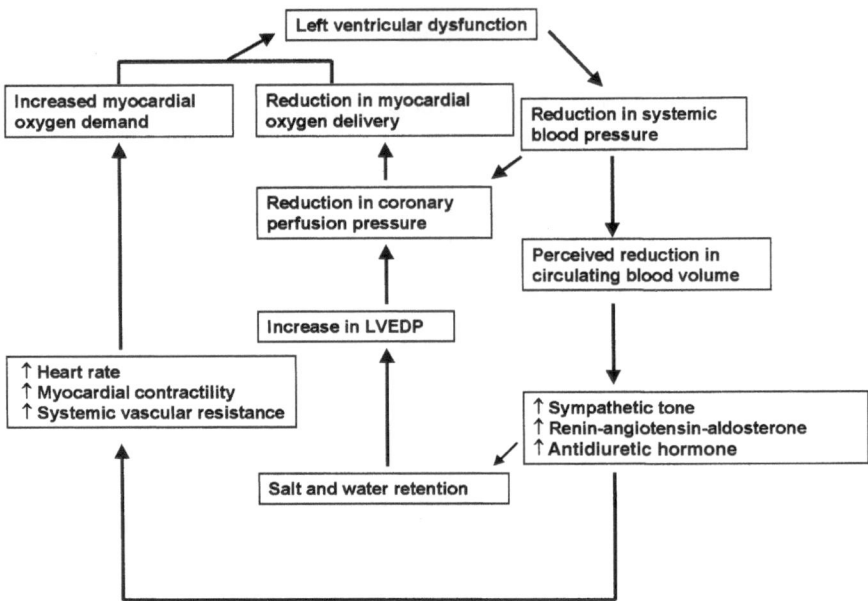

Figure 7.2. The reduction in cardiac output associated with left-ventricular dysfunction results in a series of compensatory responses that function to maintain blood pressure at the expense of aggravating any disparity in myocardial oxygen demand and supply. This imbalance increases left-ventricular dysfunction and sets up a vicious cycle. (Reprinted from Nathens AB, Maier RV. Shock and resuscitation. In: Norton JA, Bollinger RR, Chang AE, et al, eds. Surgery: Basic Science and Clinical Evidence. New York: Springer-Verlag, 2001, with permission.)

Diagnosing cardiogenic shock involves utilizing the physical exam to look for jugular venous distention, pulmonary edema, an S_3 gallop, and evidence of perfusion abnormalities. Clinical and laboratory data suggesting end-organ hypoperfusion include mottled extremities, lactic acidosis, elevation in blood urea nitrogen and creatinine, and oliguria. An immediate electrocardiogram should be obtained, and cardiac enzymes should be drawn to make the diagnosis of myocardial infarction. A chest x-ray gives information regarding the existence of pulmonary edema; arterial blood gas measurement helps determine oxygenation and acid–base status. Echocardiography is invaluable as a noninvasive method for determining ventricular function, wall motion abnormalities, valvular function, and the presence or absence of pericardial fluid. Pulmonary artery catheter placement is useful for ongoing measurement of cardiac function and to gauge the resuscitation.

The therapeutic objective in managing intrinsic cardiogenic shock is to perform general supportive measures (oxygenation/ventilation, electrolyte, and arrhythmia correction) while expediting a diagnostic workup. Intravenous fluid can improve perfusion in the hypovolemic patient. Vasodilators should be used with caution, as they may serve to reduce afterload in cardiogenic shock but also may exacerbate hypotension. Inotropes (dobutamine) or pressors (dopamine, norepinephrine) are required in the hemodynamically unstable following or concurrent with volume resuscitation. These medications are administered with the understanding that they also increase myocardial oxygen demand as contractility and systemic vascular resistance are increased. There is no evidence that survival is improved with the use of inotropes or pressors, which are considered only as temporizing measures until a definitive intervention can occur.

An important adjunct to therapy for patients with intrinsic cardiogenic shock is the use of the **intraaortic balloon pump (IABP)**. The IABP device is placed in the thoracic aorta via the femoral artery. It serves to decrease myocardial oxygen demand by augmenting diastolic pressure, improving coronary blood flow, and reducing afterload. The IABP is a means of temporary support for the failing heart while definitive measures are planned.

Treatment of extrinsic cardiogenic shock is directed at relief of the underlying cause: decompression of a tension pneumothorax, repair of a diaphragmatic hernia, evacuation of the mediastinal hematoma, or drainage of the pericardial effusion. Early, rapid diagnosis of the condition leading to compressive cardiogenic shock is imperative in order to decrease morbidity and mortality. Echocardiography is the most sensitive, rapidly available modality to demonstrate pericardial fluid and the need for surgical intervention. In the patient at risk for extrinsic cardiac compression, an echocardiogram should be requested early in the diagnostic workup.

Neurogenic Shock (see Algorithm 7.4)

Neurogenic shock must be differentiated from spinal shock. The former comprises a group of clinical features including bradycardia and hypotension following acute cervical or high thoracic spinal cord injury. The latter term, **spinal shock**, refers to loss of spinal cord reflexes below the level of cord injury. **Neurogenic shock occurs after acute spinal cord transection and is characterized by loss of sympathetic tone, leading to arterial and venous dilatation and hypotension.** Persistent, unopposed vagal tone results in severe bradycardia. The patient is generally warm and perfused. **In a patient who presents with spinal cord injury and concomitant hypotension, a bleeding source must be ruled out before the symptom complex can be attributed solely to neurologic sources.** Pressor support frequently is required in these patients. Continuous infusions of dopamine or epinephrine provide both α- and β-adrenergic support to counteract the bradycardia and hypotension.

Diagnostic and Therapeutic Adjuncts

Pulmonary Artery Catheter

If the cause of the shock state is unclear or if it is multifactorial, the use of a **pulmonary artery catheter (PAC) can be useful to help differen-**

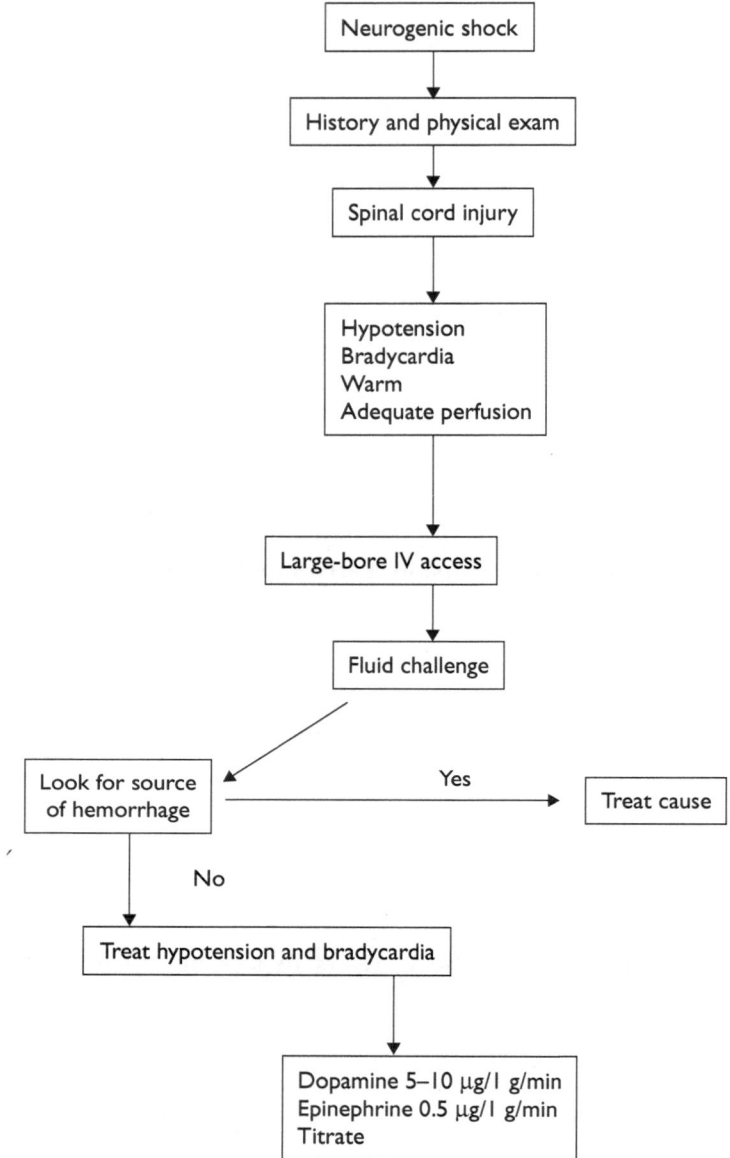

Algorithm 7.4. Algorithm for treating neurogenic shock.

tiate between etiologies and to guide resuscitation (Table 7.2).[3] The classic patient for pulmonary artery catheterization is in septic shock with myocardial depression and hypovolemia due to vasomotor dilatation and third-space fluid losses. In **Case 2**, aggressive fluid resuscitation has not corrected the hypotension and tachycardia likely due to severe sepsis. Placement of a pulmonary artery catheter may guide

[3] Parker M, Peruzzi W. Pulmonary artery catheters in sepsis/septic shock. New Horizons 1997;5(3):228–232.

Table 7.2. Differential diagnosis of shock states based on hemodynamic parameters.

Type of shock	CVP or PCWP	Cardiac output	Systemic vascular resistance	Venous O_2 saturation
Hypovolemic	↓	↓	↑	↓
Cardiogenic	↑	↓	↑	↓
Septic	↓↑	↑	↓	↑
Traumatic	↓	↓↑	↓↑	↓
Neurogenic	↓	↓	↓	↓
Hypoadrenal	↓↑	↓↑	↑↓	↓

CVP, central venous pressure; PCWP, pulmonary capillary wedge pressure.
Source: Reprinted from Nathens AB, Maier RV. Shock and resuscitation. In: Norton JA, Bollinger RR, Chang AE, et al, eds. Surgery: Basic Science and Clinical Evidence. New York: Springer-Verlag, 2001, with permission.

further fluid resuscitation if needed or guide the clinician toward other therapies, such as inotropic support. In this scenario, information gained from pulmonary artery catheterization can help guide the use of fluid, inotropes, and pressors.

Other patient groups have been shown to benefit from the use of the PAC. A frequently cited example is the traumatized elderly patient with multiple comorbidities who may have myocardial ischemia or dysfunction either preceding or secondary to the traumatic event. There is compelling evidence that the earlier invasive monitoring can be established in this high-risk patient population, the greater likelihood of improved functional outcome or reduction in morbidity.[4] Even young traumatized patients may have a complex clinical picture for which more information is required in order to direct the treatment plan.[5] Use of PACs in the critical care setting remains controversial, as there have been questions raised as to the indications for use of invasive monitoring,[6] and there have been many reports of associated complications. A meta-analysis of 16 randomized controlled trials of pulmonary artery catheterization found the greatest risk-reduction in surgical patients undergoing PAC-guided therapy.[7] Significant design flaws may have created limitations in the collection and analysis of the data in these studies; these flaws will need to be addressed in future trials using PACs. Established indications for use of invasive monitoring are summarized in **Table 7.3**.

[4] McMahon D, Schwab C, et al. Comorbidity and the elderly trauma patient. World J Surg 1996;20:1113–1120; Scalea T, Simon H, et al. Geriatric blunt multitrauma: improved survival with early invasive monitoring. J Trauma 1990;30(2):129–134.
[5] Abou-Khalil B, Scalea T, et al. Hemodynamic responses to shock in young trauma patients: the need for invasive monitoring. Crit Care Med 1994;22(4):633–639.
[6] Leibowitz A, Beilin Y. Pulmonary artery catheters and outcome in the perioperative period. New Horizons 1997;5(3):214–221.
[7] Ivanov R, Allen J, et al. Pulmonary artery catheterization: a narrative and systematic critique of randomized controlled trials and recommendations for the future. New Horizons 1997;5(3):268–276.

Table 7.3. Indications for invasive monitoring.*

Unresponsive hemodynamic instability
Elderly patient
Multiple-trauma patient
Suspicion of sepsis
Previous organ dysfunction
Cardiac
Pulmonary
Renal
Hypertensive
High-risk surgery
Use of high levels (10 cm H_2O) of peak end-
expiratory pressure (PEEP)

* Established indications for the use of arterial lines and Swan-Ganz pulmonary artery catheters. These criteria are met in approximately 15% of patients in a surgical ICU, indicating that most patients can be monitored with less invasive technology.
Source: Reprinted from Livingston D, Machiedo GW. Shock. In: Polk HC Jr, Gardner B, Stone HH, eds. Basic Surgery, 5th ed. St. Louis: Quality Medical Publishing, Inc. 1995, with permission.

Inotropes and Pressors

Under most circumstances of shock, optimal fluid resuscitation should precede the use of pharmacologic agents. Proper management of shock requires optimization of preload, afterload, and myocardial contractility. Inotropic and/or pressor support may be a necessary adjunct in the resuscitation of the patient in shock (**Table 7.4**).

Dopamine is a biosynthetic precursor of epinephrine that, at low doses (1–3 μg/kg/min), may increase renal blood flow, diuresis, and natriuresis. At higher doses (3–5 μg/kg/min), stimulation of cardiac beta receptors leads to increases in contractility, cardiac output, and, later (5–10 μg/kg/min), heart rate. Above 10 μg/kg/min, alpha activity, with peripheral vasoconstriction, is most prominent.

Dobutamine is a synthetic catecholamine whose predominant effect is to stimulate an increase in cardiac contractility with little increase in heart rate. β_2-receptor activation also leads to peripheral vasodilatation. This combination of attributes leads to improved left-ventricular emptying and a reduction in pulmonary capillary wedge pressure. In **Case 1**, hemorrhagic/hypovolemic shock is excluded, and echocardiography confirms ventricular dysfunction due to myocardial contusion. Dobutamine may be indicated to improve left ventricular function and improve blood pressure.

Epinephrine is both a strong β-adrenergic and an α-receptor stimulant. At lower infusion rates, beta responses lead to increased heart rate and contractility. At higher rates of infusion, alpha effects predominate, resulting in elevation of blood pressure and systemic vascular resistance. Use of epinephrine is limited by its arrhythmogenic properties and its capability to stimulate increased myocardial oxygen requirements.

Norepinephrine exerts both α- and β-adrenergic effects. Beta effects, stimulating myocardial contractility, occur at lower doses, while alpha

Table 7.4. Vasoactive drugs and receptor activities for the treatment of shock.

Class and drug	Blood pressure	Systemic vascular resistance	Cardiac output	Heart rate	Isotrope Low-dose	Isotrope High-dose	Renal blood flow	Coronary blood flow	MvO$_2$
Alpha only									
Phenylephrine	↑↑↑	↑↑↑	↓↓↓	↓↓↓	±	±	↓↓↓	±↑↑	↑
Alpha and beta									
Norepinephrine	↑↑	↑↑↑	↓↓	↓↓	↑	↑	↓↓↓	↑↑	↑↑
Epinephrine	↑±	↑±	↑↑	↑↑↑	↑↑	↑↑↑	↓±	↑↑	↑↑↑
Dopamine	↑↑	↑↑	↑↑	↑	±	↑↑	↑↑↑	↑↑	↑↑
Beta only									
Isoproterenol	↑±	↓↓	↑↑↑↑	↑↑↑↑	↑↑↑	↑↑↑↑	±	↑↑↑	↑↑↑↑
Dobutamine	↓↓	↓↓↓	↑↑↑	↑↑	↑↑↑	↑↑↑	±	↑↑↑	↑↑↑
Beta-blocker									
Propanolol	↑↓	±→	↓↓↓	↓↓↓↓	↓↓	↓↓↓	→	↓↓	↓↓↓
Metoprolol	↓↓↓	±→	↓↓	↓↓↓	↓↓	↓↓↓	±	↓↓	↓↓
Other									
Nitroglycerine	±↓	↓↓	±↑	±↑	±	±	±↑	→	↓↓
Hydralazine	↓↓↓	↓↓↓	↑↑	↑↑	±	±	±↑	→	↓↓↓
Prazosin	↓↓	↓↓↓	↑↑↑	±↑	±	±	±↑	→	↓↓↓
Nitroprusside	↓↓	↓↓↓		±↑	±	±	↑↑	±	↓↓

Source: Reprinted from Pettitt TW, Cobb JP. Critical care. In: Doherty GM, Bauman DS, Creswell LL, Goss JA, Lairmore TC, eds. The Washington Manual of Surgery. Philadelphia: Lippincott Williams & Wilkins, 1996. With permission from Lippincott Williams & Wilkins.

vasoconstrictor effects are noted at higher doses. Norepinephrine is becoming an earlier choice as a pressor agent used for septic shock, once adequate intravascular volume has been restored. In **Case 2**, despite adequate fluid resuscitation guided by pulmonary artery, broad-spectrum antibiotics, and surgical drainage of appendiceal abscess, the patient remains hypoperfused. Norepinephrine infusion could be initiated for persistent shock.

Multiorgan Dysfunction Syndrome

Shock is the most common precursor to multiorgan dysfunction syndrome (MODS), which is recognized as part of a continuum ranging from systemic inflammatory response syndrome (SIRS) to multiorgan dysfunction, culminating in multiple system organ failure (MSOF) and death. The process may occur with or without a known infectious source. Uncontrolled systemic inflammation plays a significant role in the development of MODS. Extensive microvascular endothelial damage leads to liberation of inflammatory mediators, with subsequent microvascular ischemia, increased permeability, decreased intravascular volume, and hypoperfusion. Without intervention, the process escalates to cause end-organ damage. Mortality ranges from 30% to 50% with single organ failure and increases to 80% with three-organ dysfunction. Mortality is nearly 100% with four dysfunctional organ systems.

Recently, **activated protein C** (Xigris, Eli Lilly) has been approved for the treatment of severe sepsis. It is the first agent to demonstrate a mortality reduction in patients with severe sepsis. Activated protein C modulates coagulation, fibrinolysis, and inflammation, thus reinstating homeostasis between the major processes driving sepsis. In certain patient populations, risk of bleeding is elevated, and careful attention to patient selection should be given.

There is no specific treatment for MODS. Therapy is directed toward minimizing any stimulus of ongoing infection, ischemia, necrosis, fracture, or other tissue injury. Supportive care includes ensuring adequate oxygenation, ensuring organ perfusion, and reducing the duration of shock. Monitoring the patient for response

Table 7.5. Criteria of adequate perfusion.

Normal mental status
Normal pulse rate (no beta-blockade)
Adequate urine output
Warm, pink skin
No core/extremity temperature gradient
Normal systemic vascular resistance
No lactic acidosis
Normal oxygen extraction ratio

Source: Reprinted from Livingston D, Machiedo GW. Shock. In: Polk HC Jr, Gardner B, Stone HH, eds. Basic Surgery, 5th ed. St. Louis: Quality Medical Publishing, Inc., 1995, with permission.

to intervention is a crucial part of management. Generally accepted criteria of adequate perfusion—end points of resuscitation—are summarized in **Table 7.5**.

Summary

Shock, by definition, is a clinical syndrome that develops due to inadequate tissue perfusion. Hypoperfusion results in insufficient delivery of oxygen and nutrients for metabolism, leading to severe vital organ dysfunction. Untreated or undertreated shock may result in multiple organ failure and death. Patients enter into the shock state due to hypovolemia, trauma, sepsis, cardiac dysfunction, or severe neurologic compromise. The physician's role in patient management is to ensure adequate hemodynamic support *first* (airway, breathing, circulation), followed by an aggressive search for the etiology of shock. With few exceptions, the first inotrope, the first pressor, should be *fluid*.

Selected Readings

Abou Khalil B, Scalea T, et al. Hemodynamic responses to shock in young trauma patients: the need for invasive monitoring. Crit Care Med 1994; 22(4):633–639.

Cobb J, Perren. Critical care: a system-oriented approach. In: Norton JA, Bollinger RR, Chang AE, et al, eds. Surgery: Basic Science and Clinical Evidence. New York: Springer-Verlag, 2001.

Ivanov R, Allen J, et al. Pumonary artery catheterization: narrative and systematic critique of randomized controlled trials and recommendations for the future. New Horizons 1997;5(3):268–276.

Leibovici L, Drucker M, et al. Septic shock in bacteremic patients: risk factors, features and prognosis. Scand J Infect Dis 1997;20:71–75.

Leibowitz A, Beilin Y. Pulmonary artery catheters and outcome in the perioperative period. New Horizons 1997;5(3):214–221.

McMahon D, Schwab C, et al. Comorbidity and the elderly trauma patient. World J Surg 1996;20:1113–1120.

Nathens AB, Maier RV. Shock and resuscitation. In: Norton JA, Bollinger RR, Chang AE, et al, eds. Surgery: Basic Science and Clinical Evidence. New York: Springer-Verlag, 2001.

Parker M, Peruzzi W. Pulmonary artery catheters in sepsis/septic shock. New Horizons 1997;5(3):228–232.

Reviewers CIGA. Human albumin administration in critically ill patient: systematic review of randomized controlled trials. Br Med J 1998;317:235–240.

Scalea T, Simon H, et al. Geriatric blunt multitrauma: improved survival with early invasive monitoring. J Trauma 1990;30(2):129–134.

8

Surgical Bleeding and Hemostasis

Gregory R. Brevetti, Lucy S. Brevetti, and Rocco G. Ciocca

Objectives

1. To describe the differential diagnosis:
   - To differentiate between surgical and nonsurgical causes of bleeding.
   - To describe the treatment options for both surgical and nonsurgical bleeding.
   - To identify the indications, risks, and benefits of blood product transfusions.
2. To describe factors that can lead to abnormal bleeding postoperatively and to discuss the prevention and management of postoperative bleeding:
   - Inherited and acquired factor deficiencies.
   - Disseminated intravascular coagulation (DIC), transfusion reactions.
   - Operative technique.
3. To discuss priorities [airway, breathing, circulation (ABC)] and goals of resuscitation:
   - To defend choice of fluids.
   - To discuss indications for transfusion.
   - To discuss management of acute coagulopathy.

Case

You are asked to evaluate a 70-year-old woman who has had a femoral-peroneal artery bypass with in-situ saphenous vein because of brisk bleeding from the incision. She is anxious and has a pulse of 109 and a blood pressure of 89/45 mm Hg.

Introduction

Coagulation relies on multiple interrelated steps. The process can be broken down into three main phases:

- Phase I (**vasoconstriction**): Vascular injury results in the constriction of vascular smooth muscle and the early decrease in local blood flow.
- Phase II (**platelet aggregation**): In the presence of disrupted endothelium, thromboplastin is released, which stimulates the adherence and aggregation of platelets to subendothelial tissue.
- Phase III (**coagulation cascade activation**): Although hemostasis may occur solely through vasoconstriction and platelet aggregation, the generation of thrombin through the coagulation cascade is critical in the formation of fibrin clot. Hemostasis and fibrin clot formation work through the intrinsic and/or extrinsic pathways. Both pathways lead to a common enzyme, factor Xa, that then is followed by the common pathway (**Fig. 8.1**).

When first evaluating a bleeding patient, two crucial questions must be addressed:

1. Is the patient hemodynamically stable?
2. Why is the patient bleeding and how can it be stopped?

Is the Patient Hemodynamically Stable?

Whether or not the patient is hemodynamically stable can be determined quickly by looking at the **patient's general appearance and by obtaining a set of vital signs**. In the case presented at the beginning of this chapter, hemodynamic instability (a heart rate of 109 and blood pressure of 89/45) is caused by hypovolemia, which can be corrected with intravenous fluids. Despite the simple treatment for hypovolemia, the initial evaluation always should begin with the **ABCs**. Assuring adequate ABCs provides stabilization and permits a full history and a physical examination, thereby allowing question 2 to be answered.

Airway

The patient's ability to maintain a patent airway should be evaluated, and rapid endotracheal intubation should be considered if the patient is unconscious or otherwise unable to maintain a clear airway. The patient in our case was "anxious," which also means conscious, probably communicative, and able to protect her airway.

Breathing

Adequate breathing should be confirmed by physical exam and pulse oximetry. Oxygen by nasal cannula, face mask, or endotracheal tube may be indicated.

Circulation

Heart rate and blood pressure are good indicators of circulatory volume. Loss of less than 15% of blood volume may result in no change in blood pressure or heart rate. Hemorrhage of 15% to 30% of blood volume results in a decreased pulse pressure and tachycardia. Loss of greater than 30% will result in a decrease in systolic pressure, reflex

Intrinsic Pathway   **Extrinsic Pathway**

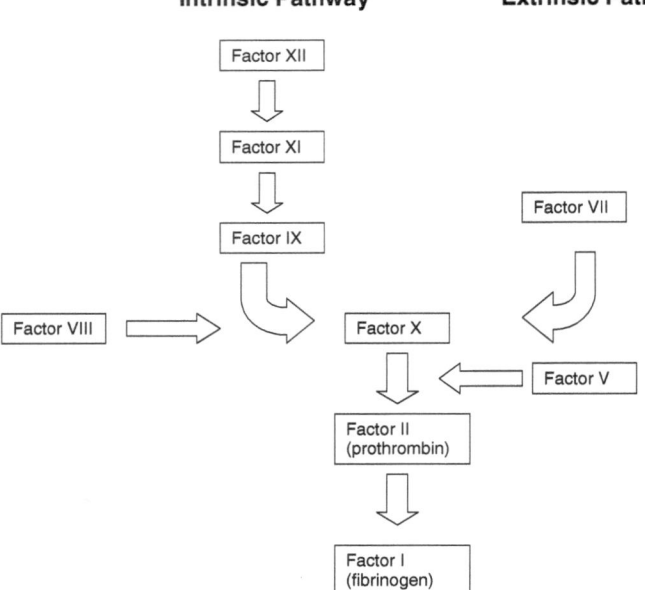

Figure 8.1. Critical steps in the coagulation cascade. The central pathway involves the activation of factors X to Xa and prothrombin to thrombin. In surgery, tissue factor (TF) generation is probably the initiating event, leading to Xa activation both through the intrinsic pathway (tenase complex) and by direct activation of X by the TR-VIIa complex. Subsequently, Xa assembles on the platelet phospholipid membrane to form the prothrombinase complex, which converts prothrombin to thrombin.

tachycardia, and possibly other signs of shock, such as acidosis, tachypnea, oliguria, and decreased sensorium. The patient in our case has lost over 30% of her blood volume. (In an average-sized woman, that would be over 1500 cc.)

If there is an obvious site of active bleeding, direct pressure is most helpful. Our patient has brisk bleeding coming from her incision. Direct digital pressure should provide temporary hemostasis, while the circulating volume can be restored easily with adequate intravenous access. The maximum rate of delivery is limited by the length and gauge of the intravenous (IV) catheter. Therefore, two large (18 gauge or larger) IVs in the antecubital veins are recommended. The antecubital veins are large and easily accessible when rapid access is needed.

Crystalloid, such as normal saline or lactated Ringer's, is indicated for the initial volume replacement. In adults, transfusion of blood products is indicated if signs of hypovolemic shock persist after approximately 2 L are infused (see Treatment, below). Laboratory tests also are done during this initial assessment (see Diagnostic Studies, below).

Why Is the Patient Bleeding and How Can It Be Stopped?

To address this question, **a complete history and a physical examination should be performed**. A few specific questions and diagnostic tests may help narrow the differential diagnosis and guide treatment. **Algorithm 8.1** addresses the emergency management of bleeding.

History

Review of Systems
Does the patient report any previous spontaneous bleeds (i.e., epistaxis) or easy bruising? Does the patient report bleeding during simple daily activities, such as brushing his/her teeth? These simple items may provide a clue to an underlying tendency to bleed.

Past Medical History
Is there a history of liver dysfunction, such as hepatitis or cirrhosis (with associated decrease in synthetic function and decrease in coagulation factors in the intrinsic pathway), **or a history of renal failure with its associated dysfunctional platelets**?

Medications
Multiple medications affect coagulation by a variety of mechanisms (Table 8.1). Many patients are unaware of the anticoagulant effect of some medications (i.e., nonsteroidal antiinflammatory drugs, NSAIDs, such as ibuprofen). The NSAIDs, including aspirin, irreversibly acetylate platelet cyclooxygenase, thus preventing the synthesis of thromboxane A_2. This effect is overcome only by new platelet synthesis over a period of 7 to 10 days.

Family History
Many coagulopathies are hereditary. Hemophilia A (factor VIII deficiency) and hemophilia B (factor IX deficiency or Christmas disease) are sex-linked recessive traits; other hereditary clotting abnormalities include factor I, V, VII, and X deficiencies and hereditary telangectasias (**Table 8.2**). Deficiencies of the various factors generally must be moderate to severe to affect clinically on bleeding.

Operative History
A complete understanding of what operation was performed and the technical details is critical in dealing with a postoperative bleeding problem. **Did the patient have adequate hemostasis at the time of surgery?** (This history should be obtained from the operating surgeon.) Diffuse microvascular bleeding and failure to form adequate clot is suggestive of an underlying clotting abnormality. Significant, bright red bleeding from a surgical wound might represent a suture line leak and require reexploration. Alternatively, if there were many adhesions that were divided at the time of surgery, these can be a source of postoperative bleeding. What medications or blood products did the patient receive while in the operating room? If the patient received large-volume transfusions with packed red cells, clotting factors and

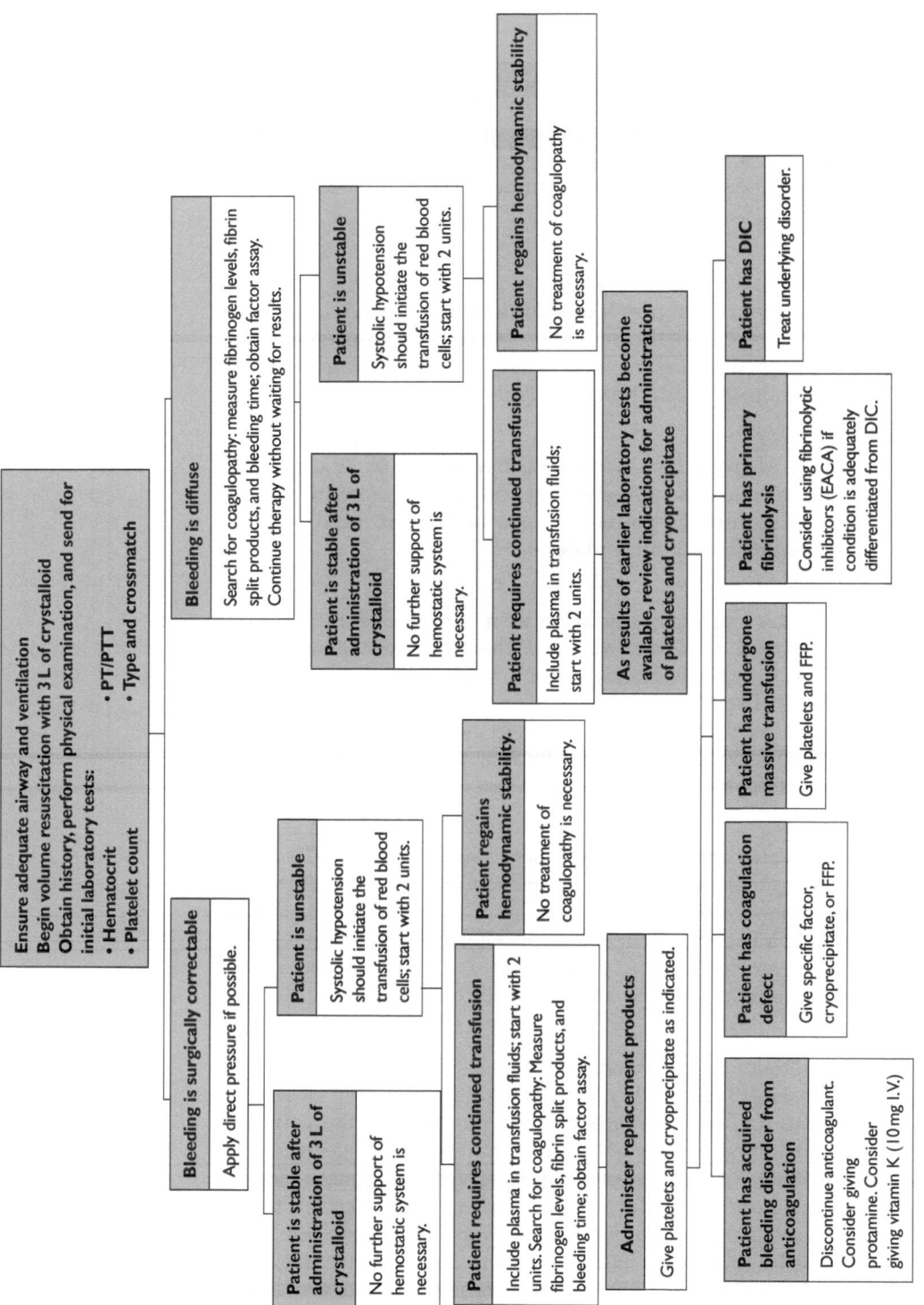

Algorithm 8.1. Algorithm for emergency management of bleeding.

Table 8.1. Alterations of hemostasis by common drugs.

Drug	Mode of action	Duration	Severity of effect
Warfarin	Inhibits synthesis of factors II, VII, IX, XI	5–7 days	Major
Heparin	Inhibits clotting factor activators; immune thrombocytopenia	4–6 hours	Major
		2–4 days	Variable
Aspirin	Blocks platelet secretion, aggregation	5–7 days	Major
Ticlopidine	Unknown	5–7 days	Major
Nonsteroidal antiinflammatory drugs	Blocks platelet section, aggregation	1–2 days	Moderate
Dipyridamole	Inhibits platelet aggregation	1–2 days	Mild
Dextran	Impairs platelet adhesion, aggregation	3–5 days	Moderate
Calcium channel blockers	Inhibits platelet aggregation (in large doses)	1 day	Mild
Vasodilators	Inhibits platelet aggregation	Short	Mild
Quinidine	Immune thrombocytopenia	2–4 days	Variable
Various antibiotics	Inhibits platelet aggregation	Few days	Variable

Source: Reprinted from Sobel M, Dyke CM. Hemorrhage and thrombotic complications of cardiac surgery. In: Baue AE, Glenn A, Geha AS, eds. Glenn's Thoracic and Cardiovascular Surgery. Stamford: Appleton and Lange, 1996, with permission.

platelets may be diluted. In addition, large-volume transfusions (over one blood volume, i.e., 5 L) may cause a patient to become calcium depleted. Citrate used to anticoagulate banked blood binds calcium, and calcium is necessary as a cofactor in multiple steps of both the intrinsic and extrinsic pathways (**Fig. 8.1**).

Physical Examination

Patients with abnormal bleeding often develop ecchymoses and hematomas at IV catheter or venipuncture sites. Bright red blood (well oxygenated) from the surgical incision suggests an arterial source. In the patient in our case, a leak from the anastomosis is possible. **If this does not resolve with local compression, reexploration may be indicated. Darker blood suggests venous bleeding or old hematoma.** Postoperative venous bleeding may cease with local compression. **Not all postoperative bleeding complications involve bleeding that is external. If bleeding is suspected, a complete physical exam may yield clues to occult bleeding.** However, in obese patients, soft tissues can mask a significant amount of bleeding. Furthermore, the chest, abdomen, pelvis, and retroperitoneum all may hold significant amounts of blood, with only subtle clues to the examining healthcare practitioner. If a thoracic operation was performed, the chest should be auscultated carefully and percussed for dullness, and the chest tube output should be inspected for quality (sanguinous vs. serosanguinous) and volume. If an abdominal operation was performed, abdominal pain, girth, and signs of flank ecchymosis should be evaluated.

Table 8.2. Hereditary hemorrhagic disorders not involving factor VIII.

Deficient factor	Inheritance	Type of bleeding	Assays	Treatment
Factor IX (Christmas disease, PTC deficiency, hemophilia B)	Sex-linked	Identical to that in factor VIII deficiency	Long PTT / Specific assay	FFP or factor IX conc / Biologic half-life 20–24hr
Factor XI (PTA deficiency)	Autosomal recessive	Less severe than that in hemophilia A or B	Long PTT / Specific assay	FFP / Biologic half-life is 60hr
Factor XII	Autosomal recessive	None	Long PTT / Specific assay	None
Factor V (parahemophilia)	Autosomal recessive	Postoperative and spontaneous bleeding, Rarely hemarthrosis, menorrhagia	Long PTT, PT / Normal P and P / Specific assay	FFP / Biologic half-life is 60hr
Factor X	Autosomal recessive (only homozygotes bleed)	Epistaxis, hemarthrosis, ecchymoses, menorrhagia	Long PT, PTT, P and P / Specific assay	FFP / Biologic half-life is 48hr
Factor VII	Autosomal recessive (only homozygotes bleed)	Epistaxis, hemarthrosis, ecchymoses, menorrhagia	Long PT, P and P / Normal PTT / Specific assay	FFP / Biologic half-life is 4–6hr
Factor II	Autosomal recessive	Epistaxis, hemarthrosis, ecchymoses, menorrhagia	Long PT, P and P / Specific assay	FFP / Biologic half-life is 72hr
Factor I	Autosomal recessive	Variable, deep tissue hemorrhage	Long PT / Low fibrinogen level	Cryoprecipitate: each bag contains 400–500 Fibrinogen; 100 mg/dL required for hemostasis / Biologic half-life is 100hr
Factor XIII	Not clear	Umbilical bleeding, posttraumatic and late postoperative bleeding, Wound heals slowly w/keloid formation	Clot solubility in 5M urea	FFP / Biologic half-life is 120hr

FFP, fresh frozen plasma; PT, prothrombin time; P and P, prothrombin proconvertin; PTA, plasma thromboplastin antecedent; PTC, plasma thromboplastin component; PTT, partial thromboplastin time.
Source: Reprinted from Addonizio VP, Stahl RF. Bleeding in emergency care. In: Wilmore DW, Cheung LY, Harken AN, et al, eds. Scientific American Surgery. New York: WebMD Corporation, 1989.

Diagnostic Studies

After taking a history and performing a physical exam, the clinician should have narrowed the differential diagnosis. **Laboratory tests will be helpful in confirming the diagnosis and managing the patient appropriately with respect to blood loss.**

Complete Blood Count (CBC)

A preoperative CBC is obtained in most patients. Postoperative levels should be compared with preoperative levels. The amount of blood loss usually is well represented by the decrease in hemoglobin and hematocrit. However, in the setting of acute blood loss, the hemoglobin and hematocrit are not accurate, as they take some time to equilibrate after acute blood loss. For example, the patient in our case may have a hemoglobin of 10 g/dL (intraoperative hemoglobin of 11 g/dL), low urine output, and significant bloody drainage from an incision site. However, once her intravascular volume has been restored and the hemodyamics are corrected with crystalloid, she will have a much lower hemoglobin.

Platelet Counts

Platelet counts are affected by a variety of causes as well as medications (Table 8.3). Heparin, ranitidine, or cimetidine cause thrombocytopenia in some patients and should be discontinued if platelet counts decline during their use. Postoperative bleeding in the setting of moderate to severe thrombocytopenia mandates platelet transfusions. However, a normal platelet count is not synonymous with normally functioning platelets. As mentioned above, aspirin affects the platelet function without a change in platelet count.

Prothrombin Time (PT) and Partial Thromboplastin Time (PTT) (Table 8.3)

Prothrombin time evaluates the **extrinsic pathway**. Elevations are caused by liver dysfunction or Coumadin use. Liver dysfunction may result in abnormal synthesis of prothrombin and factors VII, IX, and X. Coumadin inhibits synthesis of these factors, which are vitamin K dependent. The **international normalized ratio (INR)** is a method used to measure the degree of anticoagulation and is a ratio of the patient's PT to the control PT. Partial thromboplastin time tests the **intrinsic pathway**. Elevations in PTT are caused by deficiencies in factors XII, XI, IX, and VIII as well as factors in the common pathway. Also, PTT is used to monitor the degree of anticoagulation on heparin. Heparin accelerates the binding of thrombin to antithrombin III, thus potentiating its anticoagulant effect.

Bleeding Time (Table 8.3)

A very good index of a patient's coagulation is the bleeding time. A standardized injury at the skin level is created with an automatic lancet, and the amount of time necessary to clot is the bleeding time. (Ivy forearm method normal is 2 to 9.5 minutes.) The test is somewhat cumbersome to perform and probably is underutilized. It measures the adequacy of coagulation factors as well as platelet function, thus taking

Table 8.3. Common causes for abnormalities in coagulation screening tests and suggestions for initial further analysis.

Finding	Potential cause	Further test
Thrombocytopenia	Immune thrombocytopenia (ITP)	Antiplatelet antibodies, thrombopoietin
	Impaired platelet production	Complete blood cell count and bone marrow analysis
	Disseminated intravascular coagulation	aPTT, PT, fibrin degradation products
	Heparin-induced thrombocytopenia	HIT test
Prolonged bleeding time	Von Willebrand disease or thrombocytopathic	Platelet aggregation tests and von Willebrand factor
	Uremia, liver failure, myeloproliferative disorder, etc.	—
aPTT prolonged, PT normal	Coagulation factor deficiency (factor VIII, IX, XI, or XII)	Measure coagulation factor
	Use of heparin	—
PT prolonged, aPTT normal	Coagulation factor deficiency (factor VII)	Measure coagulation factor
	Vitamin K deficiency	Measure factor VII (vitamin K–dependent) and factor V (vitamin K–independent) or administer vitamin K and repeat after 1–2 days
	(Mild) hepatic insufficiency	—
Both aPTT and PT prolonged	Coagulation factor deficiency (factor X, V, II or fibrinogen)	Measure coagulation factor
	Use of oral anticoagulants	—
	Severe hepatic insufficiency	Measure coagulation factors
	Disseminated intravascular coagulation	Platelets, fibrin degradation products
	Loss/dilution caused by excessive bleeding/massive transfusion	—

aPTT, activated PTT; HIT, heparin induced thromcytopenia.
Source: Reprinted from Levi M, van der Poll T. Hemostasis and coagulation. In: Norton JA, Bollinger RR, Chang AE, et al, eds. Surgery: Basic Science and Clinical Evidence, New York: Spinger-Verlag, 2001, with permission.

into account all of the components necessary to achieve hemostasis. For example, aspirin use may affect bleeding and bleeding time, yet platelet count and PT/PTT will be normal. Also, patients with uremia may have platelets that do not function properly, yet their platelet count may be normal.

Liver Function Tests (LFTs, Including AST/ALT/Total Bilirubin/Alkaline Phosphatase)
Abnormalities in coagulation factors made in the liver (factors II, VII, IX, and XI) affect bleeding. Hepatitis, passive liver congestion, cirrhosis, and hepatic ischemia all can result in hepatic dysfunction, decreased protein synthesis, and abnormal coagulation. Abnormal LFTs can alert the physician to one of these conditions and the propensity to bleed. An elevated alkaline phosphatase may suggest biliary obstruction and an associated decrease in vitamin K–dependent factors.

Blood Urea Nitrogen (BUN)/Creatinine
Patients with uremia have dysfunctional platelets and are more likely to bleed. Platelet dysfunction in uremia is extremely complex and involves multiple qualitative defects, including defects in adhesion, aggregation, and proteins responsible for platelet contractile function.

Fibrin Degradation Products (FDP) and Fibrinogen
Disseminated intravascular coagulation (DIC) is a frequently encountered consumptive coagulopathy in which platelets and fibrinogen are consumed. It involves an activation of the coagulation system with a concomitant activation of fibrinolysis. As a result, platelet counts and fibrinogen levels decrease, and fibrin split products increase.

Treatment

As mentioned earlier, the treatment of hypovolemia occurs simultaneously with the evaluation for its cause. If a surgical etiology is identified, local pressure may result in hemostasis. Bleeding that fails control by local pressure may require a second operation for suture repair or cauterization of bleeding sites. If a nonsurgical etiology is suspected, therapy should be directed toward the specific abnormality.

Fluid resuscitation is accomplished by the use of three main types of volume expanders: **crystalloid solutions, colloid solutions, and blood products**. Each category has specific indications, advantages, and disadvantages.

Crystalloid Solutions
A wide variety of crystalloid solutions exists and constitutes the first line of therapy for patients who are hypovolemic. Lactated Ringer's solution and normal (0.9%) saline are used most frequently. These solutions are isotonic and can be given in large amounts without causing significant electrolyte aberrations (**Table 8.4**). Hypertonic saline is used occasionally in emergency situations with the intention of mobilizing interstitial fluid intravascularly, thus increasing circulating volume. Although crystalloid equilibrates with the interstitium almost immediately, it has few disadvantages other than hemodilution and fluid overload.

Table 8.4. Volume resuscitation.

	Sodium	pH	Effect on intravascular volume	Cost	Volume
Normal saline	140	5.7	+	+	1000 cc
Ringer's lactate	130	6.7	+	+	1000 cc
6% hetastarch	154	3.5–7.0	+++	++	500 cc
5% albumin	130–160	6.4–7.4	++	+++	250–500 cc
Packed red cells	135–145	6.6–7.6	+++	++++	Approx. 300 cc

Colloid Solutions

The use of colloids is common in clinical practice; however, the true value of colloid use remains controversial. Colloid is very expensive when compared to crystalloid. It has the advantage of containing larger molecules (i.e., protein or starch), and thus it remains in the intravascular space longer than crystalloid. However, despite that advantage, colloid molecules eventually do equilibrate with the interstitial space, thus that short-term advantage is lost.

Blood Products

Transfusion of blood products exposes the recipient to a number of risks, minimized by stringent blood bank protocols, but it is indicated for a number of reasons discussed in this section. Risks include febrile reactions, allergic reactions, hemolytic reactions, and infectious complications. Simple febrile reactions are thought to be due to leukocyte antigens, whereas hemolytic reactions are caused by ABO incompatibility. Allergic reactions are much less frequent. Most of these reactions occur in patients with a prior transfusion history. Hemolytic reactions may be severe and potentially fatal if the amount of infused blood is large. Thus, any suspicion of a possible transfusion reaction must result in an immediate cessation of blood product infusion and in further workup to delineate the type of reaction.

A significant degree of public anxiety is directed at the possibility of blood-borne infection. Realistically, the risk of transmitting various blood-borne infections is low with current antigen screening. The risk of hepatitis B is estimated at 16/1,000,000, hepatitis C at 10/1,000,000, and HIV at approximately 1/500,000.

Whole blood is available, but component blood products allow treatment for specific deficiencies without volume overload. Component therapy also avoids the use of scarce blood fractions that might not be needed in the specific circumstance.

Packed Red Blood Cells (PRBCs): Packed red blood cells have a typical hematocrit of about 70%. One unit measures approximately 250 cc. It is important to know that in an average-sized adult (70 kg), one unit of PRBCs raises the systemic hematocrit approximately 3%. Posttransfusion hemoglobin and hematocrit levels that do not increase appropriately may indicate ongoing, possibly occult, blood loss. In a critically ill patient, a hematocrit of about 30% to 35% is desired for optimal oxygen-carrying capacity and oxygen delivery. This is used as a general guideline to determine the amount of PRBCs necessary. PRBCs also are associated with fewer febrile and allergic reactions than whole-blood preparations.

Fresh Frozen Plasma (FFP): Fresh frozen plasma is an acellular fraction of whole blood. One unit measures approximately 200 to 250 cc. Fresh frozen plasma contains clotting factors, fibrinogen, and other plasma proteins. However, factors V and VIII are less stable, and therefore FFP is not a good source for these factors.

Platelet Concentrates: Platelet concentrates typically come in 8 to 10 packs. Each pack measures approximately 25 to 50 cc. Platelet concentrates are given when thrombocytopenia exists in the setting of bleeding or when platelet dysfunction exists even in the presence of a normal platelet count (in patients with renal failure or post–cardiopulmonary bypass). The platelet count generally will rise 5000 to 10,000 per "pack" transfused. Platelet counts that do not increase appropriately also may indicate ongoing blood loss or platelet consumption, that is, DIC.

Cryoprecipitate: Cryoprecipitate is a concentrate of factor VIII, fibrinogen, and von Willebrand factor. It is given in 10 unit "packs" that are pooled from 10 different donors. Each "pack" in the 10-pack consists of 1 cc of cryoprecipitate diluted with some saline. These factors are decreased in patients with hemophilia A (because of synthetic deficiency), in patients who have had massive transfusions (because of factor dilution), and in patients with DIC (because fibrinogen is consumed).

Factor VIII or Factor IX Concentrates: Specific factors, such as factor VIII or factor IX concentrates, should be used in patients with known deficiencies. Hematologic consultation can greatly assist in the management of these complex patients.

Calcium: Calcium is a major cofactor of both intrinsic and extrinsic pathways. As mentioned before, calcium becomes depleted after multiple PRBC transfusions. Therefore, empiric calcium supplementation with 1 g of calcium gluconate or 1 g of calcium chloride is indicated in patients with large-volume transfusions or with low calcium levels.

Case Management and Conclusion

Upon hearing the nurse's concerns regarding the incisional bleeding of the patient in our case, you immediately go to the patient's bedside to assess her. You find the above-stated vital signs, including a respiratory rate of 25, oxygen saturation of 95%, and a large puddle of bright blood in her bed. You first talk with her and establish her level of consciousness and airway/breathing. You then make sure she has adequate IV access (which she does since she just had surgery earlier that day). You ask the nurse to give her a 500-cc bolus of normal saline (NS), and you ask an assistant to insert a Foley catheter so you can monitor her urine output closely. As someone else is obtaining the laboratory values of a CBC, PT/PTT, and ABG, you continue to assess the patient by checking the site of bleeding. The groin incision is continuously draining blood during this time period; a pressure dressing is placed. However, over the next 30 minutes, the patient soaks the pressure dressing, has had minimal urine output, and has a blood pressure of 110/60. The laboratory values return with the PT/PTT minimally elevated; the hemoglobin is now 7.5 g/dL. You decide to transfuse her 1 unit of PRBCs. You call the attending surgeon to tell him of the events. You also tell him that you think this is surgical bleeding and that the patient needs to return to the operating room for a repair.

Summary

An understanding of the processes of hemostasis and thrombosis is necessary for every surgical procedure. There are a large number of biochemical events that occur in response to endothelial injury that result in the formation of a fibrin clot. Clinical bleeding may result from a defect or deficiency in any of these events or from technical error. An understanding of the specific history and physiology of a particular patient and of the intraoperative details is necessary to diagnose the etiology of postoperative bleeding. In the case discussed in this chapter, because of the large amount of bright red blood, the attending surgeon is concerned about a technical error that mandates a second trip to the operating room. The treating physician must be aware of the risks, benefits, and indications of the various treatments for postoperative bleeding.

Selected Readings

Addonizio VP, Stahl RF. Bleeding. Sci Am 1989;7:1–12.

Brettler DB, Levine PH. Clinical manifestations and therapy of inherited coagulation factor deficiencies. In: Colman RW, Hirsh J, Marder VJ, Salzman EW, eds. Hemostasis and Thrombosis: Basic Principles and Clinical Practice. Philadelphia: JB Lippincott, 1994;169–183.

Davie EW. Biochemical and molecular aspects of the coagulation cascade. Thromb Haemost 1995;74:1–6.

Davie EW, Fujikawa K, Kisiel W. The coagulation cascade: initiation, maintenance, and regulation. Biochemistry 1991;30:10363–10370.

Furie B, Furie BC. The molecular basis of blood coagulation. Cell 1988;53: 505–518.

Gill FM. Congenital bleeding disorders: hemophilia and von Willebrand's disease. Med Clin North Am 1984;68:601–615.

Greenberg CS, Orthner CL. Blood coagulation and fibrinolysis. In: Lee GR, Foerster J, Lukens J, Paraskevas F, Greer JP, Rodgers GM, eds. Wintrobe's Clinical Hematology, 10th ed. Baltimore: Williams & Wilkins, 1999:684–764.

Levi M, van der Poll T. Hemostasis and coagulation. In: Norton JA, et al, eds. Surgery: Basic Science and Clinical Evidence. New York: Springer, 2001:161–176.

Marino PL. The ICU Book, Philadelphia: Lea & Febiger, 1991.

Patrono C. Aspirin as an antiplatelet drug. N Engl J Med 1994;3:1287–1294.

Bioethical Principles and Clinical Decision Making

Candice S. Rettie and Randall S. Burd

Objectives

1. To consider the four fundamental moral principles of bioethics in developing an approach to the practice of surgery.
2. To recognize ethical dilemmas in patient care.
3. To develop an approach to resolving ethical dilemmas encountered in the practice of surgery.
4. To be aware of personal beliefs that inform the surgeon's personal approach to providing care for patients.

Case

You are a medical student in the second week of your required surgery clerkship. You have been assigned to follow a 90-year-old man, Mr. Braun, who was admitted the week before with acute cholecystitis. Following an open cholecystectomy, he has remained in the surgical intensive care unit (SICU) with progressively worsening vital signs. Before admission, he was remarkably healthy and independent, with no chronic or acute disease. The patient is pleading with anyone who will listen that he be discharged. He feels that his death is imminent and articulates that he is ready to die. He wants to die at home, in peace, surrounded by his family. The patient's surgical team, however, is focused on continuing resuscitation. Recently, they successfully treated a 94-year-old in similar circumstances who had a complete recovery. The family members say that they want all possible action taken to keep Mr. Braun alive until the birth of his first great-grandchild, expected in several weeks. On admission, the patient stated that he has a living will, but it has not been provided for the medical record. The core issues to be addressed are:

- Who is responsible for determining this patient's resuscitation status?

- What approach would you use when speaking with the patient and his family?

Introduction

The curriculum of medical students in their surgical clerkship focuses on pathophysiology and the mechanics of treatment. At first, bioethics seems a peripheral issue, outside the core curriculum of required clinical clerkships. Of necessity, students must focus on mastering the basics of medicine and on acquiring the techniques and skills that will allow them to function as physicians. The subtlety of the daily practice of bioethics is not always apparent to the novice practitioner. Outstanding physicians incorporate bioethics into their practice flawlessly, making it a regular part of their daily work by being aware of how bioethics is part of routine care. For others, the awareness of the elemental contribution of bioethics to the routine practice of medicine may come only when its absence has resulted in a crisis.

By analogy, human genomics can illustrate the role of bioethics in the practice of surgery. Components of the genome provide the code maintaining basic physiologic processes. The complex conversion from this code to the normal processes of the human body may continue seamlessly and unabated for years. Mutations are monitored and usually well contained by the body's immunologic surveillance. When mutations develop that cannot be contained, the system breaks down, and this may result in disability or death.

In a similar way, **bioethical principles** guide the process of medical decision making. **Truth telling, informed consent, autonomy, professionalism, competence, and confidentiality** are bioethical principles that are inherent in every physician–patient interaction. For the skilled physician, these principles are applied effortlessly and provide the foundation for interacting with colleagues, applying biomedical science at the bedside, and maintaining the academic mission of the medical school. **Algorithm 9.1** shows how to incorporate these principles into your decision-making process.

Occasional, minor lapses in the application of bioethics may have little impact, but repeated or egregious lapses in the practice of bioethics may result in a breakdown of the system or a crisis that is not resolved easily. Ineffectual practice of bioethics can have many consequences. The physician must attempt to understand the patient's values and to determine issues relevant to the patient when making decisions about the patient's healthcare. Failure to take these steps may adversely affect patient outcome and can harm the physician–patient relationship, possibly leading to legal actions against the physician.

The core objective of this chapter is to show the relevance of bioethics to the practice of surgery. Although the application of ethical principles acquired during the career of a skilled physician cannot be conveyed in a brief chapter, basic principles of bioethics are presented so that the student can recognize and respond when challenged with bioethical dilemmas in the clinics and on the ward.

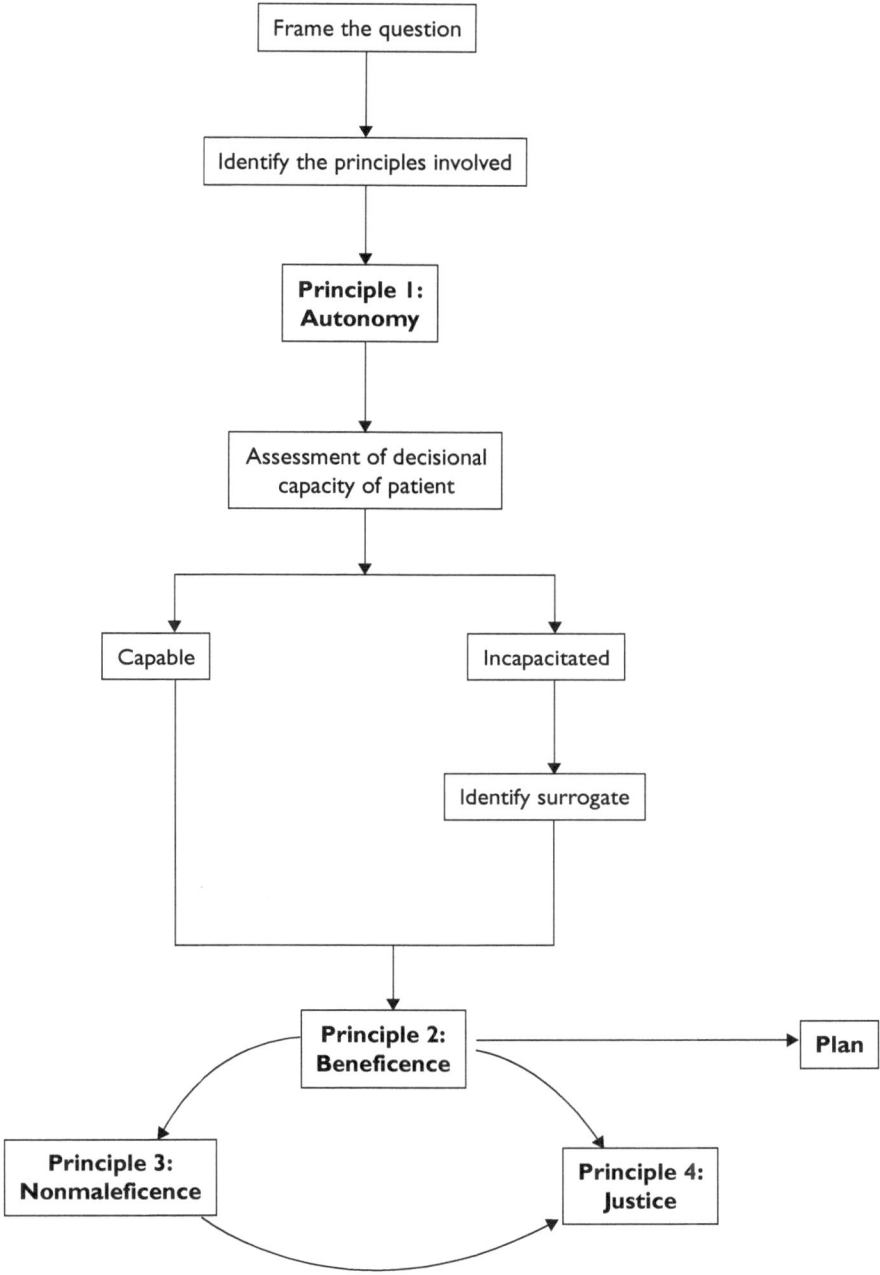

Algorithm 9.1. Determining the bioethical issues.

Surgeons regularly may encounter the following bioethical situations:

- Informed consent and patient autonomy, e.g., refusal of care
- Triage of resources: macro- and microallocation
- Confidentiality, e.g., HIV status

- DNR/no code issues
- Impact of care provider beliefs/attitudes on patient care

These situations are addressed briefly in this chapter.

Four Core Moral Principles

Biomedical ethics has been described as applied ethics—the use of theory, principles, and rules to resolve problems that arise in the practice of medicine. The four basic principles of bioethics—**autonomy, beneficence, nonmaleficence,** and **justice**—are the foundation for medical decision making. Nonmaleficence and justice are derived directly from the first two principles of autonomy and beneficence. The four principles are described below.

The goal in providing surgical care is to recognize situations that require application of these principles. By preparing for such situations before they occur, one can have a thoughtful and organized approach to resolving difficult questions of surgical care. These dilemmas usually are complex and often cannot be resolved by simultaneously honoring the four principles equally.

Autonomy

Maxim: Do not do to others that which they would not have done unto them, and do for them that which one has contracted to do.

The first principle of bioethics is **autonomy, which is derived from the principle of mutual respect. A person is autonomous if he or she is self-governing, that is, has self-determination without undue constraint from external forces. If one is to say that a patient's autonomy is being respected in a decision-making process, the patient should give informed consent or assent to his care.**

The focus is on what the patient wants, not on what the care provider wants. This concept is in direct contrast to the commonly taught maxim: Do unto others as you would have them do unto you. The emphasis in bioethics is on identifying the patient's values and desires before determining the best course of action.

Algorithm 9.2 describes the process for gathering information and creating a plan, in the context of bioethical principles. If the patient is capable, autonomy is the guiding principle. If the patient is incapacitated, the guiding principle in reaching a decision or in creating a plan of action is beneficence, defined as weighing the benefits, risks, and burdens of an intervention in the contest of the individual.

In the case of the 90-year-old patient presented above, his current values about his life and death center on attaining a peaceful death at home. Prolongation of life is not a central value for him. In obtaining informed consent for discontinuation of hospital care, the medical team would need to address difficult issues, including:

- Whether the patient is capable of giving informed consent
- What standards of disclosure should be met (how much information should be provided)

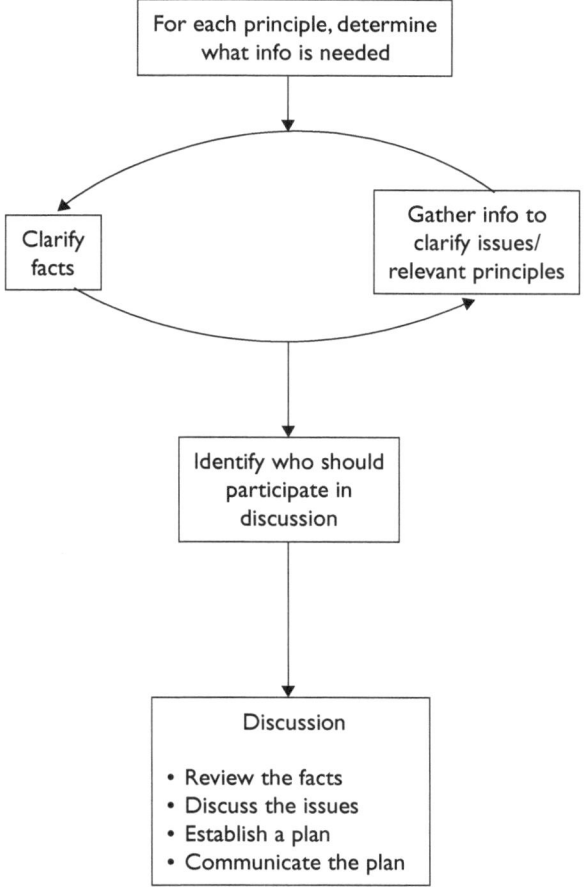

Algorithm 9.2. The process of gathering information and creating a plan.

- What level of understanding is necessary
- The "voluntariness" (freedom from controlling influence) of his consent

Beneficence

Maxim: Do to others *their* good.

The second principle of bioethics is **beneficence, which is derived from the morality of the community and is applied by focusing on the individual's desires in the context of that community**. For the physician, there is not only a commitment to do good, but also, more importantly, **a duty to do good**. Implicit in the concept of beneficence is the duty to avoid harm. The principle of beneficence makes explicit society's common commitment to do good, even when an understanding of "good" is community-dependent and divergent. For example, in some societies, the knowledge that a patient has a terminal illness is concealed from the patient, since the shared belief system is that such knowledge unnecessarily hastens death and diminishes the individual's quality of life.

To the case of Mr. Braun, his "good" is a peaceful death at home. His desire is in direct conflict with the surgery team's "good," which is prolongation of life and return to health. Application of the principle of beneficence requires that Mr. Braun's wish for discharge be honored. Discharging a patient against medical advice or a patient's refusal of care confronts physicians with a challenge to their medical authority and their commitment to assist the patient to return to health. Application of the principle of beneficence, however, requires that Mr. Braun be discharged to in-home hospice care.

Nonmaleficence

Maxim: Do no harm/evil.

The third principle of bioethics is **nonmaleficence, which is derived directly from the principle of beneficence and is made explicit in a line from the Hippocratic oath: "I will apply dietetic measures for the benefit of the sick according to my ability and judgment; I will keep them from harm and do justice."**

Mr. Braun died in the SICU. Until his final hours, he was lucid and adamant that he did not want heroic medical measures to be taken to save his life. But Mr. Braun's desires are likely to be in direct conflict with the goal of the healthcare team—to restore him to health. The focus of the dilemma is on how one determines or defines harm. The issues to be addressed include:

- What does the patient consider harmful?
- When is allowing cessation of life and allowing death harmful?
- Is providing invasive treatment against the wishes of the patient harmful?
- Is death in the SICU more harmful than death at home?

Mr. Braun was a practicing Orthodox Jew. It was his belief that his body must be buried intact to enter heaven. When it became clear that Mr. Braun's death was inevitable, the attending physician approached the family to request permission for an autopsy to determine why Mr. Braun had failed resuscitation. One question to ponder is: In this situation, is it harmful to request that the family consider an autopsy?

Justice

Maxim: Do the greatest good and the least harm.

The fourth principle of bioethics is **justice, which requires the reconciliation or balance between conflicts inherent in the principles of autonomy and beneficence. In seeking to achieve justice, the physician's obligation is to balance respect for the patient's right to self-determination with the physician's Hippocratic oath: "First do no harm."**

In Mr. Braun's case, his request for a peaceful death at home must be reconciled with the reality that discharging him from the hospital will remove him from access to the life support technology that is keeping him alive. One ethical dilemma centers on whether or not discharging him to hospice care at a nearby institution is an acceptable resolution.

Frequently Encountered Ethical Issues in the Practice of Surgery

This section reviews commonly encountered ethical challenges in the clinical practice of surgery.

Informed Consent

Patients have the right to know available treatment options and to understand the implications of their choice. Each patient can then make choices consistent with their own values and goals.[1]

The concept of informed consent is based on the principle of autonomy and the assumption that truth telling has characterized the patient–physician interaction. Respect for the patient's cultural values shapes the conversation about informed consent. As mentioned earlier, in societies in which knowledge of a terminal illness is viewed as harmful, patients may waive their right to informed consent.

Principles of Informed Consent[2]

- **Assess the patient's ability to understand consequences of the decision.** The patient's decisional capacity needs to be determined. A referral for a mental status assessment may be indicated.
- **If the patient is incapable, identify an appropriate surrogate.** Advance directives generally identify the patient's choice for a surrogate. If the surrogate is unknown, usually the next of kin are asked, with the hierarchy progressing as follows: spouse, adult children, parents, adult siblings. An adult friend/partner also may fill this role. If there is an irresolvable conflict, a legal conservator should be appointed.
- **Document the goals and values that the patient or surrogate expresses as the most important for the decision.** If the patient is incapacitated, a living will, if available, often provides sufficient examples of the patient's preferences to allow the decision-making process to proceed.
- **Explain how the goals would be affected by the benefit, burdens, and risks of the intervention.** The guiding principle here is to err

---

[1] Drickamer M. Ethics in clinical practice. In: Rosenthal RA, Zenilman ME, Katlic MR, eds. Principles and Practice of Geriatric Surgery. New York: Springer-Verlag, 2001.

[2] Modified from Drickamer M. Ethics in clinical practice. In: Rosenthal RA, Zenilman ME, Katlic MR, eds. Principles and Practice of Geriatric Surgery. New York: Springer-Verlag, 2001.

on the side of saving a life or preserving function, with the understanding that such interventions may need to be withdrawn if it later becomes clear that they are counter to the patient's wishes.

- **Document the decision and who was present for the decision.** Formal documentation describing the entire discussion should be entered into the patient record. The documentation should include an explicit description of the reasons why the patient agreed with treatment or declined intervention.

Informed consent also includes informed refusal of care:

Patients have a right to decline any and all medical interventions while they are capable of making a decision and to refuse by advance directive or proxy when they are no longer capable of decision making.[3]

Mr. Braun was aware of his treatment options and the implications of accepting or refusing life support. He chose to refuse life support. Mr. Braun's ability to form a judgment and make decisions for himself must be determined.

The limits of a patient's autonomy may be tempered by other forces, such as the lack of availability (e.g., lack of a donor organ for someone with end-stage disease), lack of accessibility (e.g., there is a donor organ, but not in the district where the patient resides), and societal demands. In medical decision making, professional judgment is an equal player to patient autonomy. The physician's role is to offer an informed judgment regarding the health of the patient. While patients have the right to refuse treatment, they do not have the right to demand treatment if it is the opinion of a trained professional that a specific treatment is not indicated.

Triage of Resources: Macro- and Microallocation

The combination of limited healthcare dollars and the rapid expansion of new and expensive medical technologies increasingly demands the triage of medical resources. In this environment, the rights that patients have when receiving healthcare remain a topic of political as well as of ethical debate. Should there be universal healthcare or a two-tiered system based on the patient's financial strength? How much money should be provided for each area of biomedical research? How should recipients be listed for organ donation?

The principle of justice demands that many difficult issues be addressed, such as the one of allocation of resources. Questions that revolve around the bioethical principle of justice usually have no simple answer. How does one mediate between two dying patients' requests for an organ transplant when only one organ is available? An ethical approach to resolving the competing priorities demands consideration of patient autonomy/self-determination and societal interests.

---

[3] Ibid.

Confidentiality

The principle of confidentiality refers to the right of patients to determine who shall have access to their personal information:

Patients have a right to privacy and to confidentiality in matters pertaining to their health and medical care.[4]

Information about a patient may be shared with the patient's family or friends only with the permission of the patient, or the patient's surrogate if the patient has lost decision-making capability. There are no exceptions to this principle. In the case of Mr. Braun, the issue of confidentiality is confronted in multiple contexts, including the decision of whom to include in the discussion of his resuscitation status. A common breach of confidentiality is the discussion of patient information in hospital cafeterias or other public places that also serve patients, families, and visitors. Another commonly encountered breach is conversation in the elevator between members of the care team that continues when others enter the elevator.

Do-Not-Resuscitate (DNR) Orders

Dealing with DNR orders is a highly charged area. **The most important caveat to remember is that the goal of the intervention in a particular clinical situation must be consistent with the patient's wishes.** If the patient stated that she did not want to be resuscitated following a cardiac arrest, it may be reasonable to rescind the DNR order if the arrest happens while the patient is under general anesthesia and is easily resuscitated. While obtaining informed consent, it is important to review the adverse outcomes so that the patient's wishes in specific clinical situations are understood.

Impact of Care Provider Beliefs/Attitudes on Patient Care

Awareness of one's personal beliefs and values with regard to bioethics is essential. To honor the principle of autonomy, care providers must be able to hear the patient and determine the patient's values. If one enters into discussions without awareness of one's own values, it is easy for the care provider's values to color his or her understanding of the patient's wishes. Physicians have the unique opportunity and challenge to influence their patients' lives by listening to patients mindfully, without imposing personal standards or expectations. Effective medical treatment is promoted by understanding the patient's knowledge of his/her current medical condition and his/her values regarding life and health.

---

[4] Drickamer M. Ethics in clinical practice. In: Rosenthal RA, Zenilman ME, Katlic MR, eds. Principles and Practice of Geriatric Surgery. New York: Springer-Verlag, 2001.

Summary

It is critical for physicians to understand the concepts underlying the four principles of bioethics (autonomy, beneficence, nonmaleficence, and justice). Bioethics should be integrated into all components of patient care. By familiarizing yourself with the principles of bioethics and thinking about how to handle frequently encountered ethical situations, you will be able to address these issues when you encounter them. By using the four principles of bioethics, patient satisfaction is enhanced, patient adherence to therapeutic regimens is increased, physician satisfaction is enhanced, and health care is ultimately improved.

Selected Readings

Beauchamp TL, Childress JF. Principles of Biomedical Ethics, 2nd ed. New York: Oxford University Press, 1983.

Drickamer M. Ethics in clinical practice. In: Rosenthal RA, Zenilman ME, Katlic MR, eds. Principles and Practice of Geriatric Surgery. New York: Springer-Verlag, 2001.

Engelhardt HT. The Foundations of Bioethics. New York: Oxford University Press, 1986.

Clerkship Survival Skills: Speed Reading and Successful Examination Strategies

Candice S. Rettie

Objectives

1. **To develop effective study strategies.**
2. **To maximize your score on standardized written exams.**
3. **To excel in standardized clinical exams.**

Case

As an MSIII, this is your second day in your 8-week surgery clerkship. Your required readings amount to hundreds of pages. In addition, you have to read for your clinical responsibilities, survive rounds, and participate in the care of your patients. There are two final exams: a standardized multiple-choice exam and a standardized clinical exam. You feel as if you will never get the reading done. You also hate multiple-choice exams: you always score 10 to 15 points lower than you think you should. You have had only one clinical exam, and it was a complete disaster. You were so nervous about being observed that you broke out in hives and had to take antihistamines. By the time you got into the exam, you were so foggy that you could not remember what the letters in the mnemonic AMPLE stood for, and you kept nodding off while your first patient told you about her history of chronic abdominal pain. What are you going to do?

Introduction

You know that the goals of the surgery clerkship are to acquire the attitudes, skills, and knowledge to function competently as an undifferentiated physician, and to master the necessary materials to competently identify patients in need of a surgical consultation. This means that you will need to

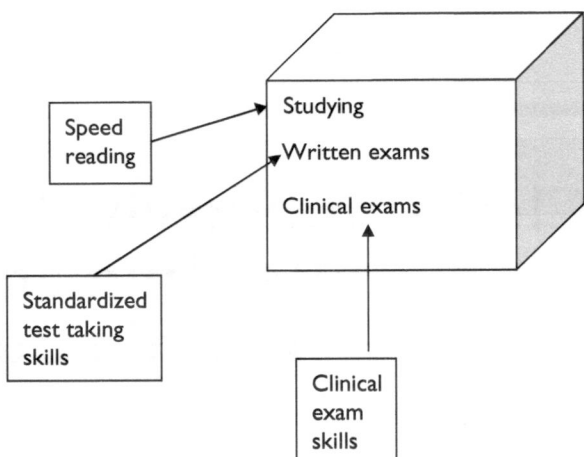

Algorithm 10.1. Components of successful academic performance.

- Master clinical reasoning
- Learn to manage patients
- Learn basic surgical knowledge, attitudes, and skills
- Learn the normative elements of surgery
- Become familiar with operative environment and the care of the acutely ill surgical patient

You also are required to keep up on your readings. You know that reading is necessary in order to master each of the above activities. But how are you going to find time to read and then study? This chapter is a very practical guide to surviving the academic part of the clerkship and to dealing with the case presented at the beginning of this chapter. Three topics are covered: mastering speed reading, excelling on standardized clinical exams, and maximizing your score on standardized written exams. See **Algorithm 10.1** covering the components of successful academic performance.

Speed Reading

Read Every Day

Regardless of whether your school uses traditional lecture series, problem-based learning, or small-group discussions, reading is an essential, daily activity. It may be very tempting and feel necessary to devote extraordinary amounts of time to your clinical experience at the sacrifice of time spent reading. Participating in "cutting to cure" is very compelling. There always is one more clinical task that needs to be done, whether it is checking up on labs, writing a note in the chart, or checking on vitals. To provide the best patient care and to remain on the cutting edge of medical science, make reading a part of your clinical practice. Brief daily reading is essential in order to

- manage the clinical problems you encounter;
- prepare for formal teaching sessions; and
- prepare for final assessments (written and performance exams).

If all goes well, you will be reading because you are fascinated by the topic.

Medical students are very pragmatic. There is no time to waste on low-yield activities. The major issue is how to make reading or studying a high-yield activity. What can you do to maximize the effectiveness of your studying—to understand, integrate, and remember the material?

What Should You Read?

Find out what the course objectives are and read to answer the objectives. Many clerkships use the Association of Surgical Education's *Manual of Surgical Objectives*. Find out if there are required textbooks or suggested readings. Ask prior students what books they have found useful. Look for books that provide diagrams, anatomic illustrations, and other supporting visual information that are useful. Last, check out whether or not supplemental materials, such as CD-ROMs, are provided. Once you have made your choices of study materials, use them judiciously. You do not have time to read cover to cover, word by word. Research has documented that the fastest readers and those who retain the most information read for concepts. This is the basic idea behind speed reading.

How Can You Maximize Your Reading?

The most effective method of studying may seem counterintuitive. The first thing to do is to turn off that little voice in your head that speaks each word out loud as you encounter it. Speed reading focuses on recognition of concepts, relationships, and important details. Basically, what you do is to read the material several times at increasing levels of specificity rather than read once, slowly, word by word. The reading algorithm—Remember-Scan-Organize-Skim-Repeat—is iterative (it repeats itself). This algorithm is remembered easily by the mnemonic R-SOS-R (See **Algorithm 10.2**). Speed reading consists of repeatedly cycling through the following sequence:

- Remember what you know: activate your prior knowledge and determine what else you want to know.
- Scan: quickly read the materials.
- Organize your previous and new knowledge into meaningful "chunks."
- Skim the reading again in order to further develop the chunks of information.
- Repeat the process until all your questions are answered.

In practice, if you use this method, it will take about the same amount of time to study the materials as if you were reading word by word, but the outcome will be different: you already will have reviewed the

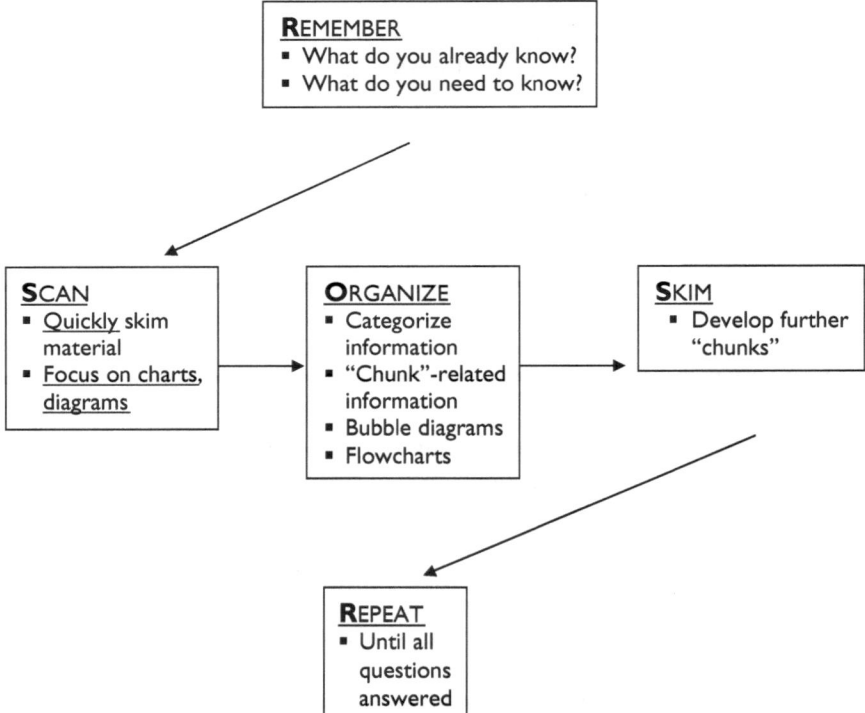

Algorithm 10.2. Mnemonic for remembering speed reading: R-SOS-R.

materials several times by the time you are done. Your understanding and retention will be greater. Try it. Each of the steps is discussed in detail below:

1. **Remember:** Your first task, **before** you start reading, is to ask yourself: **"What do I already know about the topic?"** Spend a couple of minutes remembering what you know. Jot down anything that comes to mind about the topic. This process **activates your memory and sets the stage for active learning**. As you review what you already know, **draw flow charts, create concept maps, make anatomic sketches**, and outline the concept. Keep an index card handy to **write down questions** that occur to you. **Answer the questions** on the back of each card as you encounter or figure out the answer.

2. **Scan the material:** This next step is **"pre-reading." DO NOT BEGIN TO READ YET!** Look for major headings and subtitles; note diagrams, algorithms or graphic materials, highlighted sections, etc. Spend no more than **3 minutes quickly surfing through the section**. Do not dig in and read it. The goal is to **figure out how the section is organized. What basic content is being presented?** How is it organized: organ system, chief complaint, etc.? Circle areas that you want to emphasize. Do **not** spend time carefully reading the section. You are

skimming over the surface. Do not get caught up in the depths of material or the whirlpools of facts. You will catch the necessary details later.

3. **Organize:** Spend about **3 minutes organizing what you have remembered and what you have learned** from the quick scan of the section. Figure out what additional information you need to know. **What questions do you need to have answered?**

4. **Skim:** Now you can begin an abbreviated form of reading. However, **DO NOT READ WORD FOR WORD**. Here is what you do. Guided by the questions you have just identified, spend the remaining **7 minutes repeatedly skimming the materials. Focus only on material that specifically addresses questions** that you identified above. Do not read word for word. **Read for concepts.** Look for words or phrases that are important. Focus on identifying the information that you need to learn. **Use your notecards in selecting what to read. Draw concept maps of what you read. Replicate the schematics of anatomy, etc. Revise the material on the notecards as you go along.** If you **already know the materials, skim them once**, confirming that you have sufficient knowledge of the important information. If you do not know the materials, you will skim the section three times as you read for specific information (e.g., preparing for upcoming cases, presentations, or to master the course objectives). **When you do not know the materials, quickly skim all the headings. Study the graphics, drawings, and algorithms. Next, skim the first and last sentence of each chapter. Then skim the chapter, reading or studying only the material that you do not know and that you need to know.**

5. **Repeat:** Do the process three times for each set of materials: **Remember, Scan, Organize, Skim, and Repeat**.

In general, diagrams, charts, and algorithms contain a great deal of information that supplements or restates the text. Focus on the pictorial content or the verbal, whichever is easier for you to absorb quickly; however, make sure that you have skimmed every component of the chapter regardless of whether it is pictorial, textual, or a graphic. Later in the day, take 5 minutes and review the material that you studied previously.

Let us consider strategies for applying speed reading to your reading in medical school. Here are some practical tips:

- **Read in 5 to 45-minute periods**, using any down time between cases or whenever you are waiting.
- Keep xeroxed copies of your **readings in your lab coat pocket** at all times.
- Alternatively, buy two copies of your readings: a copy for reference and a used copy to tear into readable sections that you keep in your lab coat pocket.
- **Read in 5- to 10-page segments**, then review the entire section later in the day.
- **Draw flowcharts and anatomic sketches**, create concept maps ("bubble maps"), take notes, highlight key words.

- **If you are not paying attention to what you are reading, then stop!** It is a waste of effort and time if you cannot focus on the task at hand. Take a 5-minute break and come back to it.
- If your clerkship uses the **ASE Objectives Manual, find the objectives** that relate to the topic. **Use the study questions** with each section to guide your reading and to focus your note taking.

Speed Reading Summary

Read selectively and effectively. Review the chapter headings and focus your reading on the material that is essential for your task: participating in patient care, presenting at rounds, and performing acceptably on your final exams. **Use speed-reading techniques.** The more you practice them, the better you become. Speed reading does work for scientific reading. **Always have materials with you to read.** Take advantage of any down time to read or review prior readings. **First, review what your already know about the topic. Then, quickly skim all the headings and study the graphics, drawings, and algorithms. Next, skim the first and last sentence of each chapter. Then skim it again, focusing only on the material that you do not know and need to know.**

Standardized Clinical Examinations

What is a standardized clinical examination? **Standardized clinical exams are designed to provide all examinees with equivalent clinical situations and standardized scoring procedures.** Each clinical situation is called a station. Usually, the stations are of the same duration; that is, you have the same maximum amount of time in each station. Generally, examinees are provided with a brief paper introduction that includes an opening clinical scenario and the examinee's tasks during that station. The station may have a real or standardized patient; supporting clinical information such as films and the results of previous studies; and a rater who scores your performance according to predetermined criteria. You may or may not get feedback on your performance during the exam. If the purpose of the examination is formative, that is, to provide you with feedback about your performance, you usually will get specific and immediate feedback. However, if the purpose of the examination is summative, that is, to determine your grade, feedback usually is in the form of a total grade for the entire examination, not station specific, and the feedback generally does not occur during the exam.

Standardized clinical examinations have become a preferred method for generating a clinical grade in clerkships. The standardization of the clinical experience and of the scoring procedures reduces subjectivity. Standardized clinical examinations make it feasible to test examinees' knowledge, skills, and attitudes in clinical situations while controlling for factors such as the complexity of the cases, the individual differences in expectations of examiners, and the variability of clinical settings. There are many versions of standardized clinical examinations.

Some use standardized patients, some use standardized paper cases (e.g., films and labs that need to be interpreted), but all **standardized clinical examinations have the common characteristic of reducing the variability that is inherent in clinical settings through the standardization of the clinical presentations and the scoring.**

The key to success in standardized clinical examinations is to be prepared, professional, and confident. Whether you are taking a history, conducting a physical examination, or interpreting labs, **follow a logical sequence.** If you are being rated by an observer, **you must "think out loud" to get full credit.** Arriving at the correct diagnosis usually is a small portion of material that the rater is scoring. The rater also is scoring the specific questions or maneuvers, the reasoning process, your attitude and communication skills, and your ability to synthesize the information that you have collected. If you state only the diagnosis without "thinking out loud," the observer will have no basis for awarding you the points that you deserve, because you have not provided data that can be scored. **It is critical that you talk your way through the station if you are to get full credit for what you know.**

Know the basic clinical skills listed in your clerkship's objectives. Identify the major clinical scenarios that were emphasized during your clerkship. **Know the basic sequence of taking a focused surgical history. Know how to conduct a focused physical examination.** The ASE Objectives Manual provides a symptom-based listing of many competencies. Check the standard surgical textbooks for overviews of the focused surgical history and physical examination. Most standardized clinical examinations have stations that require a focused history and/or a focused physical examination. The next section summarizes how to effectively demonstrate your skills in these two areas.

The Focused Surgical History and the Focused Surgical Physical Examination

The evaluation of the patient is systematic. **The classic order is identification of the chief complaint, obtaining the histories (history of the present illness, past medical history, and social history), conducting a review of systems, conducting the physical examination, and requesting labs and imaging studies or evaluations.** However, for practical purposes (as when treating trauma patients) and to set patients at ease by conversing with them, elements of the history may be obtained during the physical examination (PE). The physical findings on the PE may suggest additional questions to the clinician, and the patient may offer additional information that should be followed up.

The Focused Surgical History
A successful surgical history provides a working hypothesis about the etiology of the patient's symptoms. The **components of the history are the chief complaint (CC), the history of the present illness (HPI), the past medical history (PMH), the family history (FH) and social history (SH), and the review of systems (ROS).** See **Algorithm 10.3** covering conducting a focused surgical history.

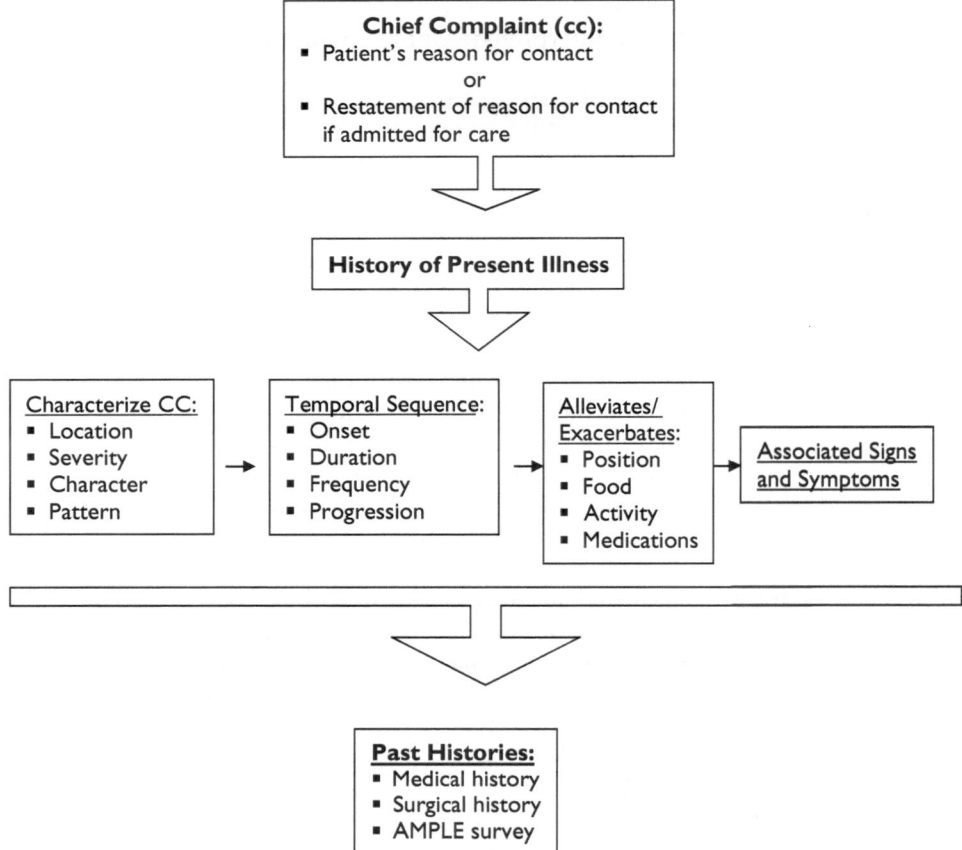

Algorithm 10.3. Conducting a focused surgical history.

The **chief complaint (CC) should include the age and gender of the patient, a description of the chief complaint, and the duration of the complaint.** Frequently, pain is part of the CC for patients who are referred to a surgeon. **Table 10.1** presents the **PPQRSTA** mnemonic that provides a systematic approach to gathering information about symptoms of pain.

The **history of the present illness (HPI) describes the exact nature and duration of each symptom.** The HPI **begins with the first event** that is likely to be associated with the current chief complaint. The HPI should **include previous treatment and the onset of various symptoms.** Reviewing the medical record (when feasible) can provide invaluable information about the HPI and the past medical history.

The **past medical history (PMH) provides a context for the chief complaint and is a listing of the patient's medical problems.** The **AMPLE** survey (**Table 10.2**) provides one method for covering allergies, medications, previous surgeries, and significant illnesses or injuries.

Table 10.1. Focused history for pain symptoms: PPQRSTA.

PP: Precipitating and palliating factors
Q: Quality of the pain (e.g., constant, boring, crampy)
R: Radiation of the pain (e.g., location and movement)
S: Severity of the pain as rated on a scale of 1 (low) to 10 (high)
T: Timing of the onset (frequency, duration, and progression)
A: Associated symptoms

The **family history (FH)** should include queries about medical problems and causes of death for all first-degree relatives and information about familial disorders that may be surgically significant. The **social history (SH)** should include queries about employment, travel, recreational preferences, and health risk factors, such as smoking, excessive alcohol intake, unprotected sexual activity, and illicit drug use.

The final step in the focused surgical history is the **review of systems (ROS)**. Queries for the ROS are obtained by using an organ system approach, **searching for pertinent positives and negatives**. To **evaluate operative risk**, the pulmonary, cardiac, and renal systems and metabolic abnormalities must be assessed, since they are affected directly by anesthesia and surgery.

The Focused Surgical Physical Examination
The **focused surgical physical examination provides the surgeon with the opportunity to combine the art of medicine with the technology of medicine.** Setting the patient at ease, to minimize anxiety or tension that can be expressed as spasms or rigidity, is essential if an adequate physical examination is to be obtained. Also, touch is an essential component of the exam. Careful, precise, skillful, and gentle technique while palpating provides useful data and contributes to the patient's perception of being treated in a respectful and professional manner by a caring physician.

The first step in the focused surgical PE is to **obtain an overall impression** of the patient. The **vital signs** are confirmed or obtained, and then the PE proceeds **systematically from head to toe, proximal to distal**. Rectal and pelvic examinations are part of every complete physical examination. As with any PE, there are **four primary components**:

Table 10.2. Focused surgical history: the AMPLE survey.

A: Allergies
M: Medications (current)
P: Past medical history
L: Last meal
E: Events preceding the emergency

- **Inspection**
- **Palpation**
- **Auscultation**
- **Specific physical examination maneuvers**

This combination of activities should proceed in **a logical sequence** that allows the generation of a useful set of differential diagnoses. **Comparison of normal and abnormal findings** suggests whether or not specific diagnoses should be considered. There are many books and study manuals available that tailor generic algorithms to specific chief complaints. See the selected readings list at the end of this chapter for some suggestions.

Organization Is Key

Throughout the history and physical examination, proceed in an organized manner. You may miss a detail, but you should identify the important elements that allow you to proceed to effectively treat the patient. There are endless aids to organizing a patient interaction. For example, in a simulated trauma resuscitation, complete the ABCs (assess the airway, control life-threatening bleeding, assess circulation, etc.), while simultaneously completing a primary and then a secondary survey. For the past medical history, obtain an AMPLE history (**Table 10.2**) and so on.

Professionalism

Effective Communication: **Knock on the door** of the exam room and, as soon as you enter, **introduce yourself** and **confirm the identity** of the patient. While you are **washing your hands**, you can open the discussion with some phrase such as, "Mrs. Jones, what brings you here today?" **Make eye contact** with the patient. A good rule of thumb is to maintain eye contact long enough to determine the color of the patient's eyes. This brief period of eye contact upon meeting the patient is sufficient for the patient to feel that you have connected and to confirm that you are paying attention to the patient as a person, not just as a chief complaint.

　　Talk in everyday language. Use words that someone you meet at the grocery store who does not have formal training in healthcare would understand. Words like *syncope, claudication,* or *dysuria* have meaning for you, but may sound like musical rhythms or a new kind of insult to the uninitiated. **Use an iterative pattern of open and closed questions. Start with the open question:** "What brings you here today?" **Progress to increasingly closed questions as you narrow your focus:** "Where was the pain?" "Please point to it." "How long did it last?" Then return to the open question as you go to the next section of your history or exam: "Has anything else been troubling you?" "What else happens when you . . . ?" The final question should be "Is there anything else that you think I should know?" or "Do you have any other questions for me?" While ending on this note may take an extra 2 or 3 minutes, the information that you obtain can be critical to successfully and quickly addressing the patient's complaint. Further, in reality, patients will perceive that you are taking the time to care for them.

Follow-up appointments can be scheduled to deal with the additional topics. The important point is that patients know that you are available and that you are paying attention to what they say. At the completion of a series of questions, make sure that you **summarize the key points** so that patients can confirm your understanding of their situation. Demonstrating this approach in a standardized clinical examination indicates that you take the clinical assessment seriously and that you have mastered the basic approach to interacting with patients.

Appearance: Whether you are completing a standardized examination or whether you are on the hospital floor or in the office, you should look *clean* and *presentable*. Wear a clean, pressed lab coat with your name tag clearly visible. Have a pen and pad of paper in your pocket. Carry a stethoscope. Being unshaven, looking unwashed, or appearing disheveled is not professional. Looking sloppy or wearing a soiled lab coat suggests lack of attention to detail and a lackadaisical approach to cleanliness. Patients expect their physicians to pay attention to detail as necessary and to have an orderly, hygienic approach to patient care. Especially in surgery, there is an expectation of attention to personal hygiene consistent with the emphasis on aseptic technique. There is an unwritten assumption that sloppiness and lack of precision lead to mistakes, whether in patient care or personal appearance. Look the part of a professional, competent physician.

Confidence: Demeanor is important. Your patients expect you to **be realistically confident** in your skills. Patients are looking for someone who has the skills to treat them. Patients do not want to be treated by a physician who appears uncertain of his or her abilities. In a standardized examination, the rater likely will be assessing your demeanor and your ability to realistically inspire confidence and trust.

Be confident. You know a great deal. You always have more to learn, but at this point the emphasis is on demonstration of basic skills. You are well practiced in history taking and conducting a physical examination. If you are uncertain about an algorithm, talk to someone and find out what you need to know. Projecting a realistic sense of confidence and competence is an essential requirement for success in a clinical examination.

Research indicates that individuals who **project an air of confidence** are perceived by others as more competent. Further, behavior has a strong influence on beliefs. If you act with confidence, you inspire trust in your patients and colleagues. If observers in the standardized clinical exam see that you are confident, they will expect you to perform acceptably. However, if you look ill-at-ease and uncertain, the observer may expect you to make mistakes and may be more sensitive to any errors that you do make. Of course, this is not to say that one should be arrogant or condescending. Arrogance alienates patients, colleagues, and support staff alike. It is very difficult to sustain a viable patient practice if patients do not return, colleagues do not refer, and support staff do not provide the expected backup.

Confidentiality: The patients are placing their trust in you that any discussion and findings of your encounter will not be shared with others without their knowledge or permission. Recent regulations to this effect have only heightened the importance of this element of the "patient-physician" relationship.

Think Out Loud

When you are taking a standardized clinical examination, **if you are thinking something, say it out loud**. You get credit for observable behavior and, unfortunately, thinking is not observable. The rater will not be able to give you credit for observing your patient's pallor unless you state that you have observed the pallor of the patient's skin. Thinking out loud can be disconcerting if you are not used to it. Once again, practice thinking out loud. An additional benefit of judiciously saying what you are doing (or observing) is that you are providing patient education. With effective physician–patient communication, patients learn to become better observers of their own health and, subsequently, more effective partners in their own care.

Standardized Clinical Examinations Summary

Be prepared: know the basic algorithms for a focused surgical history and physical examination and practice them. Be professional, organized, and confident in your approach to the patient. Look the part. Communicate in everyday language, using a sequence of open and closed questions. Summarize key points during the history. Think out loud so you can be given credit for knowing what you know.

Standardized Written Examinations

It takes two things **to get a good score** on standardized written examinations: **basic knowledge of the topics and good test-taking skills**. This section discusses how to maximize your score on standardized examinations, such as the National Board Subject Examination. Acquiring the basic knowledge is up to you. Read. Review. Take practice tests. Talk with people who already have taken the test and find out what content areas were covered on the exam.

We focus here on test-taking skills. People who have good test-taking skills get higher scores on tests. Read on and find out why.

Pace Yourself

Figure out how much time you have, on average, per question. For example, if there are 100 questions on the exam and you have 2 hours to complete it, then you have an average of 1.2 minutes per question. **Plan on no more than 60 seconds per question.**

The First Time Through the Test: Get Credit for What You Know

Make sure that you **answer all the questions you know**. How do you do that? Go through the exam three times. Each time you focus on a different set of questions. The first time you go through the exam, you are going to answer only the questions of which you are immediately certain that you can select the correct answer. Once again, you want to get full credit for everything that you know. Skip items that you have to think about or that take a long time to read. If you think you probably know the answer, mark the item and skip it. You will return to it during your second pass through the test.

Once again, **the first time through the test, focus on items that you can answer quickly and correctly**. Using this process, you have automatically gotten credit for your basic knowledge. In contrast, if you answer each item in sequence, spending extra time reading long items or sorting out answers that you are not sure about, you may not have the time to complete the test, thereby missing some items that you could have answered. By completing each item in sequence, you are likely to miss points that you should have gotten! So, go through the test quickly, **answer what you know, and get the baseline number of points that you deserve**.

The Second Time Through the Test: Maximize Your Score

The second time through the exam, you will focus on the items that you can probably answer correctly—the ones you marked previously. Your goal this time is to increase your score through the use of probabilities. With a five-option item, purely through random chance, you will select the right answer 20% of the time. If you can narrow your choice to two options (assuming that the correct answer is one of the two), you have increased the probability of a correct response to 50%.

It is important to remember that in professionally produced examinations, all options are present because they contain some element of plausibility. Consequently, each item has some clue to the correct answer. Use this information to increase your odds: find the clues through the principle of convergence—the overlap of themes.

Here is a simple illustration:

Which of the following authors have won the greatest number of Abby Awards?
  a. Jones and Smith
  b. Smith and White
  c. White and Allen
  d. Smith and Taylor[1]

The right answer is the one with the greatest overlap of themes, topics, or facts: where there is convergence. So you analyze the names in the answers. You notice immediately that there are repetitions in the names: Smith is used three times and White is used two times. It is likely that these two names are the "themes." Furthermore, there is only one Jones, one Taylor, and one Allen. You eliminate the options with the names that occur only once. Only option b is left. When you look at option b, you see that it contains Smith (three hits) and White (two hits). Smith and White converge.

Let's do a slightly more complicated item:

---

[1] S. Case, Personal correspondence with the author regarding materials used to teach test-taking, 1998.

Which of the following individuals is most closely associated with the Jones Act?
  a. Robert E. Lee
  b. Stephen E. Douglas
  c. Abraham Lincoln
  d. James Madison[2]

You know nothing about the Jones Act. For all you know, it could be a theater performance. However, you review the options and figure out that there is some relationship to history and government. Already you have two themes: history and government. Let us look at history first: Lee, Douglas, and Lincoln were alive during the Civil War era. Then look at government: Lee was a general, Douglas was an orator, Lincoln was a president, and Madison was a president. You can now refine your government theme to presidents. The final step is to look for the overlap of presidents and the Civil War. The answer has to be c, Abraham Lincoln.

Here is a further refinement:

How many pounds of pressure is exerted by a callam?
a. 260
b. 2.6
c. 150
d. 2600[3]

An obvious theme is the repetition of the number sequence 2 to 6. You need to find the second theme, and you also wonder why have 150 as an option. Remember, every option provides you with a clue to the correct answer. All of the options with 2 to 6 are of a different magnitude. Option c, 150, is a repetition of magnitude. The convergence of 2 to 6 and a number in the hundreds points to option a, 260, as the correct answer.

The Third Time Through the Test: Use Chance to Increase Your Score

If you are *not penalized* for an incorrect answer, always mark an answer for each question. Most professionally developed examinations have a "balanced" answer key. A balanced answer key indicates that an effort has been made to have approximately the same percentage of correct answers assigned to each option to increase the likelihood that the test is measuring knowledge. The test makers want to avoid the situation where an ill-prepared examinee receives a test score that matches a well-prepared examinee. For example, if an examinee figured out that the right answers to the first five items were always option d, the examinee's first choice on any subsequent items would be option d. The examinee would receive a high score, but it would be meaningless. An examination with a balanced answer key reduces the probability that an examinee will achieve a spuriously high score. For example, if the test is composed of 50 items with five options, approximately 10 items

---

[2] Ibid.
[3] Ibid.

will have option a as the correct answer, approximately 10 items will have option b as the correct answer, and so on. So, for an examination that uses mostly five-option items, the chance of getting an item right by randomly selecting one of the five options is about 20%. For items that you have no idea what the right answer is, there is some evidence to suggest that the probability of getting more items correct is further increased by selecting only one option (e.g., option b) for all those items. If you *are penalized* for wrong answers, double check your answers when going through the test for the third time. Leave the ones that are less than a 50/50 chance blank. Of course, you only use these tricks if you cannot use knowledge to arrive at the right answer. Two other axioms to remember: Options that use absolutes such as "always" or "never" rarely are right. "Never is never right; always is always wrong"; The more detail provided, the more likely it is that the answer is right.

Standardized Written Examinations Summary

Your goal on standardized written examinations is to get the maximum number of points possible. To achieve this:

- Go through the test three times.
- Answer what you know.
- Answer what you can figure out using the test-taking tricks described above.

If you combine knowledge, common sense, and these test-taking skills, it is likely that your scores will improve.

Summary

Read every day, but do not read everything: read selectively. For examinations, be prepared, be confident, and use common sense. For standardized clinical exams, know the basic algorithms and practice them; be presentable, be organized, and think out loud. For standardized written examinations, go through the exam three times:

- The first time, answer only the items that you know immediately.
- The second time, use the principle of convergence to maximize your score for items for which you can narrow the options to three or fewer.
- The third time, fill in blank items if there is no penalty for incorrect answers; regardless of the penalty for incorrect answers, double check your answers.

Selected Readings

Bell R, DaRosa D. Introduction: strategies for effective learning and retention during a surgical clerkship. In: Polk HC, Gardner B, Stone HH, eds. Basic Surgery, 5th ed. New York: Springer-Verlag, 1995.

Curriculum Committee of the Association for Surgical Education, eds. The Manual of Surgical Objectives: A Symptom and Problem-Based Approach, 4th ed. Springfield, IL: Association for Surgical Education, 1998.

DaRosa D, Dunnington G. How to survive and excel in a surgery clerkship. In: Lawrence PF, ed. Essentials of General Surgery, 2nd ed. Philadelphia: Williams & Wilkins, 1992.

Kaiser S. Recording and presenting patient data. In: Bauer JJ, ed. Mount Sinai Handbook of Surgery: A Case-Oriented Approach. Baltimore: Williams & Wilkins, 1998.

Levien DH. The history and physical examination. In: Introduction to Surgery, 3rd ed. Philadelphia: WB Saunders, 1999.

II

Management of Surgical Diseases During the Clerkship

Head and Neck Lesions

James J. Chandler and Doreen M. Agnese

Objectives

1. To provide a survey of head and neck surgery, designed as an introduction to this field.
2. To help the physician, surgical resident, or medical student develop an understanding of the diagnosis and treatment of primary cancers of various head and neck sites.
3. To enable the reader to develop an approach to a neck mass and to be able to discuss diagnostic methods and treatment.
4. To be able to answer such questions as: What are the more common neck masses in children and their embryonic origins? What is the relationship of alcohol and tobacco products to cancer? How is the risk of cancer of the thyroid assessed?
5. To develop an understanding of thyroid malignancies and their cells of origin.
6. To be able to develop a plan for diagnosis and treatment of salivary gland tumors and of primary hyperparathyroidism.
7. To develop an understanding of thyroiditis.

Case

A 48-year-old man is seen at your office. He noted a lump in the anterior neck while shaving a week ago; the lump is not painful or tender and has not changed. He has been completely well. On examination, you find a 2-cm-diameter lump just to the left of the midline, at the anterior margin of the sternocleidomastoid muscle. The lump is moderately firm, and it moves up when he swallows. The lump seems to be in the edge of the thyroid lobe. See **Algorithms 11.1** and **11.2**.

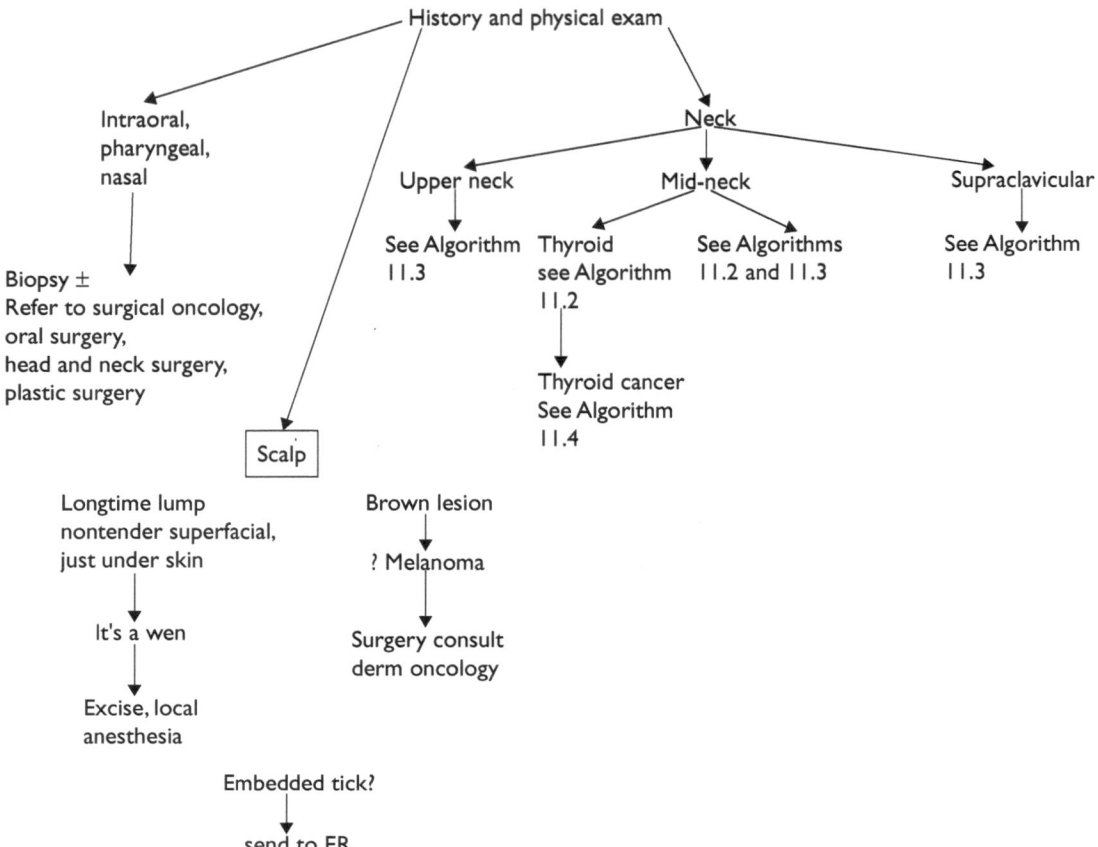

Algorithm 11.1. Algorithm for approach to a patient with a mass in the head or neck.

Introduction

Problems presented that are centered in the region of the head and neck are best addressed while simultaneously considering the regional anatomy (which is reliable, with minimal anatomic variation between patients) and the patient's medical and social history. For example, the patient in the case presented above stated that he never smoked and that he drank only an occasional glass of wine. **There is a close relationship of high alcohol intake or the use of smokeless tobacco with cancers of the oral cavity and pharynx, and there is a close relationship of tobacco smoking and alcohol intake with cancers of the esophagus and the entire respiratory tract.**

The patient in our case would not be expected to have a cancer primary in any of these areas, given his social history.

Risk Factors

Tobacco, in its various forms, is a risk factor for the development of head and neck cancer. These forms include inhaled tobacco, chewing tobacco, and snuff (often referred to as "snoose" in the western states), which is held against the cheek or gums. Betel nut chewing, common in the western Pacific basin and South Asia, also is associated with increased risk. **Most cases of head and neck cancer are associated with a significant history of alcohol consumption coupled with a history of tobacco use. Marijuana use and some viruses have been implicated to play a causative role in the development of head and neck malig-**

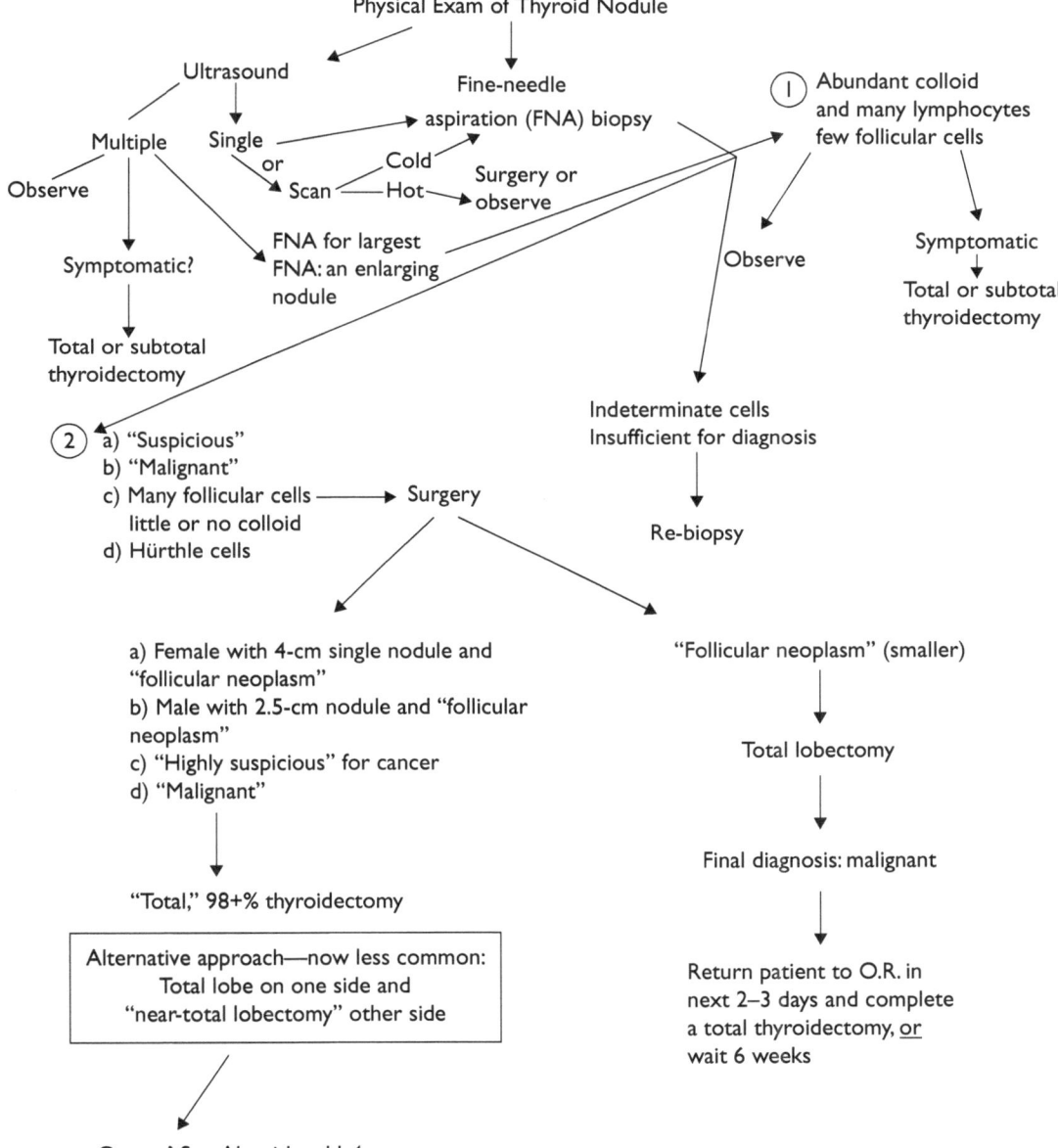

Algorithm 11.2. Algorithm for the evaluation and diagnosis of a thyroid nodule.

nancies. Radiation therapy for acne or skin warts can be followed by skin or thyroid cancers years later.

History

Important points to elicit in the history of the patient presenting with a mass in the head and neck region are:

- **the exact location of the lesion**
- **the length of time the lesion has been present**
- **the rate of growth of the lesion:** rapid enlargement implies infection or malignancy
- **the presence of pain or tenderness:** cancer usually is not painful unless there is a superimposed infection or nerve invasion
- **the presence of an unpleasant odor:** bacterial tonsillitis, a foreign body in a child's nasal passage, and squamous cell carcinoma of the tonsil or base of tongue with superimposed bacterial infection all are noteworthy for the associated odor
- **history of difficulty swallowing**
- **painful or tender persistent lesion in the mouth**
- **referred pain to the ear**
- **hoarseness**
- **weight loss**
- **history of radiation exposure.**

A thorough **family history** can be helpful. Specific questions regarding family members with goiter, multiple endocrine neoplasia syndrome, or a high incidence of skin cancers should be asked.

In addition to **a history of the use of tobacco and alcohol, a history of the use of other nonprescription substances** should be sought. For example, cocaine use may result in intranasal lesions.

A complete **sexual history** should be obtained. Oropharyngeal sexually transmitted diseases have been reported. Risk factors for HIV and AIDS may be identified that may alter the differential diagnosis.

The patient in our case was asked about these points, but nothing contributory was found. This was a neck lump without symptoms, discovered suddenly during a morning shave.

Head and Neck Examination

Inspection (see Algorithm 11.3)

Many lesions in the head and neck can be identified using simple inspection. On the scalp, **epidermal inclusion cysts** (known as "wens") easily can be appreciated; a puncta often is not visible, and skin color is normal. The external ear protrudes and especially is prone to damage from sun exposure. A horn-like, hard little lesion that can be torn off, producing a shallow ulcer, is referred to as **actinic keratosis**. This lesion is a precursor of squamous cell carcinoma. Patients with these lesions are managed appropriately by referral to a dermatologist or head and neck surgeon for treatment. **Any ulcerated skin lesion demands**

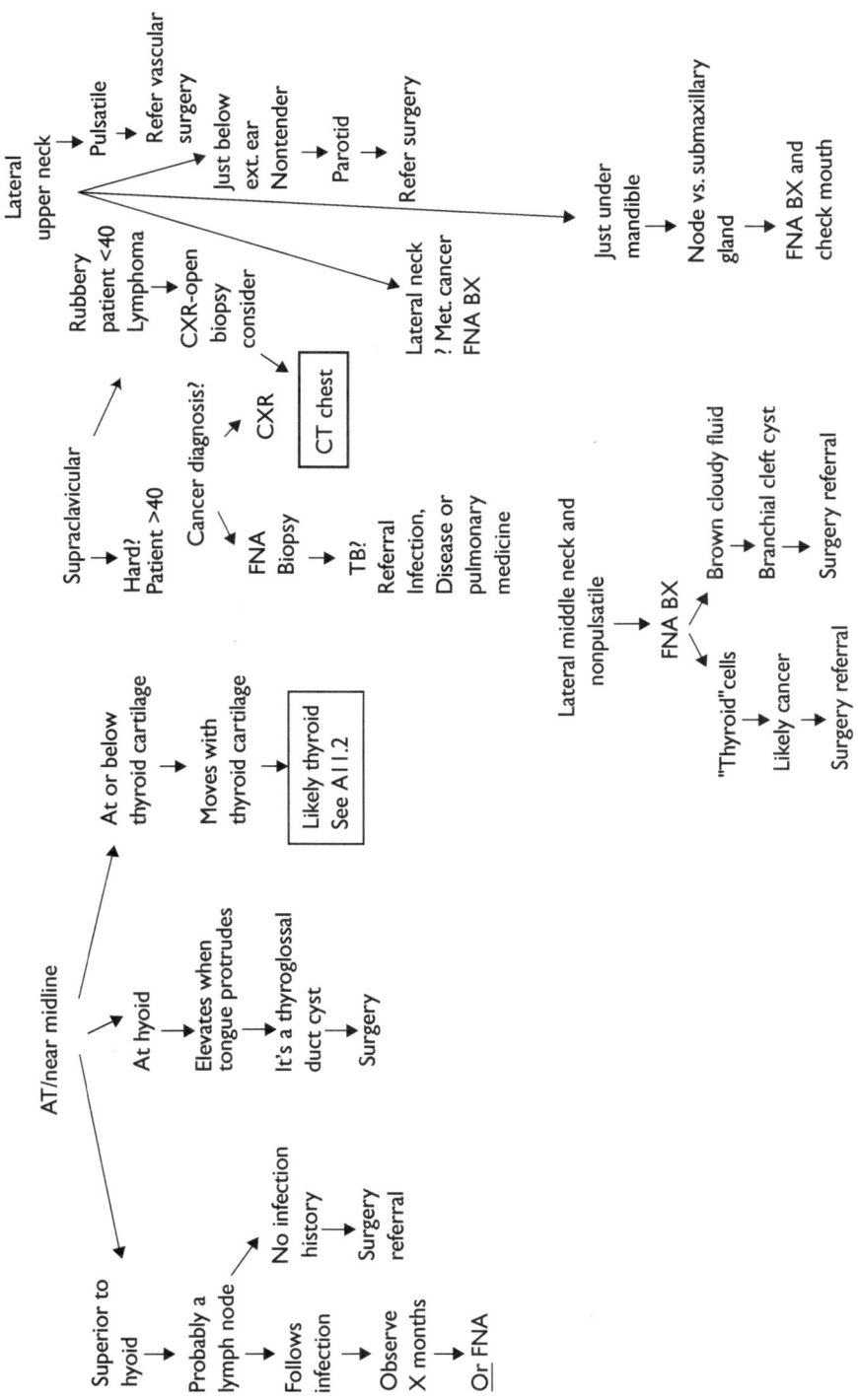

Algorithm 11.3. Algorithm for the evaluation and management of a neck mass.

biopsy so that a diagnosis can be made and appropriate treatment given. **Skin lesions that have changed during a period of observation, have irregular borders, display variegated pigmentation, or bleed when rubbed must be referred for excision or biopsy.** These may be melanomas, requiring complete removal with curative intent.

Gray-white plaques on the lower lip may be seen. These lesions are called **leukoplakia**, and a small percentage subsequently develop cancer. **Squamous cell carcinomas of the tongue** usually are firm, tender, and painful. They often are raised and on the side of the tongue. **Cancers of the gums, tonsillar pillars, and inner surfaces of the cheeks** generally are redder than the adjacent surfaces. A patient who seems sick and shows a swollen tonsil near the midline may have a **peritonsillar abscess**, which requires urgent drainage. A bluish cyst in the floor of a child's mouth is rare and is a **ranula**.

Brown patches on the lips signal **Peutz-Jeghers syndrome**, associated with intestinal polyps that can bleed or obstruct. Skin tumors of various size consisting of tiny blood vessels, **hemangiomas**, can be found anywhere in the head and neck region. **Epidermal inclusion cysts** or **sebaceous cysts** commonly are found behind the lower external ear, in areas of acne activity, the posterior neck, and the earlobes (especially at the site of skin or ear piercing). **The pink or red skin blotches on sun-exposed skin** may be malignant or premalignant and generally require diagnosis and possible treatment from a specialist in skin conditions. Darkly pigmented spots or skin blotches that leave a gray, roughened zone when the surface is lightly scraped are **seborrheic keratoses, related to skin aging.**

Cervical lymph nodes that are obvious on inspection or palpation mandate a complete examination of the head and neck. A firm unilateral neck mass in an adult is cancer until proven otherwise (see Algorithm 11.3). Many of these are cervical metastases from squamous cell carcinoma of the head and neck. Deviation of the tongue to the side of the lesion may be appreciated when the patient protrudes the tongue, suggesting 12th cranial nerve invasion by cancer.

A painless, hard mass in the lower neck in a patient who lives in crowded conditions or is immunocompromised, with or without another known to have tuberculosis, may be **scrofula**, a tuberculosis lymph nodal mass.

A **lump** in the upper midline of the **anterior neck** may be a **thyroglossal duct cyst** (see **Algorithm 11.3**). If located further up, under the chin, it will be an enlarged **submental lymph node**. If you stand to the side and ask that the tongue be put out, **elevation of this lump with tongue protrusion is diagnostic of a thyroglossal duct cyst.** **Branchial cleft cyst** presents at the anterior border of the sternocleidomastoid muscle or just in front of the external ear's tragus. **Thyroid enlargement**, diffuse or nodular, has been termed **goiter**. The swelling in the thyroid often is easily visible, as in our case.

When inspecting the thyroid, try sitting lower than the patient, with your eyes at the level of her/his midneck, using some light from the side. Ask the patient to swallow. When the patient swallows, the thyroid slides up and down and the thyroid nodule or **multinodular goiter** easily is seen.

Palpation

A **thyroid nodule** often can be appreciated moving up and down under the sternocleidomastoid muscle, as you palpate more deeply lateral to the trachea. **Lipomas** may present in the supraclavicular areas. These lesions have well-defined borders and are relatively soft. **Masses in the neck may represent malignant or inflammatory disease.** Enlarged lymph nodes tend to be found along the course of the jugular vein and are termed **high-jugular lymph nodes** when located in the upper neck, below the angle of the jaw. Firm, nontender masses in the neck that are not easily moved are likely **cancer metastatic to cervical lymph nodes.**

Infections of the tonsils or teeth also can result in enlargement of neck lymph nodes, but these nodes are tender. When **cancer metastasizes to the upper jugular nodes, the most common primary sites are the base of the tongue, the nasopharynx, and the tonsillar areas.** Cancer metastatic to mid-jugular nodes—lymph nodes in the central lateral neck under the muscle—**most commonly originates from the thyroid lobe on that side. Supraclavicular lymph node metastases** generally are from **cancer sites below the clavicles.** Keep in mind, however, that lung cancer can and does spread anywhere (see **Algorithm 11.3**).

Palpation of the thyroid gland is best performed by facing the patient, placing the index finger on the thyroid cartilage (Adam's apple) to stabilize it while curling the fingers of the opposite hand around the sternocleidomastoid muscle, resting the thumb on the thyroid isthmus. The neck muscles should be relaxed. When the patient is asked to swallow, the thyroid lobe slips up and down between your fingers and thumb, allowing you to appreciate a nodule in that thyroid lobe. The neck lump in our case patient was firm. It moved up with the thyroid lobe when he swallowed.

Examination of the oral cavity requires palpation for completeness. A moistened, gloved finger gently sweeps over the gum surfaces, the floor of the mouth, and the tongue, searching for rough or tender areas. With the patient breathing through the mouth, one quickly can sweep across the base of the tongue to the epiglottis. **Bimanual** examination especially is useful for the floor of the mouth and can be used for cheek surfaces and for the tongue.

Special Examination Techniques

Special examination techniques are performed by surgical oncologists and head and neck surgical specialists. **Fiberoptic laryngoscopes** are passed through the nose for direct examination of the vocal cords and nearby areas. **Pediatric (3.6 mm in diameter) and anesthesia (4.0 mm) bronchoscopes**, both fiberoptic, also are useful for this examination. **A complete examination, searching for a primary cancer site, requires general anesthesia. The examination relies on the use of fiberoptic instruments to look into and at all surfaces that can be reached,** including the nasopharynx and sinuses, and the performance of appropriate biopsies. Esophagoscopy and bronchoscopy are added when the primary cancer site has not been found: about 3% of patients with metastatic cancer found in a cervical lymph node will have a final unknown primary classification.

Imaging studies also play an important diagnostic role. Computed tomography **(CT) scan with contrast is most useful in evaluating suspicious cervical lymph nodes. For suspected or known supraclavicular nodes involved with cancer or for lymphoma anywhere above the clavicles, CT of the chest with contrast is used.** Adenocarcinoma diagnosed by cervical lymph node biopsy indicates the need for further studies, possibly including mammography and endoscopy. **Magnetic resonance imaging (MRI) is superior to CT for evaluating neural elements.** Positron emission tomography (PET) scanning may supplant the use of some modalities, but currently the cost factor argues against its use except in special circumstances. **Ultrasound is used to assess the entire thyroid gland (see Algorithm 11.2).** Ultrasound can determine whether a lesion is cystic or solid: a **thyroid lesion demonstrated on ultrasound is benign if it is entirely cystic.** Radioisotope scanning also may be useful; nodules that take up less isotope than the surrounding thyroid tissue are termed "cold" and have a much higher chance of being malignant than "hot" nodules (1% incidence of cancer in "hot" nodules). **Sestamibi scan** often is able to locate a parathyroid benign tumor (adenoma).

Biopsy Techniques

Fine-needle aspiration (FNA) is the initial biopsy technique used for the diagnosis of thyroid lesions and neck masses, with few exceptions (see Algorithm 11.2). In the case presented, FNA was the first step chosen by the thyroid surgeon to whom this 48-year-old healthy man with a suspected thyroid nodule was referred. Using local anesthetic, the lump (nonpulsatile) is fixed between fingers of the nondominant hand, and a needle attached to a small syringe (for best suction) is passed into the lesion, then quickly passed in and part way out of the mass, "chopping" firm tissue to free cells to be aspirated. An experienced cytopathologist should evaluate this specimen.

Fine-needle aspiration for diagnosis of a thyroid nodule may not be definitive. If the material is deemed "insufficient for diagnosis," a repeat FNA should be performed. **The presence of abundant colloid or lymphocytes suggests benign disease, with the indication for surgery resting on factors other than suspicion of malignancy. "Papillary cancer," "suspicious for papillary cancer," and "follicular neoplasm" are phrases in the pathology report that argue for surgical removal, since a significant number of these patients will have a malignancy.**

Biopsy of an intraoral lesion can be taken with a scalpel or using a dermal "punch" biopsy technique. Biopsy for suspected lymphoma (see Algorithm 11.3) requires open surgical biopsy of some or all of the lymph node. The complete diagnosis requires more tissue than can be obtained with needle aspiration or **needle core biopsy.** An open biopsy in the neck always is done by a surgeon familiar with the planning for possible neck dissection, because a **diagnosis of squamous cell cancer in a node mandates the excision of the biopsy incision site** as part of a curative operation.

On the face, surgeons plan to take a little normal-appearing skin with the biopsy, while cosmetically planning the best approaches for removal of a suspected cancer. In assessing a pigmented lesion anywhere on the skin, a possible melanoma, **"shave" biopsy is never appropriate because the depth of invasion determines the plan for surgical cure. Punch biopsy at the thickest part of the lesion or excisional biopsy with a tiny margin is preferred as the initial diagnostic biopsy when melanoma is suspected.**

The case patient's biopsy was sufficient for diagnosis. The pathologist described the cytology as "follicular neoplasm," and an operation was recommended to the patient. He concurred, after learning about the options, the procedure, and the significant risks. A preoperative ultrasound study of the neck revealed no abnormality except for a left thyroid lobe solid nodule, 1.8 cm in diameter.

Benign Lesions of the Head and Neck

Congenital

Thyroglossal duct cysts are in the midline, may enlarge quickly with infection, and elevate with tongue protrusion (see **Algorithm 11.3**). These lesions are removed completely (including the central portion of the hyoid bone) with general anesthesia. A midline mass in a baby or young child may be lingual thyroid tissue. These masses may require excision if they cause obstruction. It is important to recognize that this might be the only functional thyroid tissue present; this means that normal thyroid must be identified by scanning technique before any surgical intervention is planned.

Dermoid cysts, consisting of elements from all three germ cell layers, are rare in the head and neck.

First branchial cleft sinus or cyst presents in the preauricular skin, lying close to the parotid gland. This lesion always is deep and difficult to remove completely. Incomplete removal is followed by recurrence. **Second branchial cleft cyst** presents at the anterior border of the sternocleidomastoid muscle in the middle or lower neck or as a large tender infected mass under the muscle. Diagnosis is made by aspirating brown turbid fluid. After treatment of the acute infection, the child or young adult returns for elective surgical removal. A **cystic hygroma** is a large, soft mass in the side of the neck above the clavicle. These complex, cystic lesions present in infancy and are difficult to remove; suspected cases should be referred to a pediatric surgeon for definitive management.

In older patients, the differential diagnosis of a mass presenting in the upper neck must be considered: metastatic cancer, carotid body

tumor, carotid artery aneurysm, branchial cleft cyst, or a primary cancer (see Algorithm 11.3).

Salivary gland tumors are most common in the parotid gland, and the majority of these are benign (75–85%). Most parotid tumors are "mixed tumors" or pleomorphic adenomas. All parotid tumors are removed by surgeons experienced in dissecting parotid tissue off the seventh cranial nerve. In the case of malignant tumors of the parotid, the nerve is no longer sacrificed (unless it is grossly involved with cancer), and the area is treated by irradiation after surgery. Tumors of other salivary glands are more likely to be malignant.

Infections

In a child or teenager, **upper neck masses usually are enlarged lymph nodes draining an infected area**. In the posterolateral neck, lateral to the sternocleidomastoid, and in the posterior triangle, these lumps almost always are **inflamed nodes draining a zone of scalp infection**. However, thyroid cancer in a node can present here. A mass in the thyroid or adjacent to the thyroid is relatively common in all ages with the exception of infancy. **Malignancy always must be considered.** Consider doing an FNA.

Scrofula (tuberculous lymphadenitis in the neck) is treated medically after diagnosis has been made. One actually might avoid the usual skin test in this case because the intermediate tuberculin test could result in a huge reaction, with skin slough of the forearm. Chest x-ray, CT of the neck and chest, sputum, or, better yet, early morning gastric washings for tuberculosis (TB) smear and culture should result in a positive diagnosis in a patient with a tuberculous infection severe enough to result in scrofula.

Ludwig's angina is a severe, spreading, acute infection that arises from mixed mouth bacterial flora. It involves the floor of the mouth and produces pain and tenderness under the jaw in the midline. Immediate referral is essential because some patients require emergency drainage in addition to antibiotics to protect the airway.

Vincent's angina ("trench mouth") develops from poor hygiene and ulcerations in the gums, and is noted by fetid odor, acute infection, and rapid spreading. This condition is managed with antibiotics as well. Referral usually is indicated, because differentiation from Ludwig's angina is important.

Vascular (see Algorithm 11.3)

A **carotid body tumor** easily can be mistaken for a low, lateral parotid gland tumor. If a hard lump is right over the likely site of the carotid bulb, Doppler color flow study and possibly CT should precede any needle biopsy or surgical removal. **Aneurysms of the carotid artery** and a **tortuous innominate artery** present as pulsatile masses in the lateral neck. While color flow Doppler clarifies these diagnoses, consultation with a vascular surgeon should be strongly considered.

Parathyroid

The two superior parathyroid glands arise from the fourth branchial pouches, along with the lateral thyroid lobes. The two inferior glands arise from the third branchial pouches and normally lie more anterior than the superior two. **Primary hyperparathyroidism (pHPT)** results in elevated serum calcium (Ca^{2+}) levels and usually is picked up on a routine blood serum laboratory study. Confirmation of pHPT comes from finding elevated serum Ca^{2+} with elevated parathyroid hormone (PTH). This condition can result in bone demineralization, fractures, severe arthritis, renal failure, ureteral stones, acute pancreatitis, peptic ulcer, and mental changes. However, most patients are asymptomatic at the time of diagnosis.

Cure for pHPT is surgical. Since the majority of cases are caused by a single parathyoid adenoma, identification of the site of the adenoma, if possible, allows a more rapid procedure that usually requires only a short stay after surgery. Thus, **with pHPT diagnosed with a radioisotope scan (sestamibi scan) demonstrating the site of the single adenoma, the surgeon can remove the enlarged gland and check the probability of cure with a rapid PTH level intraoperatively.** Bloods for this test are drawn before and after removal of the adenoma. The PTH level falls within 5 minutes to a level consistent with cure after removing the single adenoma responsible for pHPT. In about 4% of cases there are two adenomas; in about 15% the cause of pHPT is hyperplasia, which usually involves all four glands. In the event that the sestamibi scan is not able to find a single adenoma or rapid PTH assay is not helpful or available, the surgeon plans a more elaborate procedure, requiring finding all parathyroids before removing any. To aid in locating these glands, some use intravenous methylene blue dye preoperatively. To aid locating a single adenoma, one can use a sestamibi scan preoperatively and then use a gamma-detecting probe to pick up the radioactive emissions in the operating room.

Thyroid

Diffuse enlargement and nodular masses of the thyroid are the most common neck masses. History and physical examination should be done first, before laboratory evaluation, imaging studies, or biopsy (see **Algorithm 11.2**).

Thyroiditis

Chronic lymphocytic (Hashimoto's) thyroiditis is found virtually only in women, can be nodular, and leads to **hypothyroidism**. Surgery is reserved for those with the late fibrosis that can develop, causing tracheal or esophageal compression symptoms, and for cases in which cancer is suspected. **Subacute thyroiditis** produces a swollen and tender thyroid. Medical endocrinologists treat these cases with antiinflammatory medication.

Hyperthyroidism

A diffuse goiter with signs and symptoms of hypermetabolic activity, elevated thyroxine, and low thyroid stimulating hormone levels is consistent with **primary hyperthyroidism—Graves' disease**. The treatment for this condition is medical, with an antithyroid agent used initially, sometimes with a beta-blocker added, and radioactive iodine used for recurrence. **Women who are pregnant or anticipate the possibility of pregnancy should not receive antithyroid drugs or radiation therapy due to the risk of resultant fetal hypothyroidism.** In these cases and some others, surgical intervention may be warranted. Medical follow-up is necessary, both to assess thyroid function and to decide on hormone replacement therapy.

Before any surgery on the thyroid, one must be certain either that the patient is euthyroid or that the hyperthyroid state is controlled to avoid the potentially lethal complication of "thyroid storm." This dangerous condition is caused by release of thyroid hormone from the thyroid gland during surgical manipulation and results in severe tachycardia, fever, and other signs of hypermetabolism. For this reason, antithyroid drug plus a beta-blocker are given to "cool off" the thyroid and stop the symptoms and signs of Graves' disease before surgery. If the thyroxine level in the serum has not fallen to a safe level for surgery, beta-blockers are continued for 4 or 5 days postoperatively. Iodine usually is given in an oral form for a week before operating on a hyperactive thyroid so as to block the release of thyroid hormone and to make the gland firmer and less vascular.

Thyroid Nodules (see Algorithm 11.2)
Multinodular goiters usually are benign, with nodules composed of colloid. These goiters may enlarge and compress the trachea and/or esophagus. **It is important to remember that an individual nodule in a multinodular goiter may be malignant.** If a nodule is notably larger than others or enlarges during a period of observation, biopsy is recommended. Finding a **"follicular" lesion** indicates the need for surgical referral. Finding a **solitary thyroid nodule** indicates the need for further evaluation if the diameter is greater than 0.8 cm on ultrasound. Fine-needle aspiration, often with guidance by ultrasound, is the best initial diagnostic modality. Radioisotope scan then may be indicated to discover a "cold" nodule. If a nodule is large enough to be seen easily or if symptoms are present, surgical intervention is considered, regardless of the results of FNA. If the biopsy yields primarily thyroid follicle cells, surgical referral is indicated.

While attempted "suppression" of a possibly malignant thyroid nodule through the administration of oral thyroid hormone formerly was a popular first step, the recommendation by a majority of medical and surgical endocrinologists today is surgical removal and evaluation by the pathologist. Some simple rules of thumb indicate the risk of malignancy in a thyroid nodule:

1. **Most thyroid lesions and problems occur in women;** a woman with a single nodule at age 40 is least likely, compared with women of other ages, to have a malignancy (about 10% likelihood in the surgical literature).
2. **The chance of cancer increases as the age of the patient increases or decreases from age 40.** A woman at age 20 or age 60 with a single

nodule has about a 25% chance of having cancer in the single nodule.

3. **A male, for reasons unknown, has a two to three times greater likelihood of thyroid cancer as compared with a female of the same age** with the same size thyroid nodule.

4. **The larger the follicular neoplasm of the thyroid, the more likely it is cancer.** A 4-cm thyroid tumor composed of thyroid follicular cells has a more than 50% likelihood of being cancer.

5. **Firm neck lymph node, hoarse voice, lung nodule, bone pain or lesion, and hard and fixed thyroid mass are some of the signs of aggressive cancer.**

The patient in our case had a left thyroid lobe resection. This tissue was sent to the pathologist with request for rapid section diagnosis. The pathologist, via intercom into the operating room, reported that there was a 1.8-cm-diameter follicular lesion in the left thyroid lobe. She could not see any definite sign of malignancy in the sections studied. The surgeon closed the neck, and the patient went home 6 hours later; he was able to swallow and felt only some mild discomfort.

Salivary Glands

Parotid tumors are much more frequent than tumors in the other salivary glands, and most are benign. All tumors are removed under general anesthesia, dissecting the gland containing the tumor off the facial nerve. **The tumor is never just lifted out of the glandular tissue because doing so leads to a high rate of recurrence, with difficulty of cure thereafter. Pleomorphic adenoma**, the most common benign parotid tumor, can become very large, and removal should be undertaken early when cure and safe removal are much easier. **Submandibular (also termed "submaxillary") gland enlargement** is less common. Fine-needle aspiration is useful. **Tumors of submandibular, sublingual, and minor salivary glands** are more likely malignant, and all are treated by complete removal of the gland.

Be warned—the submandibular gland can be enlarged because of blockage of the orifice of Stensen's duct by a "stone" or by cancer of the floor of the mouth. Check the area behind the teeth, below the tongue.

Sites of Head and Neck Cancer

Skin

Premalignant and low-grade skin cancers are common, but melanoma is the more feared lesion, and we constantly must be on the lookout for it. Therefore, plan biopsy for any pigmented lesion that has changed, is asymmetric, has irregular borders, has variegated color pattern, or is ulcerated. Seborrheic keratoses are the "age spots" seen on the skin; some of these are difficult to differentiate from melanoma. The **scalp** may be hiding a malignancy, a wen, a buried tick, or the site of a Lyme disease–carrying tick bite. Check for these.

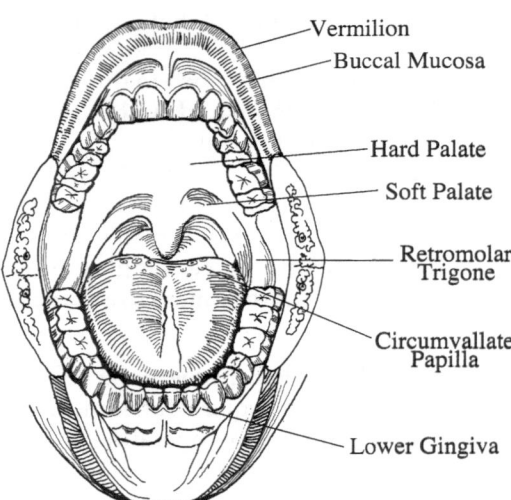

Figure 11.1. Oral Cavity includes lips, floor of mouth, anterior two thirds of tongue, buccal mucosa, hard palate, upper and lower alveolar ridge, and retromolar trigone. (Reprinted from Bradford CR. Head and neck malignancies. In: Norton JA, Bollinger RR, Chang AE, et al, eds. Surgery: Basic Science and Clinical Evidence. New York: Springer-Verlag, 2001, with permission.)

Oral Cavity

The oral cavity includes the lips, buccal mucosa, oral tongue (anterior two thirds), floor of mouth, hard palate, upper and lower alveolar ridges, and retromolar trigone (Fig. 11.1). Virtually all malignancies here are squamous cell in origin. They often are painful, generally raised or ulcerated, and firmer to the touch than surrounding tissue. The pain from superficial infection often can be relieved through antibiotic treatment. A patient with a suspected lesion is referred immediately for early biopsy, and, if necessary, a multidisciplinary treatment plan for cancer cure can be instituted. Cancers of this region affect speech and swallowing patterns. A new onset of hoarseness or painful or difficult swallowing, especially when coupled with a history of tobacco or alcohol use, should prompt a thorough evaluation to identify a primary cancer. The therapy for oral cavity cancers is dependent on the site and cancer stage at presentation.

Squamous cell carcinoma of the **lip**, almost always the lower lip, is the most common oral cavity malignancy. Early lesions are treated with wide excision. Neck dissection is indicated when neck metastases are present or when the primary cancer is large. Additional treatment is given in cases in which a margin is involved, if there is perineural, vascular, or lymphatic invasion, and for large primary tumors (>3 cm). Carcinoma of the **buccal mucosa** is rare, often arising from areas of leukoplakia. Early-stage lesions not involving bony structures are well treated with radiation therapy. More advanced lesions are treated with resection, followed by radiation.

Cancers of the **oral tongue** often are associated with occult cervical lymph node metastases. Selective neck dissection is combined with primary resection (usually hemiglossectomy) in all but the most superficial lesions. Forty percent to 70% of patients with cancers of the **floor of the mouth** larger than 2 cm have occult lymph node metastases. Because of this, surgical resection includes selective neck dissection or cervical lymph node irradiation. Early cancers of the **retromolar trigone** or **alveolar ridge** are treated effectively by transoral resection. More advanced lesions may require mandibulectomy and neck dissection, followed by postoperative radiation. Lesions of the **palate** and all abnormal-appearing lesions need biopsy.

Pharynx

The **pharynx** is a muscular tube that extends from the base of the skull to the cervical esophagus. It consists of three subdivisions—**the nasopharynx, the oropharynx, and the hypopharynx** (**Fig. 11.2**). The **nasopharynx** extends from the nose openings to the soft palate, and about 2% of the squamous cell cancers of the head and neck begin in this part of the pharynx. These may present with nose bleed, nasal obstruction, headache, or unilateral hearing loss. The majority of these cancers are associated with enlarged cervical lymph nodes at the time of presentation. Due to the difficulties of surgery in this region, early

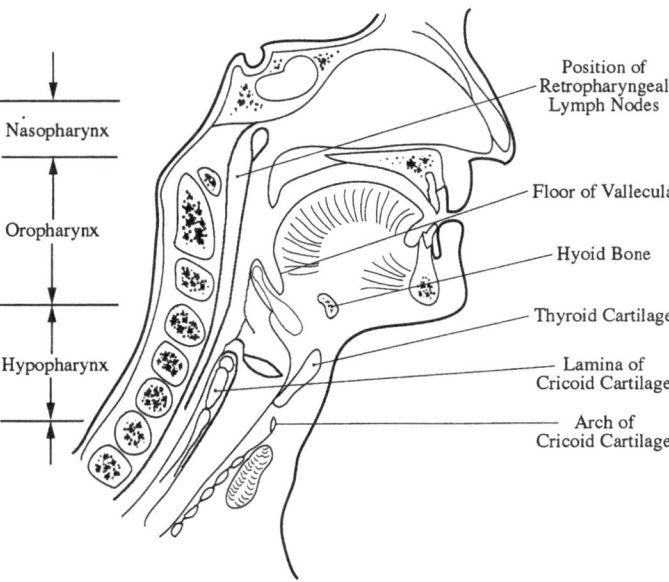

Figure 11.2. Sagittal view of the face and neck depicting the subdivisions of the pharynx as described in the text. (Reprinted from Bradford CR. Head and neck malignancies. In: Norton JA, Bollinger RR, Chang AE, et al, eds. Surgery: Basic Science and Clinical Evidence. New York: Springer-Verlag, 2001, with permission.)

cancers are treated most appropriately with primary radiation therapy. In more advanced lesions, chemotherapy is added.

The **oropharynx** includes the tonsillar fossa and anterior and posterior tonsillar pillars, tongue base, uvula, and lateral and posterior pharyngeal walls. Cancers of the oropharynx commonly present with chronic sore throat and ear pain, and later-stage patients may notice voice change, difficulty swallowing, or pain upon opening the mouth. Small cancers without cervical lymph node involvement can be treated equally well with surgical excision or primary radiation therapy. Advanced cancers require multimodality therapy. Cancers of the base of the tongue are very challenging. These often are diagnosed late, metastases are more common, and there is significant morbidity associated with treatment. Early cancers are treated best with radiation in order to preserve function.

The **hypopharynx** extends from the hyoid bone to the level of the cricoid cartilage. Cancers in this zone are very aggressive and generally have poor outcome irrespective of the therapy chosen.

Larynx

The **larynx** is composed of three parts—**the supraglottis, the glottis, and the subglottis (Figs. 11.3 and 11.4)**. The **supraglottic larynx** consists of the epiglottis, the aryepiglottic folds, the arytenoids, and the false vocal cords. The **glottis** includes the true vocal cords and the anterior and posterior commissures. The **subglottic larynx** extends from the lower portion of the glottic larynx to the hyoid bone. The primary symptom associated with laryngeal cancer is hoarseness, but airway obstruction, painful swallowing, neck mass, and weight loss may occur. In general, early-stage disease can be managed with radiation therapy or conservation surgery. More advanced cancers require laryngectomy, with or without neck dissection, and postoperative radiation therapy or induction ("neoadjuvant") chemotherapy plus radiation therapy.

Sinuses and Nasal Cavity

These cancers are rare, and most are squamous cell cancers. Multiple other cell types, including melanoma, occur. Most cancers present late and all suspected cases should be referred early. Biopsy and careful staging studies by CT, MRI, and possibly PET are essential for planning treatment.

Salivary Glands

Cancers of the **salivary glands** can arise in **major glands (including the parotid, submandibular, and sublingual) and minor glands**. Surgery is the main form of treatment. Malignant tumors of the parotid gland are treated with total parotidectomy with preservation of the facial nerve, unless the nerve is involved directly. If the cancer is "high grade," selective or modified radical neck dissection is added, then usually followed by postoperative radiation therapy.

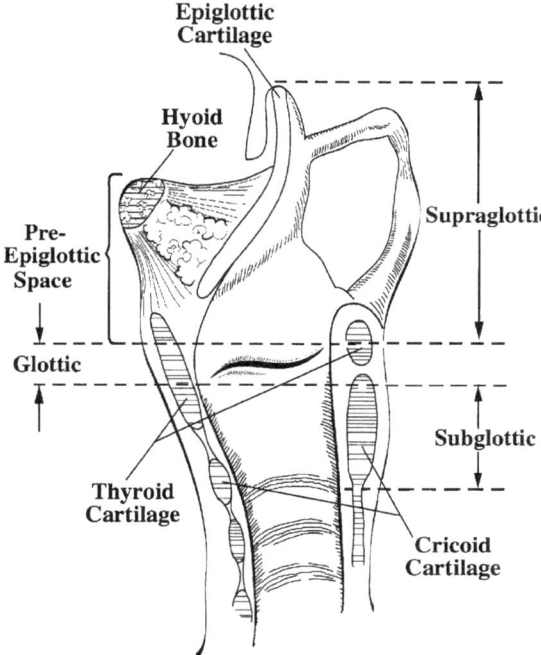

Figure 11.3. Sagittal view of the larynx depicting the subdivisions of the larynx. The preepiglottic space is that area anterior to the epiglottis bordered by the hyoid bone superiorly and the thyrohyoid membrane and superior rim of the thyroid cartilage anteriorly. (Reprinted from Bradford CR. Head and neck malignancies. In: Norton JA, Bollinger RR, Chang AE, et al, eds. Surgery: Basic Science and Clinical Evidence. New York: Springer-Verlag, 2001, with permission.)

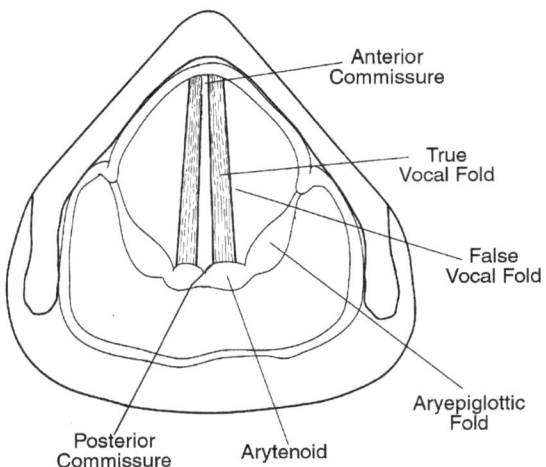

Figure 11.4. Laryngoscopic view of endolarynx. Relevant structures are identified. (Reprinted from Bradford CR. Head and neck malignancies. In: Norton JA, Bollinger RR, Chang AE, et al, eds. Surgery: Basic Science and Clinical Evidence. New York: Springer-Verlag, 2001, with permission.)

Thyroid (see Algorithm 11.4)

Because intraoperative frozen section analysis of thyroid tissue cannot always distinguish benign from malignant follicular lesions, the experienced thyroid surgeon must plan the surgical procedure based on the operative findings, size of the tumor, and all of the factors noted earlier indicating the risk of cancer. **Whether to remove all or most of the thyroid gland has been controversial (Tables 11.1 and 11.2). An excellent discussion of the evidence for these approaches is found in** R.J. Weigel's chapter on thyroid surgery in Surgery: Basic Science and Clinical Evidence, edited by J.A. Norton et al, published by Springer-Verlag,

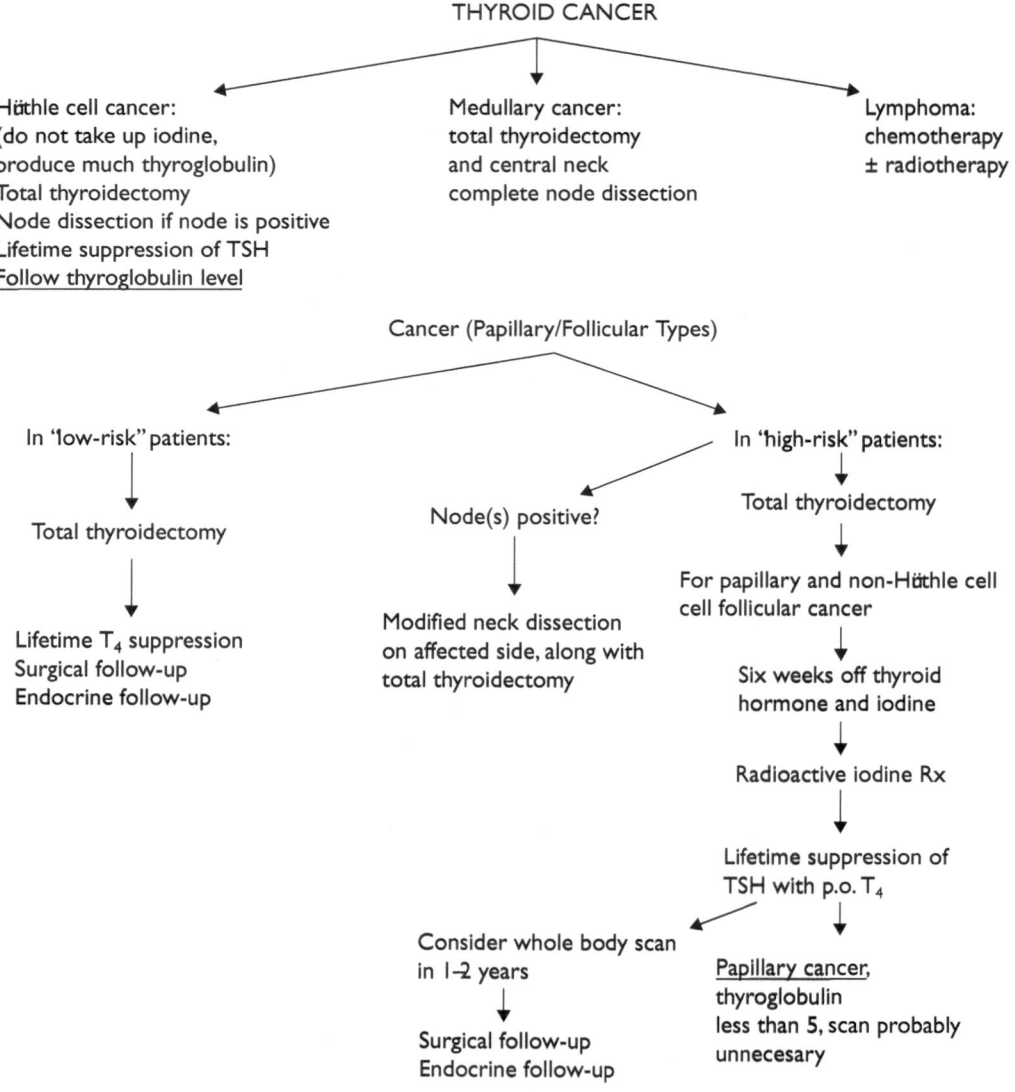

Algorithm 11.4. Algorithm for the treatment of thyroid cancer.

Table 11.1. Proponents supporting less than total thyroidectomy (level II evidence).

Authors	Total patients	Risk stratification (basis)	Mean follow-up (years)	Outcome	Conclusions
Nguyen and Dilawari 1995[a]	155	(AMES) 141 low	9	Mortality TT vs. <TT; 2.3% vs. 1.85% (NS)	For low-risk patients, conservative resection is adequate
Shaha et al 1997[b]	1038	(AMES) 465 low	20	Local recurrence, Lob vs. <Lob; 27% vs. 4% ($p = .005$) Local recurrence, TT vs. Lob; 1% vs. 4% ($p = .1$) Overall failure, TT vs. Lob; 8% vs. 13% ($p = .06$)	Avoid less than lobectomy; for low-risk patients, no advantage in recurrence or survival for total thyroidectomy vs. lobectomy
Sanders and Cady 1998[c]	1019	(AMES) 790 low	13	Recurrence TT vs. Lob: Low risk; 5% vs. 5% High risk; 29% vs. 34% (NS)	For low-risk (AMES) patients, lobectomy is adequate
Wanebo et al 1998[d]	347	(Age) 216 low 103 intermediate 28 high		10-yr mortality TT vs. Lob: Low; 16.5% vs. 12.4% (NS) Intermediate; 75.4% vs. 33.5% (NS) High; 65% vs. 20% (NS)	No benefit of total thyroidectomy in any risk group

TT, total thyroidectomy; Lob, lobectomy.

[a] Nguyen KV, Dilawari RA. Predictive value of AMES scoring system in selection of extent of surgery in well differentiated carcinoma of thyroid. Am Surg 1995;61:151–155.

[b] Shaha AR, Shah JP, Loree TR. Low-risk differentiated thyroid cancer: the need for selective treatment. Ann Surg Oncol 1997;4:328–333.

[c] Sanders LE, Cady B. Differentiated thyroid cancer: reexamination of risk groups and outcome of treatment. Arch Surg 1988;133:419–425.

[d] Wanebo H, Coburn M, Teates D, Cole B. Total thyroidectomy does not enhance disease control or survival even in high-risk patients with differentiated thyroid cancer. Ann Surg 1998;227:912–921.

Source: Reprinted from Weigel RJ. Thyroid. In: Norton JA, Bollinger RR, Chang AE, et al, eds. Surgery: Basic Science and Clinical Evidence. New York: Springer-Verlag, 2001, with permission.

Table 11.2. Proponents supporting total thyroidectomy (level II evidence).

Authors	Total patients	Risk stratification (basis)	Mean follow-up (years)	Outcome	Conclusions
DeGroot et al 1990[a]	269	I: 128 II: 89 III: 29 IV: 20 (class)	12	Recurrence TT/NT vs. ST/Lob; ($p < .016$) 20-yr mortality TT/NT vs. ST/Lob; 10% vs. 20% ($p < .004$) (tumors > 1.0 cm)	Decreased risk of recurrence for TT/NT vs. ST/Lob Decreased mortality for tumors > 1.0 cm for TT/NT vs. ST/Lob
Samaan et al 1992[b]	1599	I: 670 II: 563 III: 271 IV: 95 (class)	11	Mortality TT vs. Lob vs. <Lob: 9% vs. 15% vs. 19% ($p < .003$)	In patients not receiving RAI, decreased recurrence and mortality for TT Trend for improved outcome with TT for patients receiving RAI
Mazzafferi and Jhiang 1994[c]	1355	I: 170 II: 948 III: 204 IV: 33 (class)	15.7	30-yr recurrence (class II, III) TT vs. Lob; 26% vs. 40% ($p < .002$) 30-yr mortality TT vs. Lob; 6% vs. 9% ($p = .02$)	Total thyroidectomy results in lower recurrence and mortality compared to lesser resections
Loh et al 1997[d]	700	I: 516 II: 57 III: 104 IV: 23 (TNM)	11.3	10-yr recurrence TT vs. Lob: 23% vs. 46% ($p < .0001$) 10-yr mortality TT vs. Lob: 5% vs. 11% ($p < .01$)	Patients undergoing less than total thyroidectomy had higher recurrence and mortality

TT, total thyroidectomy; Lob, lobectomy; ST/Lob, subtotal thyroid lobectomy; NT, near-total thyroidectomy; RAI, radioactive iodine.

[a] DeGroot LJ, Kaplan EL, McCormick M, Straus FH. Natural history, treatment and course of papillary thyroid carcinoma. J Clin Endocrinol Metab 1990;71:414-424.

[b] Samaan NA, Schultz PN, Hickey RC, et al. The results of various modalities of treatment of well differentiated thyroid carcinoma: a retrospective review of 1599 patients. J Clin Endocrinol Metab 1992;75:714-720.

[c] Mazzaferri EL, Jhiang SM. Long-term impact of initial surgical and medical therapy on papillary and follicular thyroid cancer. Am J Med 1994;97:418-428.

[d] Loh K-C, Greenspan FS, Gee L, Miller TR, Yeo PPB. Pathological tumor-node-metastasis (pTNM) staging for papillary and follicular thyroid carcinomas: a retrospective analysis of 700 patients. J Clin Endocrinol Metab 1997;82:3553-3562.

Source: Reprinted from Weigel RJ. Thyroid. In: Norton JA, Bollinger RR, Chang AE, et al, eds. Surgery: Basic Science and Clinical Evidence. New York: Springer-Verlag, 2001, with permission.

2001. **The majority of thyroid cancers are the papillary type.** Even those lesions classified as "follicular" will behave similar to "papillary" lesions if papillary elements are identified.

The final pathology report for our patient was available in the afternoon of the first postoperative day. The diagnosis was **papillary carcinoma of the thyroid**. The surgeon discussed the case with you and advised returning the patient to the operating room for completion **total thyroidectomy**. The patient had been forewarned about this possibility and reentered the hospital for the procedure, which was carried out without complication 72 hours after the first operation. No abnormal lymph nodes were found during the procedure; none were biopsied.

Papillary thyroid carcinomas are highly curable, spreading locally and into nearby lymph nodes before becoming blood-borne and metastatic to lung, bone, or other sites. Residual disease or metastases usually can be controlled using radioactive iodine (^{131}I); chemotherapy is not effective. Most often, the surgeon does a total thyroidectomy, performing a lymph node dissection only when metastases are identified; modified radical neck dissection preserves the sternocleidomastoid muscle, spinal accessory nerve, and jugular vein while cleaning out the lymph nodes lateral to the thyroid and along the trachea.

For **follicular cancers**, the surgical approach is similar; however, these lesions are more likely to spread via the bloodstream and are not as easily controlled with ^{131}I when metastatic. **Anaplastic carcinomas** are rare thyroid neoplasms that are highly aggressive, extensive (almost impossible to remove), and resistant to therapy. The surgical approach is to try to clear the anterior wall of the trachea and remove all cancer locally, if possible; tracheostomy may be necessary. The **rare thyroid lymphoma** responds to chemotherapy or radiotherapy. Rarely, emergency operation is necessary to free the trachea.

Medullary thyroid cancer exists in "sporadic" and familial forms— part of the multiple endocrine neoplasia (MEN) syndrome, an autosomal-dominant disease. Early diagnosis through calcitonin determination is very important, because in the MEN syndrome this cancer may cause death before age 25. More recently, the *ret* proto-oncogene has been used to determine the presence of this cancer prior to changes in the calcitonin levels, allowing even earlier surgical intervention. The surgical approach is aggressive, consisting of total thyroidectomy with meticulous "central compartment" dissection and ipsilateral modified radical neck dissection.

In determining the management of papillary and follicular thyroid cancer, the relative risk of recurrence and death is evaluated so as to plan the most effective treatment. In patients with thyroid cancer, a man over 40, a woman over 50, and anyone with distant metastases or cancer involving both lobes or invading adjacent tissues is classified as "high risk." If all other factors are "low risk," the size of the primary cancer can increase the risk of recurrence; recurrence carries a significant possibility of death from the thyroid cancer in 10 years. Involvement of one or two nearby lymph nodes may increase the risk slightly but does not have the same significance as in breast or colon cancer. Most physicians treating high-risk thyroid cancer and cancer with any node positive advocate **total thyroidectomy, ablation of remaining viable thyroid cells with radioactive iodine, followed by lifelong suppression of the thyroid-stimulating hormone (TSH), giving enough oral thyroid hormone to accomplish that**. This was the treatment program planned for our case patient.

In a lower risk patient, the ^{131}I may not be necessary, but the TSH suppression is thought to be essential. These patients should be **followed with periodic neck examinations and determination of the serum thyroglobulin levels**. A very low thyroglobulin level is evidence against papillary cancer (or "Hürthle cell cancer") recurrence.

Parathyroid

Parathyroid cancer is rare. This is fortunate, because cure may be difficult to obtain. Surgery is the only treatment for a patient with this cancer. These patients present with high serum calcium levels and usually a hard mass in the neck.

Perils and Pitfalls

In any surgery of or near the thyroid, there is a **risk of temporary or permanent injury to the recurrent laryngeal nerve and to the external branch of the superior laryngeal nerve. Removing or destroying too much parathyroid tissue carries the risk of producing severe hypoparathyroidism, which is difficult to manage and very unpleasant for the patient.** An extremely important complication, because it is life threatening, is an unrecognized postoperative compression of the trachea from an expanding hematoma after thyroid surgery. All surgeons must be aware of this possibility. **When called to see a postoperative thyroid patient who has difficulty breathing, the responding physician must not hesitate to open the incision and spread the closed muscles to relieve the pressure on the trachea by releasing the trapped blood.**

Summary

An overview of this complex topic has stressed diagnostic techniques, lesions, and cancers most frequently encountered in the head and neck. Appropriate referral, careful evaluation, and biopsy of suspicious lesions has been encouraged.

We have stressed the need for careful, logical progression from detailed history-taking to choice of appropriate diagnostic testing, only after careful physical examination. Referral to those with special training and experience often is needed. Oropharyngeal and neck lesions, in smokers, are especially worrisome because of the greatly increased risk of cancer in these individuals. Thyroid conditions, nodules, and cancer have been discussed in greater detail. Abnormalities of the thyroid cause most lumps of the neck that trigger a visit to a physician's office.

Selected Readings

Bradford CR, Head and neck malignancies. In: Norton JA, Bollinger RR, Chang AE, et al, eds. Surgery: Basic Science and Clinical Evidence. New York: Springer-Verlag, 2001, 1179–1794.

Dackiw AP, Sussman JJ, Fritsche HA Jr, et al. Relative contribution of technetium-99 m sestamibi scintigraphy, intraoperative gamma probe detection, and the rapid parathyroid hormone assay to the surgical management of hyperparathyroidism. Arch Surg 2000;135:550–557.

Le HN, Norton JA. Parathyroid. In: Norton JA, Bollinger RR, Chang AE, et al, eds. Surgery: Basic Science and Clinical Evidence. New York: Springer-Verlag, 2001, 857–877.

Levin KE, Clark OH. The reasons for failure in parathyroid operations. Arch Surg 1989;124:911–915.

Potter DD Jr, Kendrick ML. An elderly woman with recurrent hyperparathyroidism. Contemp Surg 2002;58(11):555–559.

Stojadinovic A, et al. Thyroid carcinoma: biological implications of age, method of detection, and site and extent of recurrence. Ann Surg Oncol 2002;9(8);789–798.

Weigel RJ. Thyroid. In: Norton JA, Bollinger RR, Chang AE, et al, eds. Surgery: Basic Science and Clinical Evidence. New York: Springer-Verlag, 2001, 879–895.

Wise RA, Baker HW. Surgery of the Head and Neck, 3rd ed. Chicago: Year Book Medical Publishers, 1968.

12

Swallowing Difficulty and Pain

John P. Sutyak

Objectives

1. To distinguish between dysphagia and odynophagia.
2. To discuss the anatomy and physiology of the swallowing structures and mechanism, including the physiologic lower esophageal sphincter.
3. To discuss pertinent clinical history and physical examination findings as they relate to structural and functional pathology.
4. To develop a focused evaluation plan based on history and physical exam findings.
5. To describe various therapeutic options for patients with neurologic, neoplastic, reflex-mediated, and dysmotility-mediated disorders.

Cases

Case 1

A 58-year-old man presents to your office complaining of difficulty in swallowing. He has sustained a weight loss of 15 pounds over the past 3 months.

Case 2

A 39-year-old woman presents to your office with burning chest pain, rapidly worsening over 3 years. Recent treatment with an H2 blocker has relieved her symptoms.

Case 3

A 72-year-old woman presents to your office with difficulty in swallowing for decades. She describes a recent, worsening sensation of substernal fullness.

Introduction

The swallowing mechanism is a complex interaction of pharyngeal and esophageal structures designed for the seemingly simple purpose of propelling food to the stomach and of allowing the expulsion of excess gas or potentially toxic food out of the stomach. Initial evaluation of a patient complaining of difficulty (dysphagia) or pain (odynophagia) with swallowing involves a thorough, focused **history** and a **physical examination. Appropriate diagnostic tests** then can be employed. The advent of **esophageal motility and pH studies has permitted correlation of physiologic data to the anatomic information obtained through radiographic and endoscopic studies.** Myriad primary and secondary processes may affect the swallowing mechanism. Some may be pathologic and the cause for the patient's symptoms. Others may only confuse the diagnosis, having no relationship to the patient's complaints. **In evaluating swallowing difficulty and pain, it is extremely important to relate symptoms to diagnosis, as inappropriate therapy actually may worsen the patient's symptoms or initiate new complications.**

Anatomic Considerations

The esophagus is a muscular tube extending from the cricoid to the stomach. It is composed of a mucosal layer, a submucosa, and a double outer muscular layer (**Fig. 12.1**). **No serosa is present on the esophagus, resulting in a structure that has less resistance to perforation, infiltration of malignant cells, and anastomotic breakdown follow-**

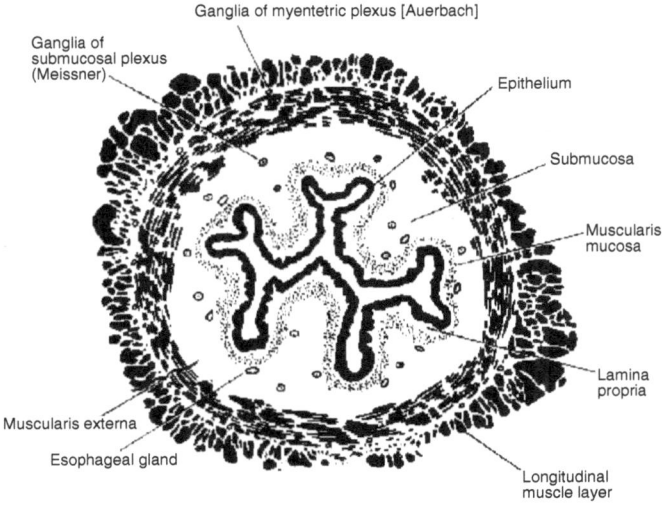

Figure 12.1. Cross section of the esophagus showing the layers of the wall (Reprinted from Jamieson GG, ed. Surgery of the Esophagus. Edinburgh: Churchill Livingstone, 1988. Copyright © 1988 Elsevier Ltd. With permission from Elsevier.)

ing surgery. Three layers compose the esophageal mucosa: a stratified, nonkeratinizing squamous epithelial lining; the lamina propria (a matrix of collagen and elastic fibers); and the muscularis mucosae. The squamous epithelium of the esophagus meets the junctional columnar epithelium of the gastric cardia in a sharp transition called the Z-line, typically located at or near the lower esophageal sphincter (**Fig. 12.2**).

Although the upper third of esophageal muscle is skeletal and the distal portion is smooth, the entire esophagus functions as one coordinated structure. Contraction of the longitudinal muscle fibers of the esophageal body produces esophageal shortening. The inner circular muscle is arranged in incomplete rings, producing a helical pattern that, on contraction, produces a corkscrew-type propulsion. Muscle layers are of uniform thickness until the distal 3 to 4 cm, where the inner circular layer thickens and divides into incomplete horizontal muscular bands on the lesser gastric curve and oblique fibers that become the gastric sling fibers on the greater curve. **Although no complete circular band exists as an anatomic lower esophageal sphincter (LES), it is the area of rearranged distal circular fibers that corresponds to the high-pressure zone of the LES.** In an adult, the cricopharyngeal muscle is located approximately 15 cm from the incisors, and the gastroesophageal junction is located approximately 45 cm from the incisors.

The esophagus has abundant lymphatic drainage within a dense submucosal plexus. **Because the lymphatic system is not segmental, lymph can travel a long distance in the plexus before traversing the muscle layer and entering regional lymph nodes.** Tumor cells of the

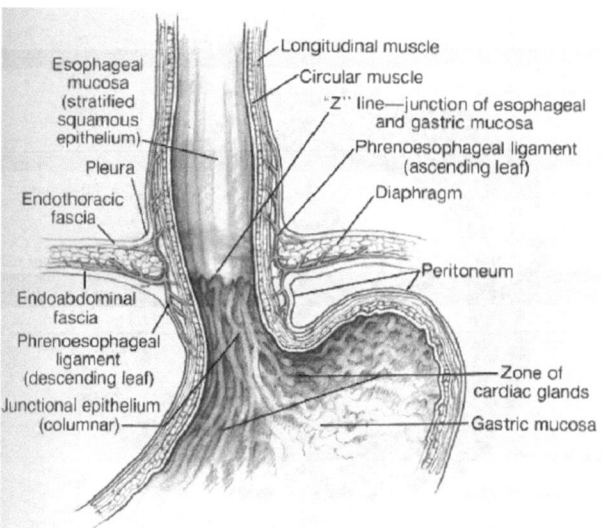

Figure 12.2. Anatomic relationships of the distal esophagus and phrenoesophageal ligament. (Reprinted from Gray SW, Skandalakis JE, McClusky DA. Atlas of Surgical Anatomy for General Surgeons. Baltimore: Williams & Wilkins, 1985, with permission.)

upper esophagus can metastasize to superior gastric nodes, or a cancer of the lower esophagus can metastasize to superior mediastinal nodes. More commonly, the lymphatic drainage from the upper esophagus courses into the cervical and peritracheal lymph nodes, while that from the lower thoracic and abdominal esophagus drains into the retrocardiac and celiac nodes.

The esophagus has both sympathetic and parasympathetic innervation. The sympathetic supply is through the cervical and thoracic sympathetic chains as well as through the splanchnic nerves derived from the celiac plexus and ganglia. Parasympathetic innervation of the pharynx and esophagus is primarily through the vagus nerve. The vagal trunks contribute to the anterior and posterior esophageal plexi. At the diaphragmatic hiatus, these plexi fuse to form the anterior and posterior vagus nerves. A rich intrinsic nervous supply called the myenteric plexus exists between the longitudinal and circular muscle layers (Auerbach's plexus) and in the submucosa (Meissner's plexus).

Physiology of Swallowing

Passage of food from mouth to stomach requires a well-coordinated series of neurologic and muscular events. The mechanism of swallowing is analogous to a mechanical system consisting of a piston pump (tongue) filling and pressurizing a cylinder (hypopharynx) connected to a three-valve (soft palate, epiglottis, and cricopharyngeus) system that propels material into a worm drive (esophagus) with a single distal valve (LES). Failure of the pump, valves, or worm drive leads to abnormalities in swallowing such as difficulty in propelling food from mouth to stomach or regurgitation of food into the oral pharynx, nasopharynx, or esophagus.

The LES acts as the valve at the end of the esophageal worm drive and provides a pressure barrier between the esophagus and stomach. Although a precise anatomic LES does not exist, muscle fiber architecture at the esophagogastric junction explains some of the sphincter-like activity of the LES. The resting tone of the LES is approximately 20 mm Hg. With initiation of a swallow, **LES pressure decreases, allowing the primary peristaltic wave to propel food into the stomach.** A pharyngeal swallow that does not initiate peristaltic contraction also leads to **LES relaxation, permitting gastric juice to reflux into the distal esophagus.** The coordinated activity of the pharyngeal swallow and LES relaxation appears to be in part vagally mediated. The intrinsic tone of the LES can be affected by diet and medications as well as by neural and hormonal mechanisms (**Table 12.1**).

History and Physical Examination

A precise medical history is essential to obtaining an accurate diagnosis of swallowing difficulties. Does the patient suffer from difficulty in swallowing (dysphagia) alone, or is pain with swallowing (odynophagia) a primary or associated complaint? If pain is the primary complaint, elucidate its nature (squeezing, burning, pressure), aggravating factors (temperature and type of food, liquids and/or solids, medications, caffeine, alcohol, position, size or time of meals), relieving factors (medications, position, eructation, emesis), time course (lifelong, several years, slow progression, worsening, stable, episodic, constant), and associated factors (patient age, weight gain or loss, presence of a mass in the neck, preexisting disease processes, chronic cough, asthma, recurrent pneumonia, tobacco and alcohol use). When dysphagia is not associated with pain or with pain as a minor complaint, questioning should still follow the pattern above (nature, aggravating factors/relieving factors/time course/associated factors) and include questions focusing on disease progression (difficulty with solids at first, then difficulty with liquids, or difficulty with both solids and liquids).

Appropriate identification and evaluation of esophageal abnormalities rely on a thorough understanding of the patient's symptoms and of how these symptoms relate to various disorders. Table 12.2 lists symptoms that may be attributable to esophageal disorders. Occasional symptoms are common and of no pathologic significance. However, frequent and persistent symptoms should prompt further investigation. **A useful method is to determine how much the symptoms have affected the patient's lifestyle in terms of activity, types of food eaten, interruption of employment, and effects on family life.** A precise relationship of symptoms to diagnosis is essential in order to avoid inappropriate and dangerous treatment.

Table 12.1. Neural, hormonal, and dietary factors thought to affect lower esophageal sphincter (LES).

Increase LES pressure
Cholinergics
Prokinetics
α-Agonists
β-Blockers
Gastrin
Motilin
Bombesin
Substance p
Decrease LES Pressure
α-Blockers
β-Blockers
Calcium channel blockers
Cholecystokinin
Estrogen
Progesterone
Somatostatin
Secretin
Caffeine (chocolate, coffee)
Fats

Source: Reprinted from Smith CD. Esophagus. In: Norton JA, Bollinger RR, Chang AE, et al, eds. Surgery: Basic Science and Clinical Evidence. New York: Springer-Verlag, 2001, with permission.

Table 12.2. Patient symptoms and likely etiologies.

Symptom	Definition	Likely etiology
Heartburn	Burning discomfort behind breast bone Bitter acidic fluid in mouth Sudden filling of mouth with clear/salty fluid	Gastroesophageal reflux (GER)
Dysphagia	Sensation of food being hindered in passage from mouth to stomach	Motor disorders Inflammatory process Diverticula Tumors
Odynophagia	Pain with swallowing	Severe inflammatory process
Globus sensation	Lump in throat unrelated to swallowing	
Chest pain	Mimics angina pectoris	GER Motor disorders Tumors
Respiratory symptoms	Asthma/wheezing, bronchitis, hemoptysis, stridor	GER Diverticula Tumors
ENT symptoms	Chronic sore throat, laryngitis, halitosis, chronic cough	GER Diverticula
Rumination	Regurgitation of recently ingested food into mouth	Achalasia Inflammatory process Diverticula Tumors

Source: Reprinted from Smith CD. Esophagus. In: Norton JA, Bollinger RR, Chang AE, et al, eds. Surgery: Basic Science and Clinical Evidence. New York: Springer-Verlag, 2001, with permission.

Although the majority of preliminary diagnostic information is obtained through a focused history, **physical examination can add important clues to the diagnosis, particularly when malignancy is of concern.** Signs of chronic or acute weight loss, lymphadenopathy, tobacco abuse, ethanol abuse, portal hypertension, and any abnormal neck or abdominal masses should be noted on physical examination. Further history and examination findings are covered under the specific diagnoses that follow later in this chapter.

Diagnostic Tests for Evaluation of Esophageal and Swallowing Disorders

Several diagnostic tests are available to evaluate patients with dysphagia/odynophagia. These tests, listed in **Table 12.3**, can be divided into **tests to assess structural abnormalities, tests to assess functional abnormalities, tests to assess esophageal exposure to gastric content, and tests to provoke esophageal symptoms.** Gastric motility and biliary disease may need to be evaluated as well to rule out gastroparesis or gallbladder disease. See **Algorithm 12.1** for swallowing evaluation.

Assessment of Structural Abnormalities

Radiographic Studies
Plain chest x-ray films may reveal changes in cardiac silhouette or tracheobronchial location, suggesting esophageal disorders. Herniation of

Table 12.3. Assessment of esophageal function.

Condition	Diagnostic test
Structural abnormalities	Barium swallow
	Endoscopy
	Chest x-ray
	CT scan
	Cinefluoroscopy
	Endoscopic ultrasound
Functional abnormalities	Manometry (stationary and 24 hour)
	Transit studies
Esophageal exposure to gastric content	24-hour pH monitoring
Provoke esophageal symptoms	Acid perfusion (Bernstein)
	Edrophonium (Tensilon)
	Balloon distention
Others	Gastric analysis
	Gastric emptying study
	Gallbladder ultrasound

Source: Reprinted from Smith CD. Esophagus. In: Norton JA, Bollinger RR, Chang AE, et al, eds. Surgery: Basic Science and Clinical Evidence. New York: Springer-Verlag, 2001, with permission.

the stomach and other structures above the diaphragm often is identified by abnormal gas patterns on chest radiographs. A simple and often specific diagnostic test for esophageal disease is a **contrast esophagogram or barium swallow**. Structural abnormalities, including diverticula, narrowing or stricture, ulcers, and hiatal or paraesophageal hernias, all can be demonstrated. **Use of fluoroscopy with videotaped recordings of both a liquid and solid contrast swallow** increases accuracy in identifying subtle abnormalities. Abnormalities of esophageal motility or gastroesophageal reflux can be seen during a barium swallow, but these disorders are more appropriately diagnosed using other tests. The value of attempting to elicit reflux is questionable because 20% of normal individuals have radiologic reflux. The **timed barium esophagogram** is a simple test of esophageal function. After ingestion of a premeasured amount of barium, spot films are taken at 1-, 2-, 5-, 10-, and 20-minute intervals. This test allows quantification of esophageal emptying and is useful for the evaluation of motility disorders. Computed tomography (**CT**) **scan of the chest** also may be useful in assessing lesions identified with barium swallow or endoscopy thought to be malignancies and in assessing the presence of complex paraesophageal hernias. A **modified fluoroscopic barium study in the lateral projection** may be useful in identifying mechanical disorders of the pharyngeal swallowing mechanism.

Endoscopy
Most patients with swallowing disorders or pain should undergo esophagoscopy. Patients with dysphagia should undergo esophagoscopy, even in the presence of a normal barium swallow. A barium swallow performed before esophagoscopy helps the endoscopist to focus on any subtle radiographic findings and helps to prevent

endoscopic misadventures with anatomic abnormalities such as esophageal diverticula.

For the initial assessment, the **flexible esophagoscope** allows a safe, thorough assessment that can be performed quickly in an outpatient setting with high patient tolerance and acceptance. The mucosa of the entire esophagus, stomach, and duodenum should be inspected carefully. Any areas of mucosal irregularity or abnormality should be photodocumented and biopsied. Retroflex views within the stomach of the gastroesophageal junction should note the presence of hiatal hernia. The location of the transition from squamous mucosa to columnar gastric mucosa (Z-line) should be noted as the distance from the incisors to this point of transition. Known esophageal diverticula can be investigated endoscopically; however, great care should be taken because diverticula can be perforated easily.

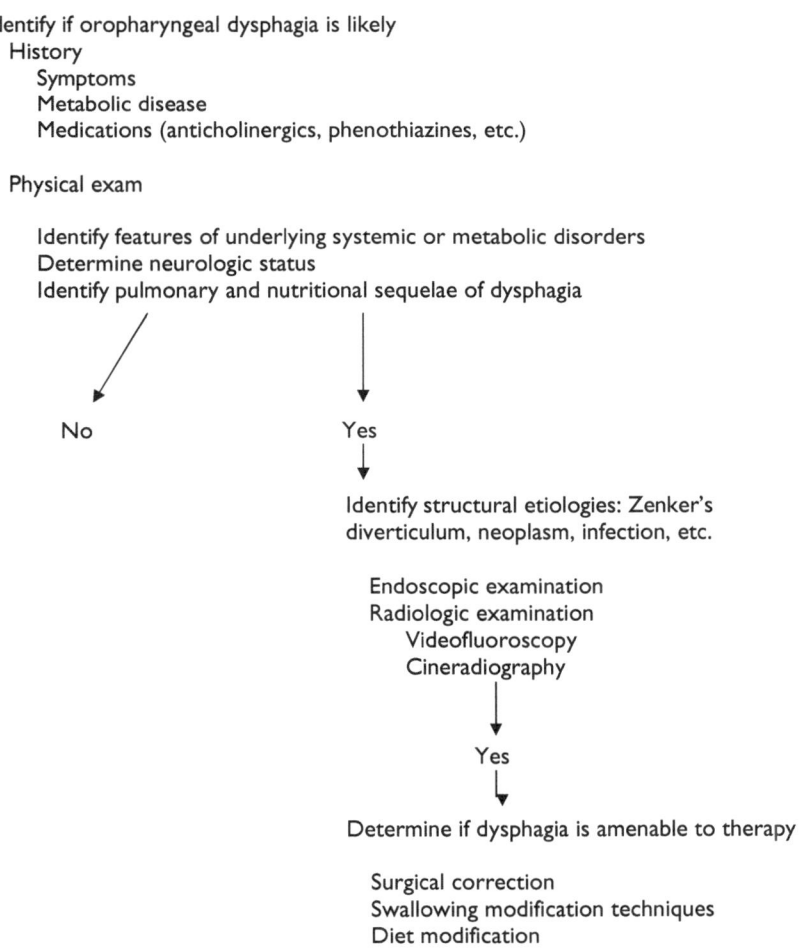

Algorithm 12.1. Algorithm for swallowing evaluation (dysphagia).

Rigid esophagoscopy rarely is indicated and remains a tool used primarily in the operating room when cricopharyngeal or cervical esophageal lesions prevent passage of a flexible scope, when biopsies deeper than those obtainable with flexible endoscopy are needed to stage disease and plan resective therapy, and for the removal of foreign bodies.

Endoscopic ultrasound (EUS) is a newer technique. It allows characterization and staging of esophageal lesions by imaging the layers of the esophageal wall and surrounding structures in order to identify depth of tumor invasion and periesophageal lymphadenopathy, and it allows EUS-guided fine-needle aspiration of lymph nodes.

Assessment of Functional Abnormalities

Esophageal Manometry
Esophageal manometry has become widely available to examine the motor function of the esophagus and the LES (**Fig. 12.3**). **Manometry is indicated when a motor abnormality is suspected on the basis of symptoms of dysphagia or odynophagia and when the barium swallow and esophagoscopy do not show an obvious structural**

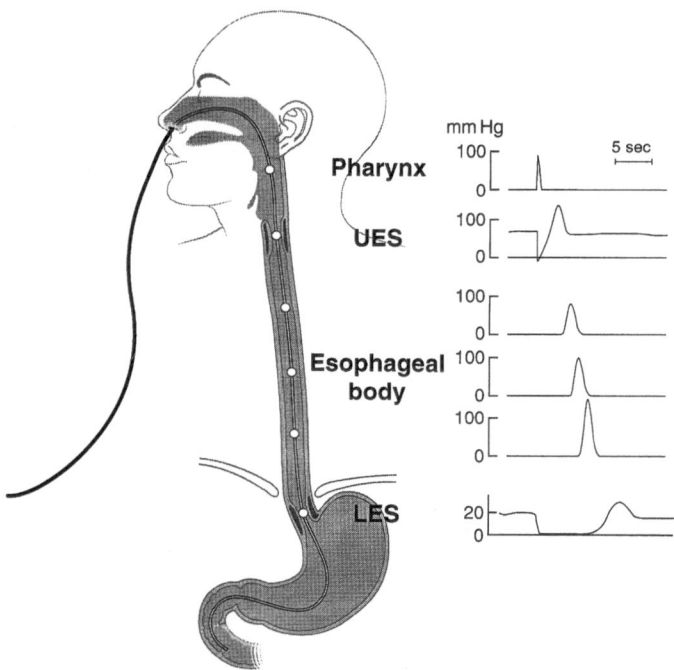

Figure 12.3. Esophageal manometry. Swallowing requires coordinated relaxation and contraction of the upper and lower esophageal sphincters (*UES, LES*) and adequate peristalsis of the esophageal body. (Reprinted from Rice TW. Esophagus. In: Norton JA, Bollinger RR, Chang AE, et al, eds. Surgery: Basic Science and Clinical Evidence. New York: Springer-Verlag, 2001, with permission.)

abnormality. **Manometry also is indicated when esophageal dysmotility or LES dysfunction is either associated with or a consequence of other structural abnormalities such as hiatal and paraesophageal hernias. Manometry is essential to confirm diagnosis of primary esophageal motility disorders such as achalasia, diffuse esophageal spasm, nutcracker esophagus, and hypertensive lower esophageal sphincter.** It may be useful in identifying nonspecific esophageal motility disorders and motility abnormalities secondary to systemic diseases of scleroderma, dermatomyositis, polymyositis, or mixed connective tissue disease. In patients with symptomatic gastroesophageal reflux, manometry is useful particularly in confirming inadequate function of the LES, assessing preoperative esophageal clearance mechanisms, and determining operative or nonoperative therapy. Esophageal manometry is performed by passing a catheter nasally into the stomach while measuring pressure through a pressure-sensitive transducer. Pharyngeal, esophageal body, and LES function can be recorded and assessed using computer-based analysis software.

Assessment of Esophageal Exposure to Gastric Content

Ambulatory 24-hour esophageal pH monitoring has become the standard for quantitating esophageal exposure to acidic content and relating symptoms to esophageal pH. A multichannel pH electrode is positioned with at least two sensors proximal to the manometrically identified LES. Gastric pH can be measured along with esophageal pH. While the patient continues a normal routine, including eating and the usual activities, the pH is recorded throughout a 24-hour cycle. The patient maintains a diary, recording body positions, meals, and symptoms, so that esophageal pH can be correlated with symptoms. At the completion of the test, the results are tallied and compared to normal values for esophageal acid exposure. The study can be performed in the presence or absence of acid-reducing medications in order to determine the effectiveness of the medication.

Twenty-four-hour pH monitoring is indicated for patients who have typical symptoms of gastroesophageal reflux, for patients for whom other diagnostic tests are equivocal, for patients with atypical symptoms of gastroesophageal reflux such as noncardiac chest pain, persistent cough, wheezing, and unexplained laryngitis, or for patients with previously failed esophageal or gastric surgery with recurrent symptoms.

Provocation of Esophageal Symptoms

Three tests previously were used to identify a relationship between symptoms and esophageal exposure to acid or motor abnormalities: the acid perfusion test (Bernstein, 0.1 N HCl infusion), edrophonium (Tensilon, acetylcholinase inhibitor precipitates contractions), and balloon distention tests. Perfusion tests are placebo controlled. Ambulatory pH testing and esophageal manometry have made these tests primarily of historical and academic interest.

Evaluation of Gastric Motility and Biliary Disease

In evaluating a patient with esophageal symptoms, it also is important to consider the impact of gastroduodenal dysfunction on lower esophageal function as well as other common gastrointestinal problems that can mimic esophageal disease. A gastric emptying study and/or right upper quadrant ultrasound may be indicated in patients with symptomatology suggestive of esophageal disorders in order to rule out gastroparesis or gallbladder disease.

Specific Conditions

Tumors

Malignant Esophageal Tumors

Overview: **The majority of esophageal neoplasms are malignant.** Less than 1% of tumors are benign. Esophageal cancer is among the top 10 leading causes of cancer deaths in the United States and is increasing in incidence. Late presentation and early spread lead to a poor prognosis. The overall 5-year survival rate is 8% to 12%. Although squamous cell carcinoma previously accounted for 90% to 95% of reported esophageal malignancies, the incidence of adenocarcinoma has increased dramatically in the past two decades and now accounts for at least 40% of all malignancies. This relative change may reflect the increased use of flexible endoscopy and closer surveillance of asymptomatic patients who are at risk of developing esophageal carcinoma. Other cell types of esophageal malignancy are extremely rare.

Squamous cell carcinomas are distributed equally among the upper, middle, and lower thirds of the esophagus. **Adenocarcinomas** most commonly are found in the lower third of the esophagus. Most adenocarcinomas are thought to arise in columnar cell Barrett's mucosa. Alcohol consumption and tobacco use are well-established factors for the development of esophageal carcinoma. Other risk factors for esophageal cancer include achalasia, radiation esophagitis, caustic esophageal injury, infection (human papilloma virus), Plummer–Vinson syndrome, leukoplakia, esophageal diverticula, ectopic gastric mucosa, and the inherited condition of familial keratosis palmaris et plantaris (tylosis).

Diagnosis: **The vast majority of esophageal carcinomas are clinically occult and present well after disease progression prevents cure.** As in **Case 1**, the classic history is a patient who presents with dysphagia and weight loss; chest pain, abdominal pain, and gastrointestinal (GI) blood loss are described less frequently (**Table 12.4**). Most patients experience dysphagia an average of 2 to 4 months before presentation. Unfortunately, dysphagia almost uniformly indicates extensive disease and incurability.

The initial study should be a **barium swallow**; this most frequently reveals distinct mucosal irregularity, stricture, a shelf in the lower esophagus, or rigidity. **Upper esophageal endoscopy** allows visualization of the affected area and biopsy to confirm the diagnosis.

Table 12.4. Presenting symptoms of esophageal carcinoma.

Symptom	Incidence (%)
Dysphagia	87
Weight loss	71
Substernal or epigastric pain/ burning	46
Vomiting or regurgitation	28
Aspiration pneumonia	14
Palpable cervical nodes	14
Hoarseness	7
Coughing and choking	3

Source: Reprinted from Smith CD. Esophagus. In: Norton JA, Bollinger RR, Chang AE, et al, eds. Surgery: Basic Science and Clinical Evidence. New York: Springer-Verlag, 2001, with permission.

Staging: The **stage** of esophageal cancer is determined by the **depth of penetration of the primary tumor (T) and the presence of lymph node (N0, N1) and distant organ metastasis (M0, M1).** The TNM descriptors can be grouped into stages with similar behavior and prognosis. Clinical (cTNM) preoperative staging determines the intent and extent of subsequent treatment, either curative or palliative. Initial staging includes a **careful physical examination for the sequelae of esophageal cancer (weight loss, supraclavicular adenopathy, pleural effusion), routine blood tests, and CT scan of the chest and abdomen. Bronchoscopy** is indicated for midesophageal tumors because of their propensity to invade the trachea and left mainstem bronchus.

The recent development of **EUS has improved staging by allowing the depth of invasion into the esophageal wall to be determined accurately and by allowing the surrounding lymph node involvement to be identified and biopsied.**

Weight loss greater than 10% has been shown to be associated with a significantly poorer outcome in patients with operable esophageal cancer. Clinical staging categorizes patients into two groups: those with potentially curable disease and those with metastatic disease (disease outside of the local or regional area) in whom palliation is currently the only treatment option.

Treatment: The overall prognosis for esophageal carcinoma is bleak. An overall 5-year survival for esophageal cancer patients was reported in only 4% after surgical resection (surgical mortality, 29%) and in only 6% after radiation therapy. **The treatment of esophageal cancer is generally a palliative practice, and cure is a chance occurrence.** However, precise clinical staging allows treatment modification of patients with carcinoma of the esophagus. **Surgical, radiation, and chemotherapy therapies** are possible, with optimal outcomes often utilizing a combination approach.

Based on reviews of current literature available on the multimodality management of patients with esophageal carcinoma, treatment pro-

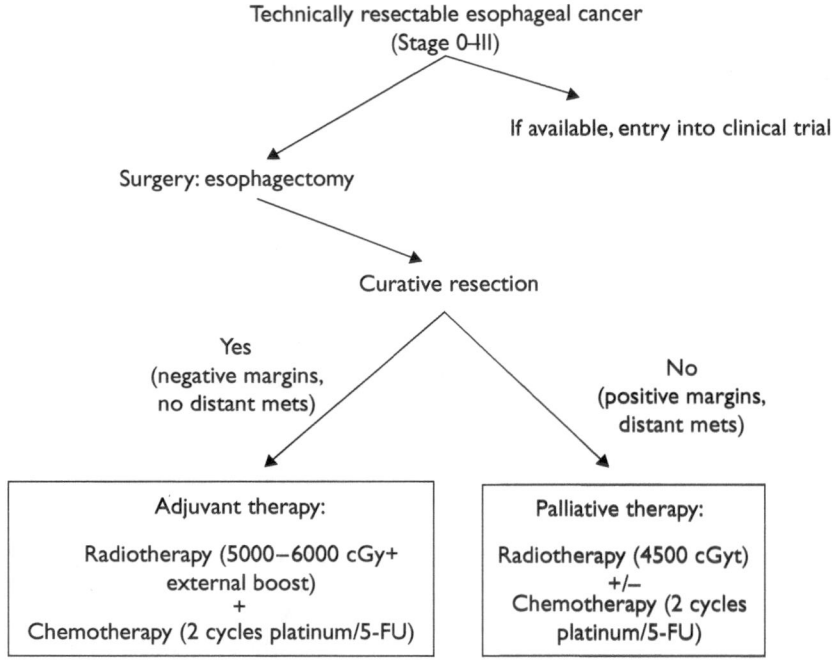

Algorithm 12.2. Management of technically resectable esophageal cancer, 5-Fu, 5-fluorouracil; mets, metastases. (Reprinted from Smith CD. Esophagus. In: Norton JA, Bollinger RR, Chang AE, et al, eds. Surgery: Basic Science and Clinical Evidence. New York: Springer-Verlag, 2001, with permission.)

tocols have been developed and are the basis of published practice guidelines for esophageal cancer (see **Algorithms 12.2 and 12.3**).[1]

Surgery: **Esophagectomy with gastric or colon replacement** is the treatment of choice for small tumors confined to the esophageal mucosa or submucosa. Surgical treatment for resectable esophageal cancers results in 5-year survival rates of 5% to 20% and an operative

---

[1] DeMeester TR, Bonavina L, Albertucci M. Evaluation of primary repair in 100 consecutive patients. Ann Surg 1986;204:9–20. Donohue PE, Samelson S, Nyhus LM, et al. The Nissen fundoplication. Effective long-term control of pathologic reflux. Arch Surg 1985;120:663–667. Ellis FH. The Nissen fundoplication. Ann Thorac Surg 1992;54:1231–1235. Grande L, Toledo-Pimentel V, Manterola C, et al. Value of Nissen fundoplication in patients with gastro-oesophageal reflux judged by long-term symptom control. Br J Surg 1994;81:548–550. Johansson J, Johnsson F, Joelsson B, et al. Outcome 5 years after 360 degree fundoplication for gastro-oesophageal reflux disease. Br J Surg 1993;80:46–49. Luostarinen M, Isolauri J, Laitinen J, et al. Fate of Nissen fundoplication after 20 years. A clinical, endoscopical, and functional analysis. Gut 1993;34:1015–1020. Macintyre IM, Goulbourne IA. Long-term results after Nissen fundoplications: a 5–15-year review. J R Coll Surg Edinb 1990; 35:159–162. Martin CJ, Cox MR, Cade RJ. Collis-Nissen gastrooplasty fundoplication for complicated gastrooesophageal reflux disease. Aust N Z J Surg 1992;62:126–129. Mira-Navarro J, Bayle-Bastos F, Frieyro-Segui M, et al. Long-term follow-up of Nissen fundoplication. Eur J Pediatr Surg 1994;4:7–10.

mortality of 2% to 7%. Once symptoms appear, most esophageal cancers have invaded adjacent structures or have spread to distant organs. In those cases in which significant obstructive symptoms exist, operative management often is the most effective means of relieving dysphagia and providing long-term palliation. In general, because esophageal cancer can have extensive and unpredictable spread longitudinally, it seems prudent to perform **total esophagectomy**, especially for those proximal- and middle-third lesions. Distal small lesions may be approached through the abdomen only, or resection for palliation alone can avoid total esophagectomy and its associated morbidity.

Nonsurgical Therapy: A randomized phase III study of chemotherapy with cisplatin, fluorouracil, and radiotherapy versus radiation therapy alone in patients with T1–3, N0–1, M0 esophageal carcinoma has demonstrated a **survival advantage for patients receiving combined therapy (Table 12.5)**. Long-term follow-up of these patients reported a 5-year survival of 26% for combined therapy, while no patient receiving radiation alone survived 5 years. A 5-year survival of 14% was seen

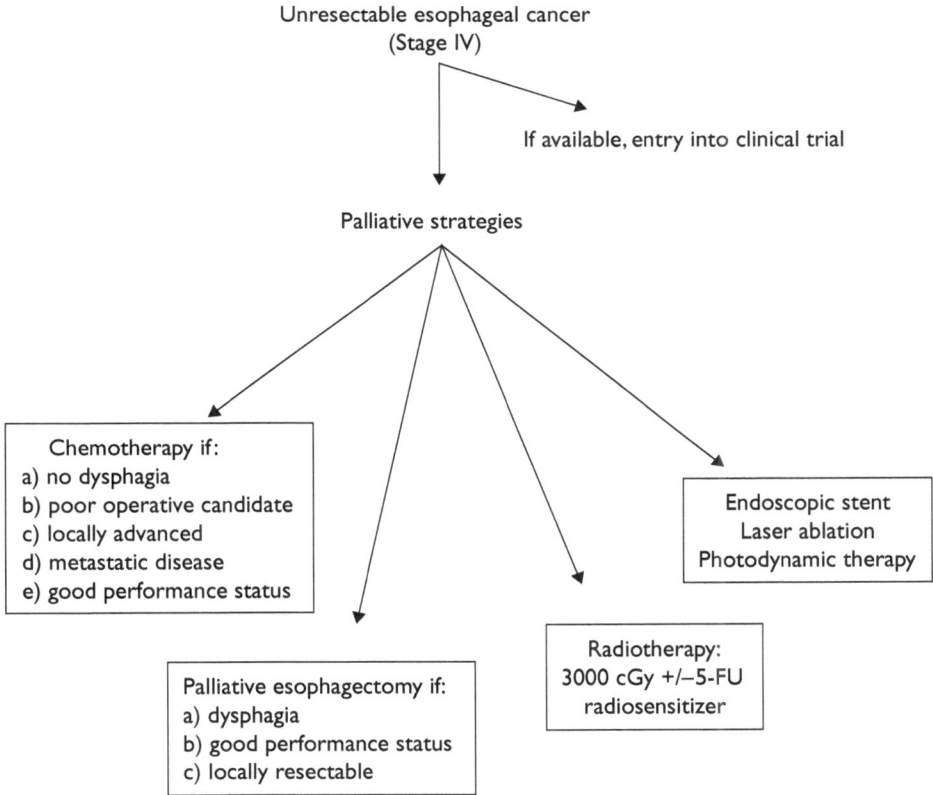

Algorithm 12.3. Management of stage IV esophageal cancer. (Reprinted from Smith CD. Esophagus. In: Norton JA, Bollinger RR, Chang AE, et al, eds. Surgery: Basic Science and Clinical Evidence. New York: Springer-Verlag, 2001, with permission.)

Table 12.5. Phase III treatment trials for esophageal carcinoma.

Author	Cell type	R1	R2	Survival	Positive findings
Cooper et al[a]	Both	Rad	Che/Rad	0% vs. 26% (5 years)	↑ Toxicity, R2
Law et al[b]	Squ	Surg	Che/Surg	Same	↑ Downstaging, R2 ↑ Curative resection, R2
Kelsen et al[c]	Both	Surg	Che/Surg	Same	
Walsh et al[d]	Adeno	Surg	Che/Rad/Surg	6% vs. 32% (3 years)	↓ N_1 and M_1 R2
Bosset et al[e]	Squ	Surg	Che/Rad/Surg	Same	↑ DF survival, R2 ↑ Curative resection, R2
Ando et al[f]	Squ	Surg	Surg/Che	Same	

Adeno, adenocarcinoma; Che, chemotherapy; Rad, radiation therapy; Squ, squamous cell carcinoma; Surg, surgery.
[a] Cooper JS. Guo MD. Herskovic A, et al. Chemoradiotherapy of locally advanced esophageal cancer. Long-term follow-up of a prospective randomized trial (RTOG 85-01). JAMA 1999;281:1623–1627.
[b] Law S, Fok M, Chow S, et al. Preoperative chemotherapy versus surgery alone for squamous cell carcinoma of the esophagus: a prospective randomized trial. J Thorac Cardiovasc Surg 1997;114:210–217.
[c] Kelsen DP, Ginsberg R, Pajak TF, et al. Chemotherapy followed by surgery compared to surgery alone for localized esophageal cancer. N Engl J Med 1998;339:1979–1984.
[d] Walsh TN, Noonan N, Hollywood D, et al. A comparison of multimodality therapy and surgery for esophageal adenocarcinoma. N Engl J Med 1996;335:462–467.
[e] Bosset JF, Gignoux M, Triboulet JP, et al. Chemoradiotherapy followed by surgery compared with surgery alone in squamous cell cancer of the esophagus. N Engl J Med 1997;337:161–167.
[f] Ando N, Iizuka T, Kakegawa T, et al. A randomized trial of surgery with and without chemotherapy for localized squamous cell carcinoma of the thoracic esophagus. J Thorac Cardiovasc Surg 1997;114:205–209.
Source: Reprinted from Rice TW. Esophagus. In: Norton JA, Bollinger RR, Chang AE, et al, eds. Surgery: Basic Science and Clinical Evidence. New York: Springer-Verlag, 2001, with permission.

in patients receiving combined therapy after randomization was closed.[2]

Palliation: **Patients with distant metastases or contraindications to chemoradiotherapy or surgery should be considered for palliative interventions.** Local and regional treatment modalities are the cornerstones of symptomatic control. **Palliative radiation therapy** is a key component and is associated with significant, albeit short-term, success in maintaining adequate swallowing. The value of **systemic chemotherapy** is limited. **Concurrent chemotherapy and radiation** have been used in the palliation of patients with metastatic tumors.

---

[2] Cooper JS, Guo MD, Herskovic A, et al. Chemoradiotherapy of locally advanced esophageal cancer. Long-term follow-up of a prospective randomized trial (RTOG 85-01). JAMA 1999;281:1623–1627. Law S, Fok M, Chow S, et al. Preoperative chemotherapy versus surgery alone for squamous cell carcinoma of the esophagus: a prospective randomized trial. J Thorac Cardiovasc Surg 1997;114:210–217. Kelsen DP, Ginsberg R, Pajak TF, et al. Chemotherapy followed by surgery compared to surgery alone for localized esophageal cancer. N Engl J Med 1998;339:1979–1984. Walsh TN, Noonan N, Hollywood D, et al. A comparison of multimodality therapy and surgery for esophageal adenocarcinoma. N Engl J Med 1996;335:462–467. Bosset JF, Gignoux M, Triboulet JP, et al. Chemoradiotherapy followed by surgery compared with surgery alone in squamous cell cancer of the esophagus. N Engl J Med 1997;337:161–167. Ando N, Iizuka T, Kakegawa T, et al. A randomized trial of surgery with and without chemotherapy for localized squamous cell carcinoma of the thoracic esophagus. J Thorac Cardiovasc Surg 1997;114:205–209.

While efficacious in improving local and regional control, this treatment comes with a significantly increased risk of toxicity and may not be appropriate in most patients.

A number of local measures can preserve swallowing and avoid the toxicity of chemotherapy and radiotherapy. **Dilation of malignant strictures with bougies or endoscopic balloon dilators** temporarily can relieve dysphagia. Dilation is typically performed not as a sole therapy but as a prelude to other, more definitive measures. **Injection with alcohol** causes tumor necrosis and a decrease in the exophytic portion of the tumor. However, dysphagia usually recurs within 30 days, necessitating retreatment.

Laser therapy is reserved for patients with severe obstruction of the esophagus requiring palliation until chemotherapy and radiotherapy take effect. It also is used in patients who are not candidates for prosthesis placement because of an anticipated short life expectancy. **Photodynamic therapy** provides longer relief of dysphagia than neodymium:yttrium-aluminum-garnet (Nd:YAG) laser therapy, but patients must avoid sunlight up to 30 days after injection because of dermal photosensitivity. This is not a desirable method of palliation for patients whose life expectancy is measured in weeks or months.

Newer, self-expanding metal stents are easier to place and require much less tumor dilation before placement. Varied lengths and configurations are available. Silicone-covered stents prevent tumor ingrowth but are more apt to migrate than noncovered stents; they are the prostheses of choice in the treatment of malignant fistula between the airway and esophagus. Stent placement after chemotherapy or radiotherapy may be associated with increased complications. Modern stents provide effective, long-lasting palliation with little morbidity and are the first mode of palliation considered for patients with esophageal carcinoma.

Benign Esophageal Tumors

Leiomyomas, Cysts, and Polyps: **Benign tumors of the esophagus are uncommon**, with three histologic types accounting for 87% of benign esophageal tumors: **leiomyomas, cysts, and polyps**. These three tumors have distinct locations in the esophagus that reflect their cells of origin.

Polyps occur almost exclusively in the cervical esophagus, while leiomyomas and cysts tend to occur in the distal two thirds.

Leiomyomas constitute 50% of benign tumors of the esophagus, with an average patient age at presentation of 38 years, in contrast to esophageal malignancy, which typically presents at a more advanced age.

Esophageal cysts are commonly congenital and are lined by columnar epithelium of the respiratory type, glandular epithelium of the gastric type, squamous epithelium, or transitional epithelium. Enteric and bronchogenic cysts are the most common. Treatment is similar to that for leiomyoma, with resection for large or symptomatic lesions. The cyst wall should be removed completely. Search for a fistulous tract to the respiratory tract should be carried out, especially in patients who have had recurrent respiratory tract infections.

Gastroesophageal Reflux Disease (GERD)

Overview

Gastroesophageal reflux (GER) is defined as failure of the antireflux barrier, allowing abnormal reflux of gastric contents into the esophagus. It is a mechanical disorder that is caused by an inadequate LES, which may be associated with a gastric emptying disorder or failed esophageal peristalsis. These abnormalities result in a spectrum of symptoms and diseases ranging from "heartburn" to esophageal tissue damage with subsequent complications of ulceration and stricture formation. A host of extraesophageal manifestations of GER, such as asthma, laryngitis, and dental breakdown, also are being increasingly identified. Gastroesophageal reflux is an extremely common condition, accounting for nearly 75% of all esophageal pathology. Nearly 44% of Americans experience monthly heartburn, and 18% of these individuals use nonprescription medication directed against GER.

Pathophysiology

Antireflux Mechanism: Although our understanding of the antireflux barrier is incomplete and has evolved over many years, a current view is that the LES, diaphragmatic crura, and phrenoesophageal ligament are key components, and **LES dysfunction is the most common cause of GER**. Three factors determine the competence of the LES: resting LES pressure, resting LES length, and abdominal length of the LES. Lower esophageal sphincter dysfunction may be either physiologic and transient or pathologic and permanent. Nearly everyone experiences physiologic reflux, most commonly related to gastric distention following a meal. Postprandial gastric distention results in pressure against the LES, which stretches and pulls the sphincter open while shortening the LES length. The resulting incompetence of the LES leads to transient periods of reflux. These transient episodes of reflux are relieved with gastric venting (belching) or when the stomach empties normally. Overeating exacerbates these episodes, and a high-fat Western diet may delay gastric emptying, thereby extending the duration of these transient episodes. **Evidence is accumulating that chronic, gastric-related, transient physiologic reflux leads to sufficient esophageal injury to cause dysfunction of the antireflux barrier; this then progresses to more permanent and pathologic reflux.**

Consequences of Reflux: Gastroesophageal reflux may lead to symptoms related to the reflux of gastric content into the esophagus, lungs, or oropharynx, or to damage to the esophageal mucosa and respiratory epithelium with subsequent changes related to repair, fibrosis, and reinjury. Manifestations of GER typically are classified as esophageal and extraesophageal. **Esophageal symptoms of GER include heartburn, chest pain, water brash, or dysphagia. Dysphagia often implicates complicated GER with esophagitis and ulceration, stricture, or Barrett's metaplastic changes. Extraesophageal manifestations gener-**

ally are pulmonary, resulting from pulmonary aspiration or bronchospasm induced when reflux stimulates a distal esophageal vagal reflex. Extraesophageal symptoms and signs include chronic cough, laryngitis, dental damage, and chronic sinusitis. With a better understanding of GER and new therapies for eliminating symptoms, fewer patients are presenting with severe complications of GER. However, those with complicated GER (high-grade esophagitis, stricture, or Barrett's mucosa) have more severe reflux, suggesting a mechanically defective LES as a major etiologic factor. Reconstruction of the defective LES has been the basis of offering operative therapy for complicated GER.

Diagnosis

The clinical diagnosis of GER is fairly straightforward if the patient reports the classic symptom of heartburn that is readily relieved after ingesting antacids. As in **Case 2**, many patients with this classic presentation will have been treated with an **empiric trial of H2 blockers or proton pump inhibitors (PPIs). Other typical symptoms of GER include regurgitation or dysphagia. Chest pain, asthma, laryngitis, recurrent pulmonary infections, chronic cough, and hoarseness may be associated with reflux.** Increasing numbers of patients with these atypical GER symptoms are being evaluated for reflux.

A careful history should confirm both typical and atypical symptoms of GER and any response to medical therapy. **Atypical symptoms, no response to high-dose medication, dysphagia, odynophagia, GI bleeding, or weight loss suggests complications of GER or another disease process entirely and should prompt a more thorough evaluation.** In a patient with typical symptoms, **endoscopic findings of esophageal erosions, ulcers, or columnar-lined esophagus are fairly specific for GER.** During **esophagogastroduodenoscopy (EGD)**, an esophageal mucosal biopsy should be obtained to confirm esophagitis, and esophageal length and the presence of a hiatal hernia or stricture can be assessed. This eliminates the need for a confirmatory barium swallow. With typical findings, no other tests beyond EGD are necessary to diagnose GER. However, in many patients, the EGD will be normal due to empiric treatment of symptoms. In this setting, 24-hour pH testing is necessary to objectively establish the diagnosis of GER.

Ambulatory 24-hour pH monitoring has been regarded as the gold standard in diagnosing GER and is of unquestionable benefit in patients where the diagnosis is unclear or in those with nonerosive esophagitis on EGD. Ambulatory pH monitoring is not mandatory in patients with typical reflux symptoms and erosive esophagitis on EGD. **Barium swallow is the test of choice in evaluating the patient with dysphagia, suspected stricture, paraesophageal hernia, or shortened esophagus.** Other studies may be helpful in difficult cases, such as **gastric emptying studies in patients with significant bloating, nausea, or vomiting**.

Treatment

There is considerable debate regarding optimal treatment of GER. With many Americans experiencing daily heartburn and the established impact this condition has on an individual's quality of life, there is tremendous amount of interest and effort devoted to understanding this condition and establishing treatment algorithms that are effective and cost efficient. See **Algorithms 12.4** and **12.5** for treatment algorithms for uncomplicated and complicated GER.

Medical: The principles of nonoperative management of GER include lifestyle modifications, medical therapy for symptomatic control, and identification of those who would be best served with an antireflux operation. Although lifestyle modifications always have been the initial step in therapy, only those patients with mild and intermittent symptoms seem to benefit from lifestyle changes alone. Most patients who seek medical advice are best treated with either medication or an operation. **Selection of a particular medical regimen depends on the**

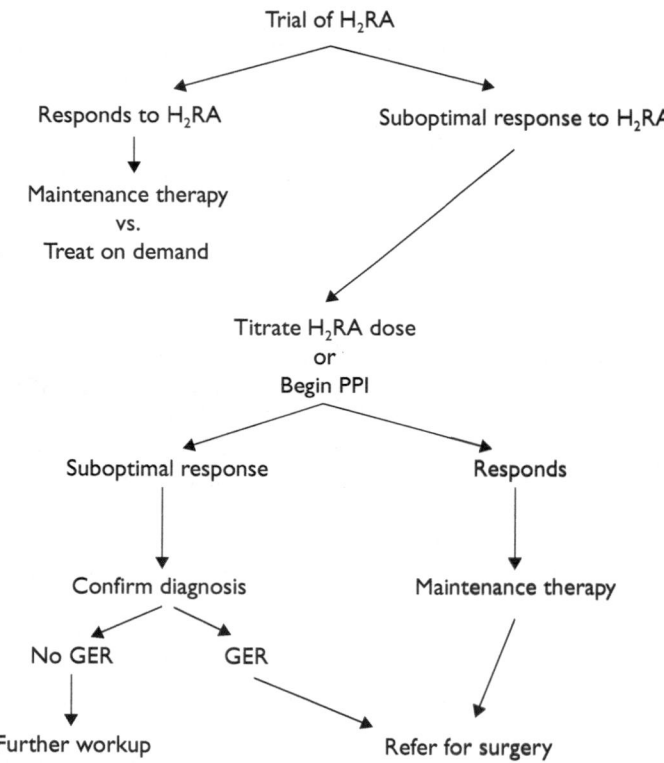

Algorithm 12.4. Management algorithm for treatment of uncomplicated gastroesophageal reflux (based on endoscopic findings). H2RA, H2 receptor antagonist; *PPI*, proton pump inhibitor; *GER*, gastroesophageal reflux. (After Fennerty MB, Castell D, Fendrick AM, et al. The diagnosis and treatment of gastroesophageal reflux disease in a managed care environment. Suggested disease management guidelines. Arch Intern Med 1996;156:477–484, with permission. Copyright © 1996 American Medical Association. All Rights Reserved. Reprinted from Smith CD. Esophagus. In: Norton JA, Bollinger RR, Chang AE, et al, eds. Surgery: Basic Science and Clinical Evidence. New York: Springer-Verlag, 2001, with permission.)

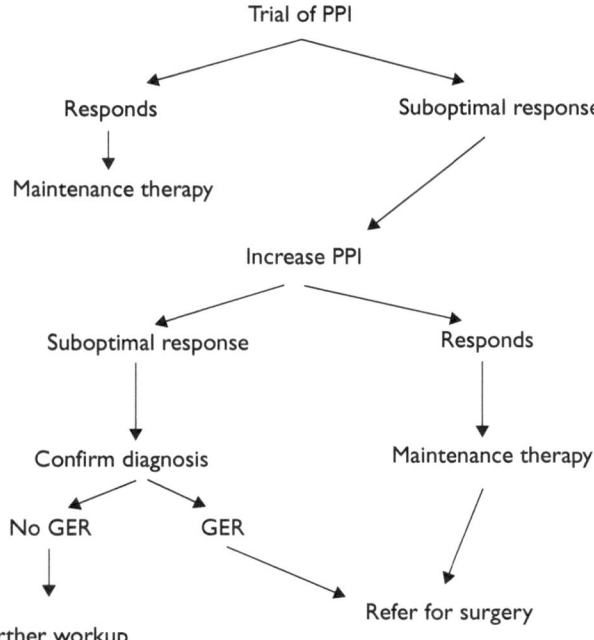

Algorithm 12.5. Management algorithm for treatment of complicated gastro-esophageal reflux (based on endoscopic findings). PPI, proton pump inhibitor; GER, gastroesophageal reflux. (After Fennerty MB, Castell D, Fendrick AM, et al. The diagnosis and treatment of gastroesophageal reflux disease in a managed care environment. Suggested disease management guidelines. Arch Intern Med 1996;156:477–484, with permission. Copyright © 1996 American Medical Association. All Rights Reserved. Reprinted from Smith CD. Esophagus. In: Norton JA, Bollinger RR, Chang AE, et al, eds. Surgery: Basic Science and Clinical Evidence. New York: Springer-Verlag, 2001, with permission.)

severity of GER, effectiveness of the proposed therapy, cost, and convenience of the regimen.

Numerous trials have shown that short-term treatment of GER with acid-suppression regimens can effectively relieve symptomatic GER and heal reflux esophagitis in approximately 90% of cases with intensive therapy. Levels of success depend on the type, duration, and dosage of antisecretory therapy. The PPIs have profoundly changed the medical treatment of GER. Rates of healing of esophagitis have improved dramatically with PPIs when compared to H2 receptor antagonists. The cost of PPIs has led many to recommend their use in only complicated or refractory GER. It appears that reflux symptoms permanently disappear only in a minority of patients with GER when they are taken off medications. Recurrence of symptoms and esophagitis is observed frequently, and thus treatment strategies based on effectiveness and outcome must be based on long-term follow-up. In fact, reflux disease must be considered a lifelong disease that requires a lifelong treatment strategy.

Surgical: Treatment algorithms for both uncomplicated (see **Algorithm 12.4**) and complicated (see **Algorithm 12.5**) reflux esophagitis begin with medical therapy. The expense and psychological burden of a lifetime of medication dependence, undesirable lifestyle changes, the uncertainty as to the long-term effects of some newer medications, and the potential for persistent mucosal changes despite symptomatic control all make surgical treatment of GER an attractive option. **Surgical therapy, which addresses the mechanical nature of this condition, is curative in 85% to 93% of patients.** Chronic medical management may be most appropriate for patients with limited life expectancy or comorbid conditions that would prohibit safe surgical intervention.

Historically, antireflux surgery was recommended only for patients with refractory or complicated gastroesophageal reflux. Recent developments have affected the long-term management of patients with GER. The rapid postoperative recovery seen with laparoscopic surgery is now feasible following antireflux procedures. The widespread availability and use of ambulatory pH monitoring has improved recognition of true GER and selection of patients for long-term therapy. Physicians now recognize that patients with GER have a greatly impaired quality of life, which normalizes with successful treatment.

The management goals of GER have changed. Rather than focusing therapy only on controlling symptoms, modern treatment aims to eliminate symptoms, improve a patient's quality of life, and institute a lifelong plan for management. **Controlled trials that compared medical and surgical therapy of GER have favored surgical therapy.** Surgical treatment was significantly more effective in improving symptoms and endoscopic signs of esophagitis for as long as 2 years. Other longitudinal studies report good to excellent long-term results in 80% to 93% of surgically treated patients (**Table 12.6**).

Table 12.6. Medical versus surgical treatment of Barrett's esophagus.

Author	No. patients		Symptom control		Stricture/esophagitis	
	Medical	Surgical	Medical	Surgical	Medical	Surgical
Attwood 1992[b] (p)[a]	26	19	22%	81%	38%	21%
Oritz 1996[c] (pr)	27	32	85%	89%	53%/45%	5%/15%
Sampliner 1994[d] (p)	27	—	70%	—	50%	—
Csendes 1998[e] (pr)	—	152	—	46%	—	64%

pr, prospective randomized; p, prospective; ret, retrospective.
[a] Before availability of proton pump inhibitors.
[b] Attwood SE, Barlow AP, Norris TL, et al. Barrett's oesophagus: effect of antireflux surgery on symptom control and development of complications. Br J Surg 1992;79:1050–1053.
[c] Ortiz A, Martinez de Haro LF, Parrilla P, et al. Conservative treatment versus antireflux surgery in Barrett's oesophagus: long-term results of a prospective study. Br J Surg 1996;83:274–278.
[d] Sampliner RE. Effect of up to 3 years of high-dose lansoprazole on Barrett's esophagus. Am J Gastroenterol 1994;89:1844–1848.
[e] Csendes A, Braghetto I, Burdiles P, et al. Long-term results of classic antireflux surgery in 152 patients with Barrett's esophagus: clinical, radiologic endoscopic, manometric, and acid reflux test analysis before and late after operation. Surgery (St. Louis) 1998;126:645–657.
Source: Reprinted from Smith CD. Esophagus. In: Norton JA, Bollinger RR, Chang AE, et al, eds. Surgery: Basic Science and Clinical Evidence. New York: Springer-Verlag, 2001, with permission.

Indications: **Antireflux surgery should be considered in patients in whom intensive medical therapy has failed.** With the advent of proton pump inhibitors, true medical failures are unusual. **Antireflux surgery also should be offered to patients whose symptoms recur immediately after stopping medications and who require long-term daily medication.** Many patients want to avoid the cost, inconvenience, and side effects of long-term medication and want to preserve their quality of life. Complications of GER, such as Barrett's esophagus and esophageal stricture, should not alter the approach to long-term management. However, patients with these complications usually have more severe disease, require more intensive medical therapy, and are referred for surgical evaluation. Occasionally, GER presents atypically with chest pain, asthma, chronic cough, or hoarseness. Patients with these atypical symptoms usually improve with surgery. However, appropriate patient selection can be very difficult. Ambulatory pH monitoring has been thought to provide the most objective way to select these patients for surgery, but an abnormal pH study does not correlate well with symptom relief following antireflux surgery. Therefore, a trial of medical therapy with resolution of symptoms remains the best way to prove an association between GER and an individual's atypical symptoms. When such an association exists, antireflux surgery is indicated.

Preoperative Evaluation: The preoperative evaluation should both justify the need for surgery and direct the operative technique to optimize outcome. At a minimum, all patients being considered for surgery should undergo **a thorough history and a physical exam, EGD, and esophageal manometry**. Esophageal manometry allows evaluation of the lower esophageal sphincter and is diagnostic in differentiating GER from achalasia. Equally important is its use in assessing esophageal body pressures and identifying individuals with impaired esophageal clearance who may not do as well with a 360-degree fundoplication.

Procedures: To establish an effective antireflux barrier, **operative procedures for GER are designed to restore adequate LES pressure, position the LES within the abdomen where it is under positive (intraabdominal) pressure, and to close any associated hiatal defect.** Advances in laparoscopic technology and technique allow the reproduction of "open" procedures while eliminating the morbidity of an upper midline incision. Open antireflux operations remain indicated when the laparoscopic technique is not available or is contraindicated. Contraindications to laparoscopic antireflux surgery include uncorrectable coagulopathy, severe chronic obstructive pulmonary disease (COPD) such that CO_2 elimination is impeded during laparoscopy, and advanced pregnancy. Only a very experienced laparoscopic surgeon should attempt the minimally invasive approach in the presence of previous upper abdominal operation or prior antireflux surgery.

In patients with normal esophageal body peristalsis, **laparoscopic Nissen fundoplication (Fig. 12.4)** has emerged as the most widely accepted and applied antireflux operation. Thousands of laparoscopic Nissen fundoplication patients have been reported in the world litera-

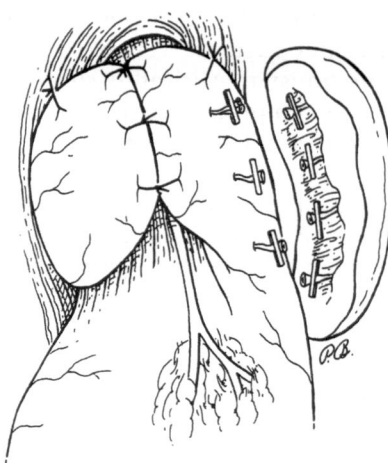

Figure 12.4. Depiction of Nissen 360-degree fundoplication. (Reprinted from Smith CD. Esophagus. In: Norton JA, Bollinger RR, Chang AE, et al, eds. Surgery: Basic Science and Clinical Evidence. New York: Springer-Verlag, 2001, with permission.)

ture, with 93% of patients symptom free at 1 year postoperatively. Only 3% require some medical therapy for symptom control. Overall, 97% of patients are satisfied with their results. Transient dysphagia occurs in nearly 50% and resolves within 3 weeks of surgery.

Summary: **Antireflux surgery is indicated in any patient with GER refractory to medical management or in any patient who has symptom recurrence when medicine is withdrawn.** In many patients with classic symptoms, an EGD and esophageal manometry are all the preoperative testing necessary. Additional tests are confirmatory in difficult cases. The laparoscopic Nissen fundoplication is both safe and effective in the long-term management of nearly all patients with chronic GER. The Toupet fundoplication may be best used in patients with impaired esophageal body peristalsis.

Hiatal Hernias: Sliding and Paraesophageal Hernias

Overview

The majority of patients with hiatal hernia are asymptomatic, and the diagnosis often is made incidentally during investigation of other gastrointestinal problems. The underlying etiology of hiatal hernias remains unclear.

Hiatal hernias can be classified into four types. A **type I hiatal hernia** (**Fig. 12.5**) also is known as a **sliding hiatal hernia**. It consists of a simple herniation of the gastroesophageal junction into the chest. The phrenoesophageal ligament is attenuated, and there is no true hernia sac. This is the most common hiatal hernia and is frequently diagnosed in women and in the fifth and sixth decades of life. **Type II hiatal hernias** (**Fig. 12.5**) are commonly referred to as **paraesophageal hernias**. The gastroesophageal junction remains at the esophageal hiatus while the gastric fundus herniates alongside the esophagus, through the hiatus, and into the chest. **Type III hiatal hernias are a combination of type I and type II hernias**, with the esophagogastric junction being displaced into the chest along with the gastric fundus and body. Paraesophageal hernias (types II and III) have a true hernia sac accompanying the herniated stomach. **Type IV hernias are an advanced stage of paraesophageal hernia** in which the entire stomach and other intraabdominal contents (colon, spleen) are herniated into the chest. As in **Case 3**, paraesophageal hernias are found predominantly in older individuals.

Diagnosis

When symptoms are present, **sliding hernias have a different presentation from paraesophageal hernias**. Paraesophageal hernias tend to produce more dysphagia, chest pain, bloating, and respiratory problems than do sliding hernias. Symptoms associated with a sliding hernia more often are related to LES dysfunction and include classic reflux symptoms, heartburn, regurgitation, and dysphagia.

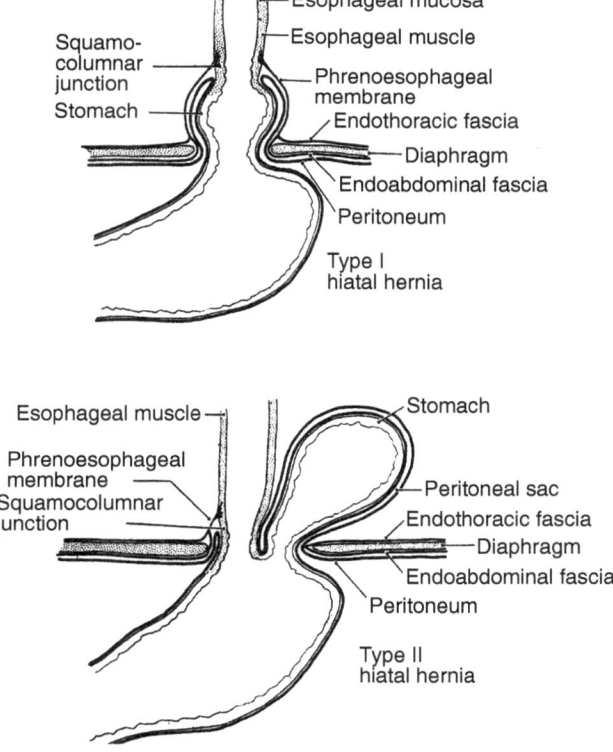

Figure 12.5. Classification of hiatal hernia. (Reprinted from Smith CD. Esophagus. In: Norton JA, Bollinger RR, Chang AE, et al, eds. Surgery: Basic Science and Clinical Evidence. New York: Springer-Verlag, 2001, with permission.)

Treatment

Because a hiatal hernia is a purely mechanical abnormality, nonoperative treatment does not exist. The risk of bleeding, incarceration, strangulation, perforation, and death with paraesophageal hernias is such that **when a type II or greater hernia is identified, operative repair should be performed.** In contrast, a significant number of patients with type I hiatal hernias are asymptomatic and remain so throughout the remainder of their life. Therefore, the presence of a sliding (type I) hiatal hernia alone does not mandate intervention. However, **patients with a type I hernia and gastroesophageal reflux, chest pain, dysphagia, regurgitation, or other symptoms referable to their hernias should undergo symptom-specific workup and may be best treated with an operative repair.** Occult gastrointestinal bleeding is a complication of hiatal hernia thought to result from the mechanical trauma of the stomach moving into and out of the chest, causing subtle erosions in the stomach that slowly bleed and lead to anemia.

The operation can be performed through the chest or abdomen and via "open" or minimally invasive techniques. Most sliding type I hernias are repaired on the basis of GER symptoms, and an antireflux procedure is critical to successful treatment. Routine addition of a fundoplication to the repair of the other three types of hiatal hernia is controversial. Most patients with type II hernias do not have reflux symptoms, and an antireflux operation for these patients may add little benefit. With careful questioning, patients with type II hernias may give a history of GER symptoms that spontaneously abated, suggesting an anatomic change (perhaps hernia development) leading to symptom resolution.

Barrett's Esophagus

Overview

Barrett's esophagus is a condition in which the normal squamous epithelium of the esophagus is partially replaced by metaplastic columnar epithelium, placing patients at risk for developing adenocarcinoma. Intestinal metaplasia (not gastric-type columnar changes) constitutes true Barrett's esophagus, with a risk of progression to dysplasia and adenocarcinoma. **Barrett's esophagus occurs in 7% to 10% of people with GER and may represent the end stage of the natural history of GER.** Barrett's esophagus is associated with a more profound mechanical deficiency of the LES, severe impairment of esophageal body function, and marked esophageal acid exposure.

Only a small number of patients with Barrett's esophagus develop carcinoma. The estimated incidence of adenocarcinoma in patients with Barrett's esophagus is 0.2% to 2.1% per year. Only patients with specialized columnar epithelium are at an increased risk of developing Barrett's adenocarcinoma. The presence of epithelial dysplasia, particularly high-grade dysplasia, is a risk factor for adenocarcinoma, and the progression of specialized columnar epithelium to dysplasia and invasive carcinoma is well documented.

Diagnosis
Heartburn, regurgitation, and—with stricture formation—dysphagia are the most common symptoms. Heartburn is milder than in the absence of Barrett's changes, presumably because the metaplastic epithelium is less sensitive than squamous epithelium. The diagnosis often is suggested by the esophagoscopic finding of a pink epithelium in the lower esophagus instead of the shiny gray-pink squamous mucosa, but every case should be verified by biopsy. Radiographic findings consist of hiatal hernia, stricture, ulcer, or a reticular pattern to the mucosa—changes of low sensitivity and specificity.

Treatment
Treatment goals for patients with Barrett's esophagus are relief of symptoms and arrest of ongoing reflux-mediated epithelial damage. Patients with Barrett's have more severe esophagitis and frequently require more intensive therapy for control of reflux. Regardless of medical versus surgical treatment, patients with Barrett's esophagus require **long-term endoscopic surveillance with biopsy of columnar segments for progressive metaplastic changes or progression to dysplasia**. Esophagectomy, if performed with a low operative mortality, is indicated in patients with a diagnosis of high-grade dysplasia. Several studies have compared medical and surgical therapy in patients with Barrett's esophagus.

Current evidence suggests that neither medical nor surgical therapy result in regression of Barrett's epithelium. There is evidence suggesting that antireflux surgery may prevent progression of Barrett's changes and protect against dysplasia and malignancy. **These are very strong data in support of the favorable impact of operative therapy on the natural history of Barrett's esophagus.**[3]

Achalasia

Overview
This idiopathic degenerative disorder results in aperistalsis of the esophageal body and abnormal to absent LES relaxation. It has been described in all age groups. The majority of patients present at between 20 and 40 years of age. There is no gender partiality. Achalasia is a risk factor for esophageal malignancy. Squamous cell carcinoma is estimated to develop in approximately 5% of patients at an average of 20 years after initial diagnosis. Carcinoma presents approximately 10

---

[3] Ortiz A, Martinez de Haro LF, Parrilla P, et al. Conservative treatment versus antireflux surgery in Barrett's oesophagus: long-term results of a prospective study. Br J Surg 1996;83:274–278. Martinez de Haro LF, Ortiz A, Parrilla P, et al. Long-term results of Nissen fundoplication in reflux esophagitis without strictures. Clinical, endoscopic, and pH-metric evaluation. Dig Dis Sci 1992;37:523–527. Sagar PM, Ackroyd R, Hosie KB, et al. Regression and progression of Barrett's oesophagus after antireflux surgery. Br J Surg 1995;82:806–810. Putnam JBJ, Suell DA, Natarajan G. A comparison of three techniques of esophagectomy for carcinoma of the esophagus from one institution with a residency training program. Ann Thorac Surg 1994;57:319–325.

years earlier than in the general population and is associated with a worse prognosis, possibly due to delayed diagnosis.

Diagnosis

Patients typically describe **dysphagia** for solids and, to varying degrees, for liquids. Exacerbation of dysphagia may occur with ingestion of cold liquids or during emotional stress. Symptoms onset is gradual. The average duration of dysphagia before presentation is 2 years. **Regurgitation** is reported in 60% to 90% of patients and **chest pain** in about 50%. **Recurrent respiratory infections, aspiration pneumonia, and lung abscess** also may be initial presentations.

Barium swallow reveals the typical distal esophageal bird's-beak deformity and proximal esophageal dilatation in 90% of patients (**Fig. 12.6**). This typical esophagogram also may be found with **"pseudoachalasia,"** typically seen with gastroesophageal malignancies or as part of a paraneoplastic syndrome. **Vigorous achalasia**, a very early stage of achalasia, may present with strong tertiary esophageal contractions resulting in a radiographic appearance similar to diffuse esophageal spasm. Even with a typical presentation, **esophagoscopy** is essential to investigate the esophageal mucosa and exclude a malignancy. **Esophageal manometry** is diagnostic and demonstrates absent peristalsis in the distal esophagus with incomplete or failed LES relax-

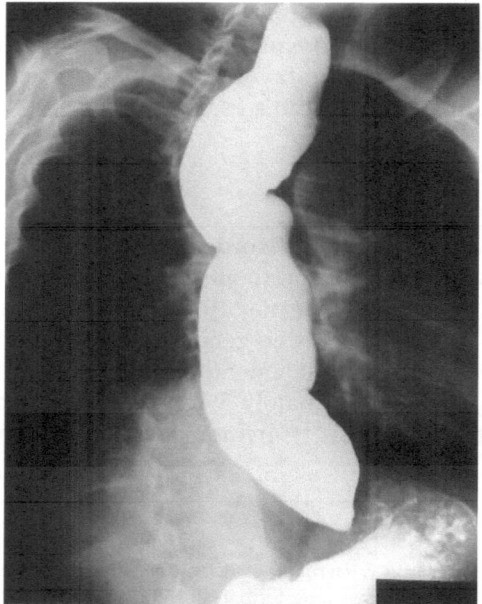

Figure 12.6. Barium esophagogram. Contour: multiple rapid swallows of low-density barium provide a full-column technique that demonstrates esophageal contour in a patient with achalasia. (Reprinted from Rice TW. Esophagus. In: Norton JA, Bollinger RR, Chang AE, et al, eds. Surgery: Basic Science and Clinical Evidence. New York: Springer-Verlag, 2001, with permission.)

ation. Normal esophageal motility should prompt an aggressive search for a tumor causing pseudoachalasia. A **CT scan of the chest or endoscopic ultrasound** usually identifies the cause of pseudoachalasia.

Treatment

The treatment of achalasia is **palliative** and directed at decreasing LES resistance and increasing esophageal emptying.

Pharmacotherapy: Calcium channel blockers (nifedipine, verapamil), opioids (loperamide), nitrates (isorsorbide dinitrate), and anticholinergics (cimetropium bromide) relax smooth muscle and have been used to treat achalasia. They provide transient and incomplete relief of symptoms and may produce unpleasant side effects. **With the excellent results obtained by other modes of therapy, pharmacotherapy is best reserved as an adjunct or for patients who are not candidates for more effective treatments.**

Endoscopic Botulinum Toxin Injection: Botulinum toxin (BoTox) is a potent inhibitor of acetylcholine release from presynaptic nerve terminals. It has been used with minimal side effects in the management of skeletal disorders such as blepharospasm and dystonias. Endoscopically injected into the LES, **BoTox has been used in the management of achalasia by decreasing the resting LES tone. It appears to be a fairly effective short-term therapy**, with results lasting at least 6 months in less than 50% of patients. Advantages include safety, ease of administration, and minimal side effects. BoTox injection may be useful in patients who are not candidates for other more efficacious therapies.

Esophageal Dilation: **Pneumatic dilation with modern instruments is highly successful in controlling symptoms.** The objective is to break muscle fibers of the LES and decrease LES tone. Dilatation carries a risk of esophageal perforation. Decreasing LES pressure does not always correspond to symptom improvement. Up to 50% of patients with initial good response to dilation have recurrence of their symptoms within 5 years. Fortunately, patients who respond to dilatation appear to respond equally well to a second session.

Surgical Myotomy: Operative esophageal myotomy divides the muscle layers of the LES without entering the esophageal mucosa. **From the available data, it appears that the long-term effectiveness of operative myotomy is better than that seen with dilatation.**

Esophageal Diverticula

Defined as an epithelial-lined mucosal pouch that protrudes from the esophageal lumen, esophageal diverticula are an acquired disorder, with most occurring in adults. Most are pulsion diverticula, the consequence of elevated intraluminal pressure causing mucosal and submucosal herniation through the musculature. Traction diverticula occur as a periesophageal inflammatory process adheres, scars, and retracts, pulling the esophageal wall. Diverticula found in the pharyngoesophageal and epiphrenic locations are pulsion diverticula associated with abnormal esophageal motility. Midesophageal diverticula usually are traction diverticula resulting from mediastinal lymph node inflammation.

Motor Disorders

Disordered motor function of either the pharyngeal or esophageal phase of swallowing leads to a variety of swallowing disorders, with the primary clinical manifestation being dysphagia. The development and widespread use of esophageal manometry has allowed the characterization of both normal and abnormal motor function of the esophagus.

Disordered Pharyngeal Swallowing
Diseases affecting pharyngoesophageal function produce a characteristic type of dysphagia. Patients experience the more universally understood symptom of "difficulty in swallowing." Neurologic and muscular disorders such as stroke, amyotrophic lateral sclerosis, and muscular dystrophies may present with dysphagia and esophageal dysfunction. **Table 12.7** lists conditions that can disrupt the carefully coordinated steps in the pharyngeal phase of swallowing. Aspiration or nasopharyngeal regurgitation can occur frequently.

Primary Esophageal Motor Disorders

Overview: Spastic disorders of the esophagus are primarily disorders defined by manometric abnormalities in the smooth muscle segment of the esophagus. These smooth muscle "spasms" typically consist of tertiary contractions that are simultaneous, repetitive, nonperistaltic, and often of prolonged duration and increased power. **Spastic disorders of the esophagus classically are discussed as four distinct entities: diffuse esophageal spasm, nutcracker esophagus, hypertensive LES, and nonspecific esophageal motility dysfunction (Table 12.8).** Reports of evolution of one motility pattern into another suggest that these separate disorders may be within a single spectrum of motor dysfunction.

Diagnosis and Treatment Overview: **Dysphagia and chest pain are the dominant presenting symptoms,** with chest pain occurring in 80% to 90% of patients and dysphagia in 30% to 60%. Symptoms often are

Table 12.7. Classification of disordered pharyngeal phase of swallowing.

Muscular diseases (dermatomyositis, polymyositis, etc.)
Central nervous system disease (CVA, MS, AMLS, brainstem tumor, etc.)
Miscellaneous
  Structural lesions
  Cricopharyngeus dysfunction

AMLS, amyotrophic lateral sclerosis; CVA, cardiovascular accident; MS, multiple sclerosis.
Source: Reprinted from Smith CD. Esophagus. In: Norton JA, Bollinger RR, Chang AE, et al, eds. Surgery: Basic Science and Clinical Evidence. New York: Springer-Verlag, 2001, with permission.

Table 12.8. Manometric criteria for spastic motor disorders of the esophagus.

Diffuse esophageal spasm	Simultaneous contractions (>10% of wet swallows)
	Intermittent *normal* peristalsis
Nutcracker esophagus	High-amplitude contraction (>180 mm Hg)
	Normal peristalsis
Hypertensive LES	High resting LES pressure (>45 mm Hg)
	Normal LES relaxation
	Normal peristalsis
Nonspecific motor dysfunction	Frequent nonpropagated or retrograde contractions
	Low-amplitude contractions (<30 mm Hg)
	Abnormal waveforms
	Body aperistalsis with normal LES

LES, lower esophageal sphincter.
Source: Reprinted from Smith CD. Esophagus. In: Norton JA, Bollinger RR, Chang AE, et al, eds. Surgery: Basic Science and Clinical Evidence. New York: Springer-Verlag, 2001, with permission.

brought on by psychological or emotional stress. Before the widespread availability of esophageal motility testing, many patients carried psychiatric diagnoses before their esophageal condition was identified. Often, the diagnosis of a spastic esophageal disorder becomes one of exclusion as cardiac causes or acid reflux explanations for the symptom complex are ruled out. **Esophageal manometry** remains the gold standard for diagnosing spastic esophageal disorders.

Approaches to the treatment of esophageal spastic disorders are aimed at ameliorating symptoms. After a thorough workup and exclusion of other conditions, **a trial of pharmacotherapy with smooth muscle relaxants** (calcium channel blockers, nitrates, and anticholinergics) is reasonable. Favorable responses to **dilation and BoTox** have been reported in patients with diffuse esophageal spasm and hypertensive LES. **Operative myotomy** may be particularly effective in those with hypertensive LES and less so in patients with segmental spasm and nutcracker esophagus.

Diffuse Esophageal Spasm: **Diffuse esophageal spasm (DES) is characterized by simultaneous, nonperistaltic, repetitive high-amplitude contractions of the esophageal body.** These contractions may occur spontaneously or with swallowing. The cause is unknown. Patients complain of chest pain and dysphagia and may have had extensive cardiac evaluation. **Barium esophagogram** demonstrates a normal upper esophagus with a corkscrew pattern in the distal esophagus (**Fig. 12.7**). **Esophageal manometry** is diagnostic, but the classic pattern of diffuse spasm is uncommon in patients presenting with chest pain.

Diffuse esophageal spasm has similarities to spastic bowel, and psychiatric abnormalities are present in up to 80% of patients. **The use of mild sedatives is currently the first treatment.** Calcium channel blockers and nitrates have been used to control symptoms.

Nutcracker Esophagus: **Nutcracker esophagus is characterized by hyperperistalsis of the distal esophagus with esophageal contraction pressures at least 2 standard deviations above normal.** Psychiatric disturbances also are present. Chest pain and dysphagia are managed

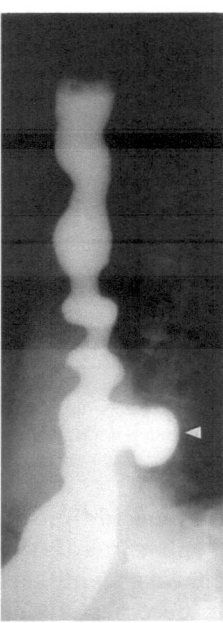

Figure 12.7. Barium esophagogram. Function: single swallows of low-density barium every 20 to 30 seconds to assess esophageal function in a patient with diffuse esophageal spasm and an epiphrenic diverticulum (*arrowhead*). (Reprinted from Rice TW. Esophagus. In: Norton JA, Bollinger RR, Chang AE, et al, eds. Surgery: Basic Science and Clinical Evidence. New York: Springer-Verlag, 2001, with permission.)

with **medical therapy**. Myotomy has unpredictable results, and surgical treatment should be avoided.

Hypertensive LES: Manometry characterizes the disorder of hypertensive lower esophageal sphincter. Resting pressure is more than 45 mm Hg. Lower esophageal sphincter relaxation and esophageal peristalsis are normal. **Medical therapy and bougie dilation** are the treatments of choice. Myotomy rarely is required.

Nonspecific Motor Disorder: Despite all attempts to classify motility disorders, many patients present with functional abnormalities of the esophageal body or sphincters that do not follow patterns. These are classified as nonspecific motility disorders and **should not be assumed to be part of a named abnormality in order to avoid a false diagnosis and incorrect therapy**. Diagnosis is by exclusion of the named motility disorders following manometry. Therapy must be individualized.

Esophageal Manifestations of Scleroderma

Scleroderma, a systemic collagen-vascular disease, impinges upon esophageal function in approximately 80% of patients. Fibrosis, collagen deposition, and patchy smooth muscle atrophy can be identified. Skeletal muscle is unaffected. Symptoms of GER are common. Esophageal smooth muscle destruction produces diminished esophageal peristalsis and a hypotensive LES. Esophageal stricture and shortening can be significant problems.

Esophageal Strictures

Diagnosis

Injury or destruction of the esophagus can result in narrowing that restricts swallowing and produces dysphagia. The patient may not perceive difficulty swallowing until the esophageal lumen is one-half the normal 20 to 25 mm diameter. Because the obstruction is structural, dysphagia associated with esophageal stricture is constant, reproducible, and predictable.

Barium esophagogram is the initial investigative tool in the evaluation of dysphagia and suspected esophageal stricture. Barium esophagogram provides a guide for **esophagoscopy**, which is the crucial invasive investigation in the diagnosis of esophageal strictures. **Endoscopy, biopsy, and dilatation** can be performed safely as one procedure.

For **benign dilatable strictures, the injuring agent must be removed and the stricture treated by dilatation as necessary**. Nondilatable benign strictures and resectable malignant strictures are treated by resection and reconstruction.

Esophageal stricture is a late **complication of severe, uncontrolled GER**. Most peptic strictures are located in the distal esophagus above a hiatal hernia and are smooth, tapered areas of concentric narrowing. Occurrence of the stricture well above the esophagogastric junction is predictive of Barrett's mucosa. Barrett's mucosa has been reported in 44% of patients with peptic esophageal strictures.

Aggressive control of acid reflux and dilatation are applied for long-term control of peptic strictures. **Both medical and surgical options are available for reflux control.** Medical management should be started in all patients after dilatation. The most potent acid suppression medications (proton pump inhibitors) also are the most successful and provide the best results in the medical treatment of peptic strictures. Surgery should be considered in young patients who will require lifelong medication and in patients who cannot tolerate medication.

Summary

The patient presenting with swallowing problems represents a significant challenge to the clinician. The complex physiology and diverse etiologies of swallowing disorders require a thorough history and a physical examination, as well as physiologically based investigations of the esophageal and upper gastrointestinal tract function. Thorough investigation should provide information sufficient to make a decision about the initiation and/or continuation of medical therapy or the need for surgical intervention.

Selected Readings

Attwood SE, Barlow AP, Norris TL, et al. Barrett's oesophagus: effect of anti-reflux surgery on symptom control and development of complications. Br J Surg 1992;79:1050–1053.

Csendes A, Braghetto I, Burdiles P, et al. Long-term results of classic antireflux surgery in 152 patients with Barrett's esophagus: clinical, radiologic, endoscopic, manometric, and acid reflux test analysis before and late after operation. Surgery (St. Louis) 1998;126:645–657.

DeMeester TR, Bonavina L, Albertucci M. Evaluation of primary repair in 100 consecutive patients. Ann Surg 1986; 204:9–20.

Donohue PE, Samelson S, Nyhus LM, et al. The Nissen fundoplication. Effective long-term control of pathologic reflux. Arch Surg 1985;120:663–667.

Ellis FH. The Nissen fundoplication. Ann Thorac Surg 1992;54:1231–1235.

Grande L, Toledo-Pimentel V, Manterola C, et al. Value of Nissen fundoplication in patients with gastro-oesophageal reflux judged by long-term symptom control. Br J Surg 1994;81:548–550.

Johansson J, Johnsson F, Joelsson B, et al. Outcome 5 years after 360 degree fundoplication for gastro-oesophageal reflux disease. Br J Surg 1993;80:46–49.

Lairmore C, Multiple endocrine neoplasia. In: Norton JA, Bollinger RR, Chang AE, et al, eds. Surgery: Basic Science and Clinical Evidence. New York: Springer-Verlag, 2001.

Lau CL, Harpole DH Jr. Lung neoplasms. In: Norton JA, Bollinger RR, Chang AE, et al, eds. Surgery: Basic Science and Clinical Evidence. New York: Springer-Verlag, 2001.

Luostarinen M, Isolauri J, Laitenen J, et al. Fate of Nissen fundoplication after 20 years. A clinical, endoscopical and functional analysis. Gut 1993;34:1015–1020.

Macintyre IM, Goulbourne IA. Long-term results after Nissen fundoplications: a 5–15-year review. J R Coll Surg Edinb 1990; 35:159–162.

Martin CJ, Cox MR, Cade RJ. Collis-Nissen gastroplasty fundoplication for complicated gastroesophageal reflux disease. Aust N Z J Surg 1992;62:126–129.

Martinez de Haro LF, Ortiz A, Parrilla P, et al. Long-term results of Nissen fundoplication in reflux esophagitis without strictures. Clinical, endoscopic, and pH-metric evaluation. Dig Dis Sci 1992;37:523–527.

Mira-Navarro J, Bayle-Bastos F, Frieyro-Segui M, et al. Long-term follow-up of Nissen fundoplication. Eur J Pediatr Surg 1994;4:7–10.

Ortiz A, Martinez de-Haro LF, Parrilla P, et al. Conservative treatment versus antireflux surgery in Barrett's oesophagus: long-term results of a prospective study. Br J Surg 1996;83:274–278.

Putnam JBJ, Suell DA, Natarajan G. A comparison of three techniques of esophagectomy for carcinoma of the esophagus from one institution with a residency training program. Ann Thorac Surg 1994;57:319–325.

Rice TW. Esophagus. In: Norton JA, Bollinger RR, Chang AE, et al, eds. Surgery: Basic Science and Clinical Evidence. New York: Springer-Verlag, 2001.

Sagar PM, Ackroyd R, Hosie KB, et al. Regression and progression of Barrett's oesophagus after antireflux surgery. Br J Surg 1995;82:806–810.

Sampliner RE. Effect of up to 3 years of high-dose lansoprazole on Barrett's esophagus. Am J Gastroenterol 1994;89:1844–1848.

Smith CD. Esophagus. In: Norton JA, Bollinger RR, Chang AE, et al, eds. Surgery: Basic Science and Clinical Evidence. New York: Springer-Verlag, 2001.

Way LW. Current Surgical Diagnosis and Treatment, 10th ed. New York: Appleton and Lang, 1994:411–440.

Hemoptysis, Cough, and Pulmonary Lesions

John E. Langenfeld

Objectives

Hemoptysis

1. To know how to assess whether a patient has life-threatening hemoptysis.
2. To list the differential diagnosis of a patient with hemoptysis.
3. To discuss the initial stabilization of a patient presenting with hemoptysis.
4. To know the different diagnostic modalities available in the assessment of pulmonary bleeding.
5. To understand the risk and benefits of surgery versus pulmonary embolization in the treatment of hemoptysis.

Pulmonary Nodule

1. To discuss the differential diagnosis of nodules presenting in the lung and mediastinum.
2. To describe the common risk factors for lung cancer and the presenting symptoms.
3. To know the algorithm for the evaluation of a patient with a lung nodule.
4. To be able to discuss the prognosis of patients with different stages of lung cancer and how surgical and medical therapies affect on survival.
5. To understand which patients do not benefit from a surgical resection.
6. To know how to evaluate a patient's risk when considering a pulmonary resection.
7. To discuss the surgical management of metastatic tumors to the lung.

Cases

Case 1

A 57-year-old man presents to the emergency room with the complaint of hemoptysis. What is the initial workup of this patient and how should he be treated?

Case 2

A 62-year-old man is referred to you because a routine chest x-ray demonstrated a 1.2-cm asymptomatic nodule in the right upper lobe. How should this patient be evaluated?

Hemoptysis

Hemoptysis most often is caused by **bronchogenic carcinomas** and **inflammatory diseases of the lung.** Hemoptysis also can be caused by **interstitial lung disease, pulmonary embolism, cardiac disease, coagulopathy, trauma, and iatrogenic causes.** The most commonly associated cardiac disease to cause hemoptysis is **mitral stenosis.** The **Swan-Ganz catheter** is the most common iatrogenic cause of massive hemoptysis in the hospital. See **Table 13.1** for a thorough listing of causes of hemoptysis.

Immediate Evaluation

The **assessment of stability** is the most important determination in the initial evaluation of a patient who presents with hemoptysis. Massive hemoptysis generally is defined as more than 250 mL of expectorated blood within 24 hours and is associated with higher mortality rates. Patients rarely exsanguinate from hemoptysis, but rather they asphyxiate from aspirated blood. Aspiration of even a small amount of blood into the airways can lead to asphyxiation. See **Case 13.1.**

Table 13.1. Causes of hemoptysis.

Bronchogenic carcinoma	Iatrogenic
Inflammatory diseases	Swan-Ganz catheter
Tuberculosis	Bronchoscopy
Aspergillosis	Pulmonary embolism
Cystic fibrosis	Arteriovenous fistula (rare)
Lung abscess	Chest trauma
Pneumonia	Pulmonary contusion
Bronchiectasis	Gunshot wound
Bronchitis	Stab wound
Cardiovascular	Transected bronchus
Mitral stenosis	Miscellaneous
Congestive heart failure	Coagulopathy
Congenital heart disease	Epistaxis
Interstitial lung disease	Broncholithiasis
Goodpasture's syndrome	
Wegener's granulomatosis	

The initial immediate assessment should determine quickly whether the patient has life-threatening hemoptysis. Patients should be considered to have potentially **life-threatening hemoptysis if they have an altered mental status, diminished blood pressure, rapid or slow pulse, or labored breathing; give a history of aspiration or massive hemoptysis; or have a room air O$_2$ saturation below 90%.** These patients should be evaluated and treated emergently.

Fortunately, most patients do not present with massive hemoptysis or with evidence of aspiration of blood. Most patients can be worked up on a more elective basis, but they should be admitted to the hospital for close observation. Consultants, who typically consist of a pulmonologist and a thoracic surgeon, should be called upon early in the patient's evaluation.

Evaluation of a Stable Patient

The initial evaluation of a stable patient with hemoptysis consists of a good history and physical. **It is important when taking a history to establish clearly that the bleeding is occurring from the lungs.** Bleeding from the nose or upper gastrointestinal tract at times can be confused with hemoptysis. A good history usually can distinguish whether the blood was coughed up from the lungs or whether it was regurgitated or vomited from the gastrointestinal tract.

History

The following information, obtained from a good history, can help determine the etiology of the hemoptysis, help guide the diagnostic evaluation, and help direct therapy:

1. The **amount** of bleeding (greater than 250 mL/24 hours is massive)
2. **Smoking** or other risk factors for cancer
3. Fever, chills, productive cough (**infectious**)
4. Acute onset of shortness of breath prior to hemoptysis (**pulmonary embolism**)
5. History of previous hemoptysis and **pulmonary diseases**
6. **Cardiac** history
7. **Medications**: Coumadin and platelet inhibitors; patients taking immunosuppressive drugs (e.g., steroids, chemotherapy) are at risk of developing fungal opportunistic infections
8. **Alcohol** use (patient at risk for aspiration pneumonia)
9. Prior history or exposure to **tuberculosis**
10. **Travel history**: (coccidioidomycosis in the Southwest, tuberculosis, common in many countries, histoplasmosis in Mississippi, Missouri, Ohio River Valley)
11. **Trauma history**

Physical Examination

Vital Signs
Heart rate, blood pressure, temperature, and respiratory rate should be determined immediately. The **oxygen saturation** also should be

determined using a pulse oxymeter (90% or below demonstrates severe hypoxia).

Head, Eyes, Ears, Nose, Throat

Assess the presence of **enlarged lymph nodes**, which may signify metastatic lung carcinoma. A **carotid bruit** suggests the presence of cardiovascular disease. Examine the **nose for evidence of bleeding**.

Chest/Lung

Assess whether **breathing is labored**, which may indicate pneumonia, presence of blood in the tracheobronchial tree, or pulmonary embolus. The presence of diminished **breath sounds and vocal fremitus** suggests consolidation of the lung. The presence of **rales** suggests congestive heart failure.

Cardiovascular

The **rhythm**, presence of a **cardiac murmur or a jugular venous distention**, and the **point of maximal impact** should be determined.

Abdomen

Examine for the presence of an **enlarged liver**, which can occur in right-sided heart failure.

Extremities/Skin

Assess for the presence of a **coagulopathy** (petechia, bruises). **Unilateral leg swelling** suggests deep venous thromboses. **Bilateral leg edema** is more consistent with lymph edema or congestive heart failure.

Diagnostic Evaluation (Table 13.2)

The history and physical help determine which diagnostic tests are needed and the urgency with which you need to proceed. In general,

Table 13.2. Diagnostic evaluation for hemoptysis.

Vital signs
Arterial blood gas
Portable chest radiograph
Blood work
CBC
Electrolytes
BUN/creatinine
Liver function
PT/PTT
Type and crossmatch
Sputum cultures
Pulmonary function test
Computed tomography (CT) of the chest
Bronchoscopy
Flexible
Rigid (massive hemoptysis)
Echocardiogram
IF heart disease is suspected

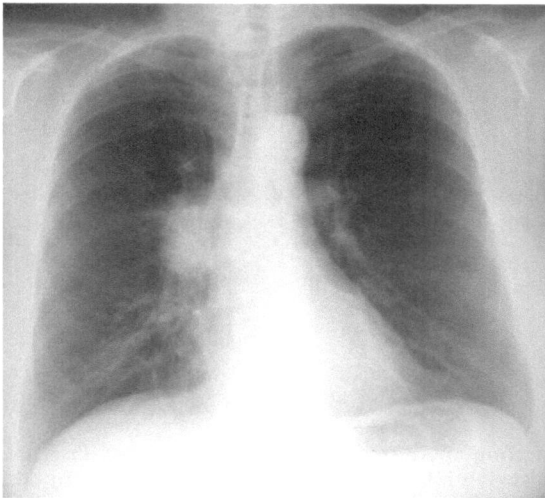

Figure 13.1. Chest radiograph of a patient with non–small-cell lung cancer discloses right hilar enlargement.

all patients should receive a **chest x-ray, an electrocardiogram (ECG), arterial blood gases, and blood work consisting of a complete blood count (CBC), electrolytes, blood ureanitrogen (BUN)/creatinine, liver function tests, prothrombin time/partial thromboplastin time (PT/PTT), and a type and crossmatch. Sputum cultures for bacteria and fungus should be obtained on all patients.**

A **chest radiograph is the first diagnostic test that should be done (Fig. 13.1).** A chest x-ray may demonstrate the presence of an abscess, lung nodule, consolidation, or atelectasis representing the possible source of bleeding. It also can suggest the presence of heart disease, showing enlargement of the ventricle or atrium and the presence of Kerley B lines. Massive pulmonary hemorrhage may occur from an area that appears normal on routine chest radiograph.

Computed tomography (CT) of the chest helps to delineate the cause of hemoptysis (Fig. 13.2). In patients with bronchiogenic carcinoma, a CT scan may demonstrate the presence of a pulmonary mass, determine the extent of local invasion, and assess metastatic spread to the mediastinal lymph nodes, liver, or adrenal glands. A CT scan also can identify a lung abscess, bronchiectasis, lung consolidation, and an arteriovenous malformation.

A **flexible bronchoscopy** frequently is used in the evaluation of a patient with hemoptysis. A flexible bronchoscopy can identify the site of the bleeding, which is critical if surgery is contemplated as a means of controlling the bleeding. A flexible bronchoscope can detect the presence of a tumor obstructing a lobar bronchus. Bronchial washings should be sent for cultures, and a cytology specimen should be examined for the presence of cancer cells. A **rigid bronchoscopy** most often

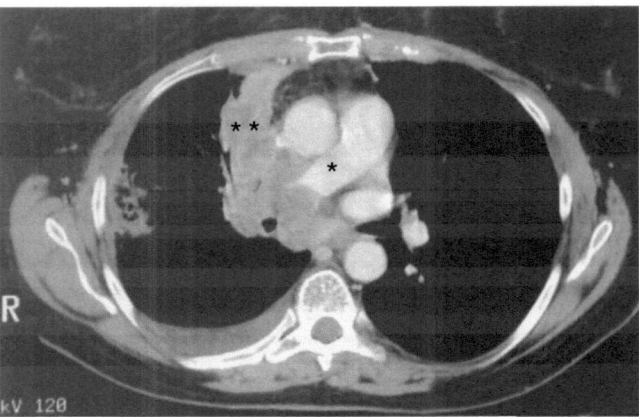

Figure 13.2. Accompanying computed tomography (CT) scan confirms the presence of extensive hilar and mediastinal adenopathy. In addition, a focal peripheral lung opacity is present: the primary lung neoplasm. Atelecfic changes also are seen in the right upper lung (**). The tumor invades the main pulmonary artery (*). A right pleural effusion is seen. This is too small to be visible on the posteroanterior (PA) chest radiograph.

is used in patients with massive hemoptysis. A rigid bronchoscope basically is a hollow metal tube with a light source and a side port for anesthesia. A rigid bronchoscopy is performed most frequently in the operating room under general anesthesia. The larger size of the rigid bronchoscope allows for better suctioning and control of the airway than a flexible bronchoscope.

Management (Table 13.3)

The treatment options for controlling bleeding originating from the lung include **medical management, bronchial lavage, embolization of bronchial arteries, and surgery. The management of patients with hemoptysis is dependent on the amount of hemoptysis, the etiology of the hemoptysis, the number of recurrent bleeding episodes, and the general medical condition of the patient.** The initial goal is to control bleeding so the workup can proceed in an organized manner.

Table 13.3. Management of patients with hemoptysis.

Medical management
Bed rest
Antitussive agent
Postural drainage and antimicrobials
Correct coagulopathies
Prevent aspiration
Ice-cold bronchial lavage
Bronchial artery embolization
Surgical resection of the bleeding lung

Fortunately, **bleeding in most patients is not massive and can be controlled with conservative measures**, which include bed rest and controlling the cough. Patients with pulmonary infections should be treated with postural drainage and started on the appropriate antimicrobial agent. Any coagulopathies should be corrected. A flexible bronchoscopy should be performed to assess for the presence of a bronchogenic carcinoma. Surgery should be considered in patients who present with recurring hemoptysis.

The objectives in treating patient with massive hemoptysis are to prevent asphyxiation, localize the site of bleeding, and arrest the hemorrhage. Medical therapy should be initiated promptly. Patients are placed with the bleeding side down to prevent aspiration of blood into the contralateral lung. A large-bore intravenous (IV) line is secured; typed and crossmatched blood is made available. Prophylactic antibiotics have been recommended, but this remains controversial. Patients with tuberculosis are treated with antituberculosis therapy. Effective antituberculin therapy can control hemoptysis, and, if surgery becomes necessary, the complication rate is reduced. Bronchodilators are not used because they may cause vasodilatation. Patients with a violent cough are treated with antitussives (codeine). However, the cough should not be suppressed completely, because this may lead to accumulation of blood in the airways.

The treatment options for a patient presenting with massive hemoptysis include continued medical management, embolization of the bleeding bronchial arteries, and a surgical resection of the lung. There are no controlled studies demonstrating superiority of one modality over another; however, the literature does support the recommendations discussed below.

Bronchial lavage has been reported to temporarily control massive hemoptysis in 97% of patients. The procedure is performed by irrigating the major bronchi of the bleeding lung with ice-cold saline using a rigid bronchoscope. Following a brief period of lavage, the nonbleeding lung is ventilated using the rigid bronchoscope. Bronchial lavage is considered a temporizing measure, and definitive therapy should not be delayed if required. The bleeding segmental bronchus can be controlled by passing a Fogarty catheter (bronchial blocker) into the appropriate segmental bronchus using a flexible bronchoscope. The bronchial blocker can tamponade the bleeding and prevent blood from accumulating into the nonbleeding lung.

Embolization of a bleeding bronchial artery is being used more frequently as the initial treatment to control massive hemoptysis. The morbidity and mortality of bronchial artery embolization is significantly less than that of an emergent pulmonary resection. Arterial embolization is 87% to 94% successful in achieving effective homeostasis. A major criticism of systemic embolization is the rate of rebleeding. Some consider embolization only a temporizing measure. Control of hemoptysis following bronchial artery embolization is 77% at 1 year and 50% to 60% at 5 years. Patients presenting with massive hemoptysis from a fungal infection or abscess are thought to be at highest risk of rebleeding. While the rate of rebleeding at 5 years is relatively high, bronchial artery embolization may represent the preferred method to control bleeding in a critically ill patient. After controlling the hemoptysis by embolization, a decision can be made as to whether a lung resection should be performed as a more elective procedure.

A surgical resection of the involved lung also has been used to control massive hemoptysis. The most commonly performed operation is a lobectomy. The site of bleeding must be localized, which usually can be achieved by bronchoscopy. Pulmonary resection has been shown to be an effective method to control and prevent recurrent bleeding. Emergency pulmonary resection has substantial mortality and morbidity rates. Spillage of blood or pus into the dependent lung contributes to the morbidity and mortality. Major complications, which include respiratory failure, bronchopleural fistula, empyema, pulmonary edema, and pneumonia, occur in up to 60% of patients. Adequate pulmonary reserve, which can be determined by a bedside spirometer, must be assessed prior to surgery. The morbidity and mortality rates following surgical resection are significantly lower when pulmonary resection is performed as an elective procedure.

Conservative measures using medical treatment and/or bronchial artery embolization should be used initially to control bleeding. An elective pulmonary resection then can be performed on medically fit patients in order to prevent recurrent hemoptysis. Patients who are typically considered for surgery are those with resectable lung carcinomas and patients with recurrent bleeding from benign disease.

Solitary Pulmonary Nodules

Evaluation of a Solitary Pulmonary Nodule (Table 13.4)

Solitary pulmonary nodules typically are found as an incidental finding on a routine chest radiograph. See Case 13.2 and Algorithm 13.1. The incidence of a solitary pulmonary nodule being malignant varies, ranging from 3% to 50%. The most common benign lesions are hamartomas and granulomas. Although metastatic tumors to the lung are frequently multiple, they can present as solitary lesions, representing 5% to 10% of resected nodules. The noninfectious granulomatous diseases sarcoidosis and Wegner's granulomatosis typically present with multiple pulmonary lesions but occasionally can present as solitary pulmonary nodules.

If the nodule contains a central nidus of calcification, diffuse calcification, or ring-like calcification, it is most likely a granuloma. Lumps of calcification throughout the lesion (popcorn calcification) suggest a hamartoma. All old chest radiographs should be reviewed if available. If the nodule had increased in size compared to a previous radiograph, this is strongly suggestive of a malignancy. Typically, if no growth is observed for 2 years, it is considered benign. However, some tumors, especially bronchioloalveolar cell carcinoma, exhibit no growth for over 2 years.

Table 13.4. Solitary pulmonary nodules.

Neoplasms
  Malignant
    Bronchial carcinoma
    Carcinoid tumor
    Metastasis
    Other rare primary lung tumor: sarcomas,
      lymphoma, melanoma, plasmacytoma
  Benign
    Hamartoma
    Other benign lung tumors (uncommon)
Inflammatory
  Infectious granulomas
    Histoplasmosis
    Tuberculosis
    Aspergillosis
    Cryptococcosis
    Blastomycosis
    Coccidioidomycosis
  Noninfectious (usually multiple)
    Sarcoidosis
    Embolus
    Rheumatoid nodule
    Wegener's granulomatosis
    Bronchiolitis obliterans-organizing pneumonia
      (BOOP)
    Mucoid impaction
Granuloma
Benign lung tumor (hamartoma)
Metastasis
Arteriovenous malformation

History

When evaluating a patient for possible lung cancer the following factors are of particular importance:

1. **Symptoms**
2. **Prior history of cancer**
3. **Smoking history**
4. **Family history of cancer**
5. **Prior medical history**

Physical Examination

Since a solitary pulmonary nodule may represent a metastatic nodule, a complete physical should be performed. Female patients should be asked whether a recent mammogram and Pap smear have been performed. Patients should be assessed for the presence of metastatic disease.

Head and Neck
Lymph nodes should be carefully examined for metastatic disease.

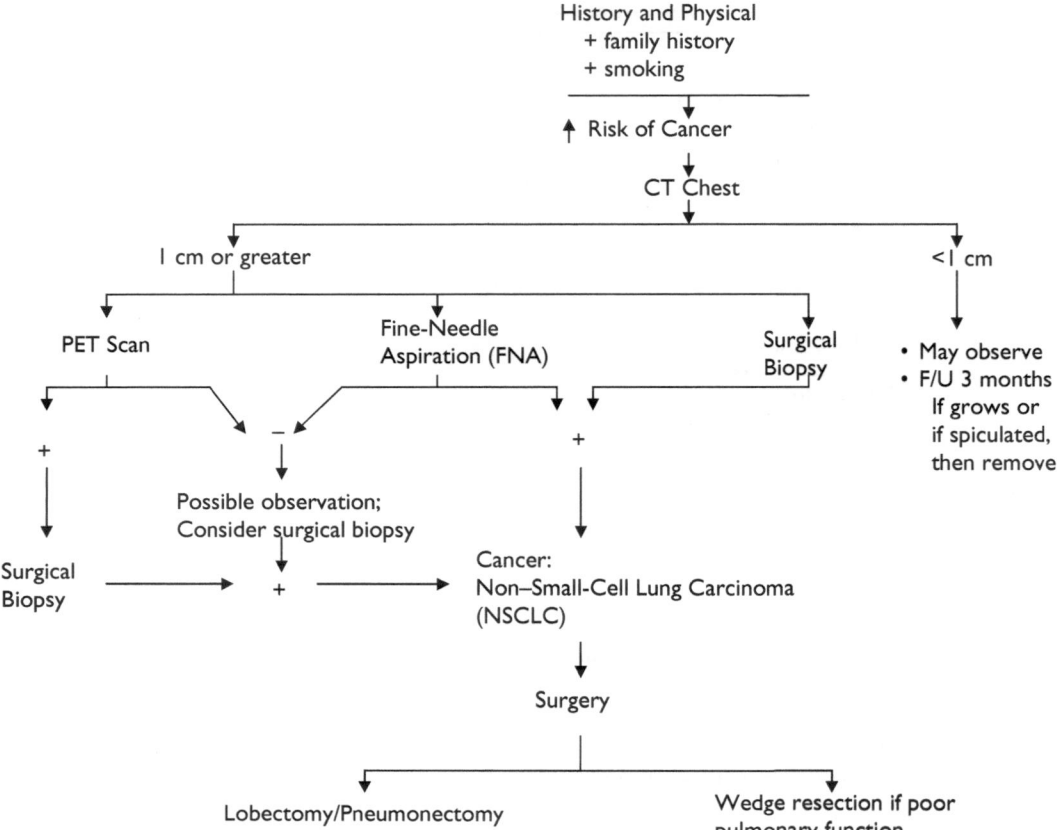

Algorithm 13.1. Algorithm for the evaluation of a solitary pulmonary module.

Cardiac
Assess **risk of cardiac disease, murmurs, enlarged heart, and jugular venous distention.**

Lungs
Examine for **accessory muscle use, wheezing, chest wall tenderness, pleural effusion, consolidation, and presence of a barreled chest from severe chronic obstructive pulmonary disease (COPD).**

Extremities
Determine the **presence of clubbing, peripheral vascular disease, and bone pain.**

Neurologic
Assess **focal neurologic deficits** from metastatic disease.

Imaging Studies

All patients with pulmonary nodules should have a CT scan of the chest (Fig. 13.2). A more recently introduced imaging modality to assess a patient's risk of having lung cancer is a **positron emission tomography (PET) scan** (Fig. 13.3); see Lung Neoplasms, below. Since diagnostic studies cannot predict absolutely which pulmonary nodules are cancerous, a **histologic evaluation** is required. **The radiographic studies can guide the physician in determining which patients should have more invasive procedures to confirm a diagnosis.** Small nodules (less than 1 cm) are observed frequently with serial CT scans. Larger lesions should have a confirmatory histologic diagnosis.

Histologic Diagnosis of a Solitary Lung Nodule

Although not commonly used today, a diagnosis of lung cancer can be made by **examining the sputum cytologically** for the presence of cancer cells. **Bronchoscopy** can make the diagnosis of lung cancer for central lesion by direct biopsy, brushing and washings. A **transthoracic fine-needle aspiration (FNA) can yield a diagnosis in 80% to 95% of patients.** Patients with intermediate FNA results have a 20% to 30% chance of having cancer. Therefore, patients with a nondiagnostic FNA should have a **lung biopsy.** The main complication with FNA is a pneumothorax, which occurs in 25% of patients. More invasive methods include a **wedge resection via video-assisted thoracoscopic surgery (VATS) or a thoracotomy. Surgery is being used more frequently to make the diagnosis of a solitary pulmonary nodule** since the VATS procedure is less invasive than a thoracotomy incision, which had been used previously.

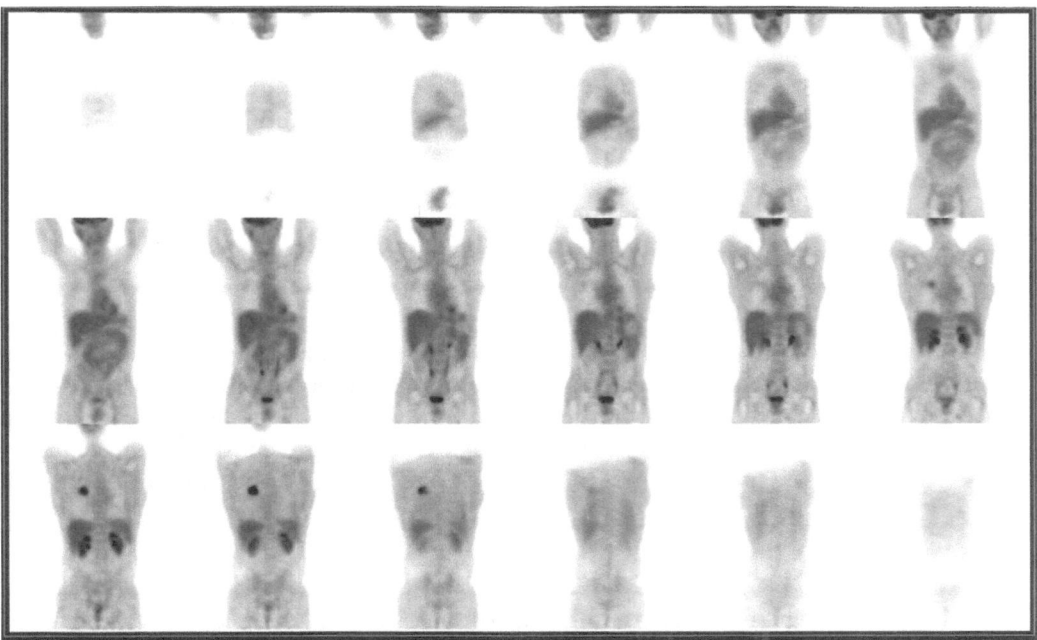

Figure 13.3. Positron emission tomography (PET) scan of patient with lung lesion.

The decision to proceed with an FNA or a lung biopsy is largely based on physician preference. There are no studies proving one evaluation strategy is better than another. The proponents of early surgery argue that VATS can be performed with a low morbidity and a short hospital stay, and will always obtain a diagnosis. An FNA does carry a lower risk and usually does not require hospitalization, but it is not always diagnostic. An FNA should be encouraged strongly in patients with multiple medical problems. Another important consideration is patients with central tumors. Due to their location to hilar vessels, central tumors may require a lobectomy instead of wedge resection in order to obtain a diagnosis.

Lung Neoplasms

Lung cancer is the leading cause of cancer deaths in the United States among both men and women. Approximately 180,000 patients are diagnosed with lung cancer per year in the United States. The average age at the time of diagnosis is 60 years. The long-term survival for lung cancer remains poor, with only a 14% overall 5-year survival. **High cure rates following resection can be expected with patients who present with early disease.** It is imperative for physicians treating lung cancer to properly evaluate their patients to determine which patients may benefit from surgical resection and which may benefit from multimodality therapy.

Epidemiology

Studies have confirmed that 80% to 90% of lung cancers are caused by **tobacco use**. Risk factors include **the age at which smoking is started, the frequency, and the duration**. The duration of smoking is the most important risk factor. Studies have demonstrated an increased risk of lung cancer in people exposed to **secondhand smoke**. Several studies also have demonstrated an increased risk of lung cancer in **uranium miners**. Occupational exposure linked to lung cancer includes **inhalation of asbestos and polycyclic aromatic hydrocarbons, and exposure to arsenic, chromates, and bis(chloromethyl)ether.**

Cancer Prevention

Studies have linked **diets high in fruits and vegetables** to lower incidence of lung cancer, suggesting that **vitamin A** may help prevent lung cancer. However, the vitamin A derivative beta-carotene did not show an improvement in survival or in the prevention of lung cancer in prospective randomized studies. Ongoing studies are evaluating other agents that may reduce the risks of lung cancers.

Malignant Tumors

The majority of lung tumors that are malignant consist of **adenocarcinoma, squamous cell carcinoma, large-cell carcinoma, or small-cell lung carcinoma (Table 13.5).** The first three are referred to as

Table 13.5. Histologic classification of malignant epithelial lung tumors.

Squamous cell carcinoma
  Variant:
    Papillary
    Clear cell
    Small cell
    Basaloid

Small-cell carcinoma
  Variant:
    Combined small-cell carcinoma

Adenocarcinoma
  Acinar
  Papillary
  Bronchioloalveolar carcinoma
  Solid adenocarcinoma with mucin

Large cell carcinoma

Source: Reprinted from World Health Organization. Histo-
logical typing of lung and pleural tumours, 3rd ed.,
1999:21–22, with permission.

non–small-cell lung carcinoma (NSCLC) and present 80% of all lung
carcinomas. **The best chance for cure for NSCLC remains surgical
resection.** Adenocarcinoma is the most common cause of lung cancer,
accounting for 46% of the cases. Adenocarcinoma most frequently
presents as a peripheral lung nodule and has the tendency to spread
via the lymphatics and hematogenously. Bronchoalveolar carcinoma,
an adenocarcinoma subtype, may present as a discrete nodule, as mul-
tifocal nodules, or as a diffuse infiltrating tumor. Squamous cell carcinoma is the second most common cause of lung cancer. Squamous cell
carcinoma typically presents as a central tumor, which can occlude a
proximal bronchus.

Small-cell lung carcinomas also are known as "oat cell" carcinomas.
At times, the differentiation among carcinoids, lymphocytic tumors,
and poorly differentiated NSCLC may be difficult. Immunohisto-
chemical staining should allow for proper identification of these
tumors. Small-cell lung carcinomas have a propensity for early spread
and are typically treated by chemotherapy. However, patients with
small-cell lung carcinomas can present with a small tumor (less than
3-cm) without metastasis and have 5-year survivals of 50% following
surgical resection.

Benign Tumors

Benign tumors of the lung represent only 5% of lung tumors. The most
common cause of benign tumor is a hamartoma. Hamartoma represents 75% of all benign tumors of the lung and accounts for 8% of
pulmonary neoplasm. Other causes of benign lung tumor occur only
rarely.

Bronchial Gland Tumors

Five tumors comprise bronchial gland tumors: **bronchial carcinoid, adenoid cystic carcinoma, mucoepidermoid carcinoma, bronchial mucous gland adenoma, and pleomorphic mixed tumors.** Bronchial carcinoid constitutes 85% of this group of tumors. Ninety percent of carcinoid tumors present in the main stem or lobar bronchi, with less than 10% presenting as a solitary nodule. Because carcinoid tumors frequently present in major bronchi, patients may present with symptoms secondary to an obstructed airway.

Bronchial carcinoids are classified as neuroendocrine tumors, the amine precursor uptake decarboxylase (APUD) tumors that arise from Kulchitsky cells in the respiratory epithelium. The more common typical carcinoid tumor only metastasizes in 5% to 6% of patients. The more aggressive atypical variant metastasizes more frequently. Carcinoid tumors are a common cause of lung tumors presenting in young patients. Ninety percent of patients with typical carcinoids are cured with a surgical resection. Atypical carcinoids occur in 15% of patients and have a higher incidence of metastasis when compared to typical carcinoids.

Metastatic Tumors

Sarcomas and carcinomas arising from the breast, kidney, and colon have a propensity to metastasize to the lung. The lung may be the only site of distant spread. Although never studied in a prospective randomized trial, several **studies have suggested a survival advantage in patients whose lung metastases are surgically resected.** The recommendation for surgical resection results from the following criteria: **the lung is the only site of metastatic spread, the primary tumor is controlled, there is no effective medical treatment available, and the metastatic tumor can be resected completely.** Survival appears to be dependent on the tumor type, number of metastasis, and the latency between the diagnosis of the primary tumor and the development of metastatic spread to the lung. The best survival has been in patients with solitary tumors and a latency over 1 year. However, 5-year survivals up to 20% are reported with multiple pulmonary metastasis presenting as synchronous disease.

Tumors of the Mediastinum

Tumors presenting in the chest cavity that are not originating from the lung or pleural surface are classified according to their location within the mediastinum (**Table 13.6**). The mediastinum anatomic alley is divided into the anterior, middle, and posterior compartments. The anterior compartment extends from the undersurface of the sternum to the anterior borders of the heart and great vessels. The posterior compartment extends from the anterior border of the vertebral bodies to the ribs posteriorly. The middle mediastinum includes all structures between the anterior and posterior mediastinum. These anatomic boundaries serve as an excellent means to develop an accurate differ-

Table 13.6. Tumors of the mediastinum.

Anterior
  Thymus
    Thymoma
    Thymic carcinoma
    Carcinoid
  Lymphoma
  Germ cell tumor
  Thyroid
    Most commonly a benign goiter
  Parathyroid adenoma
Posterior mediastinum
  Neurogenic tumors
    Benign
      Schwannoma (neurilemmoma)
      Neurofibroma
      Ganglioneuroma
      Pheochromocytoma
      Paraganglioma
    Malignant
      Malignant schwannoma
      Neuroblastoma
      Malignant paraganglioma

ential diagnosis. The anterior mediastinum consists mainly of tumors of the thymus (predominantly thymomas), lymphomas, and germ cell tumors. The majority of posterior mediastinal tumors are neuroendocrine in origin and usually are benign in adults.

Clinical Presentations

Primary Tumor
Patients with lung cancer typically present with symptoms (Table 13.7). Symptoms at presentation are from the primary tumor in 27% of patients and are dependent on the location of the tumor. Central tumors may cause a cough, hemoptysis, obstructive pneumonia, or wheezing. Peripheral tumors are more likely to present with chest pain, dyspnea, or pleural effusion. The primary tumor may cause symptoms by direct extension into mediastinal structures. Patients may present with pain from direct rib involvement, or a tumor in the superior sulcus (Pancoast) can cause radicular arm pain and weakness from invasion of the brachial plexus. Invasion of the superior vena cava (superior vena cava syndrome) may cause facial and upper torso venous engorgement. Hoarseness from recurrent laryngeal nerve invasion also may occur.

Metastatic Tumor
Metastatic disease from mediastinal tumors is the presenting symptom in 32% of the cases. **The most common sites of distant lung metastasis are the adrenal gland, lung, bone, liver, and brain.** Bone pain from metastatic spread occurs in 20% to 25% of patients. Ten percent of

Table 13.7. Initial symptoms at presentation of lung cancer.

Symptoms	Percentage (%)
Cough	74
Weight loss	68
Dyspnea	58
Chest pain	49
Hemoptysis	29
Lymphadenopathy	23
Bone pain	25
Hepatomegaly	21
Clubbing	20
Intracranial	12
Superior vena cava syndrome	4
Hoarseness	18

Source: Reprinted from Hyde L, Hyde CI. Clinical manifestations of lung cancer. Chest 1974;65:300.

patients present with brain metastasis; however, 25% of patients eventually develop brain metastasis.

Paraneoplastic Syndromes

Paraneoplastic syndromes occur most commonly with small-cell carcinomas and squamous cell carcinomas (**Table 13.8**). Paraneoplastic syndromes include hypertrophic pulmonary osteoarthropathy, inappropriate secretion of antidiuretic hormone (ADH), hypercalcemia, Cushing's syndrome, and neurologic and myopathic syndromes. Inappropriate secretion of ADH and Cushing's syndrome most commonly are related to small-cell carcinomas. Hypercalcemia from the production of either a parathyroid hormone or a parathyroid-like substance is associated most commonly with squamous cell carcinomas.

Superior Sulcus Tumor

Superior sulcus tumors arise from the apex of the lung and can invade the upper ribs or brachial plexus. Patients frequently complain of arm or shoulder pain and may have T1 nerve root weakness or present with Horner's syndrome. All patients presenting with a superior sulcus tumors should have their mediastinal lymph nodes evaluated by mediastinoscopy. The survival is extremely poor when this group of patients presents with mediastinal lymph metastasis. Patients are treated with radiotherapy (30 to 45 Gy), followed by en bloc resection in 4 weeks. Recent studies suggest a benefit to neoadjuvant chemotherapy, in addition to radiotherapy.

Diagnosis and Staging

Patients who are being considered for a potentially curative resection must be properly staged clinically. Diagnostic and staging modalities include **chest radiograph, CT scan of the chest and brain, PET scan, bone scan, and lymph node sampling by mediastinoscopy or anterior thoracotomy**. The extent of the workup often is dependent on

Table 13.8. Paraneoplastic syndromes in lung cancer patients.

Metabolic
  Hypercalcemia
  Cushing's syndrome
  Inappropriate antidiuretic hormone production
  Carcinoid syndrome
  Gynecomastia
  Hypercalcitonemia
  Elevated growth hormone level
  Elevated prolactin, follicle-stimulating hormone,
    luteinizing hormone levels
  Hypoglycemia
  Hyperthyroidism

Neurologic
  Encephalopathy
  Subacute cerebellar degeneration
  Peripheral neuropathy
  Polymyositis
  Autonomic neuropathy
  Lambert–Eaton syndrome
  Opsoclonus and myoclonus

Skeletal
  Clubbing
  Pulmonary hypertrophic osteoarthropathy

Hematologic
  Anemia
  Leukemoid reactions
  Thrombocytosis
  Thrombocytopenia
  Eosinophilia
  Pure red cell aplasia
  Leukoerythroblastosis
  Disseminated intravascular coagulation

Cutaneous and muscular
  Hyperkeratosis
  Dermatomyositis
  Acanthosis nigricans
  Hyperpigmentation
  Erythema gyratum repens
  Hypertrichosis lanuaginosa acquisita

Other
  Nephrotic syndrome
  Hypouricemia
  Secretion of vasoactive intestinal peptide with
    diarrhea
  Hyperamylasemia
  Anorexia-cachexia

Source: Reprinted from Shields TW. Presentation, diagnosis, and staging of bronchial carcinoma and of the asymptomatic solitary pulmonary nodule. In: Shields TW, ed. Thoracic Surgery. Malvern, PA: Williams & Wilkins, 1994. With permission from Lippincott Williams & Wilkins.

symptoms. All patients should receive a CT of the chest that includes the liver and adrenal gland. Patients with complaints of bone pain or neurologic changes should receive a bone scan or CT of the brain, respectively. A PET scan is being used more often in the evaluation of patients with lung cancer.

Chest Radiograph

A posteroanterior and lateral chest radiograph can determine the size of the tumor, bone metastasis, collapsed lung, and pleural effusion. Mediastinal nodal involvement can be assessed if it is large, but a chest radiograph is not as sensitive as a CT scan.

Computed Tomography

A CT scan determines the size of the primary tumor, tumor growth into the chest wall and mediastinum, enlarged lymph nodes, and liver and adrenal metastasis. A mediastinal lymph node larger than 1 cm is considered suspicious for metastasis; if it is less than 1 cm, it is considered normal. The false-negative rate in assessing mediastinal metastasis is 10% to 20% when using these criteria. The false-negative rate increases the larger and more central the tumor is. The false-positive rate is 25% to 30%. Therefore, a tissue diagnosis is required to confirm the presence or absence of mediastinal metastasis.

Positron Emission Tomography

The PET scan determines the presence of tissue that has increased glucose metabolism when compared to the surrounding normal tissue. Enhanced glucose metabolism occurs with malignant tumors and inflammatory lesions. The PET scan measures the uptake of a positron emission analogue (2–18 F) fluoro-2-deoxy-D-glucose (FDG). The FDG-PET has a reported sensitivity of 95% and specificity of 80% in determining whether a solitary pulmonary nodule is benign or malignant. False-positive results can occur with inflammatory conditions. The PET scan also has been shown to be more sensitive and specific than a CT scan in detecting mediastinal metastasis. A whole-body PET scan detects unsuspected distant metastasis in 11% to 14% of patients.

Cervical Mediastinoscopy

Cervical mediastinoscopy is used extensively to examine the presence of metastasis to the mediastinal lymph nodes. (See **Algorithm 13.2.**) Mediastinoscopy examines the paratracheal, subcarinal, and tracheobronchial lymph nodes. This technique provides histology from N2 and N3 lymph nodes (see section on staging, below), which would dictate treatment. N3 lymph node metastases are considered inoperable, and N2 lymph node metastasis may require preoperative chemotherapy.

Staging of Non–Small-Cell Lung Carcinoma

The staging of lung cancer is based on the TNM classification: (see **Algorithm 13.3**). The T determines the size of the primary tumor, distance from carina, pleural involvement, and invasion into the chest wall or mediastinum. The presence and location of hilar and mediastinal lymph node metastasis and metastasis outside the involved hemithorax are assessed. The TNM descriptors are shown in **Table 13.9**.

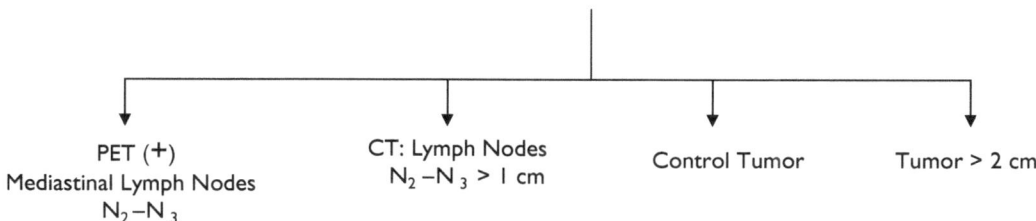

Algorithm 13.2. Algorithm for the use of mediastinoscopy.

Surgical Management of Non–Small-Cell Lung Carcinoma

Surgical resection remains the most effective treatment for NSCLC. Surgery should be performed only in patients in whom complete excision of the tumor can be performed. Patients with N1 disease and selected patients with N2 nodal metastasis are surgical candidates. Patients with contralateral mediastinal lymph node metastasis, malignant pleural effusions, or metastatic spread to other organs are not surgical candidates. Patients with N2 disease are treated with chemotherapy prior to surgery. Two small prospective randomized

Stage		Treatment
IL	⟶	Lobectomy with hilar and mediastinal lymph node dissection; postop. chemotherapy and irradiation (RT) not indicated
II	⟶	Lobectomy with hilar and mediastinal lymph node dissection; postop. chemotherapy/RT does not prolong survival
IIIA	T3N0–1 ⎫ T1–3N2 ⎭ ⟶	If clinically stage IIIA, preop. chemotherapy; possible RT followed by surgery*
IIIB	T4N0 ⎫ T4N1–2 ⎬ ⟶ Any T, N3 ⎭	Chemotherapy/RT (+surgery in highly selected cases) Chemotherapy/RT Chemotherapy/RT
IV	All other M+ ⟶	Chemotherapy/RT
Special cases		
	Pantumor ⟶	Preop. chemotherapy/RT followed by surgery

*If stage IIIA disease is diagnosed only after surgery, postoperative irradiation and chemotherapy are given; the combination yields significantly longer disease-free survival than irradiation alone. Postoperative irradiation alone improves local control but has no appreciable effect on survival.

Algorithm 13.3. Algorithm for staging of non–small-cell carcinoma of the lung. (Reprinted from Warren WH, James TW. Non-small cell carcinoma of the lung (continued). Reprinted from Saclarides TJ, Millikan KW, Godellas CV, eds. Surgical Oncology: An Algorithmic Approach. New York: Springer-Verlag, 2002, with permission.)

Table 13.9. Lung cancer TNM descriptors.

Primary tumor (T)

TX   Primary tumor cannot be assessed, or tumor proven by the presence of malignant cells in
     sputum or bronchial washings but not visualized by imaging or bronchoscopy

T0   No evidence of primary tumor

Tis Carcinoma in situ

T1   Tumor ≤3 cm in greatest dimension, surrounded by lung or visceral pleura, without
     bronchoscopic evidence of invasion more proximal than the lobar bronchus* (i.e., not in
     the main bronchus)

T2   Tumor with any of the following features of size or extent:
     >3 cm in greatest dimension
     Involves main bronchus, ≥2 cm distal to the carina
     Invades the visceral pleura
     Association with atelectasis or obstructive pneumonitis that extends to the hilar
     region but does not involve the entire lung

T3   Tumor of any size that directly invades any of the following: chest wall (including
     superior sulcus tumors), diaphragm, mediastinal pleura, parietal pericardium; or tumor
     in the main bronchus <2 cm distal to the carina, but without involvement of the carina;
     or associated atelectasis or obstructive pneumonitis of the entire lung

T4   Tumor of any size that invades any of the following: mediastinum, heart, great vessels,
     trachea, esophagus, vertebral body, carina; or tumor with a malignant pleural or
     pericardial effusion,† or with satellite tumor nodule(s) within the ipsilateral primary
     tumor lobe of the lung

Regional lymph nodes (N)

NX   Regional lymph nodes cannot be assessed

N0   No regional lymph node metastasis

N1   Metastasis to ipsilateral peribronchial and/or ipsilateral hilar lymph nodes, and
     intrapulmonary nodes involved by direct extension of the primary tumor

N2   Metastasis to ipsilateral mediastinal and/or subcarinal lymph node(s)

N3   Metastasis to contralateral mediastinal, contralateral hilar, ipsilateral or contralateral
     scalene, or supraclavicular lymph node(s)

Distant metastasis (M)

MX   Presence of distant metastasis cannot be assessed

M0   No distant metastasis

M1   Distant metastasis present‡

* The uncommon superficial tumor of any size with its invasive component limited to the bronchial wall, which may extend proximal to the main bronchus, is also classified T1.

† Most pleural effusions associated with lung cancer are due to tumor. However, there are a few patients in whom multiple cytopathologic examinations of pleural fluid show no tumor. In these cases, the fluid is nonbloody and is not an exudate. When these elements and clinical judgment dictate that the effusion is not related to the tumor, the effusion should be excluded as a staging element and the patient's disease should be staged T1, T2, or T3. Pericardial effusion is classified according to the same rules.

‡ Separate metastatic tumor nodule(s) in the ipsilateral nonprimary tumor lobe(s) of the lung also are classified M1.
Source: Reprinted from Mountain CF. Revisions in the international system for staging lung cancer. Chest 1997;111:1711, with permission.

studies have shown that patients with N2 disease who receive pre-operative chemotherapy (neoadjuvant) have a survival advantage over those who do not.[1] It remains to be determined whether neoadjuvant chemotherapy is beneficial for only selected patients with N2 disease.

---

[1] Rosell R, Gomez-Codina J, Camps C, et al. A randomized trial comparing preoperative chemotherapy plus surgery with surgery alone in patients with non-small cell lung cancer. N Engl J Med 1994;330:153–158. Roth JA, Fossella F, Romaki R, et al. A randomized trial comparing perioperative chemotherapy and surgery with surgery alone in resectable stage IIIA non-small cell lung cancer. J Natl Cancer Inst 1994;86:673–680.

The primary tumor and surrounding intrapulmonary lymphatics must be removed. Lobectomy is considered the operation of choice, but a pneumonectomy may be required to obtain negative margins. Wedge resection has a higher incidence of local recurrence and is not recommended unless the patient cannot tolerate a lobectomy. **Patients who are not considered surgical candidates because of extensive disease or general medical condition are treated with chemotherapy and/or radiation.**

Preoperative Pulmonary Evaluation

An assessment should be made to determine whether the patient can tolerate surgery. **Most patients should have a pulmonary function test prior to surgery.** (See **Algorithm 13.4.**) Patients with a forced expira-

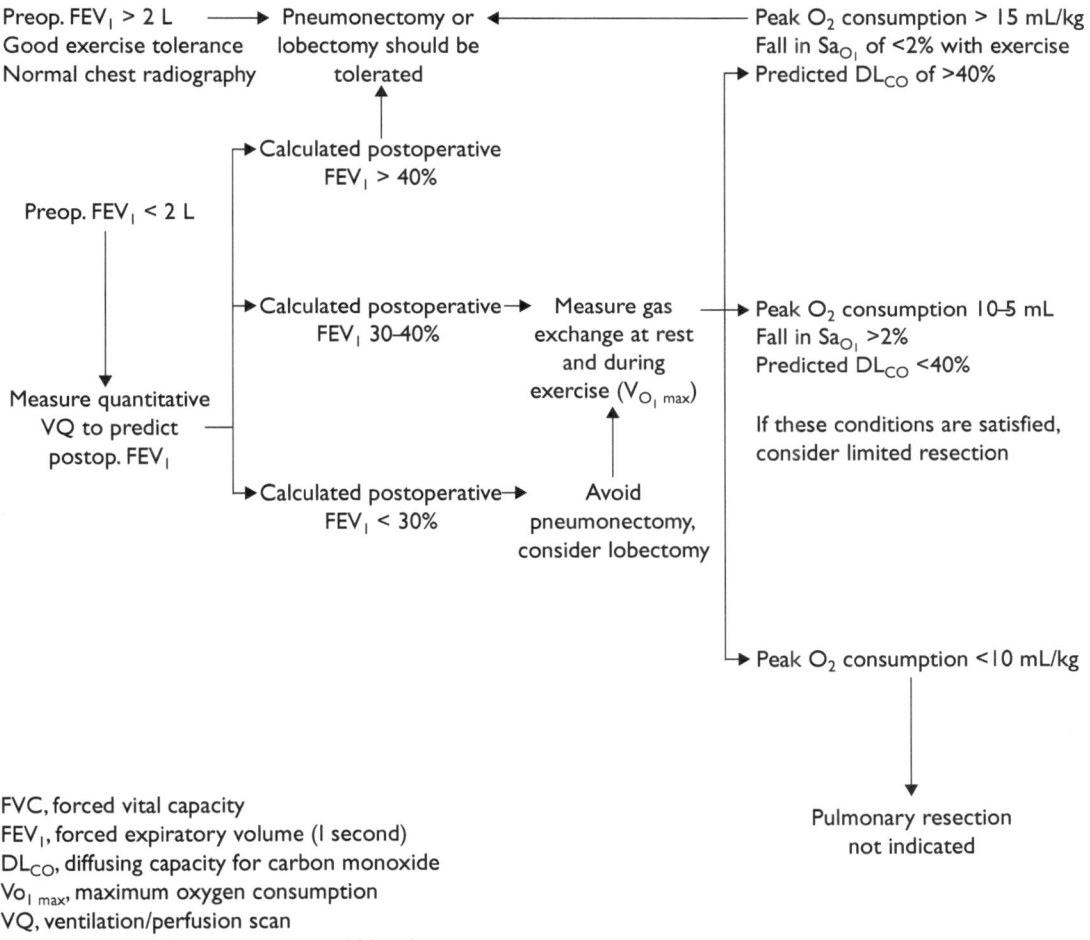

FVC, forced vital capacity
FEV_I, forced expiratory volume (I second)
DL_{CO}, diffusing capacity for carbon monoxide
$Vo_{I\ max}$, maximum oxygen consumption
VQ, ventilation/perfusion scan
Sa_{O_I}, saturation of oxygen in arterial blood

Algorithm 13.4. Evaluation of pulmonary function prior to surgery for non–small-cell carcinoma of the lung. (Reprinted from Warren WH, Jomes TW. Non-small cell carcinoma of the lung (continued). Reprinted from Saclarides TJ, Millikan KW, Godellas CV, eds. Surgical Oncology: An Algorithmic Approach. New York: Springer-Verlag, 2002, with permission.)

tory volume in 1 second (FEV₁) of greater than 2.00, or greater than 60% of predicted normal value, are thought to have sufficient pulmonary reserves to tolerate a pneumonectomy. Patients with a predicted postoperative FEV₁ of greater than 1.0, or greater than 40% of predicted, should have sufficient pulmonary reserve to tolerate a lobectomy. A quantitative ventilation perfusion scan also may be helpful to predict postoperative FEV₁. Arterial blood gases should be drawn to assess for arterial hypoxia and hypercapnia. The pulmonary status also can be assessed clinically by ambulating the patient. Patients who are short of breath at rest or upon minimal activity are considered poor surgical candidates. Patients who can walk a flight of stairs typically can tolerate a lobectomy.

Survival

The 5-year survival following resection for a stage I NSCLC is between 38% and 85% (**Fig. 13.4**). A significantly worse survival occurs in patients with tumors greater than 3 cm (stage IB) than in those patients presenting with tumors less than 3 cm (stage IA). Surgical resection of stage II tumors results in survival rates between 22% and 55%. Prior to neoadjuvant chemotherapy, patients with N2 mediastinal lymph node metastasis (stage IIIA) had a 5-year survival of only 7%. With the advent of multimodality treatment, an improvement in the 5-year survival to 25% has been reported in completely resected disease stage IIIA patients. Studies currently are evaluating which patients with mediastinal (N2) lymph node metastasis will benefit from surgical resection. Patients with clinical stage IIIB or stage IV disease are not considered surgical candidates. The 1-year survival for these patients is 20% to 37% and 5-year survival is 1% to 7%.

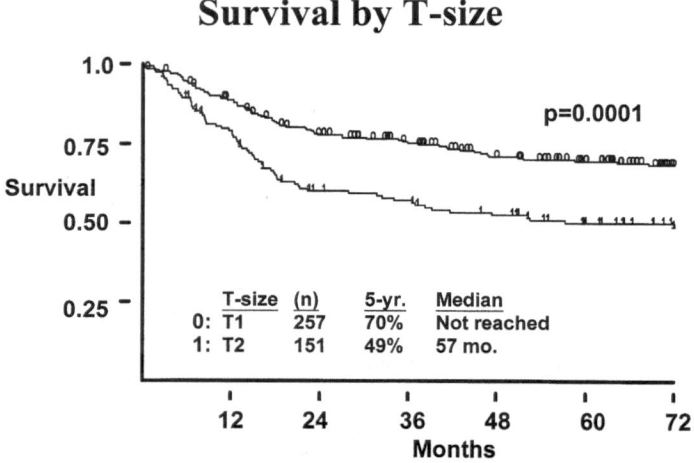

Figure 13.4. Duke University Medical Center data, 1980–1992. Survival curves for stage I NSCLC based on tumor size. Graphs truncated at 72 months with 148 patients alive. (Reprinted from Lau CL, Harpole DH, Jr. Lung neoplasms. In: Norton JA, Bollinger RR, Chang AE, et al., eds. Surgery: Basic Science and Clinical Evidence. New York: Springer-Verlag, 2001, with permission.)

Neoadjuvant and Adjuvant Therapy

Prospective randomized studies demonstrate there is no advantage of adjuvant (postoperative) chemotherapy for stage I NSCLC patients. Four prospective randomized studies have analyzed the effects of postoperative chemotherapy and/or radiotherapy for patients with stage II to III NSCLC.[2] These studies all showed that there was no survival benefit for adjuvant therapy.

Two phase III neoadjuvant trials in stage IIIA lung cancer patients demonstrated a significant improvement in survival in those patients receiving chemotherapy prior surgery.[3] The M.D. Anderson trial randomized 60 patients to preoperative and postoperative chemotherapy and surgery versus surgery alone. The 3-year survival was 56% in the neoadjuvant group compared to 15% in the control group. The Spanish trial randomized 60 patients to preoperative chemotherapy followed by surgery and postoperative radiation, or surgery followed by radiation. This study also demonstrated a significant improvement in survival in the chemotherapy-treated group.

Management of Small-Cell Lung Carcinoma

Most patients with small-cell lung carcinoma (SCLC) present with advanced disease, with 70% of patients presenting with extrathoracic metastasis. Therefore, the majority of patients with SCLC infrequently are treated with surgery. **Chemotherapy is the main therapeutic modality used to treat SCLC, although thoracic irradiation may be valuable.** Rarely, patients with SCLC present with a solitary nodule. Surgery alone provides a curative therapy in 25% of patients. With the addition of postoperative chemotherapy, 5-year survival rates up to 80% have been reported in patients with T1, N0, M0 disease. However, at present, surgery is not recommended even in patients with very limited disease.

Surveillance Following Surgical Resection

There has been no proven benefit to routine chest radiographs following a surgical resection of lung cancer. However, patients frequently are followed with chest radiographs every 4 months for the first 2 years, followed by chest radiographs every 6 months. Whether routine CT scans after surgical resection add a benefit to the patient survival remains to be determined.

---

[2] Lau CL, Harpole DH Jr. In: Norton JA, Bollinger RR, Chang AE, Lowry SF, et al. Surgery: Basic Science and Clinical Evidence, New York: Springer-Verlag, 2001.
[3] Rosell R, Gomez-Codina J, Camps C, et al. A randomized trial comparing preoperative chemotherapy plus surgery with surgery alone in patients with non-small cell lung cancer. N Engl J Med 1994;330:153–158. Roth JA, Fossella F, Romaki R, et al. A randomized trial comparing perioperative chemotherapy and surgery with surgery alone in resectable stage IIIA non-small cell lung cancer. J Natl Cancer Inst 1994;86:673–680.

Summary

When evaluating patients with hemoptysis, it is important to determine whether the bleeding is massive and if the airway is secure. The treatment options used to control bleeding originating from the lung include medical management, bronchial lavage, embolization of bronchial arteries, and surgery.

Critical in treating patients with lung cancer is determining the clinical stage. Patients with stage I and stage II non–small-cell carcinoma are best treated with surgical resection, while patients with stage IIIA non–small-cell carcinoma should receive chemotherapy prior to surgical resection. More advanced lung cancer is treated with chemotherapy with or without radiotherapy.

Basic guidelines for the evaluation, staging, and treatment of lung cancer are highlighted (see **Algorithm 13.1**).

Selected Readings

International Registry of Lung Metastases, Ginsberg RJ, et al. Long-term results of lung metastasectomy: prognostic analyses based on 5,206 cases. J Thorac Cardiovasc Surg 1997;37–49.

Kato A, Kudo S, et al. Bronchial artery embolization for hemoptysis due to begin immediate and long-term results. Cardiovasc Intervent Radiol 2000; 23(5):1–7.

Lau CL, Harpole DH Jr. In: Norton JA, Bollinger RR, Chang AE, Lowry SF, et al. Surgery: Basic Science and Clinical Evidence, New York: Springer-Verlag, 2001.

Lee TW, Wan S, et al. Management of massive hemoptysis: a single institution experiment. Cardiovasc Surg 2000;6(4):232–235.

Mal H, Rullon I, et al. Immediate and long-term results of bronchial artery embolization and life threatening hemoptysis. Chest 1999;115(4):996–1001.

Pierson FG, Deslauries J, Ginsberg RJ, et al. Thorac Surg 1995.

Rosell R, Gomez-Codina J, Camps C, et al. A randomized trial comparing preoperative chemotherapy plus surgery with surgery alone in patients with non-small cell lung cancer. N Engl J Med 1994;330:153–158.

Roth JA, Fossella F, Romaki R, et al. A randomized trial comparing perioperative chemotherapy and surgery with surgery alone in resectable stage IIIA non-small cell lung cancer. J Natl Cancer Inst 1994;86:673–680.

Rusch VW, Giroux DJ, et al. Induction chemoradiation and surgical resection for non-small cell lung carcinomas of the superior sulcus: initial results of S. Oncology Group Trial 9416 (Intergroup Trial 0160). J Thorac Cardiovasc Surg 2001;121(3):472–483.

Shields TW, LoCicero J, Ponn RB. General Thoracic Surgery, 5th ed, vol 1. 2000.

Heart Murmurs: Congenital Heart Disease

Alan J. Spotnitz

Objectives

1. To understand the significance of a heart murmur in an infant.
2. To understand the classification of congenital heart disease.
3. To understand the difference between palliative and corrective surgery for congenital heart disease.

Case

A 6-month-old baby is brought to your office by his mother. He has been having frequent upper respiratory infections. The mother says she thinks he is short of breath at times and does not eat as well as his older brother did at the same age.

Introduction

The identification of a heart murmur early in life may be indicative of a significant congenital malformation of the heart. Such malformations may be present in 0.5% to 0.8% of all live births. It is **important to be able to differentiate potentially life-threatening lesions from benign processes**. To do this, **a basic understanding of these potentially complex lesions is necessary. When the diagnosis of a significant heart murmur seriously is considered, these infants must be referred to a pediatric cardiologist and pediatric cardiac surgeon for appropriate diagnosis and corrective or palliative procedures.**

A relatively simple way to classify these potentially confusing lesions is according to categories based on the major presenting symptom: **congestive heart failure or cyanosis (Table 14.1).** Diagnosis of these lesions frequently can be made on the basis of the **history and physical examination as well as with some basic noninterventional testing,**

Table 14.1. Presentation and classification of congenital heart disease.

Congestive heart failure	
Left-to-right shunt	Obstructive lesions
(increased pulmonary blood flow)	
Patent ductus arteriosus	Aortic stenosis
Atrial septal defect	Mitral stenosis
Ventricular septal defect	Pulmonic stenosis
Atrioventricular canal	Coarctation of the aorta
Truncus arteriosus	Interrupted aortic arch
Aortopulmonary window	
Cyanosis	
Right-to-left shunt	Complex lesions
(decreased pulmonary blood flow)	
Tetralogy of Fallot	Transposition of the great arteries
	With intact ventricular septum
	With ventricular septal defect
Tricuspid atresia	Total anomalous pulmonary venous
	connection
Pulmonary atresia	Cor triatriatum
With intact ventricular septum	
With ventricular septal defect	
	Hypoplastic left heart syndrome
Miscellaneous	
Anomalous origin of the left coronary artery from the pulmonary artery	
Corrected transposition of the great arteries	
Ebstein's anomaly	
Vascular rings	

Source: Reprinted from Backer CL, Mavroudis C. Congenital heart disease. In: Norton JA, Bollinger RR, Chang AE, et al, eds. Surgery: Basic Science and Clinical Evidence. New York: Springer-Verlag, 2001, with permission.

including chest x-ray, electrocardiogram, and echocardiogram. **Cardiac catheterization** in the diagnosis of these patients is required in fewer than 20% of all cases. (See **Algorithm 14.1.**)

Congestive Heart Failure

The infant described in the case presented above is likely to be having signs of **congestive heart failure**. Infants and children with congestive heart failure are symptomatic for either of two reasons: **obstructing lesions** or **overcirculation of the lungs**.

Obstructive lesions leading to signs and symptoms of congestive heart failure involve the heart valves or the aorta. These include aortic stenosis, mitral stenosis, and various degrees of narrowing of the thoracic aorta between the aortic valve and the level of the ductus arteriosus. Initial presentation can range from a benign sounding heart murmur to life-threatening congestive heart failure. The symptoms caused by the obstructive lesion are attributed to blood backing up into the pulmonary circulation, causing pulmonary edema or congestion.

Congestive heart failure also can be caused by **left to right shunting** of arterial blood, leading to **overcirculation of the lungs**. This can occur at several levels of the heart. Abnormal communication can exist at the level of the atria (atrial septal defect), ventricles (ventricular septal defect), or in an extracardiac location (aortopulmonary window or patent ductus arteriosus signs). The most common symptoms that occur in this setting include recurrent upper respiratory infection, tachypnea, tachycardia, and failure to thrive. Oxygenated blood flows from the left side to the right side of the circulation because of the lower resistance and pressures in the right side of the heart. Excessive flow of blood through the pulmonary vasculature results in congestive heart failure and pulmonary hypertension. Enlargement of the right atrium and ventricle will occur. **Pulmonary vascular resistance gradually increases** due to this overcirculation from a complex interaction of factors. Ultimately, the pulmonary resistance becomes high and irreversible. If the resistance becomes high enough, flow reversal may occur, with right to left shunting and cyanosis (**Eisenmenger's syn-**

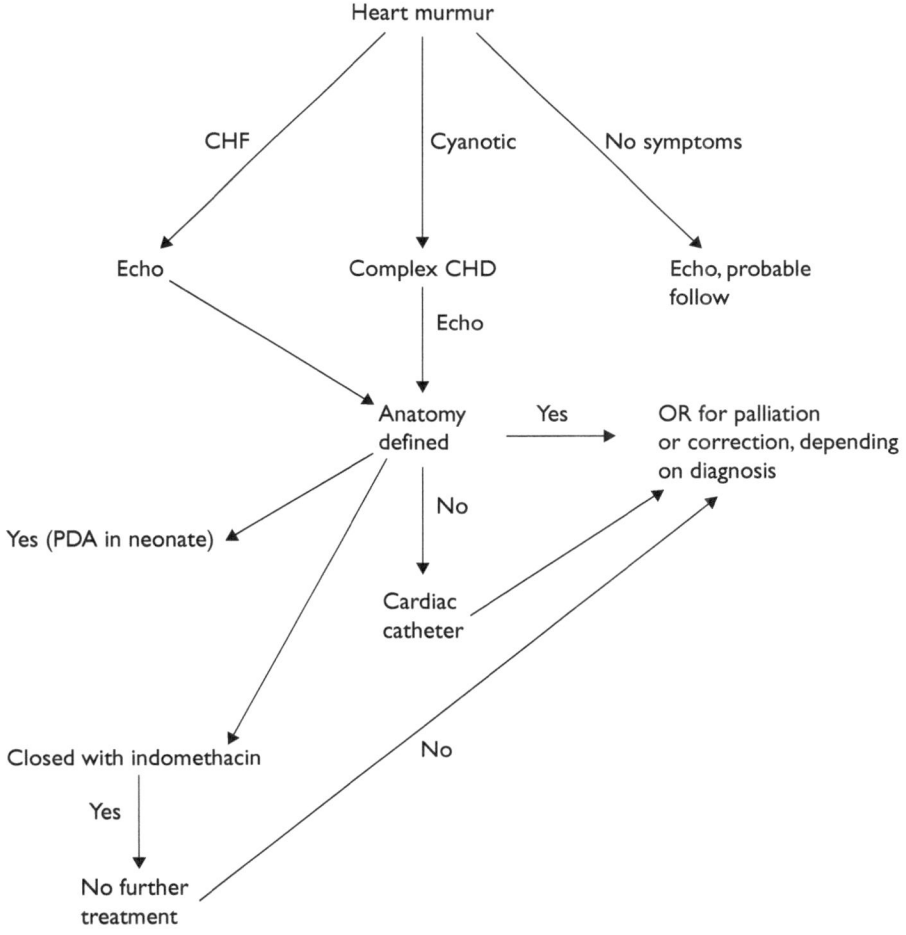

Algorithm 14.1. Algorithm for the diagnosis and treatment of a child with a heart murmur. CHD, congestive heart disease; CHF, congestive heart failure; PDA, patent ductus arteriosus.

drome). The goal of surgical therapy is to correct these lesions. Frequently, this can be accomplished with a low operative mortality. **As pulmonary resistance increases, so does the operative risk.** Even before Eisenmenger's syndrome occurs, a high fixed resistance may preclude surgical correction.

The infant in the case presented above is consistent with an infant who has either an obstructive lesion or a shunting lesion. The presence of congestive heart failure and the absence of cyanosis places the infant in this category.

Cyanosis

The cyanosis related to cyanotic congenital heart disease is due to the significant **mixing of oxygenated and nonoxygenated blood within the heart and the output of this blood to the systemic circulation.** For this to occur, either an intracardiac defect with pulmonary outflow obstruction (forcing blood to shunt right to left) or a complex congenital anomaly must exist. When the **absolute level of desaturated blood in the systemic circulation exceeds 5 g/mL, cyanosis appears.** As noted, two basic categories exist. In the first, septal defects similar to those that occur in left to right shunting are present, but these are associated with some **form of pulmonary outflow obstruction** (subvalvular, supravalvular, or atresia of the pulmonary arteries). The result is right-to-left shunting and cyanosis. The classic lesion is known as **tetralogy of Fallot (ventricular septal defect, overriding aorta, pulmonary arterial obstruction, and right ventricular hypertrophy).**

The other lesions causing cyanosis, in which markedly abnormal anatomy exists, such as transposition of the great vessels and total anomalous pulmonary venous return, are referred to as "**complex lesions.**"

History and Physical Examination

The **history** is obtained from the parent or from observations of the infant at the time of delivery. The parent usually is most observant of abnormalities in the **child's behavior**, especially if there is an older sibling with whom to compare the child's behavior, as in the case presented above. **Family history** is relevant, as there may be as much as a threefold increase in the incidence of congenital disease when a prior sibling has been born with a congenital defect. **Signs and symptoms of congestive heart failure** should be sought from the parent, especially recurrent respiratory infections or difficulties feeding (shortness of breath, sweating). Cyanosis may appear early in neonates born with transposition of the great vessels or some other complex lesion. Perfusion of the pulmonary circulation may have been dependent on a patent ductus arteriosus communicating between the descending thoracic aorta and the pulmonary artery. As the ductus begins to close in the first hours and days of life, decreased pulmonary blood flow and cyanosis, either from hypoxia or new right to left flow, occurs.

Prostaglandin may be necessary to maintain this fetal circulation (patent ductus) until diagnostic studies can be completed. Other infants do not develop signs of cyanosis until they are a few months of age. There may be a history of cyanosis related to crying. **Signs of cyanosis related to tetralogy of Fallot may not appear until several months of life as pulmonary outflow obstruction (and right-to-left shunting) increases.**

The **physical examination** is directed to a **systematic evaluation** of the infant or child. **Findings consistent with congestive heart failure or chronic hypoxemia are sought.** Low weight and poor nutrition are not uncommon. The **pulmonary exam** may reveal fine rales and rhonchi. The **cardiac exam** usually reveals the presence of a heart murmur. **With obstructive lesions, this usually is consistent with the murmurs of aortic or mitral stenosis. Ventricular septal defects usually have a continuous "machinery-type" murmur over the anterior chest. The murmur of an atrial septal defect is related to increased blood flow across the pulmonic valve and not to the flow across the atrial septum.** This murmur is thus **loudest over the pulmonary outflow tract to the left side of the sternum. A systolic murmur heard loudest in the back is suggestive of coarctation of the aorta, especially if lower extremity pulses are decreased.** It is likely to be continuous. Hepatomegaly may be a consistent finding in the presence of congestive heart failure. Examination of the periphery is crucial in looking for signs of cyanosis, clubbing, or microemboli, which may be present in right-to-left shunting.

Diagnostic Studies

Routine chest x-ray may be diagnostic, especially to a well-trained pediatric radiologist. Over- or undercirculation of the lungs may be present along with cardiomegaly and other deformities of the base of the heart. The classic "figure of eight" appearance of the heart is associated with transposition of the great vessels. When the cardiac silhouette has the appearance of a boot and the infant is cyanotic, tetralogy of Fallot will be suspected. **The electrocardiogram can reveal left or right ventricular hypertrophy as well as conduction abnormalities associated with some complex congenital deformities. Echocardiography is an accurate diagnostic tool and can be used for definitive diagnosis and planning for surgical correction in the majority of infants and children requiring surgical intervention. Cardiac catheterization and angiography may be required to confirm the diagnosis and aid in planning surgical correction in more complex situations.**

Treatment

The ultimate goal of therapy is to reverse symptoms or, alternatively, restore as normal an anatomy as possible. In the emergency setting, palliation may be all that is possible by surgical intervention. Defin-

itive correction is best performed on an elective basis. Pharmacologic methods used to maintain the patency of a patent ductus or to enhance its closure have made many surgical interventions less of an emergency. In many situations, early corrective surgery is possible. The infant is maintained by medical treatment of congestive heart failure until the proper time for surgery arrives.

In contrast to surgery in the adult, stenotic lesions in infants and children can be quite challenging due to the absence of a suitable valve substitute. Pulmonic stenosis usually is corrected transvenously by balloon dilatation in the catheterization laboratory. Any resulting pulmonic insufficiency, if the stenosis is the only lesion, is not of concern. Mitral stenosis may be amenable to open commissurotomy, but some form of shunting and correction to bypass the stenotic lesion may be necessary. Aortic stenosis, if the annulus is of adequate size, may be susceptible to open commissurotomy. Otherwise, the Ross procedure, in which the patient's own pulmonic valve is transplanted to the aortic position, seems to be the best option since there is the likelihood that the valve will continue to grow as the child grows.

Severely cyanotic infants or those in profound heart failure may require immediate diagnosis and surgical intervention. Especially in complex situations or when the remainder of the heart has not developed, palliative procedures are performed. When this is necessary, the goal is to establish sufficient blood flow to maintain life. Emergent atrial septostomy may be required for a neonate with transposition of the great vessels. Profoundly cyanotic infants may require the creation of adequate blood supply to the pulmonary circulation. This is done by the creation of a left-to-right shunt. A modification of the classic Blalock-Taussig shunt (subclavian artery to pulmonary artery) is performed and can be closed when the definitive procedure is performed. The presence of profound pulmonary overcirculation, which may occur with a large ventricular septal defect or aortopulmonary window, may require pulmonary artery banding to restrict pulmonary blood flow.

The dominant approach to many of these lesions now is one of total correction in infancy rather than palliation with later correction. Lesions that lead to overcirculation of the pulmonary vasculature must be corrected early in life or palliated before irreversible pulmonary hypertension develops. Repairs of atrial septal defects usually can be delayed until a child reaches 3 or 4 years of age and can be corrected before he/she begins school. The risk of endocarditis is increased significantly in these patients as well as in older patients with a patent ductus.

Results

With increasing refinements in the techniques of pediatric cardiac surgery, the operative mortality for many of these procedures has dropped dramatically with improved long-term survival. It is no longer uncommon to see adults who have undergone corrective surgery as children parenting their own children.

Summary

A heart murmur present in a child or an infant with signs and symptoms of congestive heart failure or cyanosis is indicative of a significant mechanical lesion within the heart. A relatively simple method of classification of these potentially complex lesions is based on the presenting symptom of the patient, either congestive heart failure or cyanosis. Prompt referrals to experts in this area result in the best outcomes possible.

Selected Readings

Backer CL, Marroudis C. Congenital heart disease. In: Norton JA, Bollinger RR, Chang AE, et al, eds. Surgery: Basic Science and Clinical Evidence. New York: Springer-Verlag, 2001.

Castaneda AR, Jonas RA, Mayer JE, Handley FL. Cardiac Surgery of the Neonate and Infant. Philadelphia: WB Saunders, 1994.

Townsend CM, Beauchamp DR, Evers MB, Mattox KL, Sabiston DC. Sabiston Textbook of Surgery, 15th ed. Chapter 54 "The Heart," Sections 3 through 13 and 15 and 16. Philadelphia: Saunders, 1997: 1961–2082, 2118–2135.

15

Heart Murmurs: Acquired Heart Disease

Alan J. Spotnitz

Objectives

1. To understand the potential significance of a heart murmur in the absence of symptoms.
2. To understand the factors relevant to the selection of a heart valve.
3. To recognize the need for anticoagulants in patients following valvular heart surgery.
4. To understand the risks of valvular heart surgery and its indications.

Cases

Case 1

A 55-year-old man presents to your office complaining of fatigue and shortness of breath after playing one set of tennis. Up until a year ago, he played three sets without difficulty. He was refused induction into the Marines because of a heart murmur. He denies chest pain and is otherwise asymptomatic.

Case 2

A 70-year-old woman presents to your emergency room. She is acutely short of breath and unable to lie flat. She is cold and diaphoretic. The symptoms began a few hours ago following some "indigestion." Her blood pressure is 80/50. She had the same feeling of "indigestion" a few days ago that lasted 3 to 4 hours. She has been in excellent health prior to this time and denies any prior cardiac or respiratory problems.

Introduction

Heart murmurs can be found at any age. They are caused by turbulent or abnormal flow in the heart. A murmur may or may not represent a critical structural abnormality. Chapter 14 described lesions that are congenital in nature and likely to cause murmurs in the neonate or child. This chapter discusses **heart murmurs related to acquired heart disease that become apparent in the adult population**.

Acquired disease of the heart valves can be a major clinical problem frequently requiring surgical correction. Despite the near elimination of rheumatic fever and rheumatic heart disease (historically, the major cause of acquired valvular heart disease in this country), valve surgery represented 15% of the cases reported in the Society of Thoracic Surgeons (STS) database from 1990 to 1999.[1] Of the four cardiac valves, **the aortic and mitral valves most commonly are involved**. Structural **changes in the tricuspid valve can occur, but the leading causes of tricuspid valvular disease are changes secondary to left-sided heart failure and pulmonary hypertension secondary to valvular disease of the aortic or mitral valve. The pulmonic valve rarely is involved**.

Onset of symptoms can be quite sudden (Case 2) when attribut**able to acute changes in structural anatomy of the valve (endocardi-tis, aortic dissection, and ruptured papillary muscle or chordae tendinae). More often, patients present with progressive symptoms, although an acute episode of heart failure or pulmonary edema may draw attention to the disease process**. In either situation, proper workup and appropriate medical and surgical therapy are crucial to the long- and short-term well-being of the patient. Symptoms are classified I to IV similar to The American Heart Association classification used for angina (see Table 16.1).

Anatomy of the Valves

Each heart valve is made of similar tissue components. The leaflets consist of endothelial cells on a thin, delicate, fibrous skeleton. Each leaflet is attached to the thicker fibrous skeleton of the valve annulus. **Figure 15.1** shows the anatomic relation of the four heart valves in a cross section taken through the base of the heart. **The aortic and mitral valves share a common fibrous skeleton. They come within greatest approximation at the noncoronary sinus of the aortic valve:** the anterior leaflet of the mitral valve can be viewed, at the time of aortic valve surgery, as lying just below the noncoronary sinus.

The normal aortic valve is a three-leaflet structure consisting of the left, right, and noncoronary leaflets. It usually is 2.5 to 3.5 cm^2 in area. Each leaflet is associated with its respective coronary sinus. Although variations can occur, the right coronary artery arises from the right

---

[1] The Society of Thoracic Surgeons National Adult Cardiac Surgery Database, 1999. Voluntary registry of results from more than 500 participating cardiac surgery programs nationwide. Data available at www.sts.org.

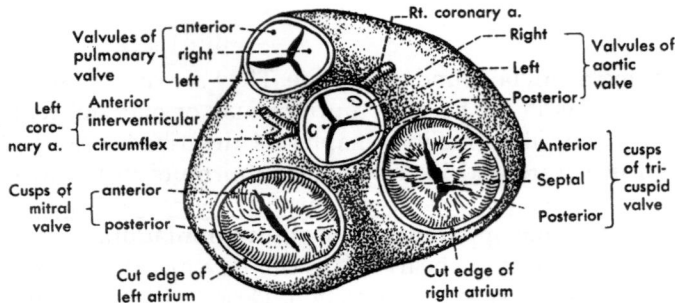

Figure 15.1. Anatomy of the cardiac valves, viewed as transverse section at the level of the base of the heart. (Reprinted with permission from Hollinshead WH. The Heart and Great Vessels. In Hollinshead WH: Anatomy for Surgeons, Volume Two, The Thorax, Abdomen and Pelvis, second edition. New York: Harper and Row: 1971:129.)

coronary sinus, which lies anatomically anterior in the aortic root. The left coronary artery arises from the left sinus and is located relatively posterior. The noncoronary sinus is toward the right side of the aortic root and lies closest to the surgeon when viewed in the operating room. The **bundle of His lies just below the aortic annulus** in the right coronary sinus adjacent to its junction with the noncoronary sinus. This relationship explains the potential for the development of heart block related to aortic valvular disease or to complications of aortic valve replacement. Often, **increasing heart block is an indication of a progressive aortic root abscess in the presence of endocarditis,** even if the patient appears to be improving otherwise, and is an indication for urgent surgery.

The mitral valve is anatomically more complex than the aortic valve. The normal valve area is 4.0 to 6.0 cm^2. In cross section, it looks like a parachute with the larger anterior leaflet and smaller posterior leaflets tethered to the papillary muscles and mitral valve annulus by the chordae tendinae. **Disruption or stretching of the chordae or papillary muscle results in mitral insufficiency due to the loss of the tethering mechanisms, which then permits prolapse of the valve leaflet back into the atrium.**

The right-sided heart valves are comparable to those on the left side but less prone to isolated structural problems. The pulmonic valve is a trileaflet valve similar in appearance to the aortic valve. It does have sinuses but no coronary ostia. The tricuspid valve has three leaflets of unequal size with a supporting apparatus similar to the mitral valve. **Significant pulmonary hypertension can lead to secondary dilatation of the tricuspid annulus and result in tricuspid insufficiency.**

Differential Diagnosis

In any adult patient presenting with new-onset congestive heart failure, exercise intolerance (**Case 1**), cardiogenic shock (**Case 2**), increasing fatigue, or angina, a significant valve problem must be considered. The differential diagnosis of an adult patient with a heart murmur can be approached in a relatively simple way. (See **Algorithm 15.1.**) **The first step is to determine if the murmur represents a significant pathologic problem.** A murmur can be totally benign and of no clinical significance. **Next, it must be determined if a heart valve abnormality is, in fact, the cause of the murmur.** Other causes do exist, such as congenital heart disease that was not recognized during childhood or an acquired ventricular defect following a myocardial infarction. The presence of a heart murmur can signify a benign or malignant tumor of the heart. Careful history and physical examination will determine the clinical significance of the murmur. **Finally, the valve involved and the cause of the murmur must be defined. Table 15.1** lists the numerous etiologies of disease of each of the heart valves.

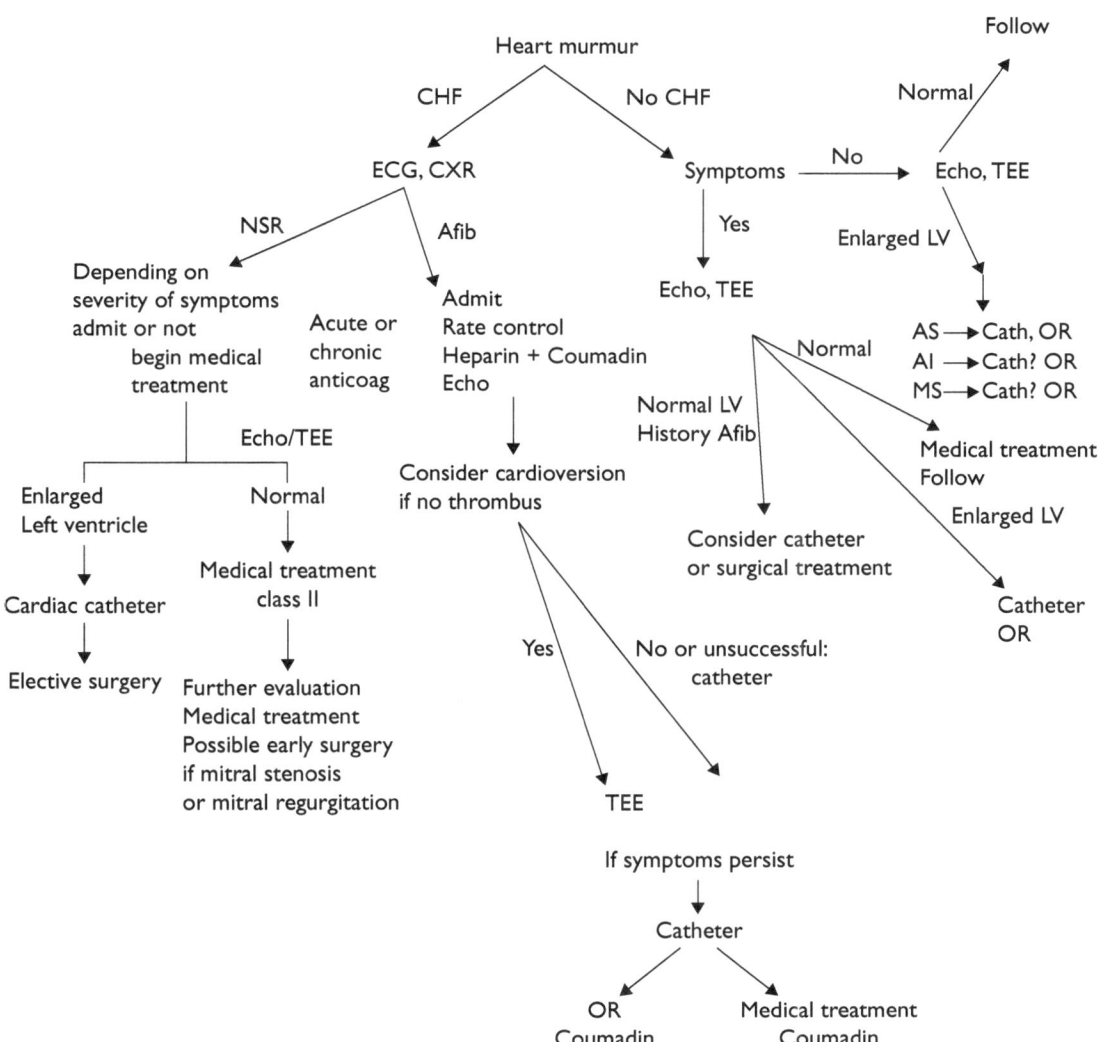

Algorithm 15.1. Algorithm for diagnosis and treatment of adults with heart murmurs. CHF, congestive heart failure; ECG, electrocardiogram; NSR, normal sinus rhythm; TEE, transesophageal echocardiography.

Table 15.1. Prevalent etiologies of valvular heart disease.

Mitral stenosis
  Valvular
    Rheumatic disease
    Nonrheumatic disease
      Infective endocarditis
      Congenital mitral stenosis
      Single papillary muscle (parachute valve)
      Mitral annual calcification
  Supravalvular
    Myxoma
    Left atrial thrombus

Mitral insufficiency
  Valvular
    Rheumatic fever
    Endocarditis
    Systemic lupus erythematosis
    Congenital
      Cleft leaflet (isolated)
      Endocardial cushion defect
    Connective tissue disorders
  Annular
    Degeneration
    Dilation
  Subvalvular
    Chordae tendinae
      Endocarditis
      Myocardial infarction
      Connective tissue disorder
      Rheumatic disease
    Papillary muscle
      Dysfunction or rupture
      Ischemia or infarction
      Endocarditis
      Inflammatory disorder
    Malalignment
      Left ventricular dilation
      Cardiomyopathy

Aortic stenosis[a]
  Acquired
    Rheumatic disease
    Degenerative (fibrocalcific) disease
      Tricuspid valve
      Congenital bicuspid valve
    Infective endocarditis
  Congenital
    Tricuspid valve with commissural fusion
    Unicuspid unicommissural valve
    Hypoplastic annulus

Aortic insufficiency
  Valvular
    Rheumatic disease
    Congenital
    Endocarditis
    Connective tissue disorder (Marfan's)
  Annular
    Connective tissue disorders (Marfan's)
    Aortic dissection
    Hypertension
    Inflammatory disease (e.g., ankylosing spondylitis)

[a] Excludes subvalvular and supravalvular processes.

Source: Reprinted from Rosengart TK, de Bois W, Francalancia NA. Adult heart disease. In: Norton JA, Bollinger RR, Chang AE, et al, eds. Surgery: Basic Science and Clinical Evidence. New York: Springer-Verlag, 2001, with permission.

Aortic Stenosis

Surgery involving the aortic valve is the second most common procedure performed in adults (isolated coronary artery bypass graft is number one) and represents approximately 60% of the valve cases reported in the STS database. **The etiology of aortic stenosis is multifactorial and often can be inferred by the age of onset of symptoms. The primary causes are a congenitally deformed bicuspid valve, rheumatic valvular disease, and degenerative disease of a three-leaflet valve. Patients who present in the fourth or fifth decade of life often have a congenital bicuspid aortic valve that becomes progressively stenotic.** The etiology is referred to as congenital in nature. **Those developing symptoms at a later age are likely to have had rheumatic heart disease and often have combined aortic stenosis and regurgitation. Patients presenting in the eighth or ninth decade usually have had a normal three-leaflet valve that has become calcified, and this etiology is referred to as "senile degenerative disease."**

Aortic stenosis has a well-recognized **triad of symptoms** that develop progressively as the area of the aortic valve drops below 1.0 cm²: **angina**, **heart failure**, and **syncope**. The obstruction to outflow from the left ventricle results in significant pressure loading and the development of ventricular hypertrophy. Intracavitary systolic pressures can reach 300 mm Hg or more. **Onset of one or all of these symptoms usually occurs after many years of an increasingly stenotic valve and is a poor prognostic sign.** Angina may be one of the first symptoms to develop. Symptoms of shortness of breath or angina are precipitated by exercise when the fixed area of the valve prevents an increase in forward cardiac output. Once frank ventricular failure occurs with increasing diastolic volumes, rapid deterioration of left ventricular function can occur, and the prognosis for the patient worsens. **Decrease in the function of the left ventricle is the leading indicator of increased operative mortality and decreased long-term survival in all patients undergoing cardiac surgery.** The exact cause of syncopal episodes remains unclear. It has been attributed to, but not proven to be related to, arrhythmias, sudden lack of ejection, or unexplained low cardiac output. **The presence of angina, heart failure, and syncope in a patient with aortic stenosis should be considered life threatening, and urgent surgical correction should be performed.**

The natural history of aortic stenosis is well recognized, with almost 100% mortality within 5 years of symptom onset without surgical valve replacement. Once symptoms occur, they should be treated appropriately with diuretics and antianginal medications while assessment of the patient progresses. Care must be taken, however, **to avoid excessive use of nitrates and diuretics, since the loss of preload can lead to hypotension and death.**

Aortic Insufficiency

Aortic insufficiency can cause symptoms of heart failure and cardiac enlargement, but the process is quite different from the process leading to aortic stenosis. Whereas pressure overload is the inciting

factor in aortic stenosis, volume overload is the culprit in aortic insufficiency. **Leakage through the valve results from one of many causes that affect the leaflets directly (rheumatic disease, endocarditis, and connective tissue disorders) or the annulus of the valve (connective tissue disorders, especially Marfan's syndrome, hypertension, and inflammatory diseases).** This volume overloading results in dilation of the ventricle followed by thickening of the ventricular wall. This compensation can be quite effective and result in a massively enlarged heart and progression of ventricular enlargement without significant symptoms. The natural history of aortic insufficiency is less clear than that of aortic stenosis, and patients may survive many years with significant regurgitation without symptoms until late in the natural course of the disease.

The scenario described in **Case 1** would not be unusual for a patient with aortic insufficiency, especially at a younger age. Symptoms usually are related to onset of congestive heart failure. In some patients, angina may be present due to reversal of flow in the coronary arteries secondary to a very low aortic diastolic pressure that may occur.

Mitral Stenosis

Mitral stenosis most commonly is caused by rheumatic valvular disease. Scarring due to endocarditis can occur. An atrial myxoma prolapsing into the mitral annulus can mimic the signs of valvular stenosis. **The major symptoms are those of congestive heart failure, but left ventricular failure per se does not occur.** Symptoms may develop when the valve area drops below $2\,cm^2$ and is related to increasing pressure in the left atrium. Pressure gradients across the mitral valve in excess of $20\,mm\,Hg$ can occur. Pulmonary congestion occurs when this pressure is transmitted back into the pulmonary circulation, especially when exercise is attempted, and the fixed output by the valve results in dramatic increases in the pulmonary artery pressure. Classically, hemoptysis would develop in late stages of the disease. Atrial dilatation is likely to occur, and subsequent atrial fibrillation will develop. **New-onset atrial fibrillation is not an uncommon presentation for mitral stenosis. Occasionally, embolization of left atrial thrombus that develops secondary to the atrial fibrillation can be the presenting sign.** Medical therapy is directed to the treatment of congestive heart failure and atrial fibrillation while the diagnostic workup progresses and a decision regarding surgery is reached.

Mitral Insufficiency

Because of the complex structure of the mitral valve, the causes of mitral insufficiency are numerous, affecting the valve leaflets, the supporting structure, or the annulus, or a combination thereof. Rheumatic valvular disease and endocarditis tend to affect the leaflet directly, but they also can affect the valve's supporting structures. Ruptured chordae tendinae or papillary muscle results in significant regurgitation, as may myocardial infarction affecting the ventricular wall at the base of the papillary muscle. Myxomatous degeneration of the valve can result as a sequela of mitral valve prolapse. Significant ventricular dilation that affects the annulus of the valve can lead to profound symptoms. **As with aortic insufficiency, significant leakage can occur through the valve without significant symptoms if onset is gradual.** Eventually, excessive volume overload affects both the left ventricle and the left atrium. Thinning of the left atrium occurs and can result in atrial fibrillation. Severe pulmonary hypertension may develop from volume and pressure overload of the pulmonary circulation. **When patients reach the later stages of this disease, operative mortalities become extremely high, and the chance for recovery of substantial ventricular function or relief of symptoms is less likely, especially in the presence of associated coronary artery disease.**

Tricuspid Regurgitation

Right-sided valvular disease, for the most part, is confined to the tricuspid valve. The typical lesion is tricuspid regurgitation secondary to pulmonary hypertension and annular dilatation. Rheumatic disease or endocarditis can affect the valve. Traumatic rupture of the supporting structures can occur, especially following blunt trauma.

Other Differential Diagnoses

The remaining causes of heart murmurs are infrequent. **Congenital anomalies** missed in childhood can prompt the need for evaluation. **Atrial septal defects** may well be missed and not become apparent until signs of congestive failure develop or a stenotic murmur (related to increased flow but no structural abnormality) occurs in the pulmonic area. **The murmur of a postinfarction ventricular septal defect** may not be recognized until a patient is in the recovery phase of a myocardial infarction (MI). Finally, **the intermittent mitral stenosis murmur related to an atrial myxoma** that intermittently obstructs diastolic flow across the mitral valve should not be missed.

Acute Changes in Valve Competency

As opposed to the gradual changes and onset of symptoms with chronic valve disease, acute changes in valve competency are not handled well by the heart. **Amounts of insufficiency tolerated in the chronic situation where the heart has been able to gradually compensate over time are not tolerated in the acute situation.** Acute aortic regurgitation associated with bacterial endocarditis or aortic dissection and acute mitral regurgitation that accompanies a ruptured papillary muscle may lead to the acute onset of severe symptoms of heart failure and shock.

    Case 2 describes a patient developing acute mitral regurgitation several days after an MI. This must be differentiated from a post-MI ventricular septal defect by echocardiography, measurements of oxygen saturation in the right heart chambers (a step up from the right atrium to the right ventricle), or left ventriculogram (or all of the above). Emergency surgery may provide the only option despite the high risk (30–75%) in these acute situations.

Diagnostic Methods

History and Physical Examination

Evaluation of a patient with a heart murmur requires a complete but focused history and physical examination. The present illness should be detailed, including a search for the onset of symptoms (if any). Subtle changes in exercise tolerance need to be explored. Factors that bring on the symptoms or relieve them should be sought. Specifics related to the etiology of the valvular disease should be sought: a **history of rheumatic fever, familial history of connective tissue disease, history of endocarditis, history of heart murmur, etc.** As in **Case 1**, a history of heart murmur described as nonsignificant in the past may be present. A **careful review of systems, past medical history, and social history** is crucial to help make decisions regarding future therapy.

The physical exam is directed toward the heart and systems that **reflect signs of valvular heart disease or secondary congestive heart failure as well as findings that might increase surgical risk.** Initial observation of the patient for presence or absence of muscle wasting is important. Many patients report weight loss in later stages of the disease because of an inability to eat related to respiratory symptoms. Examination of the head and neck for venous distention, carotid bruits, delayed carotid upstroke (aortic stenosis), water-hammer pulse (aortic insufficiency), and thyromegaly (as source of atrial fibrillation) is important.

The dentition of the patient needs to be checked. If valve surgery is contemplated, all dental work should be done prior to the implantation of a new valve to minimize the risk of prosthetic valve endocarditis. **Pulmonary exam** tries to elicit the rales and rhonchi frequently associated with congestive heart failure. **Abdominal and peripheral exams** are intended to find signs related to right-sided heart failure, including hepatosplenomegaly and peripheral edema. **Peripheral pulses are evaluated**, and the **presence or absence of varicose veins** should be noted in case bypass surgery is required.

The **cardiac exam** should note any cardiac enlargement. The presence or absence of a gallop rhythm indicative of heart failure is listened for. Last, heart murmurs are listened for and described. Murmurs are rated on a scale of I to VI, where I is barely perceptible with a stethoscope and VI describes a thrill (palpable murmur). **The typical aortic stenosis murmur is heard loudest over the second intercostal space to the right of the sternum and may radiate to the neck.** It usually is a crescendo/decrescendo murmur that may range from mid- to holosystolic. Systole may be quite prolonged. **An aortic insufficiency murmur usually is loudest in the fourth intercostal space to the left of the sternum, and is a diastolic decrescendo murmur that can be heard best with the patient leaning forward, and may be associated with a widened pulse pressure. Mitral stenosis is heard loudest at the apex of the heart, which usually is not displaced, since left ventricular enlargement is unusual.** The murmur is a low-pitched, rumbling diastolic murmur that may be accentuated by expiration. An opening "snap" may be present. **A mitral insufficiency murmur is holosystolic, blowing, loudest at the apex, and may radiate to the axilla.**

Chest X-Ray

Frequently, the history and physical give an accurate picture by which the diagnosis can be made. The **chest x-ray can be helpful for confirming signs of cardiomegaly, chamber enlargement, pulmonary congestion, etc.** An associated aortic dilatation of an ascending aortic aneurysm associated with aortic insufficiency may be present.

Electrocardiogram

An electrocardiogram clarifies any cardiac rhythm abnormalities. Conduction defects, especially in the presence of active endocarditis, should be sought. Left and right ventricular or atrial enlargement may be suggested. Other changes are suggestive of associated coronary artery disease that also must be addressed.

Echocardiogram

The easiest and currently most accurate noninvasive test used in evaluating valvular heart disease is the echocardiogram, more specifically the transesophageal echocardiogram. These studies permit a simple screening for the presence and severity of a valvular lesion. At the same time, the presence of chamber enlargement or dysfunction can be determined. A simple method thus exists to permit the ongoing evaluation of patients not yet deemed candidates for surgery. The presence or absence of calcification that might increase the complexity of surgery can be identified, and information can be provided on the suitability of a patient for mitral valve repair. If these studies indicate the need, cardiac catheterization usually is recommended. If surgery is not needed at the time of initial evaluation, echocardiogram provides a simple method for ongoing evaluation.

Cardiac Catheterization

Both left and right heart catheterizations are performed on most patients being evaluated for valve surgery. Right heart catheterization usually employs a Swan-Ganz catheter inserted via a large vein into the right heart. Measurements of right-sided chamber pressures, the pulmonary artery pressure, and the pulmonary capillary wedge pressure (which reflects the left atrial pressure) are made. Often, oxygen saturation in each location also is measured. A thermodilution cardiac output is determined. In a **left heart catheterization**, a catheter is passed from the femoral or brachial artery back though the aorta to the heart. It is used to measure pressures in the aortic root and left ventricular chamber. Any gradient indicative of stenosis across the aortic valve is measured. The gradient across the mitral valve is the difference between simultaneous measurements of pulmonary capillary wedge pressure (the equivalent of left atrial pressure) and left ventricular end-diastolic pressure. Across the aortic valve, a pullback reading is obtained on several occasions. **The valve areas then can be calculated using the Gorlin formula that relates the area of the valve to the pressure gradient across the valve and the cardiac output. Coronary angiography** is performed to look for any associated coronary disease that could be repaired simultaneously during surgery. In some younger patients and in some emergency situations, the information provided by the echocardiogram may be sufficient and heart catheterization may not be required.

Therapeutic Intervention

Indication for Surgery

Decisions regarding the management of patients with valvular heart disease are based on the recognized progression of the various lesions and the risk versus benefit of surgical intervention. Until the ideal replacement valve is developed, the inherent risks associated with prosthetic valves (limited durability, need for anticoagulation, propensity for infection, sound) must be considered along with the risk of the operation itself. One pathologic situation (the deformed valve) is being substituted with another (the prosthetic valve when needed), although with a different array of potential problems. **The surgical risk is associated with age (increases significantly by decade over 70 years of age), ventricular function (ejection fraction <40%), diabetes, renal failure or insufficiency, peripheral vascular disease, chronic obstructive pulmonary disease (COPD), etc. Associated coronary artery disease, especially in the presence of mitral regurgitation, significantly increases operative mortality. Thus, the decision is one of the benefits of preventing further deterioration in ventricular function, death, or other complications related to the valve disease versus the risk of surgery, the patient's likelihood to regain or maintain an acceptable lifestyle, and the risks inherent in the new valve substituted.**

Patients with new-onset symptoms are treated medically to relieve symptoms of congestive heart failure or angina. Congestive heart failure is treated with diuretics, digoxin, and afterload reduction when it can be tolerated. Angina is treated appropriately. Great care must be taken in patients with aortic stenosis to avoid overdiureseis or too much preload reduction (with nitroglycerine and diuretics), which can result in inadequate filling of the left ventricle and subsequent syncope or low output. Heart rate must be controlled with beta-blockers digoxin or calcium channel blockers to permit adequate chamber filling, especially when stenotic lesions are present. Anticoagulants are needed for patients in atrial fibrillation to prevent systemic embolization. There is some evidence that the use of the calcium channel blocker Procardia in asymptomatic patients with aortic insufficiency may delay their need for surgery.

Once diagnostic studies have been completed, recommendations for chronic medical therapy or surgery are made. These decisions

must be made on an individual basis and must involve an informed consent from the patient and family. Medical therapy is used for those patients when it is believed the surgical risk is too high or their long-term benefit is not sufficient for surgery. Others who are not yet ready for surgery receive medical therapy but are followed closely until indications for surgery become manifest.

As noted, the surgical management of valvular heart disease is dependent on the risk-benefit ratio for the patient. Unfortunately, this is not always so clear when the risk of the operation is high and the benefit to an individual patient not clear. However, generalized indications for surgery have evolved based on short- and long-term outcome studies. **Detailed diagnostic and therapeutic guidelines are well summarized in "Consensus Statement on Management of Patients with Valvular Heart Disease,"** developed by a combined task force of the American Heart Association and the American College of Cardiology.[2]

Aortic Stenosis and Aortic Insufficiency

In **aortic stenosis**, the rapidity with which patients deteriorate and die suddenly after the onset of symptoms has made the decision making relatively easy. **Any patient with symptomatic aortic stenosis should undergo valve replacement** unless there are significant contraindications or the patient's life expectancy is otherwise severely limited. Even those patients with significant organ dysfunction secondary to the low output state may be considered. In the past, it also was believed those asymptomatic patients with aortic stenosis and a valve area of less than 1 cm^2 or a gradient >60 mm Hg also should undergo valve replacement. More recently, **with the ability to follow patients closely with echocardiography, surgery may be delayed until symptoms develop without increased risk to the patient as long as surgery occurs rapidly following the onset of symptoms**.

In **aortic insufficiency, the decision making is not so clear**. Studies have shown that a patient with aortic insufficiency and a normal ventricle can undergo replacement with little surgical risk. On the other hand, once the ventricle begins to fail, the risk increases dramatically. Even in the absence of symptoms, increased operative mortality occurs in the presence of indicators of deteriorating ventricular function. **As a result, valve surgery is recommended for all class III and IV symptomatic patients and all patients with one of the following signs even in the absence of symptoms: increasing size of the heart, decreasing ejection fraction under observation, ejection fraction of less than 40%; or an end-systolic diameter of greater than 55 mm by echocardiography.**

At the present time, **valve replacement is the recommended treatment for surgical correction of aortic valvular diseases**. There are a few patients with aortic insufficiency in whom valvuloplasty has been successful, although replacement remains the standard.

---

[2] American Heart Disease/American College of Cardiology. Consensus Statement on Management of Patients with Valvular Heart Disease. Circulation 1998;98:1949–1984. Also available at www.americanheart.org.

Mitral Stenosis and Mitral Insufficiency

Mitral valve disease is different from aortic valvular disease in that reconstructive surgery often can be done instead of replacement of the valve. The operative mortality has been less with a repair when the long-term risks of a prosthetic valve are avoided. **Mitral stenosis** was the first valve problem approached surgically and was performed successfully in the late 1940s several years before the first successful use of the heart lung machine (by Gibbon[3] in 1953). In any case, either direct commissurotomy and reconstruction, if needed, of the subvalvular apparatus are performed, or valve replacement is done. Because of the success of mitral valvuloplasty for mitral stenosis and the detailed diagnostic images of the valves now obtainable by echocardiography, certain patients with mitral stenosis are treated using percutaneous methods in the catheterization laboratory using balloon dilators (larger balloons but similar technique to angioplasty) with good success. **The indications for surgery in the presence of mitral stenosis are class II symptoms if a commissurotomy is possible either surgically or using a balloon or all class III and IV patients even if valve replacement is likely to be needed.**

Surgical treatment of mitral insufficiency is the most difficult condition about which to make decisions. Many patients are without symptoms despite large amounts of regurgitation and decreased left ventricular function. Unlike other situations, the operative risk in patients with mitral regurgitation is related to the underlying cause of the disease and may be two to three times greater when the etiology is ischemic in nature. Ultimately, at later stages of the disease, the operative risk and the likely lack of prolongation of life or relief of symptoms make surgery inappropriate for some of these patients, although some recent investigational studies suggest certain methods of valvuloplasty may be applicable in this patient population despite the high risk. **Early surgery is indicated in patients with American Heart Association class II symptoms if repair of the valve seems likely. In all others, the recommendation is to await class III symptoms. All class III and IV patients should be considered for surgery.** On the other hand, **increasing ventricular chamber size or end systolic diameter >55 mm in the absence of symptoms is an indication for surgical correction, similar to the decision making for aortic insufficiency.**

Repair of the mitral valve has been shown to carry a lower operative mortality compared to replacement. It is the preferred operation when it can be done expeditiously. If not, valve replacement should be carried out. If replacement is performed, many surgeons recommend that as much of the subvalvular apparatus is retained at the time of valve replacement (especially if a tissue valve is used) in order to maintain the normal architecture of the ventricle following surgery. This is believed to lead to improved short- and long-term success.

---

[3] Gibbon JH Jr. Application of a mechanical heart and lung apparatus to cardiac surgery. Minn Med 1954;37:171.

Selection of Valve Prosthesis

Guidelines for the selection of prosthetic valves have been generalized but should be discussed carefully with each patient before surgery and be part of the informed consent. In general, **there are two types of prosthetic valves available: mechanical and tissue. The advantages of the former include longer durability and perhaps lower residual gradient size for size compared to stented tissue valves. The disadvantage of the mechanical valve is the requirement for lifelong anticoagulation to prevent valve thrombosis or embolization of thrombus from the valve. In addition, the closing click of the valve may be audible and objectionable to certain patients or their partners. Tissue valves do not require anticoagulation (after the first 3 months of implantation) if a patient remains in sinus rhythm. They are silent. Their durability, however, is limited.** Definitive information on durability is available only for the original first generation porcine valves and is related to the patient's age at valve implantation. In patients older than 70 years of age, a tissue valve failure is likely less than 10% of the time in the first 10 years. On the other hand, in patients younger than 35 years of age, more than 50% require replacement at a second operation within 5 years. Second-generation tissue valves have shown less of a propensity for deterioration, especially in elderly patients, and frequently outlast the patient's lifetime. The decision making, however, also is now complicated by the extended lifetime of many elderly patients. **In general, the recommendations are that a mechanical valve be used on all patients younger than 65 years of age, unless anticoagulation is contraindicated. In most patients older than 65 or 70 years of age, tissue valves are recommended, unless anticoagulation for other problems (such as chronic atrial fibrillation) is required or unless it is likely the patient will outlive a tissue valve.**

Results

For isolated **aortic valve replacement, operative mortality ranges from 2% to 5.5%. For isolated mitral valve replacement, the range is 3.5% to 7.5%.** Isolated mitral valvuloplasty has even better results. The exception is patients in later stages of mitral regurgitation, especially if ischemic in origin, in whom the 5-year survival is as low as 20%. See **Tables 15.2, 15.3,** and **15.4.**

Long-Term Care

The goals of long-term care and follow-up in these patients are aimed at minimizing those risks associated with a prosthetic valve or valve repair. In the first 6 months following surgery, **the risk of prosthetic valve endocarditis** is significantly higher than later time frames and carries a grave prognosis (mortality 50% to 80%). Beyond this time, the risks of endocarditis and methods of treatment are the same as for any deformed native valve. **Antibiotic prophylaxis is an absolute must for these patients when any dental work is performed. The same is true for any invasive procedure that might be associated with an episode**

Table 15.2. Selected series of aortic valve replacement.

Valve type	Years of enrollment	n	Operative mortality (%)	Actuarial survival	Freedom from valve-related complications	Freedom from reoperation	Source
Mechanical							
St. Jude	1982–1991	611	5.4	5yr, 78%	—	—	Fernandez[a]
St. Jude	1979–1990	254	3.9	5yr, 80% ± 3% 10yr, 47% ± 9%	10yr, 35% ± 8%	10yr, 92% ± 2%	Kratz[b]
Carbomedics	1989–1994	349	3.4	5yr, 77% ± 4%	5yr, 69% ± 4%	5yr, 96% ± 1%	Bernal[c]
Bioprosthetic							
Porcine (Carpentier-Edwards)	1979–1995	578	5	10yr, 64% ± 22% 15yr, 39% ± 3%	—	15yr, 55% ± 4%	Jamieson
Porcine (Hancock)	1982–1990	376	4	8yr, 79% ± 3%	8yr, 93% ± 3%[d]	8yr, 91% ± 4%	David[e]
Bovine pericardial (Carpentier-Edwards)	1984–1993	589	2.3	10yr, 71% ± 7%	10yr, 84% ± 6%	10yr, 76% ± 2% 15yr, 53% ± 4%	Auport[f]

[a] Purcaro A, Costantini C, Ciampani N, et al. Diagnostic criteria and management of subacute ventricular free wall rupture complicating myocardial infarction. Am J Cardiol 1997;80:397–405.

[b] Yeo TC, Malouf JF, Oh JK, et al. Clinical profile and outcome in 52 patients with cardiac pseudoaneurysm. Ann Intern Med 1998;128:299–305.

[c] Schwarz CD, Punzengruber C, Ng CK, et al. Clinical presentation of rupture of the left ventricular free wall after myocardial infarction: report of five cases with successful surgical repair. Thorac Cardiovasc Surg 1996;44:71–75.

[d] Freedom from thromboembolism.

[e] Komeda M, David TE. Surgical treatment of postinfarction false aneurysm of the left ventricle. J Thorac Cardiovasc Surg 1993;106(6):1189–1191.

[f] Auport MR, Sirinelli AL, Diermont FF, et al. The last generation of pericardial valves in the aortic position: ten year follow-up in 589 patients. Ann Thorac Surg 1996;61:615–620.

Source: Reprinted from Rosengart TK, de Bois W, Francalancia NA. Adult heart disease. In: Norton JA, Bollinger RR, Chang AE, et al, eds. Surgery: Basic Science and Clinical Evidence. New York: Springer-Verlag, 2001, with permission.

Table 15.3. Selected series of mitral valve replacement.

Valve type	Years of enrollment	n	Operative mortality (%)	Actuarial survival	Freedom from valve-related complications	Freedom from reoperation	Source
Mechanical							
St. Jude	1980–1996	514	7.2	8yr, 89%	—	—	Grossi[a]
St. Jude	1979–1990	397	3.5	10yr, 73% ± 6%	3.7% (pt-yr)	—	Jegaden[b]
Carbomedics	1989–1994	330	6.9	5yr, 77% ± 4%	10yr, 69% ± 4%	—	Bernal[c]
Bioprosthetic							
Porcine (Carpentier-Edwards)	1975–1995	512	9	10yr, 52% ± 2% 15yr, 24% ± 3%	—	15yr, 20% ± 4%	Jamieson
Porcine (Hancock)	1982–1990	195	6	8yr, 68% ± 4%[d]	8yr, 83% ± 5%[e]	8yr, 92% ± 5%	David[f]

[a] Grossi EA, Galloway AC, Miller JS, et al. Valve repair versus replacement for mitral insufficiency: when is a mechanical valve still indicated? J Thorac Cardiovasc Surg 1998;115:389–396.

[b] Lopez-Sendon J, Gonzalez A, Lopez de Sa E, et al. Diagnosis of subacute ventricular wall rupture after acute myocardial infarction: sensitivity and specificity of clinical, hemodynamic and echocardiographic criteria. J Am Coll Cardiol 1992;19:1145–1153.

[c] Schwarz CD, Punzengruber C, Ng CK, et al. Clinical presentation of rupture of the left ventricular free wall after myocardial infarction: report of five cases with successful surgical repair. Thorac Cardiovasc Surg 1996;44:71–75.

[d] Freedom from late cardiac death.

[e] Freedom from thromboembolic complications.

[f] Csapo K, Voith L, Szuk T, et al. Postinfarction left ventricular pseudoaneurysm. Clin Cardiol 1997;20:898–903.

Source: Reprinted from Rosengart TK, de Bois W, Francalancia NA. Adult heart disease. In: Norton JA, Bollinger RR, Chang AE, et al, eds. Surgery: Basic Science and Clinical Evidence. New York: Springer-Verlag, 2001, with permission.

Table 15.4. Mitral valve repair.

Primary repair technique	Year of enrollment	n	Operative mortality (%)	Ten-year actuarial survival	Freedom from reoperation	Comments	Study
Annuloplasty/ valvuloplasty	1972–1979	206	5.5	72% ± 4%	15yr, 87% ± 3%	Freedom from reoperation, 93% for degenerative disease/76% for rheumatic disease (p < 0.01)	Deloche et al.[a]
Annuloplasty	1980–1996	725	5.4	84%[e,f]	76%[b]	Increased complication/ failure rate with rheumatic or multivalve disease	Grossi et al.[b]
Annuloplasty/ valvuloplasty	1981–1992	184	0.5	88% ± 4%[e]	95% ± 2%	Failure risk directly related to degree of disease	David et al.[c]
Chordal replacement with e-PTFE[g]	1981–1995	324	0.6	75% ± 5%	96% ± 1%	Chordal replacement for anterior leaflet prolapse	David et al.[d]

[a] Deloche A, Jebara VA, Relland JYM, et al. Valve repair with Carpentier techniques: the second decade. J Thorac Cardiovasc Surg 1990;99:990–1002.

[b] Grossi EA, Galloway AC, Miller JS, et al. Valve repair versus replacement for mitral insufficiency: when is a mechanical valve still indicated? J Thorac Cardiovasc Surg 1998;115:389–396.

[c] Csapo K, Voith L, Szuk T, et al. Postinfarction left ventricular pseudoaneurysm. Clin Cardiol 1997;20:898–903.

[d] David TE, Omran A, Armstrong, et al. Long-term results of mitral valve repair for myxomatous disease with and without chordal replacement with expanded polytetrafluoroethylene. J Thorac Cardiovasc Surg 1998;115:1279–1286.

[e] Eight-year data.

[f] Freedom from late cardiac death.

[g] Expanded polytetrafluoroethylene.

Source: Reprinted from Rosengart TK, de Bois W, Francalancia NA. Adult heart disease. In: Norton JA, Bollinger RR, Chang AE, et al, eds. Surgery: Basic Science and Clinical Evidence. New York: Springer-Verlag, 2001, with permission.

Table 15.5. Summary of diagnosis and treatment of valvular heart disease in the adult.

	Aortic stenosis	Aortic insufficiency	Mitral stenosis	Mitral insufficiency
Etiology	Congenital bicuspid Rheumatic Degenerative	Rheumatic, congenital, endocarditis, connective tissue disease (Marfan's), aortic dissection, hypertension, inflammatory disease	Rheumatic, endocarditis, pseudostenosis due to myxoma	Rheumatic, ruptured chordae tendinae, papillary muscle dysfunction or rupture. LV dilation, ischemic cardiomyopathy
Signs and symptoms	Angina DOE followed by congestive heart failure Syncope	Indolent onset CHF symptoms; decreased exercise tolerance	Dyspnea on exertion, CHF, atrial fibrillation, embolization, hemoptysis (late)	CHF, atrial fibrillation, embolization, right-sided CHF; hepatomegaly
Physical findings	Cardiomegaly; crescendo-decrescendo mid-systolic murmur, loudest 2nd right intercostal space radiating to neck	Cardiomegaly; water-hammer pulse; decrescendo diastolic murmur loudest 4th left intercostal space	Possible RVH Diastolic rumble, loudest at apex	Possible RVH Holosystolic blowing murmur loudest at apex, radiating to axilla
Diagnostic studies	CXR, ECG, echocardiography	CXR, ECG, echocardiography	CXR, ECG, echocardiography	CXR, ECG, echocardiography
Cardiac catheterization and findings	Left and right; left ventriculogram, aortic root injection, coronary angiography age >40 or family history CAD; gradient >60 mm Hg; valve area <1.0 cm²	Left and right; left ventriculogram, aortic root injection, coronary angiography age >40 or family history CAD; 1+ to 4+ regurgitation	Left and right; left ventriculogram, coronary angiography age >40 or family history CAD; simultaneous PCW and LVEDP for mitral gradient; valve area < 2 cm²	Left and right; left ventriculogram, coronary angiography age >40 or family history CAD; 1+ to 4+ regurgitation on ventriculogram, ventricular and/or atrial enlargement
Medical management	If "asymptotic" close follow (every 3 months) Urgent surgery if symptoms develop	If asymptotic and normal LV, follow medically (Procardia)	Coumadin and antiarrhythmics for atrial fibrillation, treat early CHF	Coumadin and antiarrhythmics for atrial fibrillation, treat early CHF
Operative indications	Any symptomatic patient	Any symptomatic patient, all patients ESD >55 mm, EF <40%, decreasing EF or increasing heart size under treatment	Class II if commissurotomy likely Class III or IV	Class II if valvuloplasty likely, all class III or IV, ESD >55 mm regardless of symptoms
Operative procedure	Valve replacement	Valve replacement, rare valvuloplasty	Balloon commissurotomy, commissurotomy (open) or valve replacement	Valvuloplasty (may be complex) or valve replacement

CAD, coronary artery disease; CHF, congestive heart failure; CXR, chest x-ray; DOE, dyspnea on exertion; ECG, electrocardiogram; EF, ejection fraction; ESD, end systolic diameter; LVEDP, left ventricular end-diastolic pressure; PCW, pulmonary capillary wedge; RVH, right ventricular hypertrophy.

of bacteremia. **Patients with mechanical valves must be maintained on proper levels of Coumadin to maintain the international normalized ratio (INR) at a proper range.** The addition of aspirin in certain patients also may be warranted. The risk of valve thrombosis or embolization is a real potential for these patients, approaching 1% per patient year. In addition, the risk of anticoagulation-associated death or significant bleeding (requiring transfusion) is 1% to 2% per year. Patients who have had tissue valve replacement or annuloplasty rings inserted should receive anticoagulants for 3 months and can have it discontinued after that time.

Summary

Valvular heart disease was one of the first problems addressed by cardiac surgeons. Valve repair and replacement have become a "routine" method of treatment for symptomatic patients, relieving symptoms and prolonging life. **Table 15.5** provides a summary of much of what is discussed in this chapter.

Selected Readings

American Heart Association/American College of Cardiology. Consensus Statement on Management of Patients with Valvular Heart Disease. Circulation 1998;98:1949–1984.

Auport MR, Sirinelli AL, Diermont FF, et al. The last generation of pericardial valves in the aortic position: ten year follow-up in 589 patients. Ann Thoracic Surg 1996;61:615–620.

Csapo K, Voith L, Szuk T, et al. Postinfarction left ventricular pseudoaneurysm. Clin Cardiol 1997;20:898–903.

David TE, Omran A, Armstrong, et al. Long-term results of mitral valve repair for myxomatous disease with and without chordal replacement with expanded polytetrafluoroethylene. J Thorac Cardiovasc Surg 1998;115:1279–1286.

Deloche A, Jebara VA, Relland JYM, et al. Valve repair with Carpentier techniques: the second decade. J Thorac Cardiovasc Surg 1990;99:990–1002.

Grossi EA, Galloway AC, Miller JS, et al. Valve repair versus replacement for mitral insufficiency: when is a mechanical valve still indicated? J Thorac Cardiovasc Surg 1998;115:389–396.

Komeda M, David TE. Surgical treatment of postinfarction false aneurysm of the left ventricle. J Thorac Cardiovasc Surg 1993;106(60):1189–1191.

Lopez-Sendon J, Gonzalez A, Lopez de Sa E, et al. Diagnosis of subacute ventricular wall rupture after acute myocardial infarction: sensitivity and specificity of clinical, hemodynamic and echocardiographic criteria. J Am Coll Cardiol 1992;19:1145–1153.

Purcaro A, Costantini C, Ciampani N, et al. Diagnostic criteria and management of subacute ventricular free wall rupture complicating myocardial infarction. Am J Cardiol 1997;80:397–405.

Rosengart TK, de Bois W, Francalancia NA: Adult heart disease. In: Norton JA, Bollinger RR, Chang AE, et al, eds. Surgery: Basic Science and Clinical Evidence. New York: Springer-Verlag, 2001.

Schwarz CD, Penzengruber C, Ng CK, et al. Clinical presentation of rupture of the left ventricular free wall after myocardial infarction: report of five cases with successful surgical repair. Thorac Cardiovasc Surg 1996;44:71–75.

Society of Thoracic Surgeons National Adult Cardiac Surgery Database, 1999. Voluntary registry of results from more than 500 participating cardiac surgery programs nationwide. Circulation 1998;98:1949–1984.

Web Sites

American Heart Association: www.americanheart.org.
Society of Thoracic Surgeons: www.sts.org.

16

Acute and Chronic Chest Pain

Alan J. Spotnitz

Objectives

1. To understand the differential diagnosis of chest pain requiring cardiac surgical consultation.
2. To understand the physiology of and rationality for medical treatment of ischemic coronary artery disease.
3. To differentiate acute aortic dissection from myocardial infarction in the emergency setting.
4. To understand initial stabilization of the patient with aortic dissection.
5. To recognize the risk factors associated with open-heart surgery.

Case

A 65-year-old man presents to the emergency room complaining of "chest pain." He drove himself to the hospital. The pain has lasted about an hour and is now going away. He has a history of a hiatus hernia and esophageal reflux. He denies any other associated symptoms. He took an antacid without relief. Because he failed to get any pain relief, he took one of his 87-year-old father's nitroglycerin tablets, and the pain started to ease. He came to the emergency room. He is now pain free and wants to go home. Vital signs are normal except for a heart rate of 100. How do you proceed?

Introduction

This chapter discusses the causes of chest pain that may require intervention by a cardiac surgeon, distinguishes them from other causes that are of less concern, and provides a systematic approach by which the diagnosis and early treatment of these conditions can be begun before the cardiac surgeon arrives. (See Algorithm 16.1.) Often, these

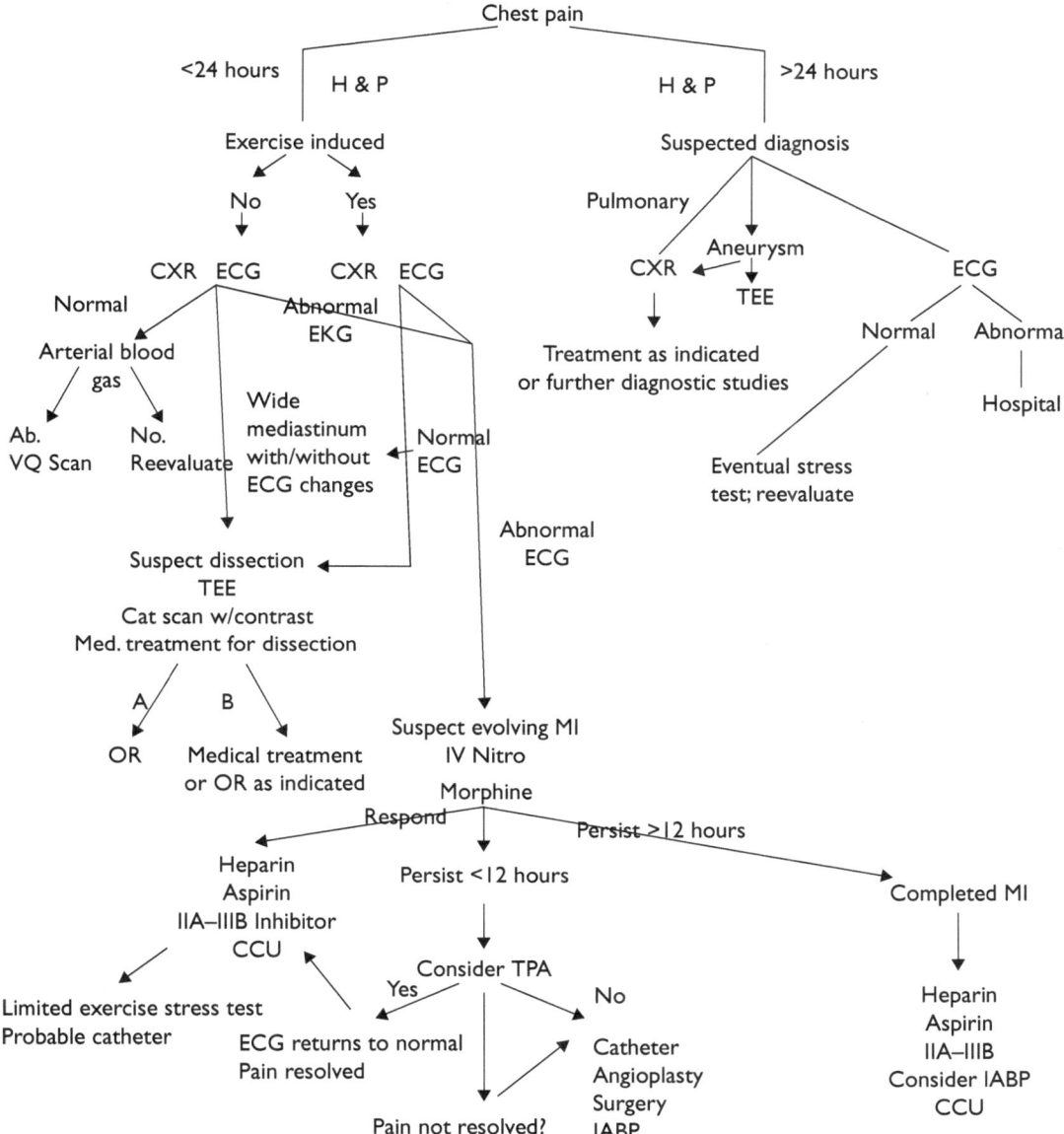

Algorithm 16.1. Algorithm for initial evaluation and treatment of patients with chest pain. CCU, cardiac care unit; CXR, chest x-ray; ECG, electrocardiogram; H&P, history and physical exam; IABP, intraaortic balloon pump; MI, myocardial infarction; OR, operating room; TEE, transesophageal echocardiography; TPA, tissue plasminogen activator.

emergencies occur at night. **Early notification of the surgical team may save precious minutes** in getting a patient through the necessary diagnostic studies and into the operating room when a lifesaving operation is required.

Differential Diagnosis

The major diagnoses associated with chest pain and treated by cardiac surgeons that should concern both medical personnel and patients include **ischemic heart disease, diseases of the thoracic aorta, diseases of the pericardium, and pulmonary embolism.** There are other diseases treated by general thoracic surgeons that are not discussed here. The case described above is relatively nonspecific, but it could describe a scenario for any of these life-threatening diagnoses.

Ischemic Heart Disease

The term **ischemic heart disease** is descriptive of a broad range of clinically significant diagnoses with a common origin. **The underlying pathogenesis in all of these is the mismatch of oxygen supply and oxygen demand of the myocardium.** The most common descriptor of the chest pain associated with this etiology is **angina pectoris.**

The most commonly recognized cause of ischemic heart disease is the occlusion of large epicardial vessels in the heart by atherosclerotic cardiovascular disease. There are other etiologies, however, including valvular heart disease, vasculitis, congenital coronary artery anomalies, episodes of coronary artery spasm related to cocaine use or other causes (Prinzmetal's angina), and dissection of the thoracic aorta when the ostia of a coronary artery are involved.

Classically, angina pectoris is characterized by substernal chest pain or pressure that may radiate down the arm. However, these symptoms may be present in less than 25% of patients with ischemic heart disease. **Other "anginal equivalents" include jaw pain, throat pain, arm pain, dyspnea on exertion, and frank pulmonary edema.** Patients with diabetes are notorious for having "silent ischemia." This means that they do not develop any symptoms of pain when ischemia occurs. They may present with previously unrecognized myocardial infarction or with an episode of acute pulmonary edema.

At one extreme of the spectrum of patients with ischemic heart disease are those with chronic stable angina. Evaluation of previous anginal episodes has resulted in this diagnosis, and the presenting problem is just another manifestation of the underlying cause. **At the other extreme are patients who die suddenly or present with an acute evolving myocardial infarction in cardiogenic shock.** In between these extremes are the patients with **new-onset angina, unstable angina, preinfarction angina, non–Q-wave myocardial infarction, and myocardial infarction without shock.**

In **chronic stable angina pectoris,** short episodes leading to ischemia of the heart muscle occur, but they reverse rapidly without significant damage to the myocardium. This pattern may go on for years, but a progressive course is more likely. **Unstable angina** is descriptive of a scenario in which new symptoms occur in a previously asymptomatic individual or in which a chronic pattern of pain associated with certain activities becomes more frequent or severe. **Rest angina**, as the term implies, **occurs in the absence of stressful activity and is an ominous sign**. **Myocardial infarction** is the end result of this process. The ischemia lasts so long that actual tissue necrosis occurs. **Q-wave myocardial infarction** is descriptive of the damage that occurs when transmural (all layers of the myocardial wall) infarction occurs and is manifest by Q-waves on the electrocardiogram (ECG). **Cardiogenic shock** results when the amount of myocardium that becomes dysfunctional due to ischemia or infarction is so large that the remaining myocardium cannot adequately maintain the systemic circulation.

To quantify the different levels of ischemia that occur before infarction and to suggest the resulting levels of risk for the patient, the **New York Heart Association Classification of Angina** (or other cardiac symptoms) was developed. It is far from accurate and is purely qualitative, but it does provide some frame of reference (**Table 16.1**).

Atherosclerosis is recognized as the major cause of coronary artery disease. It is a progressive disease that can appear microscopically even in infants. Many factors, including **genetic factors, hypertension, dietary indiscretion (including early in life), and diabetes**, have been recognized as contributing to the development of atherosclerotic cardiovascular disease. These cannot be altered. Other factors, such as **obesity, hypercholesterolemia,** and **smoking** (all major contributors to atherosclerotic disease), can be modified. **This modification can significantly alter the progressive course of the disease.** In the heart, atherosclerotic lesions tend to develop in the proximal portions of the coronary arteries and at major branch points. Patients with diabetes are

Table 16.1. New York Heart Association functional classification of angina.

Class	Description
I	Patients with cardiac disease but without resulting limitations of physical activity. Ordinary physical activity does not cause undue fatigue, palpitation, dyspnea, or anginal pain.
II	Patients with cardiac disease resulting in slight limitation of physical activity. They are comfortable at rest. Ordinary physical activity results in fatigue, palpitation, dyspnea, or anginal pain.
III	Patients with cardiac disease resulting in marked limitation of physical activity. They are comfortable at rest. Less than ordinary physical activity causes fatigue, palpitation, dyspnea, or anginal pain.
IV	Patient with cardiac disease resulting in inability to carry on any physical activity without discomfort. Symptoms of cardiac insufficiency or of the anginal syndrome may be present even at rest. If any physical activity is undertaken, discomfort is increased.

Source: Reprinted from The Criteria Committee of the New York Heart Association. Nomenclature and Criteria for Diagnosis, 9th ed. Boston: Little, Brown, 1994. With permission from Lippincott Williams & Wilkins.

likely to have more diffuse disease. Once significant stenoses have developed, symptoms may begin to manifest themselves, especially at times of stress and increased oxygen demand in the heart.

Referring to our case scenario, this patient's presentation certainly could be that of ischemic heart disease. There is a family history, he received some mild relief from nitroglycerin, and he is at the age at which atherosclerotic heart disease has a high incidence. Were you to encounter such a patient and were you to believe his pain was from acute myocardial ischemia, a **physical examination** needs to be done and **further history** needs to be obtained (as described below). Appropriate laboratory studies need to be initiated. These should include an **electrocardiogram, a chest x-ray, and cardiac enzyme screen.** Electrocardiogram may be normal at this point, but it also may be suggestive of some ongoing ischemia or previous injury to the heart. A chest x-ray might reveal signs of cardiac enlargement and may be suggestive of signs of heart failure, should there be any. Finally, cardiac enzymes drawn at this point may or may not be positive, even in the presence of ischemic disease. At the present time, **troponin levels are the most sensitive laboratory study to do for signs of myocardial injury. Creatinine phosphokinase (CPK-MB) levels specifically attributed to the heart also should be obtained.** Based on this information, the history, and the physical examination, a determination should be reached as to the likelihood of ischemic disease and how to proceed further.

Diseases of the Thoracic Aorta

Diseases of the thoracic aorta are **far more prevalent than commonly is recognized and should be considered in the differential diagnosis of any patient complaining of significant chest pain.** Involvement of the thoracic aorta takes two forms: **aneurysmal disease alone or aortic dissection that can occur with or without the presence of aneurysmal disease** and has potentially catastrophic consequences.

Aneurysms of the thoracic aorta are of two types: **saccular** and **fusiform.** The former occurs as an outpouching off the side of the vessel, while the latter consists of a dilatation of a segment of the aorta. **The definition of a true aneurysm requires that all three layers of the normal wall are present (intima, media, and adventitia) and that the diameter of the aorta in the diseased segment is at least twice its normal diameter. Atherosclerosis** frequently is associated with or is the etiology of these aneurysms. Others may be **idiopathic** in origin or be a manifestation of a **connective tissue disorder, the most common of which is Marfan's syndrome.**

Symptoms of aneurysms frequently are related to pressure on adjacent structures from the enlarging aorta. Chest pain may be related to the enlarging aorta itself. Complaints of back pain, hoarseness, cough, shortness of breath, and dysphagia may be present from encroachment on the thoracic spine, recurrent laryngeal nerve, trachea or bronchus, or esophagus, respectively. **Often, an aneurysm first may be discovered on a routine chest x-ray or computed axial**

tomography (CAT) scan obtained for some other reason. There may be no associated symptoms. Surgical repair of these aneurysms usually is recommended when they become large because of the risk of rupture and sudden death. **Once rupture has occurred, the likelihood of survival is low.**

Aortic dissection is far more likely to present as an emergency than is a thoracic aortic aneurysm. Aortic dissection is the cause of acute mortality almost twice as often as acute rupture of an abdominal aortic aneurysm. Although it does not fit the definition of an aneurysm as given above, the term **dissecting aortic aneurysm** frequently is applied. The underlying aorta may be normal in character or aneurysmal prior to the onset of the dissection. **Aortic dissection always must be considered in the emergency setting, as it can be difficult to distinguish from a myocardial infarction. Thrombolytic agents used to treat a myocardial infarction may lead to death when the etiology is aortic dissection.**

A dissecting aortic aneurysm frequently presents with the acute **onset of severe pain. The pain may be similar to angina with a crushing type of pressure or pain.** If the ascending aorta is involved and the dissection continues distally, the pain may migrate to the back. Some patients may describe a **tearing pain between the scapulae** and refer to it as the worst pain they have ever felt. **The pain may be localized to the upper abdomen at times and may be confused with an abdominal aneurysm rupture, perforated ulcer, or cholecystitis.** Because of the nature of the problem, **associated symptoms can be multiple and often are related to the loss of blood supply to major organs due to the shearing off or occlusion of major side branches. Patients may present with signs of stroke, renal failure, bowel ischemia, or limb ischemia. If the ostium of a main coronary artery is involved, there may be signs of ischemia present on the ECG. This is most common involving the right coronary. New-onset aortic insufficiency is the final sign that should not be overlooked in a patient suspected of aortic dissection. The association of chest pain with loss of one or more peripheral pulses or new-onset aortic insufficiency murmur is the** *sine qua non* of aortic dissection.

There are two classifications of aortic dissections commonly used. They are descriptive of that segment of the aorta involved. As the treatment of aortic dissections has evolved, the newer Stanford classification was developed as an additional aid in determining the type of treatment required. In **type A dissections, the ascending aorta is involved**. The dissection may be isolated to this segment or extend into the aortic arch and the descending thoracic aorta or even the abdominal aorta. **In type B dissections, only the descending aorta is involved.** Unless contraindicated, **all type A dissections should undergo emergency surgical repair**, as the mortality with medical treatment alone is extremely high. More than 70% of patients with a type A dissection who arrive in the emergency room die in the first 48 hours if not operated on. **Usually, type B dissections are treated medically unless a specific complication or sign develops.** Some of these complications are listed in **Table 16.2.**

Table 16.2. Relative indications for surgery in type B aortic dissection.

Evidence of free rupture into pleural space (hemothorax)
Evidence of increasing mediastinal hematoma
Ischemia of a significant vital organ
Recurrent pain after 24 hours of onset of the original episode
Inability to control pain within 24 hours
Inability to control blood pressure within 24 hours, especially if once symptoms persist

Referring again to our case, aneurysmal disease or, more likely, aortic dissection could be a tentative diagnosis in this patient. Age, once again, is appropriate, and male gender is appropriate: aortic dissection is somewhat more common in males than females. If this is one suspected diagnosis, **while history and physical examination are being completed, electrocardiogram and chest X-ray** are the initial diagnostic studies. If a dissection truly is considered, the team that performs **transesophageal echocardiography** needs to be notified immediately so that it can begin to mobilize the equipment required to perform the study (see Diagnostic and Confirmatory Studies, below). Electrocardiogram is likely to be normal, but it may show signs of ischemia, especially in the distribution of the right coronary artery. Chest x-ray could be normal in the presence of a dissection, but more likely one may see significant widening of the mediastinum, a straightening of the mediastinal stripe on the left side, and even signs of left pleural effusion or hemothorax.

Pericardial Disease

Diseases of the pericardium may present with a broad spectrum of symptoms and etiologies. These range from **simple, nonspecific acute pericarditis to larger pericardial effusions, tamponade, or constrictive pericarditis**. Constrictive pericarditis may be the ultimate sequela to acute pericarditis and appear months to years after the acute episode. This is especially true of tuberculous pericarditis.

Etiologies of pericarditis are numerous. **A nonspecific viral infection** is the most common cause in the adult, but **significant purulent pericarditis of a bacterial origin** can occur, especially in children. Other etiologies include **renal failure, dialysis, postcardiac surgery, following irradiation to the mediastinum, rheumatoid disease, sarcoidosis on rare occasions, and classically, with previous tuberculous pericarditis. Simple pericarditis represents as an inflammatory process involving the pericardium. Pericardial pain can be quite disabling, sharp, and pleuritic in nature. It usually is retrosternal, may radiate to the neck or left shoulder, and often may be relieved by the patient leaning forward.**

Significant pericardial effusions can occur from any of the etiologies described above. As fluid gradually accumulates, the pericardial sac can expand without hemodynamic compromise and accumulate **up to**

3 or 4 L of fluid. In the presence of a febrile illness, significant effusion should raise concerns about an infectious nature. **Bacterial, tuberculous, and fungal etiologies all have been recognized and may require fluid aspiration or pericardial biopsy for diagnosis. When the rate of fluid accumulation exceeds the ability of the pericardium to expand, tamponade will develop.** Characteristically, patients with tamponade present with chest fullness and may be in extremis with tachycardia, tachypnea, and agitation. **Beck's triad is classically descriptive of those patients with acute tamponade; venous distention, hypotension, and a small quiet heart are characteristic on exam. Pulsus paradoxus** is a classic finding associated with tamponade, either acute or chronic. Its etiology is complex and not fully understood. It is thought to be due to hemodynamic changes secondary to external pressure on the heart. This results in a leftward shift of the ventricular septum that, in turn, prevents adequate filling of the left ventricle during diastole and leads to a decrease in systolic blood pressure. **Clinically, pulsus paradoxus is characterized by at least a 10 mm Hg drop in systolic pressure associated with normal inspiration.** An asthmatic may show similar alteration in blood pressure that should not be confused with the pulsus paradoxus of cardiac tamponade.

Chronic constrictive pericarditis is the end stage of the spectrum of pericardial disease. The pericardium can become quite **thickened, rigid, and may be calcified**. Patients with constrictive pericarditis can present in what appears to be late stages of profound heart failure with low cardiac output. These end-stage patients have a potentially high mortality with or without surgical intervention.

Physical examination is usually nonspecific in the absence of tamponade. Frequently, **a pericardial friction rub may be heard, which is classically diagnostic of the problem, and neck vein distention may be present**. Referring to the case, the description is so nonspecific that it could be related to an episode of pericarditis. **Electrocardiogram, chest x-ray, and complete blood count (CBC)** are appropriate as initial screenings. Electrocardiogram may show significant **ST segment elevations throughout all leads of the ECG but without the T waves being affected significantly**. One must be careful if the ST segment elevations are limited only to regional myocardial coronary distribution. Suspicion of myocardial ischemia rather than pericarditis should be raised if this is the case. Chest x-ray is likely to be normal in the early stages of pericarditis. However, if large amounts of pericardial fluid have accumulated, increases in the cardiac silhouette may occur. (It often is estimated that at least 500 cc of pericardial fluid must be present for enlargement of the cardiac silhouette to be noted.) The result of the CBC will give any suggestion of infection or inflammatory processes.

Pulmonary Embolism

Pulmonary embolism is another major concern in the differential diagnosis of patients with new onset of chest pain. The embolus to the lung, however, is always a **consequence of disease elsewhere in the body**. Usually, this represents venous thrombosis involving the inferior vena cava, the pelvic veins in women, or the ileofemoral and deep veins of the leg. (See the chapter on venous disease.) Embolization can occur from upper extremities thrombosis, but it is rare. Tumor embolization also can occur from tumors involving the inferior vena cava or the right side of the heart. Multiple septic emboli from patients with tricuspid valve endocarditis also are causes of this problem.

The presentation can be variable. Classically, a patient presents with **tachycardia, tachypnea, pleuritic chest pain, hemoptysis, cyanosis, elevated venous pressure, or total cardiovascular collapse.** New-onset atrial fibrillation may be present and accompany the onset of symptoms. **Any of these findings** in a postoperative patient, a patient with prolonged bed rest, or others susceptible to deep vein thrombosis **should raise the possibility of pulmonary embolus.**

Again, look back to the case cited at the beginning of the chapter. Although, less likely with the presenting signs and symptoms, pulmonary embolism is certainly a possibility, though low on the differential diagnosis scale. Suspicion, however, especially if the patient complains of shortness of breath, should be raised. **The ECG is likely to be normal, but it may show signs of right ventricular strain with a new S wave in lead 1 and a new Q wave in lead 3. Chest x-ray** is likely to show little significant changes, but it could show a wedge-type infiltrate or even signs of decreased perfusion to one lung or one portion of the lung. In a patient in whom the diagnosis of pulmonary embolism has been raised, especially in the presence of shortness of breath, **a room air blood gas should be obtained, supplemental oxygen applied, and further diagnostic studies performed,** such as ventilation/perfusion scanning, pulmonary angiography, and spiral CAT scanning.

Diagnostic Methods

History and Physical Examination

The history and physical examination are crucial to the differential diagnosis and initial treatment of patients with chest pain. In the emergency setting, time is of the essence, and the initial diagnostic and therapeutic interventions must be begun based on this information. Without *question*, **the history remains the most valuable mode of evaluation.** The history is designed to elicit essential positive and negative information relevant to the diagnosis of the underlying cause of the patient's chest discomfort. In obtaining the history of a patient with chest pain, it is helpful to have a **mental checklist** and to ask the patient to **describe the location, radiation, and character of the discomfort; what causes and relieves it; time relationships, including the duration, frequency, and pattern of recurrence of the discomfort; the setting in which it occurs; and associated symptoms.**

Because of the nonspecific presentations of the various pathophysiologies described, care must be taken in obtaining a history. Asking a patient "Do you have chest pain?" may result in a negative answer when a patient, in fact, is having significant chest discomfort. More generalized descriptions may be required such as chest pressure, chest discomfort, respiratory pain, etc. Similarly, activities that relieve the symptoms, such as resting, changing position, taking a deep breath while leaning forward, etc., must be documented. Angina must be differentiated from other causes that may mimic its symptoms as listed in **Table 16.3.** It can be confused with the epigastric discomfort of "heartburn," the chest pain of pericarditis or pleuritis, or the discomfort of episodes of bursitis or inflammatory problems in the chest wall. Association of nausea, diaphoresis, shortness of breath, or syncope may be important clues as to etiology. Additional aspects of history should include but not be limited to **inquiries into family history; a history of prior myocardial infarction or heart murmurs; the presence of hypertension, diabetes, or connective tissue disorders; smoking, exercise, dietary habits, and other factors that might predispose the patient to one diagnosis or another or play a significant role in decisions about diagnostic studies and therapeutic interventions.**

The initial physical examination is directed toward eliciting findings consistent with or excluding a diagnosis suggested by the initial history. The **vital signs** and **general appearance** of the patient are major clues to the severity of the problem. **Cyanosis, agitation, and the level of pain and anxiety** in the patient are easy observational signs, as is obesity. **Performing the exam in a standard way to avoid missing relevant findings is crucial.** One way is to start at the head and work your way to the extremities in a systematic way. Quality of the **pulse, diaphoresis, warm or cold skin** are surmised in seconds as the history is taken. **Noting neck vein** distention, the position of the **trachea,** and the quality of the **carotid pulse,** and listening for carotid bruits should be next. Listening and quantifying **heart and breath sounds,** as a baseline, are important in what can be a rapidly changing physical exam. The **cardiac exam** needs to be complete and is directed toward signs of increased cardiac size, the presence of abnormal heart sounds suggestive of heart failure, and the existence of any cardiac murmurs. **Palpation for an abdominal aneurysm** is done rapidly, if possible, as is checking for the presence of **bowel sounds** or the presence of **hepatomegaly. Peripheral pulses** are checked and **signs of chronic or acute ischemia** are sought. Any **swelling,** either bilateral (congestive heart failure) or unilateral (possible deep vein thrombosis), is checked for. An experienced physician can complete this examination in 2 or 3 minutes.

Chest X-Ray

The chest x-ray is one of the initial studies that **should be completed and often is overlooked** as a means of rapidly differentiating the significant causes of chest pain. Findings of congestive heart failure, pleural effusion, or pneumothorax may be noted; enlarged cardiac silhouette consistent with cardiomegaly or large pericardial effusion may be present. Signs of aortic aneurysm or dissection may be present. Large pulmonary emboli may be diagnosed by the absence of pulmonary markings on the chest x-ray.

Table 16.3. Differential diagnosis of episodic chest pain resembling angina pectoris.

	Duration	Quality	Provocation	Relief	Location	Comment
Effort angina	5–15 minutes	Visceral (pressure)	During effort or emotion	Rest, nitroglycerin	Substernal, radiates	First episode vivid
Rest angina	5–45 minutes	Visceral (pressure)	Spontaneous (? with exercise)	Nitroglycerin	Substernal, radiates	Often nocturnal
Mitral prolapse	Minutes to hours	Superficial (rarely visceral)	Spontaneous (no pattern)	Time	Left anterior	No pattern, variable character
Esophageal reflux	10 minutes to 1 hour	Visceral	Recumbency, lack of food	Food, antacid	Substernal, epigastric	Rarely radiates
Esophageal spasm	5–60 minutes	Visceral	Spontaneous, cold liquids, exercise	Nitroglycerin	Substernal, radiates	Mimics angina
Peptic ulcer	Hours	Visceral, burning	Lack of food, "acid" foods	Foods, antacids	Epigastric, substernal	
Biliary disease	Hours	Visceral (waxes and wanes)	Spontaneous, food	Time, analgesia	Epigastric, ? radiates	Colic
Cervical disk	Variable (gradually subsides)	Superficial	Head and neck movement, palpation	Time, analgesia	Arm, neck	Not relieved by rest
Hyperventilation	2–3 minutes	Visceral	Emotion, tachypnea	Stimulus removal	Substernal	Facial paresthesia
Musculoskeletal	Variable	Superficial	Movement, palpation	Time, analgesia	Multiple	Tenderness
Pulmonary	30 minutes +	Visceral (pressure)	Often spontaneous	Rest, time, bronchodilator	Substernal	Dyspneic

Source: Reprinted from Christie LG Jr, Conti CR. Systematic approach to the evaluation of angina-like chest pain. Am Heart J 1981;102:897. Copyright © 1981 Mosby. With permission from Elsevier.

Electrocardiogram

The ECG is the major initial tool used to differentiate ischemic heart disease from other etiologies of chest pain. Acute ECG changes frequently are present, especially when there is ongoing pain. The presence of **Q waves** indicates myocardial cellular necrosis and cell death. These are present when chronic scarring has preceded the current event or may document an acute event in which recovery of function of the myocardium is unlikely. **ST segment elevations** are present during episodes of acute ischemia and represent ongoing cellular injury. **T-wave inversions** are related to ongoing ischemia. At times, **ST segment depression** is seen and must be differentiated as subendocardial ischemia or reciprocal changes to ST segment elevation elsewhere. **ST segment elevations** in all leads may be more suggestive of pericarditis.

Other Laboratory Studies

Additional lab work (blood work) is needed on these patients depending on the suspected etiology of the chest pain. It is probably appropriate that **cardiac enzymes, especially troponin levels,** be drawn on all of these patients. Depending on findings and history, **CBC and differential** may be performed. A **chemistry profile** may be required and, perhaps, **arterial blood gases** obtained to help make and confirm diagnosis.

Diagnostic and Confirmatory Studies

Diagnostic and confirmatory studies are now required as the list of diagnoses is developed. They are ordered on the basis of presumptive diagnosis from the initial history, physical exam, chest x-ray, ECG, and laboratory studies. In reality, findings from the history often establish the subsequent diagnostic path.

Echocardiography

Echocardiography is a superb diagnostic study performed early in the diagnostic sequence. It is simple to perform by an experienced technician. It is performed in two different methods. **Transthoracically,** this is a completely benign study requiring nothing from the patient except cooperation in positioning (perhaps a problem when severe pain or dyspnea are present). **Transesophageal echocardiography (TEE)** is more complicated, but it will often provide more detailed and accurate information, especially if the transthoracic study is insufficient due to technical reasons. The TEE can be difficult and stressful on some patients because of the need to pass the probe through the pharynx and down the esophagus. Despite local anesthesia, the gag reflex can make this impossible at times. Sedation often is used, and a cardiologist is present. Once the probe is in position, diagnostic information is readily available. In the presence of ischemia or myocardial infarction, rapid quantitation of ventricular function can be established. Any mechanical complication of myocardial infarction (ventricular septal defect, ruptured papillary muscle, ruptured free myocardial wall) should be diagnosed. **Transesophageal echocardiography has the highest accuracy and specificity of any study for the diagnosis of aortic aneurysms and aortic dissections.** It can be done rapidly in the emergency room and does not require transporting the patient, as other diagnostic studies do.

CAT Scan

The CAT scan is another **noninterventional study** that helps differentiate the causes of significant chest pain. Especially when contrast agents can be used (in normal renal function), aortic aneurysm and dissections can be diagnosed (**Fig. 16.1**), pericardial effusions and the

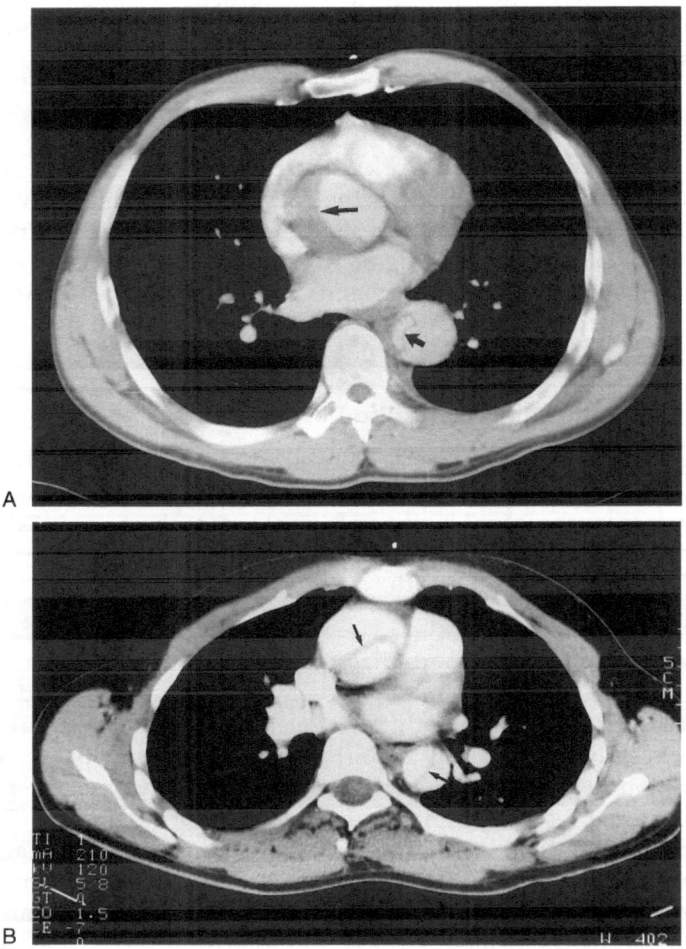

Figure 16.1. Computed tomography of acute dissection. (A) Thrombosis of the false lumen in the ascending aorta (thin arrow) and compression of the true lumen in the descending aorta (thick arrow). (B) Patency of true and false lumen with an intimal flap visible in both the ascending and descending aorta (arrows). (Reprinted from Sundt TM, Thompson RW. Diseases of the thoracic aorta and great vessels. In: Norton JA, Bollinger RR, Chang AE, et al, eds. Surgery: Basic Science and Clinical Evidence. New York: Springer-Verlag, 2001, with permission.)

thickness of the pericardium recognized, large pulmonary emboli identified, and the diagnosis of many of the other causes of chest pain not discussed in this chapter made. Because of the **simplicity and reproducibility of the study, CAT scanning often is used as the method by which patients are followed once a diagnosis of aneurysm or dissection is made or as follow-up after surgery**. The size and other characteristics of the aneurysm can be followed, and the development of false aneurysm or other complications can be recognized.

Magnetic Resonance Imaging

Magnetic Resonance Imaging (MRI) is the final diagnostic tool of a **noninvasive type** that can be very helpful in the differential diagnosis of the multiple etiologies of chest pain. However, **its very nature and the time required to obtain the study tend to make it inappropriate for the acute situation. In more chronic situations, however, especially with complex aortic dissections, it can be quite helpful in characterizing the anatomy and etiologies for chest pain.**

Cardiac Catheterization and Coronary Angiography

Cardiac catheterization and coronary angiography are the only ways presently available for the accurate diagnosis of coronary artery disease and the only way to obtain information for its definitive treatment. Certain situations may require emergency catheterization and interventional studies, primarily when the diagnosis of ischemic heart disease is made in the emergency setting and symptoms cannot be relieved easily by standard treatment methods using nitrates, beta-blockers, oxygen, and pain medication. In the early stages of an evolving myocardial infarction, acute intervention with fibrinolytic agents in the emergency room or early intervention using percutaneous techniques (angioplasty with or without stenting) or even emergency surgery may be required. An intraaortic balloon pump may be required to maximize stabilization during, prior, or even following these interventions.

In most other patients in whom the diagnosis of coronary artery disease is suspected, **exercise stress testing** is the initial diagnostic study, especially when an abnormal ECG has been obtained. The patient exercises progressively at quantified increased levels of work, usually on a treadmill, to gradually increase the heart rate and level of myocardial work. Blood pressure and electrocardiogram are monitored. The patient is questioned as to the presence of any anginal symptoms as the exercise levels increase. **Onset of symptoms, especially when associated with significant ECG changes, is considered a positive test for ischemia. The development of hypotension associated with a stress test is an ominous sign and highly suggestive of left main or critical triple vessel disease.** The accuracy of a stress test alone, however, is only about 70%. This can be improved to approximately 90% by **combining the stress test with radionuclear imaging**, where myocardial perfusion and metabolic function are evaluated at rest and exercise **(an exercise stress thallium study).**

The presence of a positive stress test or continued high suspicion for coronary artery disease even after a negative stress test usually

results in cardiac catheterization. All patients in whom ischemic heart disease is suspected ultimately undergo this test to determine the presence or absence of coronary artery or valvular heart disease. It remains the sine qua non in the diagnosis of ischemic heart disease.

Therapeutic Intervention and Results

Ischemic Heart Disease

At the present time, there are **three classifications of therapy** available to patients with ischemic heart disease. These are referred to as **medical therapy, percutaneous angioplasty**, and **coronary bypass surgery**. Decisions regarding treatment **must be individualized and based on symptoms, anatomy, and risks of the selected therapy.** Dietary management, weight loss, cessation of smoking, etc., are changes in habits and lifestyle that the patient can make; these changes contribute to both short- and long-term benefits of whichever treatment modality is selected.

The classic approach to **medical therapy** for ischemic heart disease is a **three-pronged approach to decrease oxygen demand by the heart and includes beta-blockers, nitrates, and calcium channel blockers.** As noted earlier, the prime cause of angina pectoris is the **mismatch of oxygen demand and oxygen supply** to the heart. **Oxygen demand** of the heart is determined by three major factors: **(1) heart rate; (2) wall tension**; and **(3) to a lesser extent, the level of contractility of the heart.** Wall tension is determined by **Laplace's law** of the heart, in which wall tension is directly related to pressure and volume and inversely related to the wall thickness of the chamber involved:

$$T = P \times R/2h$$

where T is the wall tension, P is the chamber pressure, R is the chamber radius, and h is the wall thickness. **Beta-blockers** are the first line of treatment. The goal of their use is first to **minimize increases in heart rate** due to response to physical and emotional demands and second to **decrease myocardial contractility. Nitrates decrease the preload** through venous dilatation and relaxation of the capacitance vessels. They also **dilate the epicardial vessels supplying the ischemic coronary beds.** Sublingual nitroglycerin, nitroglycerin paste, and other longer acting nitrates are included in this category. **Calcium channel blockers** provide **afterload reduction** (and thus, decreased wall tension) by relaxing the smooth muscle of peripheral vessels and **preventing coronary spasm.** In addition, **the oxygen-carrying capacity of the blood must be optimized.** If anemia is present, it must be corrected. In theory, **only after a patient fails to respond to the simultaneous use of all three modes of therapy at maximal tolerated doses is a patient considered to have "failed medical therapy."** The patient then becomes a candidate for another mode of treatment requiring increasing levels of intervention and risk.

The next treatment option of increasing complexity and risk to the patient is **percutaneous transluminal coronary angioplasty (PTCA).**

Developed by Andreas Grundzig[1] of Switzerland in the 1970s, PTCA has led to the development of many interventional procedures performed in the cardiac catheterization laboratory to open partially occluded coronary vessels using percutaneous techniques. These include **PTCA alone, laser angioplasty, directed atherectomy**, and, most recently, **PTCA with stenting**. Using techniques similar to cardiac catheterization, a guidewire is directed across and through the coronary lesion under fluoroscopic control. A PTCA balloon or atherectomy catheter is then passed over the guidewire and across the lesion. The balloon is inflated, compressing the lesion against the walls of the vessel, or an atherectomy is performed with actual removal of material from the wall of the vessel.

The advantage of these procedures (when they are appropriate) is that the patient suffers little in the way of disability and the hospitalization usually is quite short. Return to normal activities within a week or two is not uncommon. There are some potential disadvantages, however. Recurrence rates of 25% to 30% are not uncommon within 6 months of the procedure. In many situations, PTCA can be repeated. In 1% to 3% of all PTCAs or atherectomies, the patient requires emergency surgery due to a complication. In these situations, the surgical results are not as good as for elective surgery; perioperative myocardial infarction and mortalities both are higher. Recently, **intracoronary stents** made of fine metal mesh have been developed, and, based on limited results to date, **seem to increase the likelihood of longer patencies following angioplasty as well as to lower the risk for emergency surgery at the time of the procedure. Irradiated and drug-eluding stents** are now being tested and seem to prolong the patency even further.

Decisions on the use of **coronary artery bypass grafting (CABG)** to treat patients with ischemic heart disease are based on anatomy, symptoms, and the potential risks to the patient as well as the long-term benefits of the operation. **Certain anatomic situations (left main disease, left main equivalent, and three-vessel disease with decreased ventricular function) may warrant surgery even in the absence of symptoms** because of the large amount of myocardium in jeopardy and the recognized high mortality risk without treatment (including sudden death). **Currently, additional acceptable indications for CABG are stable angina unresponsive to medical therapy; unstable angina such as pain at rest; preinfarction or postinfarction angina; and patients with double- or triple-vessel disease with diminished left ventricular function.**[2] All patients with these conditions are likely to benefit from surgery either with **relief of symptoms, prevention of myocardial infarction, or prolongation of life.** Diabetics with two-vessel disease get better long-term results with CABG than with angioplasty. In addition, concomitant CABG may be indicated for patients under-

---

[1] Presented at the American Heart Association meeting, 1976. Transluminal dilatation of coronary artery stenosis. Letter to the editor. Lancet 1978;1:263.
[2] ACC/AHA. Guidelines for coronary artery bypass surgery, executive summary and recommendations. Circulation 1999;100:1464–1480.

going surgery for complications of myocardial infarction (acute mitral regurgitation, ventricular septal defect, or free rupture of the heart) or for patients undergoing elective valve replacement procedures with critical vessel occlusions.

The risks of surgery to certain patients may far outweigh the benefits to them. Patients with **limited life expectancy from other diseases (especially malignancies), the very elderly, or the physically impaired** might not be considered surgical candidates based on associated physical conditions. In these situations, further medical treatment or attempts at a partial revascularization utilizing PTCA for symptomatic relief may be more appropriate. Although the benefits of CABG to patients with decreased ventricular function and double- or triple-vessel disease are well recognized, **poor ventricular function adds to the mortality of patients undergoing the operation.** Other factors that increase the mortality and morbidity of CABG (as well as other open heart procedures) include **age greater than 70, morbid obesity, diabetes, chronic obstructive pulmonary disease, hypertension, history of myocardial infarction, reoperation, chronic renal failure, peripheral vascular disease, and, possibly, female gender.**

The results of CABG are excellent, but, as noted, many factors contribute to operative mortality and morbidity. Mortality at most major centers for all patients undergoing CABG ranges from 2% to 4%. **Figure 16.2** cites survival benefits of patients undergoing CABG or PTCA.

Diseases of the Thoracic Aorta

Decisions regarding treatment of patients with aortic aneurysms are dependent on the **risk/benefit ratio to the patient.** Symptomatic patients have a mean survival of approximately 2 years following onset of the symptoms. The majority of time, however, the surgeon is confronted with a patient without symptoms found to have an aneurysm on a routine chest x-ray or other study. Here, **the greatest risk to the patient is rupture of the aorta, which is more likely to occur the greater the size of the aorta. The risks of surgery are lowest when the ascending aorta needs to be approached. Surgery in the descending thoracic aorta is next in risk. The highest risk is associated with repair of the aortic arch.**

Aortic dissection is treated in a different manner because of the acuteness of the situation. **Regardless of the type of dissection (Stanford A or B), initial emergent therapy is medical, with a goal of controlling the patient's symptoms, heart rate, and blood pressure. Intravenous narcotics for pain control are used. The heart rate is controlled by intravenous beta-blockade to lower it below 70. Following beta-blockade, blood pressure control is obtained using intravenous nitroprusside of nitroglycerin.** Constant blood pressure monitoring is crucial for these patients, preferably with an arterial line in a radial artery. The extremity with the highest initial blood pressure is utilized to avoid inaccurate readings from a blocked vessel.

All patients with aortic dissection **should be admitted to the surgical service for close observation and management in consultation with cardiology or hypertension specialists. Transesophageal**

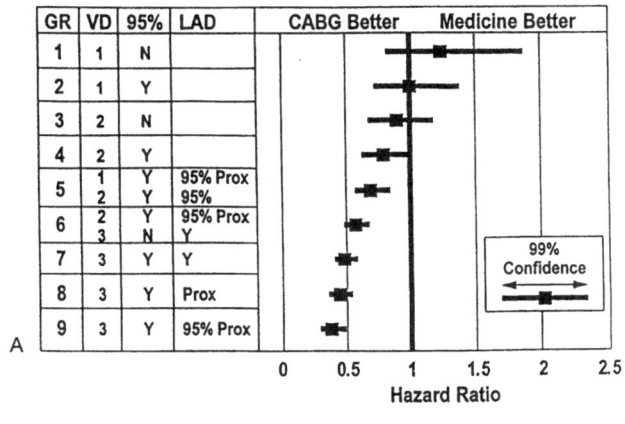

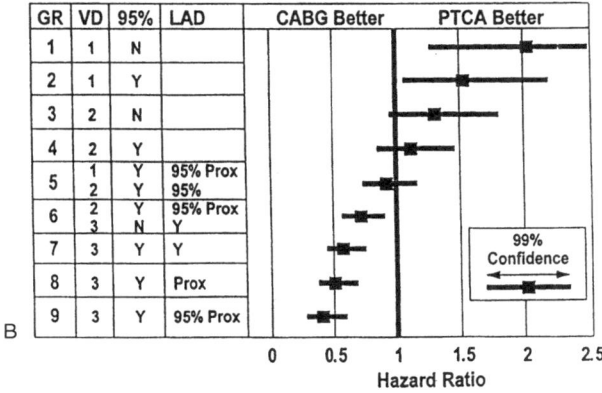

Figure 16.2. Adjusted hazard ratios comparing (A) coronary artery bypass grafting (CABG) and medicine, and (B) CABG and angioplasty, as a function of the extent of coronary artery lesions. PTCA, percutaneous transluminal coronary angioplasty; VD, number of vessels diseased; 95% ≥ 95% coronary artery stenosis; Prox, proximal; GR, group. (Reprinted from Jones RH, Kesler K, Phillips HR, et al. Long-term survival benefits of coronary artery bypass grafting and percutaneous transluminal angioplasty in patients with coronary artery disease. J Thorac Cardiovasc Surg 1996;111:1013–1025. Copyright © 1996 American Association for Thoracic Surgery. With permission from the American Association for Thoracic Surgery.)

echocardiography is the preferable diagnostic study. In type A dissections, the aortic valve can be evaluated for insufficiency, and the presence or absence of pericardial fluid (suggesting impending rupture into the pericardium and sudden death) can be evaluated. Once a diagnosis of a **type A dissection** is made and the patient is deemed a surgical candidate, **an emergency operation is performed. If there is any question of the diagnosis or if a type B dissection is identified, then aortography can be used for additional information.** Aortography can provide information on whether the dissection actually exists, what is involved, the presence of aortic insufficiency, possible identification of associated coronary disease, the site of the tear, and the involvement of major branches off the aorta. **Type B aortic dissections are normally**

treated by continuation of the initial medical therapy. This includes permanent treatment with beta-blockers and antihypertensive agents. There are certain indications, however, that require **surgery for a type B dissection (Table 16.2). These include ongoing pain, significant hemothorax, progressive mediastinal enlargement suggesting an expanding mediastinal hematoma, inability to control the blood pressure within 48 hours, and loss of blood supply to a significant branch of the distal aorta.** Loss of distal flow frequently requires surgical intervention for a repair of type B dissection. There are also methods of fenestration of the distal false lumen to permit reentry of blood flow and restoration of adequate distal circulation.

Surgery for aortic aneurysmal disease of the thoracic aorta, whether it is elective (as for most aneurysms) or emergent (as for most dissections), usually is performed in a similar fashion. Replacement of the ascending aorta requires the use of the heart–lung machine. This can be done by cross-clamping the aorta and protecting the heart in the usual techniques of ischemic arrest. The method used, especially if the aortic arch needs replacement, is that of circulatory arrest. Descending thoracic aortic surgery can be performed in many ways through a left posterolateral thoracotomy. Simple cross-clamping is possible, but the likelihood of **paralysis postoperatively is significant**, especially if more than **30 minutes** of ischemia to the spinal cord occurs. Left heart bypass, as will complete bypass and circulatory arrest, may yield some additional protection from prolonged ischemia. Whatever technique is used, there is the risk of paralysis. The artery of Adamkiewicz is thought to provide the majority of blood to the anterior spinal artery, which in turn supplies the anterior aspects of the spinal cord. The greater the extent of aorta resected and the greater the involvement of the areas distal to T6, the greater this risk.

Following treatment of the aneurysm or dissection, **careful follow-up is crucial**. One of the leading causes of death in these patients is redissection or rupture of a new aneurysm or leak from the suture line. Initial follow-up is with CAT scanning at 3 and 6 months, then every 6 months thereafter. If all remains stable after 2 years, then yearly follow-up is appropriate.

Pericardial Disease

The typical case of acute pericarditis can be treated with **antiinflammatory agents, especially salicylates**, and usually will respond rapidly. When this is not the case, concern should be raised about a different etiology other than idiopathic. Since the next level of antiinflammatory treatment for this problem requires **steroid therapies, infectious etiologies should be ruled out before steroid therapy is instituted**. The presence of a significant effusion and an ill patient should lead to **aspiration of the pericardial sac and biopsy**. Definitive therapy to prevent significant reaccumulation of fluid as well as definitive diagnosis is likely to require an **open procedure**. In patients with chronic renal failure and dialysis, initial efforts are to decrease the presence of the effusion by increasing the frequency of the dialysis episodes. If this does not work, a single simple aspiration should be performed. Repeat accumulation of fluids should lead to a **more permanent drainage procedure**. Finally, patients with chronic constrictive pericarditis require **pericardial stripping for relief of symptoms**. This pericardial stripping may be performed in any of several ways. The safest appears to be through a **median sternotomy**. Should it become necessary, cardiopulmonary bypass may be used as an adjunct for a safe procedure.

Pulmonary Embolism

Once the diagnosis of pulmonary embolus has been confirmed (or if the clinical findings are strong enough to warrant treatment), treatment and further diagnosis requires a dual approach: **treat the embolus and prevent any recurrences**. Most cases require treatment with **heparin anticoagulation and symptomatic support of the patient**. Heparin prevents the formation of additional venous thromboses (the presumed origin of the embolus) and is thought to promote dissolution of the emboli in the pulmonary circulation. Further diagnostic studies are aimed at verifying the origin of the embolus (venous thrombosis, endocarditis, tumor embolus, etc.). If anticoagulants are contraindicated or repeat embolism occurs on anticoagulants, then an **inferior vena cava umbrella** should be placed.

Summary

Several potential life-threatening diseases treated by cardiothoracic surgeons must be rapidly recognized, their pathophysiology understood, and treatment methods recognized. These major entities include coronary artery disease and dissection of and aneurysms of the thoracic aorta. Understanding Laplace's law of the heart is key to understanding both the pathophysiology and therapy for these diseases and the requirements for surgical intervention.

Selected Readings

American Heart Association/American College of Cardiology. Consensus statements on management of patients with acute myocardial infarction, Circulation 1999;99:2829–2848.

American Heart Association/American College of Cardiology. Consensus statements on management of patients with unstable angina and non-ST segment elevation myocardial infarction. J Am Coll Cardiol 2000;36: 970–1062.

Foley MI, Moneta GL. Venous disease and pulmonary embolism. In: Norton JA, Bollinger RR, Chang AE, et al, eds. Surgery: Basic Science and Clinical Evidence. New York: Springer-Verlag, 2001.

Jones RH, Kesler K, Phillips HR, et al. Long-term survival benefits of coronary artery bypass grafting and percutaneous transluminal angioplasty in patients with coronary artery disease. J Thoracic Cardiovasc Surg 1996; 111:1013–1025.

Lee RW, Zwischenberger JB. Pericardium. In: Norton JA, Bollinger RR, Chang AE, et al, eds. Surgery: Basic Science and Clinical Evidence. New York: Springer-Verlag, 2001.

Rosengart TK, de Bois W, Francalancia NA. Adult heart disease. In: Norton JA, Bollinger RR, Chang AE, et al, eds. Surgery: Basic Science and Clinical Evidence. New York: Springer-Verlag, 2001.

Sundt TM, Thompson RW. Diseases of the thoracic aorta and great vessels. In: Norton JA, Bollinger RR, Chang AE, et al, eds. Surgery: Basic Science and Clinical Evidence. New York: Springer-Verlag, 2001.

Web sites of American Heart Association: www.americanheart.org, American College of Cardiology: www.acc.org, and Society of Thoracic Surgeons: www.sts.org

Stroke

Rocco G. Ciocca

Objectives: Altered Neurologic Status

1. To describe the evaluation and management of a patient with an acute focal neurologic deficit.
2. To differentiate transient ischemic attack (TIA), reversible ischemic neurologic deficit (RIND), and cerebral vascular accident (CVA).
3. To differentiate anterior versus posterior circulation symptoms.
4. To outline the diagnostic tests and monitoring of carotid occlusive disease, including the role of angiography and noninvasive methods.
5. To discuss medical versus surgical management of carotid artery disease.

Case

A 68-year-old man with a history of hypertension, elevated cholesterol, type 2 diabetes, and a 50-pack-per-year smoking history notices that he cannot see out of his right eye. It is as if a "shade" had been pulled down over the eye.

Introduction

Stroke and its complications can be devastating. The term **stroke** and **cerebral vascular accident** (CVA) are used interchangeably in this chapter. **Approximately 500,000 people develop new strokes annually. It is the leading cause of neurologic death, and it is the third leading cause of death, preceded by myocardial infarction (MI) and cancer.** The societal costs number in the billions of dollars. While not all strokes are related to large-vessel disease, the incidence is large enough to warrant attention.

This chapter discusses the **pathophysiology of stroke, its workup, and the therapeutic options**, and presents treatment recommendations and the available evidence to support them.

Pathophysiology

Definitions

The differentiation between the aforementioned entities generally is determined by **timing and length of symptoms. A transient ischemic attack (TIA) is defined as an acute loss of cerebral function that persists for less than 24 hours.** Most of these neurologic events are brief, lasting 15 minutes or less. Generally, these events are focal and specific. Symptoms associated with anterior or carotid bifurcation disease include sensory or motor deficits affecting the contralateral face, arms, or legs, aphasia, or alterations in higher cortical dysfunction. Patients with posterior or vertebrobasilar ischemia may present with vertigo, dizziness, gait ataxia, dysarthria, nystagmus, diplopia, bilateral visual loss, drop attacks (collapse caused by loss of control of extremities without loss of consciousness), as well as bilateral or alternating motor or sensory impairment. Nonfocal symptoms, such as syncope, confusion, and "light-headedness," rarely are the result of cerebrovascular disease.

Reversible ischemic neurologic deficits (RINDs) are cerebral vascular symptoms that persist for more than 24 hours but less than 7 days. Symptoms that persist beyond 7 days usually are considered a stroke. Many would consider a stroke to have occurred if the symptoms persist beyond 24 hours. The RIND classification of symptoms seems to be used less commonly in clinical medicine.

Transient unilateral loss of vision is referred to as **amaurosis fugax**. This is the symptom described by the patient in the case presented at the beginning of this chapter. This symptom is described classically as the sensation of a shade coming down over the entire eye, half an eye, or a quadrant of an eye. This event is the consequence of a microembolus lodging in the ophthalmic artery or one of its retinal branches. A cholesterol crystal (Hollenhorst plaque) occasionally is observed on funduscopic examination as a bright refractive body in a branch of the retinal artery. The significance of the above-mentioned focal neurologic events is that they are markers of stroke potential. **While only 10% of strokes are preceded by TIAs, the patient who experiences one has a 5% to 8% per year chance of developing a stroke. Within 5 years of the onset of TIAs, the patient has a 25% to 40% chance of developing a stroke.**

A stroke also may be called a cerebral vascular accident (CVA) to distinguish it from the vascular nature of most strokes. **Thirty-four percent of strokes are the result of large-artery disease as compared with embolism, which leads to 31% of strokes, lacunar infarctions (usually associated with hypertension and small-vessel disease), which leads to 19% of strokes, and hemorrhage, which leads to 16% of strokes. Causes of stroke other than large-vessel disease rarely are associated with TIAs.**

Anatomy

A thorough **understanding of the arterial anatomy of the brain is critically important in understanding the pathology and treatment of stroke**. The anatomy is divided into **anterior and posterior, and these are connected via the circle of Willis.**

Paired internal carotid arteries that provide approximately 80% to 90% of the total cerebral blood flow feed the anterior circulation. The left common carotid artery originates directly from the aortic arch, whereas the right common carotid artery originates from the innominate artery. The common carotid arteries bifurcate at the angle of the mandible into the external and internal carotid arteries. The external carotid artery has many divisions and primarily provides circulation to the face and neck. It supplies the cerebral circulation through collaterals. The internal carotid artery can be divided into the cervical (or extracranial), intrapetrosal, intracavernous, and supraclinoid segments. The cervical, intrapetrosal, and intracavernous portions of the internal carotid artery have no branches.

The posterior circulation is composed of paired vertebral arteries that supply 10% to 20% of the total cerebral circulation. Both vertebral arteries originate from the first portion of their respective subclavian arteries and then enter the vertebral canal at the transverse foramina of the sixth cervical vertebra. The vertebral arteries unite to form the basilar artery, which then branches into the right and left posterior cerebral arteries. The posterior circulation supplies the brainstem, cranial nerves, cerebellum, and the occipital and temporal lobes of the cerebrum.

The circle of Willis (Fig. 17.1) is the term used to describe the interconnecting network of vessels that link the posterior and anterior circulations. The anterior communicating artery connects the two anterior cerebral arteries, while the posterior communicating artery connects the internal carotid arteries to the posterior cerebral arteries.

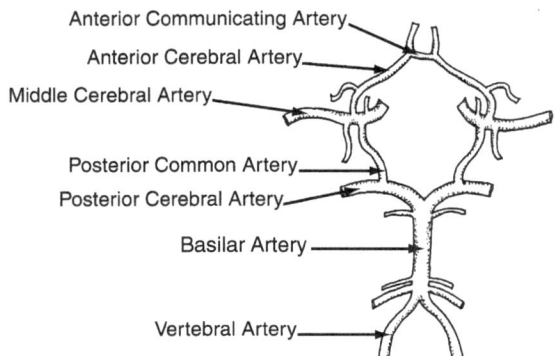

Figure 17.1. Configuration of the terminal branches of the vertebral and internal carotid arteries and their interconnections to form the circle of Willis. (Reprinted from Patel ST, Kent KC. Cerebrovascular disease. In: Norton JA, Bollinger RR, Chang AE, et al, eds. Surgery: Basic Science and Clinical Evidence. New York: Springer-Verlag, 2001, with permission.)

The circle is intact in 20% to 40% of individuals and allows for collateral flow between the hemispheres and the anterior and posterior circulation. The fact that the circle so infrequently is intact implies two things: first, there are other means of collateral circulation; second, the existence of collateral circulation cannot be assumed before surgical intervention.

Presentation

One of the most frequently misunderstood anatomic and pathophysiologic points is that carotid artery stenosis leads to atheroembolic events. The pathology usually is not secondary to decreased perfusion. The brain has a tremendously rich collateral circulation. The carotid circulation dominates the anterior circulation. The internal carotid artery is the main conduit to the brain, feeding the middle cerebral artery. The circle of Willis interconnects the anterior and posterior circulation. It is rare for people to have hypoperfusion secondary to carotid occlusive disease. The pathology is embolic and therefore focal. The "dizzies" and syncope rarely are caused by carotid disease. This is not hard to believe, since probably greater than 90% to 95% of the time carotid surgery is performed safely with a shunt.

Risk Factors and Pathology

The primary risk factors for stroke are similar to those for patients presenting with any other form of cardiovascular disease: smoking, hypertension, diabetes, hypercholesterolemia, advanced age, obesity, inactivity, and, to a lesser extent, family history.

The primary pathology leading to the development of extracranial carotid disease is atherosclerosis. This accounts for approximately 90% of lesions in the extracranial system seen in the Western world. The remaining 10% include such entities as fibromuscular dysplasia, arterial kinking because of arterial elongation, extrinsic compression, traumatic occlusion, intimal dissection, the inflammatory angiopathy, and migraines. Radiation-induced atherosclerotic change of the extracranial carotid artery has become a recognized entity. Other rare entities, usually involving intracranial vessels, include fibrinoid necrosis, amyloidosis, polyarteritis, allergic angitis, Wegener's granulomatosis, granulomatious angiitis, giant cell arteritis, and moyamoya disease. Embolization from a cardiac source also is an important contributing factor to cerebral vascular disease.

The most likely etiology of the symptoms experienced by the patient in the case presented at the beginning of this chapter is the presence of atherosclerotic plaque at the ipsilateral carotid bifurcation.

Epidemiology

Incidence/Prevalence

As previously stated, approximately 500,000 patients in the United States develop new strokes each year. It is the third leading cause of death, but perhaps more disconcerting are the **morbidity and potential loss of independence that result from stroke**.

The overall incidence of new stroke is 160 per 100,000 per year. **The incidence rises, however, as one ages.** This has been borne out by several population-based studies designed to look at the incidence of stroke. The Rochester, Minnesota, population study (from 1955 to 1969) emphasized the influence of advancing age on the progressive incidence of cerebral infarction: the 55-year-old to 64-year-old age group had a cerebral infarction rate of 276.8 per 100,000 per year; the 65-year-old to 74-year-old age group had an incidence of 632 per 100,000 per year; and the 75-year-old and over age group had a stroke rate of 1786.4 per 100,000 per year.[1]

Analysis of the cerebral infarction rate by sex distribution indicated that **the rate was approximately 1.5 times greater in men than in women of the same age**.

The prognosis after a stroke is varied, but 6 months following the survival of a stroke only 29% of the patients in the Rochester study had normal cerebral function; 71% continued to have manifestations of neurologic dysfunction. In the latter group, 4% required total nursing care, 18% were disabled but capable of contributing to self-care, and 10% were aphasic. Of the patients who suffered a fatal stroke, 38% died of the initial stoke, 10% died of a subsequent stroke, and 18% died from complications of coronary disease. The chance of recurrent stroke within 1 year of the initial stroke was 10%, and the chance of a recurrent stroke within 5 years of the initial attack was 20%.

The above data are somewhat dated, and yet, somewhat surprisingly, **the incidence of stroke actually may have increased.[2] The increased incidence may be due to greater awareness and imaging studies leading to diagnosis that is more accurate. The overall prognosis of stroke has changed little over time.**

Workup

History and Physical Examination

The history taken and the physical exam performed on a patient with a change in neurologic status are no different from any other history and physical exam. They should be thorough, and they should include a head-to-toe evaluation of the patient. It is important to **document clearly and precisely the patient's neurologic status** so that other healthcare professionals clearly can understand the neurologic status of the patient.

---

[1] Matsumato N, Whisnant JP, Kurland LT, et al. Natural history of stroke in Rochester, Minnesota, 1955 through 1969: an extension of a previous study, 1945 through 1954. Stroke 1973;4:20.

[2] Brown RD, Whisnant JP, Sicks JD, O'Fallon WM, Wiebers DO. Stroke incidence, prevalence, and survival: secular trends in Rochester, Minnesota, through 1989. Stroke 1996; 27(3):373–380.

In verbal communication with the patient regarding the patient's neurologic state, **it is helpful to speak in terms of cerebral hemispheres rather than right or left sides of the body**. Since the left cerebral hemisphere controls right-sided body function, it can be confusing as to just what a right-sided stroke means. Does it mean a right cerebral hemispheric event with associated left-sided bodily dysfunction or does it imply right-sided weakness? Therefore, speaking in terms of cerebral hemispheres provides a clearer understanding of the possible source of the problem.

The presence of a cervical bruit is an important physical finding to document in the evaluation of a patient with cerebrovascular disease. In 20% of patients with bruits, hemodynamically significant stenosis can be documented. Conversely, it is estimated that 19% to 27% of patients with notable stenotic lesions of the carotid were reported to have no bruit. It also is important to recognize that internal carotid artery plaques cause the vast majority (75–90%) of cervical bruits. The external carotid artery accounts for approximately 10% of the bruits. While the presence of a carotid bruit may denote significant carotid disease in only a small minority of patients, it is an important marker for increased risk of death from coronary artery disease. Interestingly, a bruit may disappear as the degree of stenosis increases beyond 85% to 90%.

In addition to focusing on the patient's neurologic status and whether or not a cervical bruit is present, one also must **focus attention on the overall health and physical findings** of the patient, as these are of equal, if not of more, importance. Attention needs to be paid to the patients other comorbities, and their surgical risk should be assessed.

Carotid Duplex

Duplex ultrasound (DU) is the noninvasive test of choice when evaluating a patient for the presence of extracranial carotid artery disease. It is a bimodal study employing B-mode ultrasound with Doppler waveform analysis. Evaluation of the Doppler waveform and the peak systolic and end diastolic velocities in the internal carotid artery determine the degree of internal artery within several relatively broad ranges. It is a relatively inexpensive exam that is safe and very well tolerated by the patient. It also is **accurate approximately 90% of the time in experienced vascular diagnostic laboratories**. Increasingly, DU is being used safely as the only diagnostic test in the workup of patients for carotid artery disease. Many experienced vascular surgeons have operated safely based on the results of a DU alone.

But DU does have **several limitations. First, a skilled technician must perform the DU, and it must be read properly. In addition, it may be difficult to differentiate between a very high grade stenosis and complete occlusion. Also, DU interrogates only the extracranial carotid system, and therefore tells nothing about the presence or the absence of intracranial disease.** The clinical significance of these so-called tandem lesions is open to debate. Even with these limitations, DU remains a useful diagnostic tool.

Computed Tomography Scan

Computed tomography (CT) scanning is a very useful tool in the evaluation of a patient who may have had a stroke. Axial images of the brain are obtained noninvasively, and anatomic abnormalities are visualized. **It is useful to differentiate a mass lesion from an intracranial bleed. A CT scan generally is the primary diagnostic study in evaluating an individual for a stroke. It is essential to realize, however, that a CT scan initially may be read as normal in an individual who has had a stroke. It can take anywhere from 24 to 48 hours for the stroke-induced changes to be seen on a CT scan. Therefore, it is recommended to repeat a CT scan in 48 hours if clinically indicated.**

Not too long ago in the history of carotid surgery, a CT scan was a routine study ordered prior to proceeding with surgery, even in asymptomatic patients. Prospective studies have shown that CT scans of the brain prior to carotid surgery are unnecessary and not cost-effective.[3]

Magnetic Resonance Imaging/Angiography

The advent of magnetic resonance imaging (MRI) of the brain has been a tremendous advance in neuroimaging due to increased sensitivity, flexibility, and greater variety of images. The MRI scans depend on several characteristics of body tissue being imaged. These characteristics include the density of hydrogen nuclei, whether the nuclei are moving or stationary (flow), and two magnetic properties of tissue called T1 and T2 relaxation. Scans can be generated that capitalize on tissue difference of T1, T2, hydrogen density, and flow. **Techniques that are more advanced and software allow magnetic resonance angiography (MRA), a noninvasive means of assessing vascular anatomy, to be performed, thereby noninvasively providing anatomic delineation of vascular anatomy (Fig. 17.2).**

Magnetic resonance angiography is used best in conjunction with a high-quality duplex scan. In a large study in which both techniques were evaluated, the accuracy of DU and MRA in predicting a greater than 70% carotid stenosis (86% and 88%, respectively) increased to 94% when the results of these two tests were combined.[4]

Contrast Angiography

Contrast angiography is the traditional "gold standard" for evaluating the carotid arteries and cerebral circulation. Conventional contrast

---

[3] Martin JD, Valentine RJ, Myers SI, Rossi MB, Patterson CB, Clagett GP. Is routine CT scanning necessary in the preoperative evaluation of patients undergoing carotid endarterectomy? J Vasc Surg 1991;14(3):267–270.

[4] Patel MR, Kuntz KM, Klufas RA, et al. Preoperative assessment of the carotid bifurcation: can magnetic resonance angiography and duplex ultrasonography replace contrast arteriography? Stroke 1995;26:1753–1758.

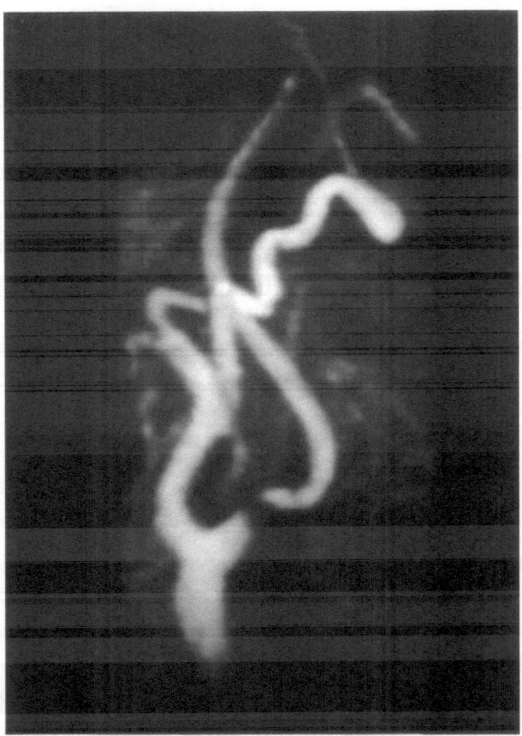

Figure 17.2. Magnetic resonance angiography (MRA) of the carotid bifurcation. MRA can provide a precise anatomic depiction of carotid bifurcation disease. (Reprinted from Patel ST, Kent KC. Cerebrovascular disease. In: Norton JA, Bollinger RR, Chang AE, et al, eds. Surgery: Basic Science and Clinical Evidence. New York: Springer-Verlag, 2001, with permission.)

angiography is performed by gaining access to the arterial system, usually through the femoral artery, and placing a catheter into the artery that needs to be studied. Radiopaque contrast material then is injected via the catheter, and x-rays are taken. **It also can provide excellent images of the aortic arch and proximal great vessels,** areas that are not imaged well by DU or MRA. The posterior and intracranial circulation can be visualized readily.

However, contrast angiography is invasive and is associated with a significant complication rate. In the Asymptomatic Carotid Atherosclerosis Study (ACAS), there was a 1.2% rate of stroke associated with angiography.[5] Contrast angiography is reserved for the rare instances in which the noninvasive studies are inconclusive and the physician is unable to make a clinical decision based on their findings.

---

[5] Executive Committee for the Asymptomatic Carotid Atherosclerosis Study. Endarterectomy for asymptomatic carotid artery stenosis. JAMA 1995;273:304–308.

Positron Emission Tomography

Positron emission tomography (PET) is a technique that utilizes radioactive tracers to visualize the extent, intensity, and rate of biologic processes occurring within the brain. Positron-emitting isotopes are produced for carbon, nitrogen, oxygen, and fluorine; these can be utilized to label a wide variety of metabolic substrates and drug analogues. When a positron decays, two photons are emitted 180 degrees apart: these photons are detected electronically by detectors that record only the simultaneously occurring photons 180 degrees apart. Input to a ring of detector is reconstructed to a tomographic image similar to those of CT.

Tracer techniques are available for measuring cerebral blood flow, cerebral blood volume, cerebral metabolic rate for oxygen, and cerebral metabolic rate for glucose; in addition, a useful derived function is the fraction of oxygen extracted by tissue (oxygen extraction fraction).

While much useful data can be acquired via a PET scan, it rarely is used for the acute evaluation of a stroke patient and rarely is necessary in preparation for carotid surgery.

Treatment

The initial therapy for a patient who presents with a change in neurologic status is supportive. It is critical to take an accurate history, with particular attention to the onset of symptoms. **There is increasing evidence that early intervention in a patient with stroke can affect the outcome positively.** A thorough physical examination needs to be performed, and clear and concise documentation of any neurologic deficit needs to be made. Comorbid conditions, such as hypertension, breathing problems, and chest pain, need to be treated aggressively.

Once it has been determined that the patient has an acute neurologic deficit, a CT scan is a very useful first study. While the study frequently is interpreted as "normal" or "unchanged" initially in the evaluation of a patient presenting with a stroke, it also is helpful in ruling out other possible causes of a change in neurologic function, particularly an intracranial bleed or mass lesion. Ruling out a bleed particularly is important if the treating physician is contemplating the use of thrombolytic therapy for the treatment of acute stroke.

There is increasing interest, growing experience, and accruing evidence to suggest that there is a role for thrombolytic therapy in the acute management of stroke. The goal is to dissolve a clot that has formed in the cerebral circulation. Successful protocols have been developed for the use of both intraarterial and intravenous thrombolytic therapy. Multicentered trials have demonstrated a significant benefit to stroke patients if the therapy can be employed within 3 to 6 hours after the onset of symptoms.[6] This benefit is at the cost of an

---

[6] Lisboa RC, Jovanovic BD, Alberts MJ. Analysis of the safety and efficacy of intra-arterial thrombolytic therapy for ischemic stroke. Stroke 2002;33(12):2866–2871.

increased rate of significant intracranial hemorrhage without a significant effect on overall mortality. In general, the benefit of thrombolysis decreases and the risks increase with time after the onset of symptoms. It is thought that, with increased awareness of the signs and symptoms of stroke and with more rapid response, employment of thrombolysis will prove to be safe and cost-effective.

The evidence does not support the use of systemic anticoagulation for either therapeutic or prophylactic treatment of stroke, the critical exception being for those patients who have cardiogenic sources of cerebral embolization (e.g., atrial fibrillation, atrial flutter, valvular disease, prosthetic valves, etc.).[7] Patients with cardiogenic sources of embolization do benefit from anticoagulation, maintaining an international normalized ratio (INR) of 2.0 to 3.0. Higher ratios are associated with increased risks of bleeding.

There is level-one evidence to support the use of antiplatelet therapy in the management and prevention of patients with stroke.[8] **Aspirin [acetylsalicylic acid (ASA)]**, secondary to its low cost, availability, and good safety profile, generally **is considered first-line antiplatelet therapy**. There is some debate as to the optimal dose, with the range being between 81 and 325 mg daily. There is good evidence that **clopidogrel (Plavix) is slightly better than ASA in preventing ischemic events, without the hematologic toxicity associated with ticlopidine (Ticlid)**. While clopidogrel is significantly more expensive than ASA, it may prove to be cost-effective if it can successfully prevent stroke and other ischemic events that carry significant morbidity.

One of the more controversial issues in the management of stroke has been the role of carotid surgery. The controversy has been abated with good evidence. The North American Symptomatic Carotid Endarterectomy Trial (NASCET) was a large prospective randomized trial designed to test the efficacy of carotid endarterectomy (CEA) in patients with symptomatic carotid stenosis.[9] Fifty centers in the United States and Canada randomized 659 patients with greater than 70% symptomatic carotid stenosis to CEA or best medical management. The study was designed as a 5-year trial, but it was concluded at 18 months due to the markedly significant benefit of CEA. The study found the 30-day mortality and stroke morbidity was 5.8% in patients randomized to CEA. The cumulative 2-year risk of ipsilateral stroke was 26% in patients treated medically and 9% in patients treated with CEA, representing an absolute risk reduction of 17% and a relative risk reduction of 65%. **The benefit of surgery has proven to be durable for at least 8 years. The benefit of surgery has shown to be greater in**

[7] VanWalraven C, Hart RG, Singer DE, et al. Oral anticoagulants vs. aspirin in nonvalvular atrial fibrillation: an individual patient meta-analysis. JAMA 2002;288(19): 2441–2448.

[8] Straus SE, Majumber SR, McAlister FA. New evidence for stroke prevention: scientific review. JAMA 2002;288(11):1388–1395.

[9] North American Symptomatic Carotid Endarterectomy Trial Collaborators. Beneficial effect of carotid endarterectomy in symptomatic patients with high-grade carotid stenosis. N Engl J Med 1991;325:445–453.

patients with higher-grade stenosis, but subset analysis has confirmed statistically significant absolute risk reduction of CEA for symptomatic patients with greater than 50% carotid artery stenosis.

See **Algorithm 17.1** for the management of extracranial carotid stenosis.

Prevention

Risk Reduction

Risk reduction is the cornerstone of prevention; it means the cessation of smoking, and the control of diabetes, hypertension, and cholesterol. In addition, as previously stated, there is good evidence to support **antiplatelet therapy with either ASA or clopidogrel** in the prevention of cerebral ischemic events. **Anticoagulation with heparin and Coumadin has been shown to reduce the incidence of stroke in patients with cardiogenic sources of embolization.**

Carotid Surgery

Just as the efficacy of CEA for the treatment of high-grade symptomatic carotid stenosis was challenged, its role in the management of asymptomatic patients with high-grade carotid stenosis required clinical trials to support its benefit. The Asymptomatic Carotid Atherosclerosis Study (ACAS) is the largest available randomized trial of patients with asymptomatic carotid stenosis.[10] The study randomized 1662 asymptomatic patients with 60% to 90% carotid stenoses to receive CEA or medical management. The 5-year risk of stroke was 5.1% in patients treated surgically and 11% in patients treated medically, yielding a statistically significant 5.9% absolute risk reduction. This beneficial effect of surgery in asymptomatic carotid disease was in large part the result of a low 30-day operative risk (2.3%) for CEA. Interestingly, only half of the strokes were related to the surgical procedure; the remainder were due to contrast angiography. This finding has led to a significant decrease in the use of routine preoperative contrast angiography for patients with carotid stenosis.

The benefit of CEA was significantly less for women. This may be accounted for partly by the fact that the perioperative stroke rate in women was higher (3.6% versus 1.7%) than for men.

Although a statistical benefit for CEA in asymptomatic patients with 60% to 99% carotid stenoses was demonstrated by ACAS, skeptics argue that 17 operations were required to prevent one stroke over 5 years. This raised questions about the cost-effectiveness as well as the sensibility of treating asymptomatic patients with CEA. Subsequent studies, however, have demonstrated the cost-effectiveness of CEA.[11] There are several caveats, however. The patient's longevity

---

[10] Executive Committee for the Asymptomatic Carotid Artherosclerosis Study. Endarterectomy for asymptomatic carotid artery stenosis. JAMA 1995;273:304–308.

[11] Back MR, Harward TRS, Huber TS, et al. Improving the cost-effectiveness of carotid endarterectomy. J Vasc Surg 1997;26:456–464.

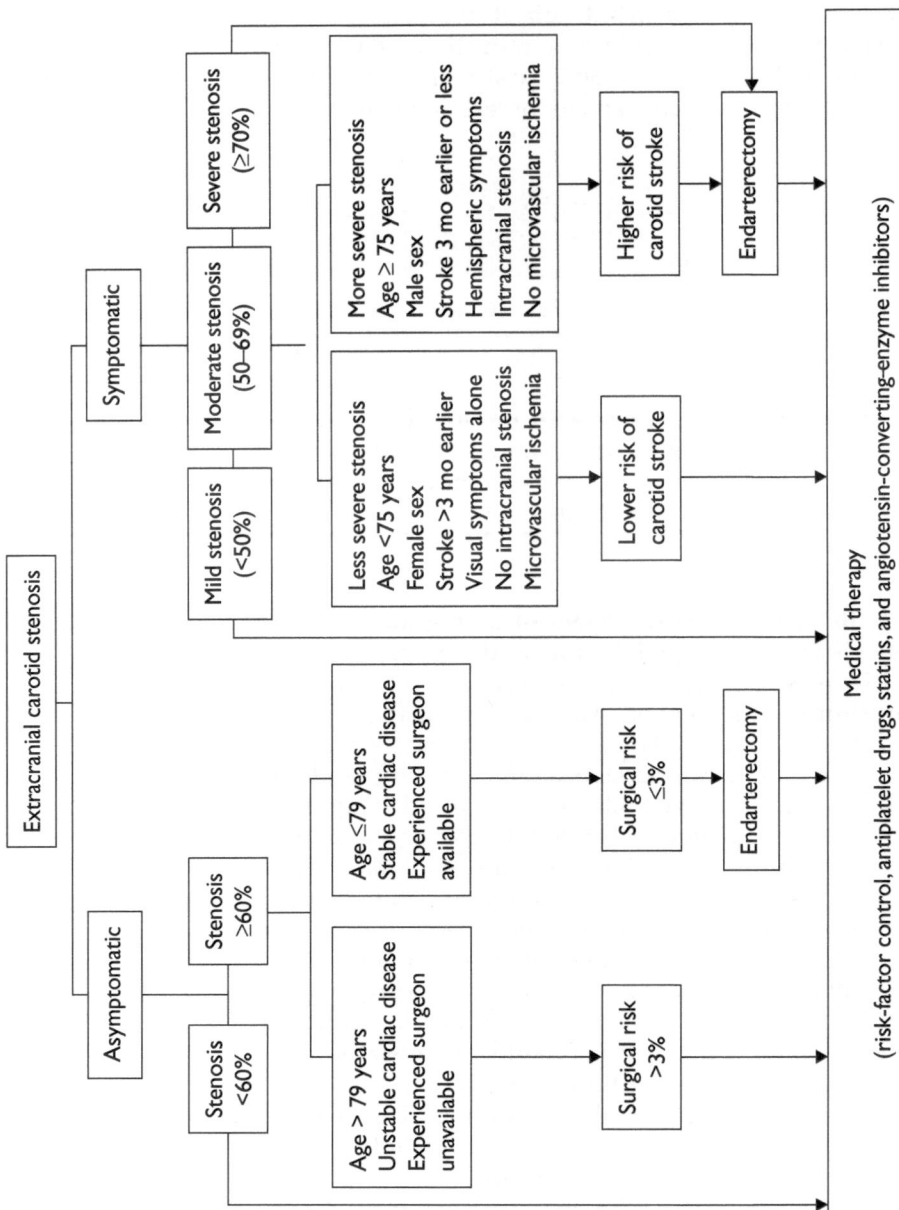

Algorithm 17.1. Algorithm for the management of extracranial carotid stenosis. The algorithm is partially based on the guidelines of the American Heart Association and the National Stroke Association.[1] Other factors not included in the figure may also be relevant in risk stratification (e.g., the results of cardiac evaluation or hemodynamic testing). (Reprinted from Sacco RL. Extracranial carotid stenosis. N Engl J Med 2001;345(15), with permission. Copyright © 2001 Massachusetts Medical Society. All rights reserved.)

must be taken into consideration. **Generally, for patients to derive a benefit from CEA, they should be expected to live 5 years; degree of stenosis also may be important, with patients with high-grade stenosis (greater than 80%) deriving the greatest benefit.**

There have been some concerns about performing CEA on patients in their 80s, the concern being that they may not live long enough to derive benefit from the surgery. There is increasing evidence to support a selectively aggressive approach in these patients as well.

While this chapter does not cover the surgical technique of carotid endarterectomy in detail, there are, however, several issues regarding this operation that do warrant brief consideration here.

The operation may be performed either under general anesthesia or via a regional block. While there are distinct advantages to both techniques, e.g., accurate cerebral monitoring under regional anesthesia, no consistent benefit has been found with either approach (**Table 17.1**).

The operation can be performed via standard operative technique or via an eversion endarterectomy. In the standard operation, the artery is opened longitudinally through the plaque, and the plaque is removed through the arteriotomy (**Fig. 17.3**). The eversion technique involves obliquely dividing the carotid bifurcation and everting the atherosclerotic plaque (**Fig. 17.4**). Both techniques have their champions. Both techniques may render excellent outcomes (**Table 17.2**).

Another hotly debated area of carotid surgery is the technique of arterial closure employed at the completion of the operation. If the carotid artery is of reasonable diameter, some surgeons advocate primary closure. Others, out of concern for restenosis, favor patch closure of the arteriotomy. The type of patch also has been debated, vein versus prosthetic material. Again, good results have been documented using any of a number of closure techniques. The evidence tends to support the bias toward patch closure.

Another issue with which the vascular surgeon must deal is cerebral protection. Surprisingly, the vast majority of patients tolerate having their carotid artery clamped for the period of the surgery. **There is a small subset of patients who do not tolerate any significant period of cerebral ischemia. Those patients needed to be shunted during the**

---

[1] (Footnote to Algorithm 17.1) Goldstein LB, Adams R, Becker K, et al. Primary prevention of ischemic stroke: a statement for healthcare professionals from the Stroke Council of the American Heart Association. Stroke 2001;32:280–299; Wolf PA, Clagett GP, Easton JD, et al. Preventing ischemic stroke in patients with prior stroke and transient ischemic attack: a statement for healthcare professionals from the Stroke Council of the American Heart Association. Stroke 1999;30:1991–1994; Albers GW, Hart RG, Lutsep HL, Newell DW, Sacco RL. Supplement to the guidelines for the management of transient ischemic attacks: a statement from the Ad Hoc Committee on Guidelines for the Management of Transient Ischemic Attacks, Stroke Council, American Heart Association. Stroke 1999;30:2502–2511; Gorelick PB, Sacco RL, Smith DB, et al. Prevention of a first stroke: a review of guidelines and multidisciplinary consensus statement from the National Stroke Association. JAMA 1999;281:1112–1120.

Table 17.1. Influence of anesthetic technique on perioperative complications in patients undergoing CEA.

Author	Year	General anesthesia			Regional anesthesia		
		CEAs	Stroke/death (%)	MI	CEAs	Stroke/death (%)	MI
Fiorani et al[b]	1997	337	5.0*	0.6	683	2.0*	0.3
Ombrellaro et al[c]	1996	126	4.8	0.8	140	2.1	2.1
Rockman et al[d]	1996	349	4.1*	1.2	1414	2.1*	0.6
Shah et al[e]	1994	419	1.9		654	2.0	
Allen et al[f]	1994	361	3.9	2.5	318	2.5	0.6
Becquemin et al[g]	1991	242	5.4	4.1*	145	4.1	0*
Bergeron et al[h]	1991	250[a]	4.4*		114	1.8*	0
Forssell et al[i]	1989	55[a]	3.6	1.8	56[a]	5.4	3.6
Godin et al[j]	1989	50	2.0		50[a]	0	
Palmer et al[k]	1989	37[a]	2.0	5.4	184[a]	1.5	1.6
Corson et al[l]	1987	242	2.9*	0.8	157	1.3*	1.3
Muskett et al[m]	1986	45[a]	0	6.7	30[a]	3.3	0
Gabelman et al[n]	1983	46[a]	6.5	2.2	54[a]	3.7	0
Pietzman et al[o]	1982	53	5.7		226	3.1	
Anderson et al[p]	1980	189	3.1		232	4.8	

CEA, carotid endarterectomy; MI, myocardial infarction.

[a] Number of patients undergoing carotid endarterectomy (number of procedures performed not indicated).

[b] Fiorani P, Sbarigia E, Speziale F, et al. General anaesthesia versus cervical block and perioperative complications in carotid artery surgery. Eur J Vasc Endovasc Surg 1997;13:37–42.

[c] Ombrellaro MP, Freeman MB, Stevens SL, et al. Effect of anesthetic technique on cardiac morbidity following carotid artery surgery. Am J Surg 1996;171:387–390.

[d] Rockman CB, Riles TS, Gold M, et al. A comparison of regional and general anesthesia in patients undergoing carotid endarterectomy. J Vasc Surg 1996;24:946–956.

[e] Shah DM, Darling RC, Chang BB, et al. Carotid endarterectomy in awake patients: its safety, acceptability, and outcome. J Vasc Surg 1994;19:1015–1020.

[f] Allen BT, Anderson CB, Rubin BG, et al. The influence of anesthetic technique on perioperative complications after carotid endarterectomy. J Vasc Surg 1994;19:834–843.

[g] Becquemin JP, Paris E, Valverde A, et al. Carotid surgery: is regional anesthesia always appropriate? J Cardiovasc Surg 1991;32:592–598.

[h] Bergeron P, Benichou H, Rudondy P, et al. Stroke prevention during carotid surgery in high risk patients (value of transcranial Doppler and local anesthesia). J Cardiovasc Surg 1991;32:713–719.

[i] Forssell C, Takolander R, Bergqvist D, et al. Local versus general anaesthesia in carotid surgery: a prospective, randomized study. Eur J Vasc Surg 1989;3:503–509.

[j] Godin MS, Bell WH, Schwedler M, et al. Cost-effectiveness of regional anesthesia in carotid endarterectomy. Am Surg 1989;55:656–659.

[k] Palmer MA. Comparison of regional and general anesthesia for carotid endarterectomy. Am J Surg 1989;157:329–330.

[l] Corson JD, Chang BB, Shah DM, et al. The influence of anesthetic choice on carotid endarterectomy outcome. Arch Surg 1987;122:807–812.

[m] Muskett A, McGreevy J, Miller M. Detailed comparison of regional and general anesthesia for carotid endarterectomy. Am J Surg 1986;691–694.

[n] Gabelman CG, Gann DS, Ashworth CJ, et al. One hundred carotid reconstructions: local versus general anesthesia. Am J Surg 1983;145:477–482.

[o] Peitzman AB, Webster MW, Loubeau J, et al. Carotid endarterectomy under regional (conductive) anesthesia. Ann Surg 1982;196:59–64.

[p] Andersen CA, Rich NM, Collins GJ, et al. Carotid endarterectomy: regional versus general anesthesia. Am Surg 1980;48:323–327.

* p value <.05 (general versus regional anesthesia).

Source: Reprinted from Patel ST, Kent KC. Cerebrovascular disease. In: Norton JA, Bollinger RR, Chang AE, et al, eds. Surgery: Basic Science and Clinical Evidence. New York: Springer-Verlag, 2001, with permission.

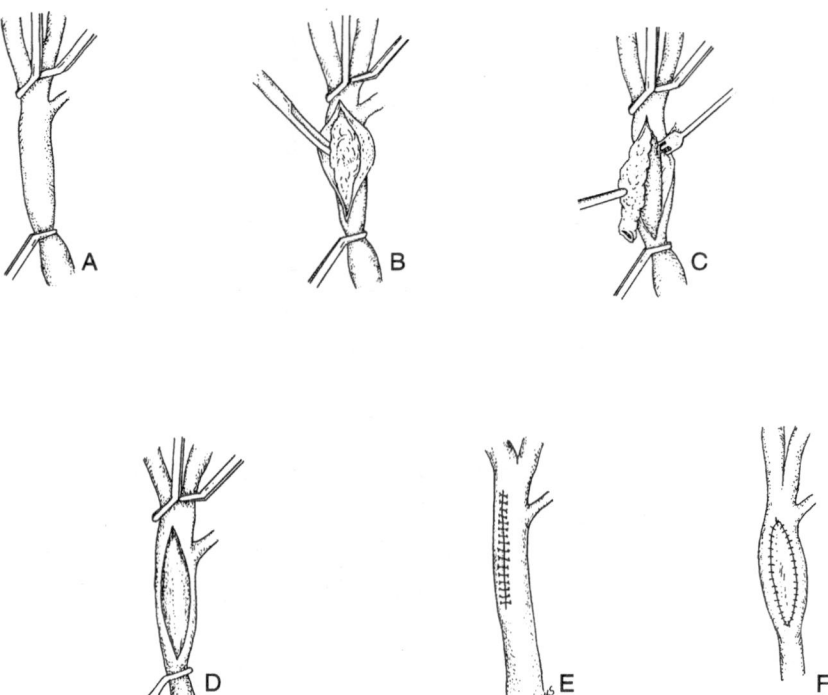

Figure 17.3. Technique of standard carotid endarterectomy. After adequate exposure is achieved, the internal, external, and common carotid arteries are clamped (A). A plane of dissection is created between the arterial wall and the atheromatous process (B). After the plaque is transected proximally, it can be reflected upward to aid in the distal portion of the endarterectomy (C). After completion of the endarterectomy, any remaining loose pieces of atheroma or strands of media are removed (D). The arteriotomy is closed primarily (E) or with a patch graft (F). (Reprinted from Patel ST, Kent KC. Cerebrovascular disease. In: Norton JA, Bollinger RR, Chang AE, et al, eds. Surgery: Basic Science and Clinical Evidence. New York: Springer-Verlag, 2001, with permission.)

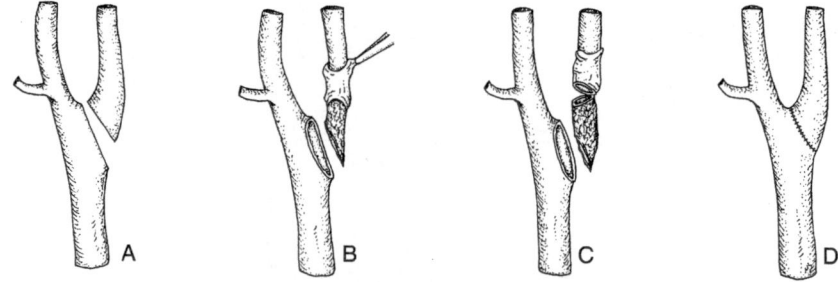

Figure 17.4. Technique of eversion carotid endarterectomy. Internal carotid artery is transected obliquely at the carotid bifurcation (A). Medial and adventitial layers of the internal carotid artery are everted over the atheromatous core (B). Completion of endarterectomy with the distal end point directly visualized (C). Internal carotid artery is reanastomosed to the common carotid artery (D). (Reprinted from Patel ST, Kent KC. Cerebrovascular disease. In: Norton JA, Bollinger RR, Chang AE, et al, eds. Surgery: Basic Science and Clinical Evidence. New York: Springer-Verlag, 2001, with permission.)

course of the procedure. There are many different types of shunts, but they all are some form of plastic tubing that is placed within the lumen of the carotid artery and maintains cerebral blood flow during the operation. The surgeon has several options regarding who needs to be shunted. The surgeon can shunt everyone. The surgeon can perform the operation under a regional anesthetic and selectively shunt only those patients who have a neurologic change upon carotid clamping. The surgical team also can monitor the patient's electroencephalogram (EEG) and selectively shunt based on changes in the EEG. Another option is to measure the backpressure in the internal carotid artery. The pressure is a measurement of cerebral collateral blood flow. Shunting generally is recommended if the carotid stump pressure falls below 45 to 50 mm Hg.

Patients who have a carotid endarterectomy generally do exceedingly well postoperatively. They must be watched closely for bleeding, acute neurologic change, hypertension, hypotension, cardiac problems, and signs of cranial nerve injury. Many patients may be discharged home on the first postoperative day. They generally are followed periodically with carotid duplex scans to check for restenosis of the operative side and to evaluate the contralateral side.

Carotid Angioplasty and Stenting

As in most aspects of vascular surgery, **endovascular techniques are being employed in the hope of decreasing patient discomfort, hospital length of stay, requirements for general anesthesia, and scarring.** There are encouraging data for and a growing experience with **balloon angioplasty for carotid stenosis.** The overall experience, however, has resulted in a **higher procedural stroke rate compared to open surgery,** with no significant decrease in length of stay and with increased costs. **With increased experience and with the advent of cerebral protection devices, the outcomes may improve.** There currently are several ongoing multicentered clinical trials designed to compare the results of carotid angioplasty to open surgery. The results of these trials will clarify the role of carotid angioplasty in the future.

Case Conclusion

The patient in the case at the beginning of this chapter presents with signs and symptoms that certainly could be attributed to atherosclerotic disease at the carotid bifurcation. After a thorough history and physical and particularly if he has a carotid bruit, he would benefit from a carotid duplex exam. If that reveals significant stenosis greater than 70%, then surgical correction of the lesion should be considered. If his carotid duplex reveals minimal disease, then other sources of arte-

Table 17.2. Influence of the technique of carotid endarterectomy on rates of perioperative stroke/death and restenosis.

Author	Year	Standard endarterectomy				Eversion endarterectomy			
		CEAs	Stroke/death (%)	Restenosis (%)	F/U (months)	CEAs	Stroke/death (%)	Restenosis (%)	F/U (months)
Ballotta et al[c]	1999	167[a]	4.2*	4.9*	34	169	0*	0*	34
Shah et al[d]	1998	474	4.2	1	18	2249	1.9	0.3	18
Cao et al[e]	1998	675	1.3	4.1	14.9	678	1.3	2.4	14.9
Entz et al[f]	1997	715[a]	4.0*			739	1.4*		
Vanmaele et al[g]	1994	98[a]	6.1	2	12	102	2.9	1	12
Kieny et al[h]	1993	156[b]		13.5	44	212	2.4	1.9	27.1

CEA, carotid endarterectomy; F/U, mean follow-up time.

[a] All CEAs performed with patch closure.

[b] All CEAs performed with primary closure.

[c] Ballotta E, Da Giau G, Saladini M, et al. Carotid endarterectomy with patch closure versus carotid eversion endarterectomy and reimplantation: a prospective randomized study. Surgery (St. Louis) 1999;125:271–279.

[d] Shah DM, Darling RC, Chang BB, et al. Carotid endarterectomy by eversion technique: its safety and durability. Ann Surg 1998;228:471–478.

[e] Cao P, Giordano G, De Rango P, et al. A randomized study on eversion versus standard carotid endarterectomy: study design and preliminary results: the Everest Trial. J Vasc Surg 1998;27:595–605.

[f] Entz L, Jaranyi Z, Nemes A. Comparison of perioperative results obtained with carotid eversion endarterectomy and with conventional patch plasty. Cardiovasc Surg 1997;5:16–20.

[g] Vanmaele RG, Van Schil PE, DeMaeseneer MG, et al. Division-endarterectomy-anastomosis of the internal carotid artery: a prospective randomized comparative study. Cardiovasc Surg 1994;2:573–581.

[h] Kieny R, Hirsch D, Seiller C, et al. Does carotid eversion endarterectomy and reimplantation reduce the risk of restenosis? Ann Vasc Surg 1993;7:407–413.

* p value <.05 (standard versus eversion endarterectomy).

Source: Reprinted from Patel ST, Kent KC. Cerebrovascular disease. In: Norton JA, Bollinger RR, Chang AE, et al, eds. Surgery: Basic Science and Clinical Evidence. New York: Springer-Verlag, 2001, with permission.

rial-to-arterial emboli must be considered. Risk management and an antiplatelet agent should be prescribed.

Summary

Stroke as a consequence of cerebral vascular disease is very prevalent, and, as the population continues to age, it most likely will become increasingly common. The individual and societal costs of strokes are very high. As a physician or healthcare provider, one must be aware of the pathophysiology as well as of the risk factors that may increase a patient's risk of stroke. The signs and symptoms of cerebral vascular disease have been discussed in detail in this chapter. An overview of appropriate diagnostic studies has been provided as well as a discussion of appropriate prophylactic and therapeutic interventions.

Selected Readings

AbuRahma AF, Robinson PA, Saiedy S, et al. Prospective randomized trial of carotid endarterectomy with primary closure and patch angioplasty with saphenous vein, jugular vein, and polytetrafluoroethylene: long-term follow-up. J Vasc Surg 1998;27:222–234.

Ballotta E, Da Giau G, Renon L, et al. Cranial and cervical nerve injuries after carotid endarterectomy: a prospective study. Surgery (St. Louis) 1999;125: 85–91.

Barnett HJ, Taylor DW, et al. Benefit of carotid endarterectomy in patients with symptomatic moderate or severe stenosis. North American Symptomatic Carotid Endarterectomy Trial Collaborators. N Engl J Med 1998;339: 1415–1425.

Dawson DL, Zieler RE, Strandness DE, et al. The role of duplex scanning and arteriography before carotid endarterectomy: a prospective study. J Vasc Surg 1993;18:673–683.

Executive Committee for the Asymptomatic Carotid Atherosclerosis Study. Endarterectomy for asymptomatic carotid artery stenosis. JAMA 1995; 273:1421–1428.

Jordan WD, Voellinger DC, Fisher WS, et al. A comparison of carotid angioplasty with stenting versus endarterectomy with regional anesthesia. J Vasc Surg 1998;28:326–334.

North American Symptomatic Carotid Endarterectomy Trial Collaborators. Beneficial effect of carotid endarterectomy in symptomatic patients with high-grade carotid stenosis. N Engl J Med 1991;325:445–453.

Patel ST, Kent KC. Cerebrovascular disease. In Norton JA, Bollinger RR, Chang AE, et al, eds. Surgery: Basic Science and Clinical Evidence. New York: Springer-Verlag, 2001.

Patel ST, Kuntz KM, Kent KC. Is routine duplex ultrasound surveillance after carotid endarterectomy cost-effective? Surgery (St. Louis) 1998;124:343–352.

Rockman CB, Riles TS, Gold M, et al. A comparison of regional and general anesthesia in patients undergoing carotid endarterectomy. J Vasc Surg 1996;24:946–956.

Salasidis GC, Latter DA, Steinmetz OK, et al. Carotid artery duplex scanning in preoperative assessment for coronary artery revascularization: the association between peripheral vascular disease, carotid artery stenosis, and stroke. J Vasc Surg 1995;21:154–162.

Shah DM, Darling RC, Chang BB, et al. Carotid endarterectomy by eversion technique: its safety and durability. Ann Surg 1998;228:471–478.

Yadav JS, Roubin GS, Iyer S, et al. Elective stenting of extracranial carotid arteries. Circulation 1997;20:S83.

18

Surgical Hypertension

Lucy S. Brevetti, Gregory R. Brevetti, and Rocco G. Ciocca

Objectives

1. To understand when to suspect surgical hypertension.
2. To describe the physiologic basis of the various forms of surgical hypertension.
3. To discuss medical and surgical management of the different types of surgical hypertension.

Case

A 36-year-old man comes to your office complaining of severe headaches, palpitations, and sweating. He gives a history of hypertension for the past 2 years. His medications include nifedipine 90 mg PO qd and atenolol 100 mg PO b.i.d. His blood pressure on exam is 220/105 mm Hg.

Introduction

Hypertension is an extremely common condition that contributes significantly to the morbidity and mortality of patients who are affected. Hypertension plays a significant role in cardiac disease, cerebrovascular disease, and other end-organ dysfunction. Its treatment can be difficult, because, unlike in the patient described, it generally is asymptomatic.

More than 95% of patients with hypertension have essential hypertension, that is, hypertension without a specifically identifiable cause. **Essential hypertension** is poorly understood. While it may occur in anybody, it is more common in certain clinical situations. Patients with a family history of hypertension or cardiac or cerebrovascular diseases may be at increased risk. In addition, patients who are obese, who smoke, and who have high sodium intake may be at increased risk. The

Table 18.1. Frequencies of the most common causes of surgical hypertension.

Endocrine	Vascular
Primary hyperaldosteronism (<1%)	Renal artery stenosis (<3%)
Cushing's syndrome (<1%)	Coarctation of the aorta (<0.1%)
Pheochromocytoma (<0.1%)	

contributing factors, pathophysiology, and treatment options are numerous and complex for essential hypertension and are beyond the scope of this chapter.

Less than 5% of patients have **secondary hypertension**, which can be **treated surgically**. Thus, one of the major goals of the history and the physical examination is to direct the clinician to a possible surgical etiology so that laboratory and radiologic evaluations can be tailored appropriately. **The differential diagnosis for surgical hypertension can be divided into two main groups: endocrine and vascular (Table 18.1).** After a complete history is taken and a physical examination is performed, a good clinician should be able to determine into which category the patient most likely falls and thus should be able to focus the diagnostic studies.

History and Physical Examination

General

The patient's age is significant because hypertension in a young patient, requiring multiple high-dose antihypertensives, should arouse the suspicion of a possible surgical etiology. The patient presented in our case is considerably younger than average for a hypertensive patient. Hypertension can occur in patients of any age; however, its prevalence increases with age. This patient has hypertension that is symptomatic. This further should increase the suspicion for a surgical etiology.

A cookbook strategy for evaluating hypertensive patients should not be used. An algorithm is useful only when there is a suspicion of a surgically correctable etiology to hypertension. (See **Algorithm 18.1**.)

Endocrine Etiology

Conn's Disease
A history of **polyuria and nocturia** may suggest **primary hyperaldosteronism (Conn's Disease)**.

Cushing's Disease
Rapid weight gain, early menopause, and oligomenorrhea are suggestive of **Cushing's disease**, which may be associated with **striking physical findings**. It is associated with the classically described "buffalo" hump, moon facies, easy bruising, and striae. Patients with Cushing's disease also suffer from **hirsutism and severe acne**. It typically occurs in middle-aged people and may be associated with **proximal muscle weakness**.

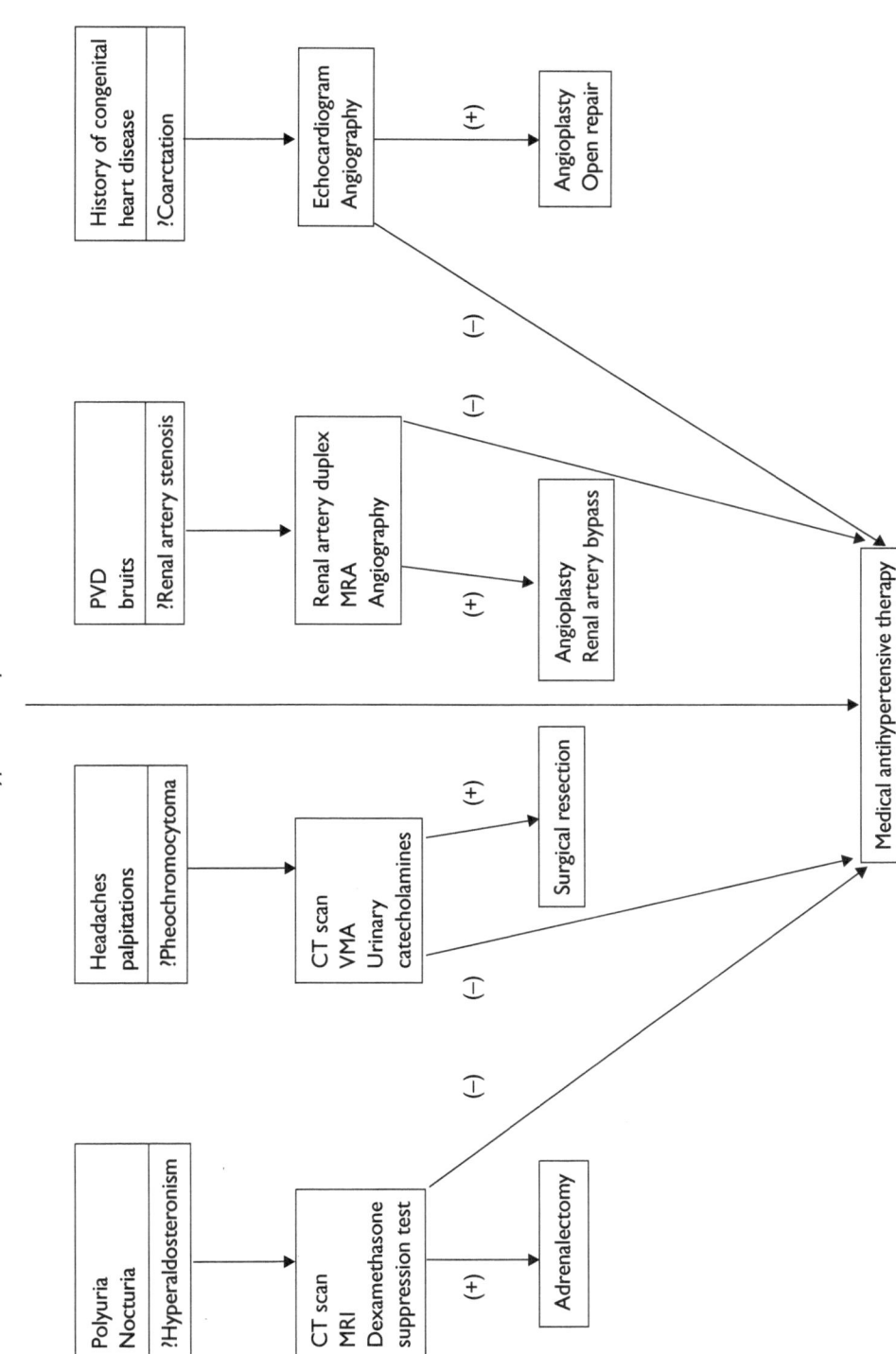

Algorithm 18.1. Algorithm for the diagnosis and treatment of the hypertensive patient. CT, computed tomography; MRA, magnetic resonance angiography; MRI, magnetic resonance imaging; PVD, peripheral vascular disease; VMA, vanillylmandelic acid.

Pheochromocytoma

Pheochromocytoma classically is associated with **refractory hypertension** along with complaints of **headaches, sweating, and palpitations**. A family history of hypertension is a helpful clue. This history usually is related to essential hypertension; however, a precise family history regarding hypertension should be sought. **Multiple endocrine neoplasia syndrome (MEN IIa)** is transmitted in an autosomal-dominant fashion. It includes **medullary carcinoma of the thyroid, pheochromocytoma, and hyperparathyroidism. MEN IIb** includes **pheochromocytoma, medullary carcinoma of the thyroid, and neuromas**. Patients with **MEN II** may have a **palpably large thyroid mass** (representing medullary carcinoma of the thyroid).

Vascular Etiology

Renal Artery Stenosis

Renal artery stenosis has been associated with a **history of peripheral vascular disease and episodes of pulmonary edema**. Hypertension due to renal artery disease may be difficult to control. **Bruits** may be noted over the renal arteries.

Coarctation of the Aorta

Complex congenital heart disease may be associated with **coarctation of the aorta**. Generally, more **complex cardiac disease** leads to **early, concomitant discovery of coarctation** (75% of cases). Only 20% present with hypertension during adulthood. However, coarctation is well described as an isolated lesion. Coarctation of the aorta in young patients may reveal a wide variety of findings depending on associated anomalies. In particular, auscultation of the precordium may reveal **murmurs consistent with atrial or ventricular septal defects, aortopulmonary shunts, or valvular stenoses**.

Case Discussion

On physical examination, the patient appears anxious and well nourished. His examination is normal except for his level of anxiety and diaphoretic skin. He has no family history of tumors or hypertension. You obtain a 24-hour urine collection for metanephrines, vanillylmandelic acid, and plasma catecholamines. You increase his atenolol and have him return to your office in 1 week.

Diagnostic Testing

Specific tests are used to rule out a diagnosis suggested by the history and physical findings.

Endocrine Etiology

Conn's Disease

Conn's disease is evaluated by **assessing plasma renin activity**. These levels remain low despite maneuvers to stimulate secretion, such as diuretic administration in the presense of Conn's disease. The most important test, however, is an **aldosterone suppression test**. In a normal individual, rapid volume expansion should cause aldosterone levels to decrease to below 10 ng/dL. In patients with Conn's disease, this suppression does not occur. Other tests that are useful in confirming this diagnosis include **magnetic resonance imaging (MRI) or computed tomography (CT) scan**. In cases in which the diagnosis is established biochemically but the imaging does not reveal the lesion, **adrenal vein sampling** can help localize the lesion or diagnose bilateral hyperplasia.

Cushing's Syndrome

Cushing's syndrome is best evaluated by **urinary free cortisol levels**. The **high-dose dexamethasone suppression test** is a useful adjunct test. A baseline cortisol level is obtained at 8 a.m., dexamethasone 1 mg is taken PO at 11 p.m., and a repeat cortisol level is drawn at 8 a.m. the next day. Cushing's syndrome is unlikely if suppression of cortisol levels occurs. If urinary cortisol is elevated or suppression does not occur, Cushing's syndrome is far more likely. The clinician next must evaluate whether **plasma adrenocorticotropic hormone (ACTH)** is involved in the cortisol elevation. **Cushing's *disease* (pituitary adenoma)** is the most common cause of Cushing's syndrome and is evaluated by **MRI or CT scan. Invasive venous sampling (for ACTH)** is useful when imaging studies are equivocal; **CT scanning** is useful to evaluate the **adrenal glands**.

Pheochromocytoma

Pheochromocytoma is an often discussed but very uncommon tumor. It can be related to the **MEN syndrome** approximately 10% of the time and is *usually* unilateral and benign. If a pheochromocytoma is suspected, the first screening tests are **urinary catecholamines, metanephrines, vanillylmandelic acid, and plasma catecholamines**. The **clonidine suppression test** is used to confirm the suspicion of pheochromocytoma when the urinary or plasma analyses are positive. A circulating catecholamine level is obtained, and clonidine 0.3 mg PO is administered. Three hours later, an additional level is drawn. If a patient has a pheochromocytoma, the circulating levels fail to suppress after 3 hours. Both **CT scanning and MRI** are very sensitive for localization. **Metaiodobenzylguanidine (MIBG) scanning** is a functional scan that can reveal the location of a pheochromocytoma not seen on CT or MRI.

Vascular Etiology

Renal Artery Stenosis

Duplex scanning usually is the first test used to screen for **renal artery stenosis**. Sensitivity may be limited by bowel gas or obesity. More specific modalities include **magnetic resonance angiography (MRA)**. Obtaining **renal vein samples** for renin levels quantitates the physiologic significance of the stenosis to the specific kidney. A ratio of 1.5 to 1 is significant and indicates that a stenosis is functionally significant.

The sensitivity of renal vein renin sampling is increased by the administration of captopril prior to venous blood sampling.

Coarctation of the Aorta

Coarctation of the aorta usually is diagnosed in early childhood and is associated with more complex cardiac anomalies. Either **angiography or echocardiography** can confirm its presence in the **neonatal population.** In **adults** presenting with unequal pulses in upper and lower extremities, a **CT scan or MRA** may be used to evaluate for coarctation. In **middle-aged adults and older patients,** serious consideration should be given to **angiography** to evaluate a coarctation and to rule out concomitant coronary artery disease.

Case Discussion

The urinary catecholamines and metanephrines are grossly positive. You proceed with a clonidine suppression test, and it, too, is positive. You obtain an abdominal CT scan with 2-mm cuts through the adrenals, but no tumor is identified. Next, you get an MIBG scan, and the area just anterior to the aortic bifurcation "lights up." You discuss this case with your attending, and he congratulates you on your finding of the pheochromocytoma in the organ of Zuckerkandl.

Treatment

Essentially, all cases of hypertension are managed with medications. The number of classes of medications, types within each class, and dosing regimens are among the most numerous of any type of medication. All types of hypertension are treated with an antihypertensive medication (**Table 18.2**).

Endocrine Etiology

Conn's Disease
Treatment of **Conn's disease** depends on whether it is caused by an **adrenal adenoma or bilateral adrenal hyperplasia.** Once chemically characterized and localized by radiologic studies, these tumors can be treated successfully either by **laparoscopic excision** (primarily left-sided tumors) or **open surgical technique.** In addition, **chemical adrenalectomy** has been described.

Cushing's Disease
Cushing's disease can be treated by **transsphenoidal resection of the pituitary gland.** If there is an **exogenous tumor that is secreting ACTH,** the condition can be treated by **excision of that tumor** (i.e., small-cell lung cancer). Treatment of **cortisol secreting adrenal tumors** is similar to that for Conn's disease: **laparoscopic excision or open surgical excision.**

Pheochromocytoma
Pheochromocytoma is treated by **surgical extirpation,** either **open or laparoscopic.** It usually is in the **adrenals,** but it can be found

Table 18.2. Antihypertensive drugs.

Class	Drug	Trade name	Initial/ maximum dose (mg/day)	Frequency of dosage	Relative cost (dose in mg)
Diuretics					
	Thiazides				
	Chlorothiazide	Diuril	500/1500	bid	1.60 (1000)
	Hydrochlorothiaxide	Esidrix	50/150	bid	1.00 (100)
		Hydro Diuril			
		Oretic			
		Thiuretic			
	Hydroflumethiazide	Saluron	100/150	bid	2.30 (50)
	Bendroflumethiazide	Naturetin	10/15	qd	3.20 (5)
	Trichlorothiazide	Naqua	4/8	qd	2.70 (4)
		Metahydrin			
	Methylclothiazide	Enduron	10/15	qd	1.90 (10)
	Benzthiazide	Exna	100/150	bid	2.60 (100)
		Aquatag			
	Polythiazide	Renese	2/8	qd	4.80 (4)
	Cyclothazide	Anhydron	1/6	qd	4.20 (4)
	Phthalimidine derivatives				
	Chlorthalidone	Hygroton	50/100	qd	2.90 (50)
	Metolazone	Zaroxolyn	2.5/5	qd	1.90 (5)
	Loop diuretics				
	Bumetanide	Bumex	0.5/1.0	qd	1.20 (0.5)
	Furosemide	Lasix	40/160	qd	1.30 (40)
	Ethacrynic acid	Edecrin	50/200	qd	2.40 (50)
	Distal tubular diuretics				
	Amiloride	Midamor	5/10	qd	2.60 (5)
	Spironolactone	Aldactone	50/100	tid	7.60 (100)
	Triamterene	Dyrenium	50/100	qd	2.10 (100)
	Combination drugs				
	Amiloride and hydrochlorothiazide	Moduretic	1 tablet (5 mg amiloride, 50 mg HCTZ)	qd	2.70 (tablet)
	Spironolactone and hydrochlorothiazide	Aldactazide	1–4 tablets	bid	2.23 (2 tablets)
	Triamterene and hydrochlorothiazide	Dyazide	1–2 tablets	bid	1.60 (2 tablets)

Continued

Table 18.2. *Continued*

Class	Drug	Trade name	Initial/maximum dose (mg/day)	Frequency of dosage	Relative cost (dose in mg)
Sympatholytics	Beta blockers				
	Atenolol	Tenormin	25/100	qd	4.40 (50)
	Metoprolol	Lopressor	50/300	bid	4.60 (100)
	Nadolol	Corgard	20/480	qd	3.05 (40)
	Pindolol	Visken	10/60	bid	3.50 (10)
	Propranolol	Inderal	40/480	bid to qid	4.40 (80)
	Timolol	Blocadren	10/60	bid	5.90 (20)
	Acebutalol	Sectral	400/1200	qd/bid	6.30 (800)
	Oxyprenolol		60/480	tid	
	Beta and alpha blocker				
	Labelalol	Normodyne Trandate	200/1200	bid	5.10 (400)
	Alpha blocker				
	Prazosin	Minipress	2/20	bid to tid	5.10 (4)
	Centrally acting				
	Clonidine	Catapres	0.1/2.4	bid	3.60 (0.4)
	Guanabenz	Wytensin	4/32	bid	5.10 (8)
	Methyldopa	Aldomet	250/2000	qd to tid	4.20 (500)
	Reserpine	Serpasil Sandril	0.1/0.5	qd	0.50 (0.1)
Vasodilators	Hydralazine	Apresoline	50/300	bid to qid	9.40 (200)
	Minoxidil	Loniten	5/100	bid	5.20 (10)
Angiotensin-converting enzyme inhibitors	Captopril	Capoten	25/150	bid	9.00 (100)
	Enalapril	Vasotec	10/40	qd to bid	10.20 (20)
	Lisinopril	Zestril Prinovil	10/40	qd	8.09 (20)
Calcium channel blockers	Diltiazem	Cardizem	120/240	tid to qid	15.50 (240)
	Nifedipine	Procardia Adalat	30/180	tid to qid	17.70 (60)
	Verapamil	Calan Isoptin	240/480	tid to qid	11.10 (320)

Source: Reprinted from Eagle KA, Haber E, DeSanctis RW, Austen WG. The Practice of Cardiology, 2nd ed. Philadelphia: Lippincott Williams & Wilkins, 1989. With permission from Lippincott Williams & Wilkins.

wherever adrenergic tissue is found. **General anesthesia can be dangerous in these patients. Preoperative treatment with alpha- and beta-blockade** is necessary prior to surgery to diminish the state of increased vascular tone. Furthermore, the anesthesiologist must be ready to deal with **extremely labile blood pressure using intravenous vasodilators and vasopressors**.

Vascular Etiology

Renal Artery Stenosis

Renovascular hypertension may be treated **surgically** in patients who are good candidates. A stenosis in the renal artery can be **bypassed** with either **saphenous vein or prosthetic graft**. More recently, **percutaneous transluminal balloon angioplasty and stenting** have become safe and less invasive methods of treatment. The long-term results of these techniques are not yet known.

Coarctation of the Aorta

Coarctation in neonates usually is **repaired at the time of surgery for other cardiac anomalies**. It can be approached either by a median sternotomy or left thoracotomy. Various surgical techniques exist, including **resection with end-to-end anastomosis, resection with tube graft interposition, subclavian artery flap repair, and patch angioplasty**. Significant **problems have arisen from balloon angioplasty of native aortic coarctation**. These include aneurysm formation, increased risk of paraplegia following open repair for "failed" angioplasty, and a high rate of restenosis. However, **balloon angioplasty is useful for recurrent stenosis following open repair** (5–10%).

Case Discussion

Your patient with the pheochromocytoma gets medically alpha blocked and then undergoes a successful laparoscopic excision of the tumor. He did well and had a stable postoperative course. He was able to be discontinued from all of his antihypertensive medications.

Summary

Hypertension is an extremely morbid condition affecting tens of millions of individuals in the United States. The vast majority (95%) of patients have primary, or idiopathic, hypertension. Treatment of these patients is an ongoing process that requires close follow-up and frequent adjustments in medications and risk-factor management. A very small percentage of individuals afflicted with hypertension may be amenable to a surgical cure.

This chapter outlined surgical causes of hypertension and their presentation, workup, and treatment. The underlying tenet in the diagnosis and treatment of surgical hypertension includes a complete history, a complete physical exam, and a high index of suspicion on the part of the clinician. After clinical presentation and suspicion suggest a particular etiology, the clinician has a variety of biochemical and radiologic studies to help confirm or rule out the diagnosis. These tests are not indicated in all patients with hypertension. Rather, they should be used selectively, when a reasonable chance of identifying a surgical etiology exists.

Selected Readings

Backer CL, Mavroudis C. Congenital heart disease. In: Norton JA, Bollinger RR, Chang AE, et al, eds. Surgery: Basic Science and Clinical Evidence. New York: Springer-Verlag, 2001.

Belli AM. New approaches to the diagnosis and management of renal artery stenosis. J Hum Hypertens 1993;8:593–594.

Hall WD. Diagnostic evaluation of the patient with systemic arterial hypertension. In: Alexander RW, Schlant RC, Fuster V, eds. Hurst's The Heart, 9th ed. New York: McGraw-Hill, 1998:1651–1672.

Joint National Committee on Detection, Evaluation, and Treatment of High Blood Pressure (fifth report). Arch Intern Med 1993;153:154–183.

Kaplan NM. Clinical Hypertension, 6th edition. Baltimore: Williams & Wilkins, 1994.

Lairmore TC. Multiple endocrine neoplasia. In: Norton JA, Bollinger RR, Chang AE, et al, eds. Surgery: Basic Science and Clinical Evidence. New York: Springer-Verlag, 2001.

Manger WM, Gifford RW Jr. Clinical and Experimental Pheochromocytoma. Cambridge, MA: Blackwell, 1996.

Novick AC. Renal revascularization for atherosclerotic ischemic renal disease. In: Calligaro KD, Dougherty MJ, Dean RH, eds. Modern Management of Renovascular Hypertension and Renal Salvage. Baltimore: Williams & Wilkins, 1996:117–123.

Rossi GP, Chiesura-Corona M, Tregnaghi A, et al. Imaging of aldosterone secreting adenomas: a prospective comparison of computed tomography and magnetic resonance imaging in 27 patients with suspected primary aldosteronism. J Hum Hypertens 1993;7:357–363.

Trainer PJ, Grossman A. The diagnosis and differential diagnosis of Cushing's syndrome. Clin Endocrinol 1991;34:317–330.

Udelsman R. Adrenal. In: Norton JA, Bollinger RR, Chang AE, et al, eds. Surgery: Basic Science and Clinical Evidence. New York: Springer-Verlag, 2001.

Winterskin BA, Baxter BT. Diseases of the abdominal aorta and its branches. In: Norton JA, Bollinger RR, Chang AE, et al. eds. Surgery: Basic Science and Clinical Evidence. New York: Springer-Verlag, 2001.

Yee ES, Soifer SJ, Turley K, et al. Infant coarctation: a spectrum in clinical presentation and treatment. Ann Thorac Surg 1986;42:488–493.

19

Breast Disease

Thomas J. Kearney

Objectives

1. To develop a differential diagnosis and a management plan for a woman with a palpable breast mass.
2. To develop a management plan for a woman with an abnormal screening mammogram.
3. To develop a management plan for a woman with a nipple discharge.
4. To develop a management plan for a woman with a swollen, tender breast.
5. To understand the role of imaging, fine-needle aspiration, core needle biopsy, and surgical biopsy in the evaluation of a woman with a breast complaint.
6. To understand the staging system for breast cancer, the surgical options for treatment, the role of radiation therapy, and the role of adjuvant systemic therapy.
7. To understand the current guidelines for breast cancer screening and the management options for "high-risk" women.

Cases

Case 1: Cysts and Fibroadenomas

A 25-year-old woman presents with a 2-cm discrete, palpable, smooth, movable mass that developed 2 months ago. The mass is slightly tender. The patient thinks that the mass is larger and more tender during the days prior to menstruation.

Case 2: Fibrocystic Condition

A 44-year-old woman presents to her gynecologist with a palpable breast mass. It has been present for several months. It occasionally is tender, particularly prior to her menstrual period. Examination reveals diffuse, bilateral tenderness. There is no dominant mass, but there is a definite thickening in one area that stands out. Her breasts feel "lumpy" throughout.

Case 3: Early-Stage Breast Cancer

A 57-year-old woman noticed a mass in her breast 3 months ago. It felt hard. Examination reveals a mass about 2 cm in diameter with no skin changes. The mass is hard, but it moves freely with respect to the chest wall. The remainder of her physical exam is unremarkable. There is no axillary or supraclavicular lymphadenopathy. Screening mammography the year before was normal, but a mammogram now shows an irregular, spiculated mass corresponding to the palpable lesion. No other abnormalities are imaged.

Case 4: Breast Abscess versus Locally Advanced Breast Cancer

A 38-year-old woman noticed a red, swollen, tender, and painful area in her left breast. She is 6 months postpartum and is breast-feeding her child. Her gynecologist prescribed dicloxacillin, which initially improved her symptoms, but now they are worse. Examination reveals a swollen, pink breast with some skin edema.

Case 5: Ductal Carcinoma in Situ, DCIS

A 54-year-old woman has an abnormal screening mammogram. She is called back for additional diagnostic views and told she has suspicious microcalcifications. A biopsy is recommended. Physical exam reveals no abnormality. Last year's mammogram is normal.

Case 6: Papilloma versus Malignancy

A 59-year-old woman is undergoing an annual breast cancer screening. Bilateral mammograms are normal. Squeezing of the right nipple expresses three drops of blood from a single duct at the 11 o'clock position. No masses are palpated. The patient states that she has noted small blood stains on her nightgown on four occasions over the past 3 months.

Case 7: Atypical Hyperplasia and Lobular Carcinoma-in-Situ

A high-risk 49-year-old woman presents with suspicious microcalcifications. Her physical examination is normal. She has a 53-year-old sister with breast cancer. She undergoes a wire localized excisional biopsy that reveals atypical ductal hyperplasia.

Introduction

The discovery of a new breast complaint is an extremely upsetting event for most women. The possibility that the new complaint represents breast cancer is foremost in their minds. Anxiety concerning severe illness, disfigurement, and the possibility of a fatal illness must be acknowledged and dealt with in an empathic manner by the patient's physician.

Almost always, a surgeon is consulted as the initial step in patient evaluation. **The surgeon must evaluate the patient appropriately and develop a management plan.** The majority of patients with a breast complaint do not have cancer. **The primary goal in breast evaluation is to decide if further evaluation is needed based on initial findings.** A final diagnosis does not need to be made at the initial visit. Normal physiologic variations related to hormonal cycling or benign breast conditions require patient education and reassurance. Occasionally, simple symptom-based interventions are required. Findings that are clearly benign may require periodic reexamination, but they may not require any further evaluation or treatment.

A surgeon also must evaluate findings that are possibly malignant. Treatment options often are complex and involve physicians from multiple disciplines. **The surgeon should be an expert in the surgical management of breast cancer. The surgeon also should be prepared to act as the coordinator of initial and follow-up care.**

The evaluation and management of patients with breast complaints and breast cancer are aided by a large body of evidence that has been derived from well-designed clinical trials conducted over the past few decades. While there are areas of legitimate disagreement among experts, there are many areas for which level I evidence is available to guide patient management.

General Evaluation

The two most common breast complaints are a palpable mass and an abnormal mammogram. These two entities, along with nipple discharge and a swollen, tender breast, represent almost all of the patient scenarios that a surgeon is likely to encounter (Table 19.1).

The surgeon must take an **appropriate history focused on the complaint**. The **duration of the complaint** as well as any **fluctuation of the complaint with the monthly menstrual cycle** are important to note. The surgeon should inquire about the **presence of breast pain and the nature of any nipple discharge**. An evaluation of **risk factors** for breast

Table 19.1. Common breast complaints.

Palpable mass
Abnormal mammogram
Nipple discharge
Swollen, tender breast

cancer is important. The **primary risk factors are increasing age and family history**. Risk factors related to **menstrual history and childbearing** are thought to represent the risk of exposure to endogenous estrogen. **Although family history is important, one must remember that the majority of breast cancer patients do not have a family history.**

Physical examination of the breast and axillary areas is mandatory. The surgeon should inspect the breast for any skin changes or retraction. Palpation should be thorough and performed in a relaxed, unhurried manner. The examination must be performed efficiently and with respect for the patient. **A general examination of the patient focused on the lungs, chest wall, and abdomen also must be performed.**

The surgeon personally should review any mammograms and ultrasound examinations. Insist upon original films. Copies often do not have the adequate resolution needed to detect minute changes. If available, several years of images should be compared side by side in order to appreciate any subtle changes over time.

The surgeon should be familiar with various **diagnostic interventions that can be performed in the office. These include fine-needle aspiration (FNA) of breast cysts and breast masses, the proper handling of cytology specimens, and the appropriate use of core needle biopsy.**

Once the evaluation is completed, **most patients can be classified as having findings that are clearly benign, probably benign, or suspicious.** Patients with findings that are clearly benign can return to routine screening. Patients with findings that are probably benign should be followed with a repeat clinical examination in several months. Clinical follow-up must be active. The patient should not leave the office without making a specific follow-up appointment. Patients with suspicious findings require further evaluation. Tissue diagnosis usually is required. The surgeon must be expert in the various techniques available for breast biopsy (**Table 19.2**).

The case scenarios presented at the start of this chapter and discussed in the text that follows illustrate the evaluation and management of patients with common breast complaints. In addition, diagnostic techniques, the treatment of breast cancer, breast screening, and the evaluation of "high-risk" women are discussed.

Palpable Breast Mass in a Younger Woman (Case 1)

The patient in **Case 1** has a finding that is probably benign. **Breast cancer before the age of 30 is rare. The primary differential is to determine if this lesion is a cyst or if it is a solid mass.** Cysts are benign,

Table 19.2. Biopsy techniques.

Core needle biopsy
Image-guided core biopsy (stereotactic or ultrasound guided)
Excisional biopsy
Wire localized excisional biopsy
Incisional biopsy (rarely used)

fluid-filled lesions. **In this age group, the most likely solid mass would be a fibroadenoma. Fibroadenomas represent a benign hyperplastic process. Fibroadenomas usually are single, but 10% to 20% are multiple. Other benign possibilities include juvenile fibroadenomas, hamartomas, lipomas, and fat necrosis. The possibility that this is a phyllodes tumor and the remote possibility that this represents breast cancer both must be considered.** The history and physical exam certainly suggest a cyst.

There are **two appropriate management options** for this patient. **Fine-needle aspiration** of the mass with a 23-gauge needle may result in the removal of cyst fluid, with resolution of the mass. If classic cyst fluid without any gross blood is obtained, it may be discarded, provided that the mass resolves completely. The patient should be scheduled for follow-up examination in 2 to 3 months. If the aspirate is bloody, the fluid should be sent for cytologic evaluation. A persistent mass after aspiration suggests a solid lesion, and the aspirated fluid should be sent for analysis as well. If no fluid is obtained, the needle may be passed through the lesion several times, and the resulting cellular material should be sent for cytologic evaluation. The surgeon must ensure that the appropriate fixative is available. In many multidisciplinary breast centers, on-site cytologic evaluation is available to assess adequacy of the sample and provide a quick diagnosis.

The other alternative for this patient is **ultrasound examination** of the affected breast. The finding of a simple cyst with a smooth wall, no cystic debris, and good through transmission of ultrasound establishes the diagnosis of a simple cyst. No further evaluation or follow-up is needed. If desired and if the cyst is tender or enlarges in the future, aspiration then can be performed. The finding of septations, mural nodules, or intracystic debris characterizes the cyst as a complex cyst. Further evaluation with aspiration and cytologic evaluation is required, since 0.3% of complex cysts are associated with malignancy. The finding of a smooth, homogeneous mass consistent with a fibroadenoma may be managed in several ways. In a young patient under 30 with physical exam findings as described and an ultrasound image consistent with a fibroadenoma, observation is usually appropriate. Repeat clinical and ultrasound evaluation at 6-month intervals for a year or two is suggested. The patient should be instructed to contact the surgeon if the mass appears larger during monthly breast self-exam (BSE). If the mass changes, biopsy is required. For patients over the age of 30, FNA of the solid mass is recommended. Cytologic findings consistent with a fibroadenoma combined with benign clinical and imaging characteristics constitute a negative "triple test" (**Table 19.3**).[1] These patients may be observed safely, with excision reserved for masses that grow. The finding of an irregular, heterogeneous mass on ultrasound mandates tissue diagnosis. If FNA of a palpable mass is bloody or the mass does not resolve, tissue diagnosis is required.

---

[1] Vetto JT, Pomier RF, Schmidt WA, et al. Diagnosis of palpable breast lesions in younger women by the modified triple test is accurate and cost-effective. Arch Surg 1996;131:967.

Table 19.3. The triple test.

Benign physical exam
Benign image
Diagnostic and benign cytology

Breast cancer is rare in women between the ages of 20 and 30. In a study of 951 breast biopsies performed on young women, no patients under age 21 were found to have breast cancer. However, 1.3% of biopsies in women age 21 to 25 and 4.0% of biopsies in women age 26 to 30 were positive for malignancy.[2] Image-guided core biopsy and excisional biopsy represent two equivalent options. Core biopsy guided by palpation alone may yield a false-negative result due to sampling error. **The most important pitfall in observing a solid mass in any woman is the risk of missing a cancer.**

Palpable Breast Mass in a Middle-Aged Woman (Case 2)

The evaluation of the patient in **Case 2** is more complex than that of the patient in the previous case. Her physical exam shows an abnormality that does not have typically benign characteristics. The examination is made more difficult by her lumpy breasts. **The incidence of breast cancer begins to rise after age 40**, and this patient could very well have a malignancy. The surgeon must prove that she does not. The patient had a mammogram performed that revealed dense breast tissue but no mass. **A negative mammogram does not rule out the presence of breast cancer.** An ultrasound also was negative. In this setting, the patient must be assumed to have a solid mass. Fine-needle aspiration with cytologic interpretation is the next step. However, in this case, the cytology report revealed blood and fat but no specific diagnosis could be made. This patient now needs a tissue diagnosis. An excisional biopsy performed as an outpatient is the appropriate choice. This patient's biopsy revealed sclerosing adenosis.

"Fibrocystic condition" is an imprecise term that describes a clinically diagnosed entity that is a manifestation of physiologic responses of breast tissue to normal hormonal cycles. The patient often has breasts that are painful, particularly prior to her menses. She has lumps that come and go. Her mammogram often shows a pattern of dense breast tissue. **It probably is more useful to describe benign breast disease in terms of a three-tiered pathologic classification that can be used to assess a patient's risk of future breast cancer development, particularly when family history is factored in.**[3] **Lesions are classified as nonproliferative, proliferative without atypia, and atypical hyperplasia (including lobular carcinoma in situ, LCIS) (Table**

---

[2] Ferguson CM, Powell RW. Breast masses in young women. Arch Surg 1989;124:1338.
[3] Dupont W, Page D. Risk factors for breast cancer in women with proliferative breast disease. N Engl J Med 1985;312:146.

19.4). Several retrospective and case-control studies show no increased risk of developing breast cancer with nonproliferative lesions and a small relative risk (RR <2.0) with proliferative lesions without atypia. Family history does modify the risk factors for the proliferative lesions slightly (RR 2.0–3.0). Patients with the nonproliferative lesions and low-risk proliferative lesions require routine breast screening. Patients with the higher risk atypical hyperplasia require special surveillance and possibly preventative therapy. This is discussed in more detail in a later section.

Early-Stage Breast Cancer (Case 3)

The patient in **Case 3** with a palpable mass and a suspicious mammogram almost certainly has breast cancer. Clinically, it appears to be localized to her breast. Fine-needle aspiration was performed, with a result revealing adenocarcinoma. The surgeon next must perform some basic studies to determine the stage of her cancer. A chest radiograph and basic blood work [complete blood count (CBC), liver function tests] are all that are usually required. If these are normal, there is no role for computed tomography (CT) scan or bone scan for patients with clinical early-stage breast cancer. The patient, in consultation with her surgeon, must now choose among the treatment options.

In the early 20th century Halsted model of breast cancer an orderly, predictable, lymphatic spread of breast cancer subsequently would give rise to systemic disease. Therapy was designed to encompass the tumor and "get it all out." The radical mastectomy was designed to remove the breast, all axillary nodes, and the pectoral muscles. A fair number of patients with early-stage breast cancer were cured with this procedure. However, well-designed, prospective clinical studies in the latter part of the 20th century demonstrated that breast cancer dissemination was often capricious and hematogenous. In the modern model of breast cancer, patients with clinically and pathologically negative nodes in fact already could have metastatic disease at the time of presentation. There are three major implications of the acceptance of this hypothesis:

1. **Breast cancer spreads capriciously and may do so at any time. Early detection is lifesaving (Table 19.5).** Early detection can increase the number of breast cancers identified and treated at a truly early stage, before potentially lethal micrometastases have occurred.

2. **Women die from breast cancer because of metastatic disease, not from the effects of local or regional tumor. Thus, the method of local**

Table 19.4. The pathologic classification of benign breast disease.

Nonproliferative	Proliferative w/o atypia	Atypical hyperplasia
Cysts	Moderate or florid hyperplasia	Atypical ductal hyperplasia
Mild hyperplasia	Intraductal papilloma	Atypical lobular hyperplasia
Papillary apocrine changes	Sclerosing adenosis	Lobular carcinoma in situ

Table 19.5. Results of screening mammogram trials.

Study	Reference	Date	Randomized	Accrual	Age (years)	RR of mortality screened versus nonscreened 40–49 (years)	All ages
HIP[a]	209	1963	Yes	60,995	40–64	0.77	0.71
BCDDP[b]	210	1970	No	280,000	>35	<1.0	<1.0
Utrecht	211	1974	No	20,555	50–64	<1.0	<1.0
Nijmegen	60	1975	No	20,555	50–64	<1.0	<1.0
Edinburgh	212	1976	Yes	45,130	45–64	0.78	0.82
Malmö	213	1976	Yes	42,283	45–69	0.51	0.51
Two-County, Sweden	214	1977	Yes	134,867	40–74	0.88	0.69
NBSS1[c]	215	1980	Yes	50,430	40–49	1.36	—
NBSS2[c]	57	1980	Yes	31,405	50–59	—	0.97
Stockholm	60	1981	Yes	51,107	40–64	1.04	0.72
Götenborg	216	1982	Yes	49,533	39–59	0.75	0.84
Miyagi Prefecture	217	1989	No	9,634	>50	—	20% increased detection

[a] Helath Insurance Plan.
[b] Breast Cancer Detection Demonstration Project.
[c] National Breast Screening Study 1 or 2.

Source: Reprinted from Pass HA. Benign and malignant diseases of the breast. In: Norton JA, Bollinger RR, Chang AE, et al, eds. Surgery: Basic Science and Clinical Evidence. New York: Springer-Verlag, 2001, with permission.

control does not depend upon survival. **Lumpectomy with radiation is equivalent to mastectomy with regard to patient survival (Table 19.6).**[4] This has been demonstrated in over half a dozen prospective clinical trials. The objectives of local control are to eliminate a tumor from the breast and chest wall that ultimately may become symptomatic by eroding, fungating, or bleeding and to remove a tumor that potentially may metastasize. Similarly, **the method chosen to achieve regional control (axillary lymph node dissection, radiation therapy) does not affect survival. The method of regional control should be chosen to maximize the amount of staging information obtained while minimizing patient risk and inconvenience.**

3. Systemic metastases are the cause of breast cancer deaths. **Systemic therapy (hormone blockade, chemotherapy) is potentially lifesaving. Systemic therapy should be considered in all women whose breast cancers are at significant risk of disseminating.** The roles of clinical staging and analysis of prognostic factors are to identify which tumors are and which tumors are not at significant risk for having associated micrometastases.

This patient may achieve local control of her tumor with either lumpectomy and radiation or mastectomy. There are several factors relevant to the choice of breast conservation versus mastectomy for the initial treatment of early breast cancer (**Table 19.7**). Patient preference for breast conservation, tumor size, and tumor location favorable for a good aesthetic result are important factors. The patient should have a single tumor and should not have a contraindication to radiation (pregnancy, previous radiation to the area, certain collagen vascular diseases). The patient should be willing to come for follow-up. Anticipated difficulty with future mammography due to suspicious areas is a relative contraindication to conservation. **Patient preference should be a major factor in choosing local treatment or mastectomy because, in most instances, the options are therapeutically equivalent.** Radiation therapy usually is given after lumpectomy because it reduces the in-breast recurrence rate (and therefore improves the ultimate success rate with breast conservation) approximately fourfold.

Breast reconstruction is an appropriate option for most women undergoing mastectomy and should be discussed with all women in whom mastectomy is considered. Immediate reconstruction almost always is feasible. Delayed reconstruction may be best for those women who are not certain of their preference for reconstruction and for those in whom the need for postmastectomy radiation therapy is likely. Prosthetic reconstruction with an implant generally is less physiologically stressful and less technically demanding. Autogenous reconstruction generally is more complex but usually has better final aesthetic results.

---

[4] Fisher B, Anderson S, Redmond CK. Reanalysis and results after 12 years of follow-up in a randomized clinical trial comparing total mastectomy with lumpectomy with or without irradiation in the treatment of breast cancer. N Engl J Med 1995;333:1456.

Table 19.6. Randomized trial of mastectomy versus breast conservation (level I evidence).

Trial	Reference	Year	n	Randomized	Stage	Design	Median Follow-up	Results
Guy's Hospital	218	1961–1970	376	Yes	T_1N_0 or T_1N_1	WLE + XRT vs. radical mastectomy + XRT	11 years	(1) Treatment deemed inadequate (omission of ALND and low-dose XRT) (2) Higher regional recurrence and lower survival in WLE + XRT group, especially in stage II patients
		1971–1976	250	Yes	T_1N_0	Radical mastectomy + XRT vs. WLE + XRT		
Gustave-Roussay	219	1972–1979	179	Yes	T_1N_0 or T_1N_1	Tumorectomy + XRT vs. MRM	10 years	No difference in overall survival, local control, distant metastasis, or contralateral breast cancer rate
NCI Milan	138	1973–1980	701	Yes	T_1N_0	Quadrentectomy, ALND, and XRT vs. radical mastectomy	10 years	(1) No difference in local recurrence or survival (2) BCT can be performed in lymph node-positive patients if there is adjuvant chemotherapy
NSABP-B06	140	1976–1984	1843	Yes	T < 4 cm N_0	Lumpectomy, ALND, and XRT vs. lumpectomy/ALND, vs. MRM	8 years	(1) 10% of patients assigned to BCT-negative margins could not be achieved (2) XRT critically important for local control as breast recurrence occurred in 10% of lumpectomy/XRT vs. 39% of lump alone ($p < .001$) (3) No difference in survival thus local recurrence does not predict survival
NCI Bethesda	220	1979–1987	247	Yes		Lumpectomy/ALND vs. MRM	8 years	No difference in survival or local control
EORTC	221	1980–1986	148	Yes	I	Lumpectomy/ALND + XRT vs. MRM	8 years	No difference in survival, local control, or distant recurrence
			755	Yes	II			
Danish Breast Cancer Group	222	1983–1989	905	Yes	I or II	Quadrantectomy/ALND + XRT vs. MRM	6 years	(1) Identical overall survival (2) Fewer local/regional recurrences in BCT group (NS)

NCI, National Cancer Institute; EORTC, European Organization for Research and Treatment of Cancer; ALND, axillary lymph node dissection; XRT, radiation therapy; MRM, modified radical mastectomy; WLE, wide local excision; BCT, breast conservation treatment; NS, not significant.

Source: Reprinted from Pass HA. Benign and malignant diseases of the breast. In: Norton JA, Bollinger RR, Chang AE, et al, eds. Surgery: Basic Science and Clinical Evidence. New York: Springer-Verlag, 2001, with permission.

Table 19.7. Factors favoring breast conservation vs. mastectomy.

Factors favoring breast conservation	Factors favoring mastectomy
Small tumor	Large tumor in small breast
Unifocal tumor	Multicentric disease
Negative margins	Positive margin
Able to have radiation	Unable to have radiation
Patient preference	Patient preference
	Difficulty with follow-up anticipated

At the time of lumpectomy or mastectomy, axillary nodes traditionally are removed from the lower levels of the axilla. When performed at the time of lumpectomy, a separate incision is made in the axilla. When combined with mastectomy, the procedure is termed a modified radical mastectomy; the pectoral muscle is not removed as in the Halsted radical mastectomy. A typical axillary dissection removes about a dozen nodes. **The axillary dissection itself does not directly change survival, but it is instead a staging technique that allows for the rational selection of adjuvant systemic therapy.**

The evolving technique of sentinel lymph node mapping and biopsy has the potential to eliminate the need for modern axillary dissection if current prospective trials validate the technique's apparent initial safety and effectiveness. At many centers, this technique has replaced standard axillary dissection. In this technique, a tracer [blue dye or technetium 99 (Tc-99)-labeled sulfur colloid] is injected into the breast. The tracer travels to the first draining axillary lymph node and is detected visually or with a hand-held gamma probe. That node is removed and tested. If it is free of cancer, the remainder of the axilla is presumed to be negative, and axillary dissection with its occasional side effects of lymphedema and frozen shoulder can be avoided. Patients with positive sentinel nodes receive an immediate axillary dissection. Several currently published studies with large numbers of subjects demonstrate a sensitivity of this technique ranging from 88% to 94%.[5] Large-scale prospective studies were scheduled to have completed accrual by mid-2003.

The presence or absence of node metastases allows the patient to be stratified by cancer stage (Tables 19.8, 19.9, 19.10, and 19.11). Based on the cancer stage, appropriate adjuvant therapy can be selected for patients. The sixth edition of the American Joint Committee on Cancer (AJCC) staging system is effective as of January 1, 2003. This edition differs from the previous system mainly in the consideration of sentinel lymph nodes biopsy results.[6] Prognostic factors help differentiate

[5] Giuliano AE, Kirgan DM, Guenthler JM, et al. Lymphatic mapping and sentinel lymphadenectomy for breast cancer. Ann Surg 1994;220:391. Krag D, Weaver D, Ashikaga T, et al. The sentinel node in breast cancer—a multicenter validation trial. N Engl J Med 1998;339:941.

[6] Greere FL, Page DL, Fleming ID, et al. AJCC Cancer Staging Manual, 6th ed. New York: Springer-Verlag, 2002.

Table 19.8. American Joint Committee on Cancer (AJCC) T category.

T	Description
Tis	Carcinoma in situ
T1	2 cm or less
T2	>2 cm but ≤5 cm
T3	Greater than 5 cm
T4	Skin, chest wall involvement, or inflammatory

Table 19.9. AJCC N and M categories.

N & M	Description
pN0	No node involvement
pN1	1 to 3 axillary nodes and/or microscopic IM nodes detected by SLN
pN2	1. 4 to 9 axillary nodes
	2. Clinically positive IM nodes without any positive axillary nodes
pN3	1. 10 or more axillary nodes
	2. Any infraclavicular or supraclavicular nodes
	3. Clinically positive IM nodes with positive axillary nodes
	4. Microscopic IM nodes with 4 or more axillary nodes
M0	No distant metastases
M1	Distant metastases

IM, intramuscular.

Table 19.10. Early-stage breast cancer.

Stage	Tumor	Nodes	Metastases
0	Tis	N0	M0
I	T1	N0	M0
IIA	T0–1	N1	M0
	T2	N0	M0
IIB	T2	N1	M0
	T3	N0	M0

Table 19.11. Locally advanced breast cancer.

Stage	Tumor	Nodes	Metastases
IIIA	T0–2	N2	M0
	T3	N1	M0
	T3	N2	M0
IIIB	T4	N0–2	M0
IIIC	Any T	N3	M0
IV	Any T	Any N	M1

those patients who are at high risk of developing metastatic disease subsequent to their initial local-regional breast cancer treatment from those who are at low risk. **Patients who fall into the high-risk groups benefit from systemic adjuvant therapy, whereas the risks of systemic therapy usually outweigh the benefits in low-risk patients. The three prognostic factors that have been proven useful in prospective, randomized trials of women with breast cancer are tumor size, axillary lymph node status, and estrogen receptor status.** Her-2-neu status now is measured routinely at most centers due to usefulness in certain situations. While other factors have been shown to be prognostic, their role in making clinical decisions has yet to be defined.

Multiple clinical trials for patients under age 70 are available to help guide adjuvant treatment decision making. The current standard is constantly changing. Current guidelines available from several sources represent the general consensus from national experts based on the best available levels of evidence.[7] There are honest differences of opinion concerning the appropriateness of current guidelines for individual patients. **Currently, all node-positive patients and most node-negative patients with tumors greater than 10 mm require adjuvant therapy. Patients with tumors smaller than 10 mm but with adverse characteristics also should be considered for systemic therapy. The type of systemic therapy varies, but it includes several different chemotherapy regimens and drugs (doxorubicin, cyclophosphamide, and paclitaxel) along with the hormonal agents tamoxifen and anastrozole.**

Woman with a Red, Swollen Breast (Case 4)

The patient in **Case 4** most likely has a breast abscess that almost always is associated with lactation and infection by skin organisms. If given early in the development of breast infection, antibiotics can prevent abscess formation. In this patient, the antibiotics decreased some of the inflammation from the surrounding cellulitis, but they could not penetrate into the abscess cavity that already had formed. An ultrasound is an excellent first test for evaluating this patient. If it reveals an irregular cavity, percutaneous drainage can be performed and antibiotics would be continued. Often, this needs to be repeated every several days, but most cases usually resolve. Occasionally, open surgical drainage is required.

The physician needs to be concerned about the possibility of locally advanced breast cancer in any patient with a red or swollen breast. Locally advanced breast cancer is considered operable or inoperable based on clinical characteristics. Presurgical systemic treatment is required for patients with stage IIIB inoperable disease and should be considered strongly for patients with stage IIIA operable disease. The concept of operable versus inoperable breast cancer originally was described decades ago. **Patients with extensive breast**

---

[7] NCCN. Practice Guidelines in Oncology. www.nccn.org, 2003.

edema, inflammatory cancer, skin satellites, arm edema, or parasternal or supraclavicular nodes always suffer recurrence when treated with surgery alone. Other grave signs include fixation to the chest wall, fixed nodes, large nodes, skin ulceration, or limited breast edema. Patients with these findings are considered to have inoperable stage IIIB or IIIC breast cancer. Patients with stage IIIA disease are operable (albeit usually with mastectomy) but are still considered to have locally advanced breast cancer.

Neoadjuvant (preoperative or induction) therapy in stage III disease can produce response rates of 75% or greater. This has become the standard approach for patients with stage IIIB breast cancer.[8] Following successful induction therapy, mastectomy and radiation are used. Survival rates are improved compared to a "surgery-first" approach, and local control rates are between 70% and 80%. For patients with operable stage IIIA breast cancer, a modified radical mastectomy followed by postoperative adjuvant therapy and postmastectomy radiation is a reasonable approach. An alternative is preoperative chemotherapy with possible "downstaging" of the tumor and subsequent lumpectomy with radiation. In stage IIIA breast cancer, the use of adjuvant therapy increases breast conservation rates. Survival is the same as with postoperative systemic therapy. Negative aspects of preoperative therapy include the potential loss of accurate staging information from down-staging of axillary nodes.

In addition, several reports have appeared concerning breast conserving surgery following induction chemotherapy in patients with early stage (I and II) breast cancer.[9] Response rates up to 80% are seen, and many patients who would require mastectomy can be treated adequately with breast conservation. Because these studies represent experiences with highly selected patients, many physicians consider this approach investigational.

Ductal Carcinoma In Situ, DCIS (Case 5)

The patient in **Case 5** with suspicious microcalcifications requires a biopsy. The most likely malignant finding is DCIS, although she may have benign microcalcifications.

Screening mammography has been shown to decrease death from breast cancer in screened populations. The American Cancer Society, along with many other organizations, recommend mammography beginning at age 40 for all women. This should be combined with annual physician exam and BSE. A screening mammogram is obtained on asymptomatic women. They are batch read by a radiologist. The radiologist must decide if they are normal or abnormal. Less

---

[8] Buzdar AU, Singletary SE, Booser DJ, et al. Combined modality treatment of stage III and inflammatory breast cancer: M.D. Anderson Cancer Center experience. Surg Oncol Clin North Am 1995;4:715.

[9] Fisher B, Brown A, Mamounas E, et al. Effect of preoperative chemotherapy on local-regional disease in women with operable breast cancer: findings from National Surgical Adjuvant Breast and Bowel Project B-18. J Clin Oncol 1997;15:2483.

Table 19.12. American College of Radiology's Breast Imaging and Reporting Database System (BIRADS).

Category	Description	Recommendation
1	Normal	Annual follow-up
2	Benign	Annual follow-up
3	Probably benign	Short-interval (6-month) follow-up
4	Suspicious	Biopsy recommended
5	Highly suggestive of malignancy	Biopsy mandatory

then 10% of screening mammograms would be expected to be abnormal. **The patients with abnormal mammograms then are recalled for diagnostic mammography. Diagnostic mammography is performed with the radiologist on site in order to direct the workup.** Additional views and special techniques such as spot compression or magnification are used. Ultrasound is obtained to evaluate mammographic masses to distinguish solid masses from fluid-filled cysts. At the completion of the diagnostic imaging session, the radiologist classifies the mammogram according to the American College of Radiology's Breast Imaging Reporting and Database System (BIRADS). The report classifies the mammogram and provides clear recommendations to treating physicians (**Table 19.12**). **Spiculated masses, solid masses, and indeterminate microcalcifications on mammography should be considered suspicious and almost always require biopsy.**

Microcalcifications can appear benign or may represent malignancy. **Microcalcifications that are clustered with numerous pleomorphic or linear forms often can represent DCIS.** This is the earliest form of breast cancer and is about 98% to 99% curable with appropriate treatment. This patient needs to have a biopsy. Because the abnormality cannot be felt, an image must be used to guide the biopsy. Traditionally, wire **localized excisional biopsy** has been performed. Approximately 75% of such patients have a benign biopsy. This has led to interest in less invasive biopsy techniques. Recently, **stereotactic biopsy with a large-bore core needle or a vacuum-assisted device (Mammotome)** has demonstrated accuracy equivalent to open biopsy in most patients. This patient underwent a vacuum-assisted core biopsy with a result revealing intermediate-grade DCIS.

The current standard for treatment of DCIS in patients desiring breast conservation is lumpectomy with clean margins followed by radiation. If a patient desires mastectomy or there are contraindications to breast conservation, simple mastectomy (without axillary node dissection) may be performed. Several prospective trials clearly show **a benefit to the addition of radiation therapy and systemic tamoxifen to lumpectomy.**[10] Survival is the same with either technique,

---

[10] Fisher B, Dignam J, Wolmark N. Tamoxifen in treatment of intraductal breast cancer: National Surgical Adjuvant Breast and Bowel Project B-24 randomised controlled trial. Lancet 1999;353:1993. Fisher B, Dignam J, Wolmark N, et al. Lumpectomy and radiation therapy for the treatment of intraductal breast cancer: findings from the National Surgical Adjuvant Breast and Bowel Project B-17. J Clin Oncol 1998;16:441.

but in-breast tumor recurrence (both recurrent DCIS and invasive breast cancer) is decreased with the addition of radiation and tamoxifen.

The patient in this scenario underwent wire-localized lumpectomy. The final pathology revealed DCIS with a diameter of 7mm. The patient had a clear margin greater than 10mm in all directions. While radiation would be considered standard in most patients, there is retrospective (level II) data available to support lumpectomy alone in selected patients with DCIS. Several classification systems are available to select patients who might safely skip radiation, most notably the Van Nuys Prognostic Index.[11] This patient has a small tumor with a wide margin around it, and lumpectomy alone would be a reasonable alternative to lumpectomy with radiation. She chose to have radiation, the treatment supported by level I evidence. She can expect about a 10% chance of in-breast tumor recurrence at 10 years. If this occurs, she will need a simple mastectomy at that time. Regular follow-up with mammography every 6 to 12 months is essential for this patient.

Papilloma versus Malignancy (Case 6)

The patient in **Case 6** with the bloody nipple discharge might have breast cancer, although benign illnesses also can cause bloody discharge. **The evaluation of women who present with nipple discharge is determined by the nature of the discharge.** A milky discharge can be physiologic, secondary to numerous medications that affect prolactin, or due to pathologic conditions such as a pituitary tumor or ectopic prolactin production. **Approximately one third of women who have lactated can express breast secretions.** Management by duct excision is indicated if the discharge is bothersome. A "fibrocystic discharge" is often brown, green, or black and usually is associated with duct ectasia or fibrocystic breasts. Fibrocystic discharge also can be treated by duct excision if bothersome.

In bloody discharges, malignancy is a concern. Clinical evaluation should be directed toward identifying palpable or mammographic lesions. Cytologic evaluation of nipple discharge has questionable usefulness, since decisions concerning surgery are made on clinical grounds. Likewise, galactography only occasionally is helpful, although some feel it helps guide excision. A negative galactogram should not be used as an excuse to avoid surgery when bloody discharge persists. Often, the discharge can be localized to one quadrant of the breast or even one duct, which is useful for guiding terminal duct excision. This is the procedure recommended for this patient. The bloody nature of the discharge, combined with its spontaneous expression on several occasions, raises the level of suspicion of malignancy.

The most common reason for bloody discharge is the presence of a papilloma, accounting for most cases. **Duct ectasia accounts for**

---

[11] Silverstein MJ, Lagios MD, Craig PH, et al. A prognostic index for ductal carcinoma in situ of the breast. Cancer 1996;77:2267.

additional cases of nipple discharge. Cancer is present in 5% to 20% of bloody nipple discharges. Terminal duct excision can be performed on an outpatient basis using local anesthesia with sedation. A circumareolar incision may be used, and there usually is no need to close the resultant breast cavity. Younger patients who still expect to have children should be warned that interference with successful lactation might result.

Atypical Hyperplasia and Lobular Carcinoma In Situ, LCIS (Case 7)

The patient in **Case 7** has atypical hyperplasia and a family history of breast cancer. She does not have breast cancer and does not need specific treatment for her atypical hyperplasia. However, she is not a routine patient. She has an increased risk of developing breast cancer based on her pathology findings. This risk is further increased by her family history. This risk can be quantified using a mathematical model.[12] This model takes into account patient current age, age at menarche, age at first live birth, family history, number of previous breast biopsies, and any finding of atypical hyperplasia. Her risk of developing breast cancer is approximately 5% over the next 5 years, with a lifetime risk of about 30%. **Atypical ductal hyperplasia represents a condition along the spectrum of breast cancer development.** In some cases, even expert breast pathologists find it difficult to distinguish atypical ductal hyperplasia from DCIS.

Lobular carcinoma in situ (LCIS) is a high-risk condition that does not require treatment, but, like atypical ductal hyperplasia, it is a marker of a greatly increased risk of developing breast cancer. It is usually an incidental finding at the time of biopsy for a palpable or mammographic abnormality. Physicians who treat patients with LCIS need a plan to address this increased risk. Current consensus recommendations for this patient would suggest that she be examined twice a year at a specialized breast center. She should continue with annual mammography. She should consider the use of tamoxifen as a preventative agent. High-risk women were randomized in the National Surgical Adjuvant Breast and Bowel Project (NSABP) P-1 Breast Cancer Prevention Trial to 5 years of placebo or tamoxifen.[13] The tamoxifen group had nearly a 50% reduction in the incidence of new breast cancers. **Tamoxifen is the only currently available, effective, breast cancer prevention agent for high-risk women.** Other agents such as raloxifene and anastrozole are being tested in clinical prevention trials.

---

[12] Gail M, Brinton L, Byar D. Projecting individualized probabilities of developing breast cancer for white females who are being examined annually. J Natl Cancer Inst 1989;81:1879.

[13] Fisher B, Constantin JP, Wickerham DL. Tamoxifen for prevention of breast cancer: report of the National Surgical Adjuvant Breast and Bowel Project P-1 study. J Natl Cancer Inst 1998;90:1371.

Other aspects in this patient's history might lead the clinician to consider the possibility that the patient carries a mutation in the *BRCA1* or *BRCA2* gene. If she were younger and there were several affected relatives with breast or ovarian cancer, the patient might wish to consider genetic testing. Carriers of the *BRCA* gene mutations appear to have a lifetime risk of developing breast cancer of 50% to 80%. Such women may wish to consider prophylactic mastectomy as a treatment option. Recommendations for *BRCA* gene mutation carriers constantly are evolving, since new data are released almost monthly.

Summary

Women who present with a breast complaint usually have a palpable mass, an abnormal mammogram, or both. The management of a palpable mass is summarized in **Algorithm 19.1**. Low-suspicion masses in

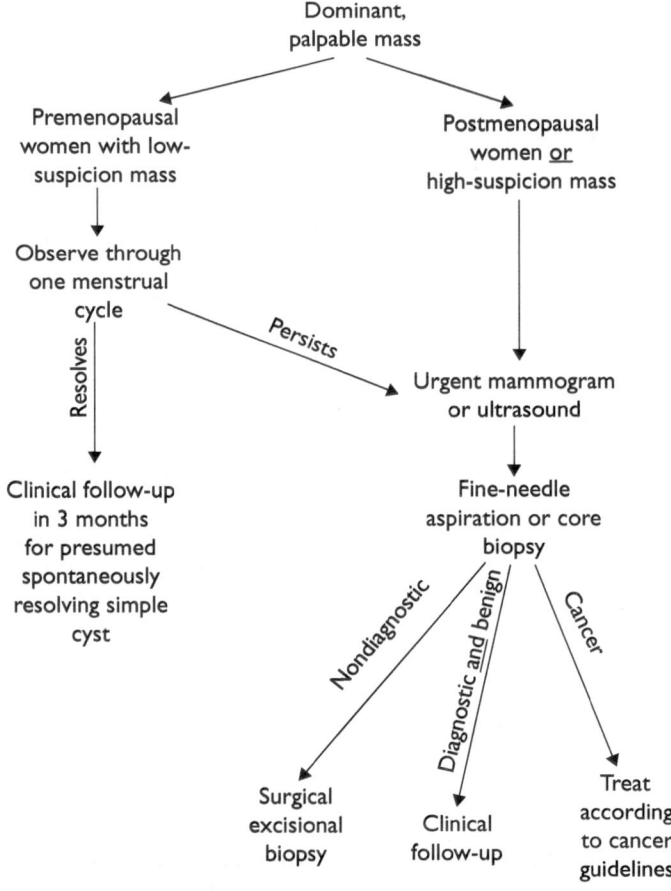

Algorithm 19.1. Algorithm for the management of palpable breast masses. (Reprinted from Pass HA. Benign and malignant diseases of the breast. In: Norton JA, Bollinger RR, Chang AE, et al, eds. Surgery: Basic Science and Clinical Evidence. New York: Springer-Verlag, 2001, with permission.)

premenopausal women may be observed through a menstrual cycle to see if they resolve. Persistent low-suspicion masses require tissue diagnosis. Suspicious masses in a premenopausal woman and virtually all palpable masses in postmenopausal women require tissue diagnosis.

Patients with probably benign mammographic abnormalities require short-interval imaging follow-up. Suspicious mammographic abnormalities require biopsy. Patients with bloody nipple discharge or a red, swollen breast may have cancer, and appropriate evaluation, including biopsy, is required.

Patients with early-stage breast cancer usually can be treated with breast-conserving surgery and radiation therapy. Most patients with invasive breast cancer benefit from systemic adjuvant therapy. Patients with locally advanced breast cancer require multimodality treatment and are best served by a multidisciplinary approach.

Finally, patients with atypical ductal hyperplasia or LCIS are at increased risk of future breast cancer and require increased surveillance and/or preventative interventions.

Selected Readings

Buzdar AU, Singletary SE, Booser DJ, et al. Combined modality treatment of stage III and inflammatory breast cancer: M.D. Anderson Cancer Center experience. Surg Oncol Clin North Am 1995;4:715.

Dupont W, Page D. Risk factors for breast cancer in women with proliferative breast disease. N Engl J Med 1985;312:146.

Ferguson CM, Powell RW. Breast masses in young women. Arch Surg 1989;124:1338.

Fisher B, Anderson S, Redmond CK. Reanalysis and results after 12 years of follow-up in a randomized clinical trial comparing total mastectomy with lumpectomy with or without irradiation in the treatment of breast cancer. N Engl J Med 1995;333:1456.

Fisher B, Brown A, Mamounas E, et al. Effect of preoperative chemotherapy on local-regional disease in women with operable breast cancer: findings from National Surgical Adjuvant Breast and Bowel Project B-18. J Clin Oncol 1997;15:2483.

Fisher B, Constantin JP, Wickerham DL. Tamoxifen for prevention of breast cancer: report of the National Surgical Adjuvant Breast and Bowel Project P-1 study. J Natl Cancer Inst 1998;90:1371.

Fisher B, Dignam J, Wolmark N, et al. Lumpectomy and radiation therapy for the treatment of intraductal breast cancer: findings from the National Surgical Adjuvant Breast and Bowel Project B-17. J Clin Oncol 1998;16:441.

Fisher B, Dignam J, Wolmark N. Tamoxifen in treatment of intraductal breast cancer: National Surgical Adjuvant Breast and Bowel Project B-24 randomised controlled trial. Lancet 1999;353:1993.

Gail M, Brinton L, Byar D. Projecting individualized probabilities of developing breast cancer for white females who are being examined annually. J Natl Cancer Inst 1989;81:1879.

Giuliano AE, Kirgan DM, Guenthler JM, et al. Lymphatic mapping and sentinel lymphadenectomy for breast cancer. Ann Surg 1994;220:391.

Krag D, Weaver D, Ashikaga T, et al. The sentinel node in breast cancer—a multicenter validation trial. N Engl J Med 1998;339:941.

NCCN. Practice Guidelines in Oncology. www.nccn.org, 2003.

Pass HA. Benign and malignant diseases of the breast. In: Norton JA, Bollinger RR, Chang AE, et al, eds. Surgery: Basic Science and Clinical Evidence. New York: Springer-Verlag, 2001.

Silverstein MJ, Lagios MD, Craig PH, et al. A prognostic index for ductal carcinoma in situ of the breast. Cancer 1996;77:2267.

Vetto JT, Pomier RF, Schmidt WA, et al. Diagnosis of palpable breast lesions in younger women by the modified triple test is accurate and cost-effective. Arch Surg 1996;131:967.

Gastrointestinal Bleeding

Siobhan A. Corbett

Objectives

1. To outline the initial management of a patient with an acute GI hemorrhage.
2. To differentiate upper versus lower GI hemorrhage.
3. To discuss the differences in evaluation and management of the patient presenting with hematemesis, melena, hematochezia, and guaiac positive stool.
4. To discuss medical versus surgical management of the common causes of GI hemorrhage.

Case

History

A 65-year-old man presents complaining of the passage of bright red blood and clots per rectum earlier that evening. This episode was preceded by mild lower abdominal cramping. The patient denies any nausea, vomiting, or abdominal pain at this time, but he states that he feels "light-headed." He reports one episode of rectal bleeding 2 months prior that was limited, and he did not seek medical advice at that time. His past medical history is significant for hypertension. The patient denies any past surgical history. He takes one baby aspirin per day and denies any allergies. He is a nonsmoker and uses only occasional alcohol.

Review of Systems

The patient denies change in bowel habits, has no history of diverticulosis, and reports no recent weight loss.

Physical Exam

Temperature 99.0℉; blood pressure 90/45; heart rate 122; respiratory rate 25. The patient appears pale and anxious. Head, ears, eyes, nose, and throat exam is normal; his neck veins are flat.

Lungs: Clear to auscultation with equal breath sounds bilaterally.
Heart: RR, sinus tachycardia, no murmurs.
Abdomen: Active bowel sounds, soft, nontender; no masses or organomegaly.
Rectal: Gross blood on digital exam, prostate is normal.
Extremities: Skin is cool and clammy. His radial pulses are equal, but they are weak and thready.

Initial Management

Assess the Severity of Bleeding

The first step in managing a patient with a gastrointestinal (GI) hemorrhage is to **assess the rate of bleeding and to estimate the blood loss (Table 20.1; Algorithm 20.1).** Patients may present in a variety of ways. For example, they may have anemia from **occult bleeding**, but they otherwise may be asymptomatic. Alternatively, patients may exhibit gradual bleeding with black or tarry stools that commonly is referred to as **melena.** Black stools occur as the result of oxidation of heme by bacterial and digestive enzymes. A major bleeding episode is likely to have occurred if there is profuse vomiting of blood (**hematemesis**) or bright red blood per rectum (**BRBPR or hematochezia**), accompanied by supine hypotension or a postural blood pressure or pulse change. Other findings indicative of **hypovolemia** include a weak, thready pulse, moist, clammy skin, decreased skin temperature of the distal extremities, tachypnea, and mental status changes (confusion, agita-

Table 20.1. Physical findings in hemorrhagic shock.[a]

	Class I	Class II	Class III	Class IV
Blood loss (mL)	<750	750–1500	1500–2000	>2000
Blood loss	UP to 15%	15%–30%	30%–40%	>40%
Pulse rate	<100	>100	>120	>140
Blood pressure	Normal	Normal	Decreased	Decreased
Pulse pressure (mm Hg)	Normal	Decreased	Decreased	Decreased
Respiratory rate	14–20	20–30	30–40	>35
Urine output (mL/h)	>30	20–30	5–15	Negligible
CNS/mental status	Slightly anxious	Mildly anxious	Anxious, confused	Confused, lethargic

[a] Alcohol or drugs (e.g., beta-blockers) may alter physical signs.
Source: Adapted from American College of Surgeons. Shock. In: Advanced Trauma Life Support Manual. Chicago: American College of Surgeons, 1997:87–107. Reprinted from Nathens AB, Maier RV. Shock and resuscitation. In: Norton JA, Bollinger RR, Chang AE, et al, eds. Surgery: Basic Science and Clinical Evidence. New York: Springer-Verlag, 2001, with permission.

Algorithm 20.1. Algorithm for initially managing a patient presenting with GI bleeding.

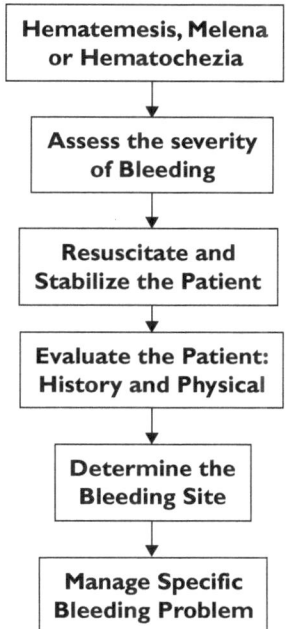

tion, or obtundation). **The overall approach to managing the patient is determined by the rate of bleeding, since this reflects the likelihood that the hemorrhage will stop spontaneously. Patients with a rapid rate of bleeding may require a laparotomy,** so it is important to involve a surgeon early.

Case Presentation: Assessment
The history of BRBPR accompanied by clots indicates that this patient may have a significant GI bleed. The patient's vital signs are indicative of **hypovolemic shock**. This diagnosis is supported by his physical findings. He appears pale and anxious. He has a weak, thready pulse, and cool, clammy skin. Taken together, this would indicate a class III/IV hemorrhage.

Resuscitate and Stabilize the Patient

Patients who have **evidence of massive blood loss should be resuscitated immediately.** The **airway is assessed** to ensure that there is no obstruction, and **oxygen administration is** required for all patients. Obtunded patients, those who cannot protect their airway, and those with massive vomiting that presents an aspiration risk should be endotracheally intubated, and ventilator support should be provided for adequate respiration. Large-bore intravenous access (×2) with 18-gauge or larger catheters should be placed. Central venous access with a Swan-Ganz introducer (8.5Fr) may be helpful for rapid infusion if peripheral access is inadequate, but it is hazardous to place it in a hypovolemic patient with empty, flat neck veins. If a central line is required, a femoral line is a reasonable alternative that can be replaced by upper extremity access once the patient is stabilized.

At the time of the insertion of the intravenous catheters, **blood should be sent for type and crossmatch, and six units of packed red blood cells should be made available. Additional laboratory evaluation should be performed to determine the complete blood count (CBC), chemistries [including electrolytes, blood urea nitrogen (BUN), creatinine, liver function tests], and a coagulation profile.** It is important to note that, in the early stages of hemorrhage, the hematocrit level may not reflect the extent of the blood loss.

Normal saline and Ringer's lactate are the fluids of choice used to resuscitate a patient suffering from class I or class II shock. The crystalloid replacement should be in a quantity sufficient to replace plasma losses plus the interstitial loss and should be on the order of 3 mL of crystalloid for each 1 mL of estimated blood loss. In a young person, up to 3 L of crystalloid may be given at the rate of 1 L every 15 to 30 minutes until the clinical signs of shock have been corrected. Adequate resuscitation can be monitored by a slowing of the heart rate and a return of urine output. However, it is important to be cautious about overloading the intravascular compartment in those patients with cardiac or renal impairment. If the bleeding has ceased, crystalloid volume replacement usually will be adequate therapy for class I or class II hemorrhage, although patients with preexisting medical conditions may require earlier transfusion at this level. **Patients presenting with class III or class IV shock who are estimated to have lost more than 35% of their circulating blood volume are given type-specific blood in addition to crystalloid until crossmatched blood is available.** (In the true emergency, O negative blood may be required.) Foley catheter placement to monitor urine output is essential in this instance.

Patients with persistent hemodynamic instability or evidence of ongoing blood loss should be monitored closely and should be prepared for possible laparotomy.

Remember: anticipate that unstable patients who have required multiple blood transfusions may become cold and develop dilutional coagulopathy that will increase the morbidity and mortality of an operative procedure. Under these circumstances, replacement of clotting factors with fresh frozen plasma is important, and it takes time for the transfusion services to make this component necessary. Therefore, think ahead. Cryoprecipitate may be required, but it should not be given unless factor VIII deficiency is demonstrated. Platelets should be administered if the platelet count is less than 50,000.

Case Discussion: Resuscitation
Immediate action is required to treat class III/IV hemorrhage. Make sure that the patient's airway is secure and provide supplemental oxygen. Start 2 large-intravenous bore (IV) lines and begin resuscitation with a 500-mL to 1-L bolus of crystalloid solution. Send blood for type and crossmatch and additional laboratory values including CBC, chemistries, and coagulation profile. Six units of packed red blood cells

(pRBCs) should be available. Place a Foley catheter to monitor urine output. Reassess vital signs frequently.

Evaluating the Patient

History

A brief, pertinent history from the patient regarding the **degree of hematemesis, melena, or hematochezia** contributes to an assessment of the degree of blood loss and the severity of the bleed. Inquiring about the **duration of the symptoms** also may help determine the rate of blood loss. As a rule, melanotic stools typically originate from the upper GI tract and maroon stools from the distal ileum or right colon, and bright red blood is indicative of bleeding from the left colon. The differential diagnoses for GI bleeding in the adult are listed in **Table 20.2.**

Additional history should include associated symptoms that may indicate the source of the bleeding:

1. A history of **nasopharyngeal lesions, trauma, or surgery** should be obtained to exclude an **oral or nasopharyngeal source** for hematemesis.

2. A history of known **ulcer disease, gastroesophageal reflux, prior epigastric pain relieved by antacids, or excessive use of aspirin, nonsteroidal antiinflammatory drugs (NSAIDs), or steroids** may implicate the **esophagus, stomach, or duodenum** as the source. Alternatively, a known history of **diverticular disease or angiodysplasia** may implicate a lower GI source.

Table 20.2. Differential diagnosis for gastrointestinal (GI) bleeding in the adult upper GI bleed: common causes.

Esophagus	Lower GI bleed: common causes
Esophagitis	Adult
Esophageal tumor	Most common cause
Esophageal varices	Upper GI bleed
Mallory-Weiss tear	Small bowel
Stomach	Vascular malformation
Gastric ulcer	Meckel's diverticulum
Gastritis	Neoplasm
Gastric neoplasm	Inflammatory bowel disease
	Ischemic bowel
Duodenum	Neoplasm
Duodenal ulcer	Large bowel/rectum/anus
Duodenitis	Angiodysplasia
Upper GI bleed: rare causes	Diverticulosis
Angiodysplasia	Hemorrhoids
Aortoenteric fistula	Rectal fissures
Hematobilia	Polyps
Crohn's disease	Neoplasms
Pancreatitis	Ischemic colitis
Marginal ulcer	Ulcerative or infectious colitis

3. A documented history of **cirrhosis** may suggest the possibility of **esophageal varices**.

4. A history of **recent vomiting** could indicate a **Mallory-Weiss tear**.

5. A history of **crampy abdominal pain and diarrhea**, accompanied by urgency, tenesmus, diarrhea, and excessive amounts of mucus, may point to **inflammatory bowel disease** in an adult.

6. A history of the **character of rectal bleeding** should be obtained along with a report of a **change in bowel habits or recent weight loss**. Bright red blood found only on the toilet paper or blood that drips into the toilet bowl most commonly is associated with an **anorectal source** of bleeding, while blood that is streaked on the stool or mixed in with the stool suggests a **proximal source**. Try to get an accurate assessment of the **amount of bleeding** that has occurred.

7. It is important also to uncover **previous episodes of bleeding** and whether there have been any **previous studies**, such as a barium enema or colonoscopy.

The physician taking the past **medical history** also should inquire about **associated major medical problems**, such as cardiac, renal, and pulmonary diseases that will influence resuscitation and determine how well the patient can tolerate anemia. For the past **surgical history**, the physician should inquire about previous **ulcer surgery**. A history of previous **gastric resection** may suggest a **marginal ulcer** as the source of bleeding. Previous **abdominal aortic aneurysm repair or aortobifemoral bypass** could indicate an **aortoenteric fistula**.

The patient's current **medication list** should be obtained, with attention to the possible use of medications that could interfere with **coagulation** (e.g., aspirin, NSAIDs, and dypiridamole) or alter the assessment of the **hemodynamic status** (e.g., beta-blockers and antihypertensive agents).

The **social history** should include relevant risk factors, including alcohol, intravenous drug, or tobacco abuse.

Physical Examination

The **physical exam** seldom provides accurate determination of the source of the bleeding. However, **the severity of the blood loss and identification of comorbid illnesses** can be assessed, and the physical exam should be performed carefully, although the results often are normal.

The physical exam should consist of the following:

1. Complete **vital signs** should be obtained to assess the severity of bleeding.
2. **Postural changes** in the **pulse and/or blood pressure** should be assessed.
3. **Sclera** should be examined for evidence of **icterus**.
4. The **mouth and the oropharynx** should be examined to exclude **nasopharyngeal causes** of hematemesis.

5. Pertinent physical findings should be sought that are indicative of comorbid disease, including signs of **chronic hepatic disease, including ascites or spider angiomata**.
6. An abdominal examination should be done, as it will reveal the presence of a **mass caused by a colonic neoplasm or the presence of an aortic aneurysm**.
7. A **rectal exam** should be performed for evidence of **frank blood or possibly a tumor mass**.
8. **Hemocult exam of any melenic-appearing stool** should be done, since the ingestion of several substances, such as iron or spinach, can impart a dark color to the stool.

Case Evaluation

The patient responds well to a 2-L infusion of lactated Ringer's. His vital signs stabilize. His blood pressure improves to 120/70, and his heart rate decreases to 90. Relevant information from this patient's history and physical include the following: There is **no history of hematemesis**, but the patient reports a **similar episode** of rectal bleeding 2 months prior for which he did not seek medical advice. This episode of bright red blood per rectum had **no antecedent symptoms**. He has no history of **diverticulosis**. He reports **no change in bowel habits** or recent weight loss. His review of systems was negative for cardiac, pulmonary, or renal symptomatology, and he denies any surgical history. He takes **no medications** and has no allergies. It seems likely that this patient is experiencing a lower **GI bleed**. However, his history and physical exam **do not exclude** an upper GI source of hemorrhage.

Determine the Bleeding Site

If hematemesis, melena, or hematochezia have not been documented, it is important to establish the site of bleeding. This can be accomplished by **placing a nasogastric tube (NGT)** (at least 18 Fr). **Remember: an upper GI source can be a common cause of a lower GI bleed. Even if the patient has massive rectal bleeding, 10% of the time the source is proximal to the ligament of Treitz.** Therefore, an NGT should be placed. If bile is aspirated from the NGT without blood, it is unlikely that a major upper GI bleed has occurred. However, about 25% of the patients with duodenal bleeding do not reflux blood into the stomach even with gagging. This group usually can be identified by lavaging the stomach with saline if blood or bile is not obtained on initial NGT placement. An attempt should be made to irrigate old blood or new bleeding from the stomach, and the NGT should be lavaged until clear. There is no advantage between iced-saline and room temperature lavage. **Over 90% of patients with bloody gastric aspirate will be found to have a lesion proximal to the ligament of Treitz.**

Case Discussion

Although an upper GI source is unlikely in this case, the NGT would help to detect one. An NGT is inserted. It returns bilious contents that are guaiac negative. The absence of blood in the NGT aspirate in the presence of bile makes upper GI bleeding very unlikely.

Management of Specific Bleeding Problems

Upper GI Bleeding

Making the Diagnosis

If the patient is stabilized in the emergency room and hematemesis or bloody nasogastric aspirate has been documented, **the first step in management is an upper endoscopy or esophagogastroduodenoscopy (EGD)** (see **Algorithm 20.2**). **An EGD is essential for managing patients with upper GI hemorrhage.** Only 10% to 20% of patients presenting with upper GI bleeding have peptic ulcers as the cause for the bleed. However, 50% of all cases of severe upper GI bleeds are caused by bleeding peptic ulcer disease. Because of the diagnostic and therapeutic potential for endoscopy, it should be included early in the management of these patients, since its utility and accuracy in identifying the bleeding source have been well documented in the literature. A patient with *a history of hematemesis in whom the rate of bleeding is high should undergo an emergent EGD* that should be performed **within 1 hour**. The stable patient with melanotic stools dictates an urgent EGD.

The EGD is an excellent diagnostic tool, and it also is **valuable therapeutically**. In skilled hands, endoscopic maneuvers, such as injection sclerotherapy, banding of varices, electrocoagulation, the use of a heater probe, the injection of ethanol or epinephrine, and laser coagulation, effectively can manage the bleeding source. Which patients require therapeutic EGD? Patients presenting with clinical scenarios listed in **Table 20.3** should be considered for therapeutic EGD. Additionally, patients at high risk for complications secondary to bleeding should be considered as candidates for therapeutic endoscopy; these would include patients over 60 years of age or those who rebleed following an initial bleeding episode.

The National Institutes of Health convened a consensus conference examining the role of EGD for upper GI hemorrhage. The panel evaluated a variety of devices used for endoscopic intervention (**Table 20.4**). Of these, **the heater probe and bipolar electrocoagulation device were determined to be the most useful**. The panel concluded that endoscopic intervention was safe and effective when performed by appropriately trained practitioners. Surgical backup was considered essential. At the time that the panel convened, long-term follow-up was not available, leaving many questions regarding the long-term efficacy for endoscopic control of bleeding.

If EGD reveals no lesions in the stomach or duodenum, there are alternative diagnostic tests that may identify the bleeding site. **Enteroclysis**, which is the direct introduction of barium sulfate into the small

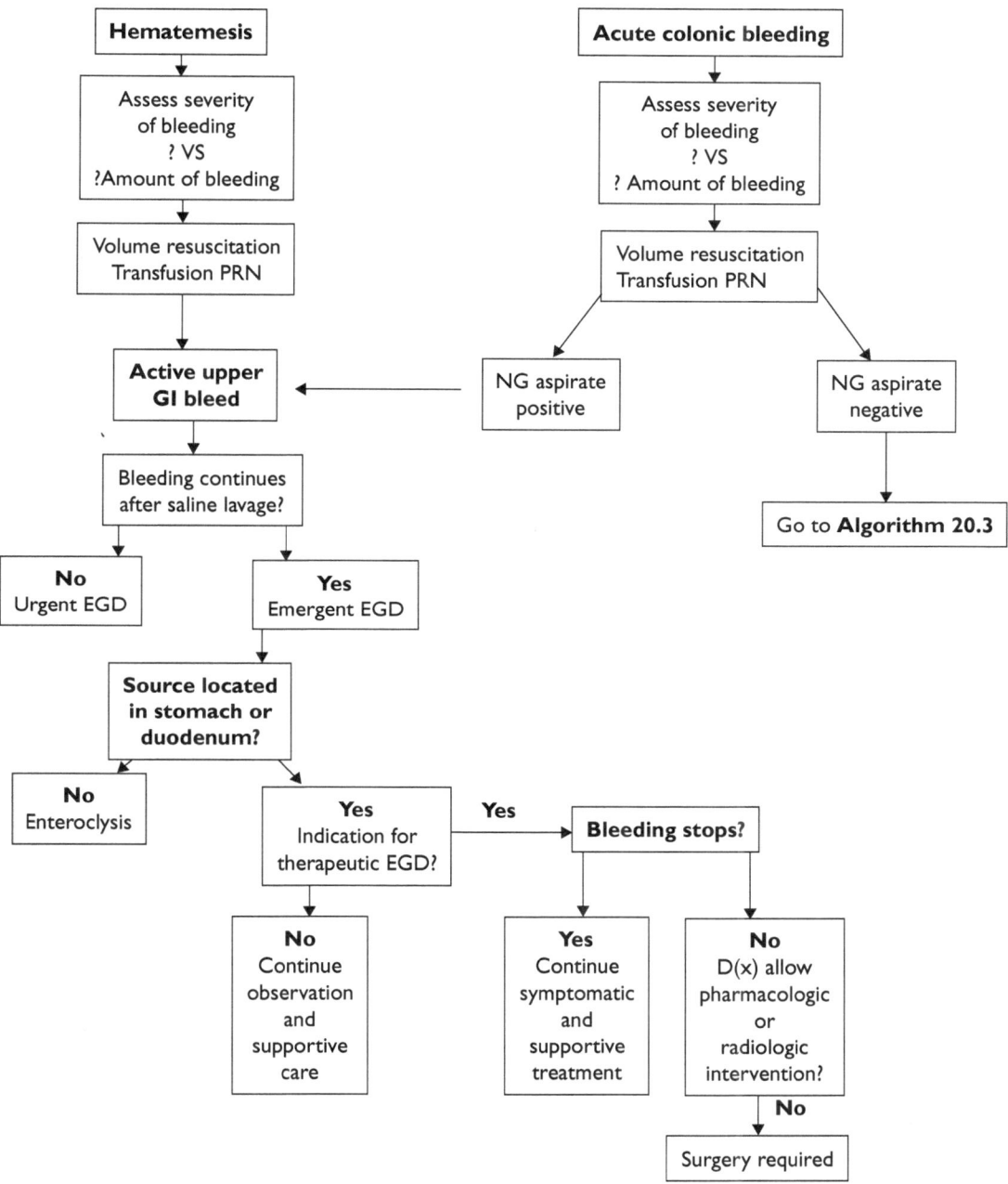

Algorithm 20.2. Algorithm for management and treatment of upper GI bleeding. EGD, esophagogastroduodenoscopy; NG, nasogastric; VS, vital signs.

Table 20.3. Predictors of peptic ulcer rebleeding.

Magnitude of bleeding
  Hemodynamic instability
  Bloody emesis or nasogastric lavage that fails to clear
  Blood-red stools

Host factors
  Anticoagulated patient
  Patient hospitalized for a related or unrelated condition

Endoscopic features
  Visible vessel
  Arterial spurting or oozing
  Raised pigmented discoloration on ulcer base
  Adherent clot on ulcer base

Source: Reprinted from Consensus conference: therapeutic endoscopy and bleeding ulcers. JAMA 1989;262:1369–1372.

bowel, followed by an **x-ray examination** of the duodenum and jejunum, should be done next. However, the absence of a lesion on this test does not rule out a bleeding source in this area. **Tagged red cell scans** may confirm the presence of active bleeding, but these are not helpful in determining the exact anatomic location of the bleeding site. This important information is extremely helpful if the bleeding episode necessitates surgical intervention. If the tagged red cell scan is positive, **arteriography** then may be considered. For arteriography to be successful in identifying the location of the hemorrhage, the bleeding must be brisk (>1 mL/min). If a lesion such as an arteriovenous malformation is identified, however, arteriography does offer the potential of therapeutic intervention through **embolization**.

What are the options for a patient who has persistent or recurrent bleeding that is believed to originate in the small bowel? In this instance, **intraoperative endoscopic exploration** may be warranted. A pediatric colonoscope may be introduced either orally or through a

Table 20.4. Comparison of endoscopic devices for the control of GI bleeding.

Device	Requires en face application?	Advantages/disadvantages	Use?
Bipolar electrocoagulation	No	Portable; depth easily controlled	Yes
Heater probe	No	Portable; depth easily controlled	Yes
Nd:YAG laser	Yes	Not portable	Maybe
Injection therapy	No	Inexpensive; simple technique	Maybe
Topical therapy	Yes	Not effective	No
Argon laser	Yes	Not effective long term; better techniques are now available	No
Monopolar electrocoagulation	Yes	Depth of tissue damage difficult to control; multiple cleanings of probe required	No

Nd:YAG, neodymium:yttrium-aluminum-garnet.
Source: Reprinted from Livingston EH. Stomach and duodenum. In: Norton JA, Bollinger RR, Chang AE, et al, eds. Surgery: Basic Science and Clinical Evidence. New York: Springer-Verlag, 2001, with permission.

distal jejunal enterotomy, and the small bowel mucosae then may be examined.

Peptic ulcers, acute gastritis, esophageal varices, and Mallory-Weiss tears account for >90% of all upper GI bleeds. The management options for these problems are reviewed briefly below.

Peptic Ulcer Disease: Bleeding from *peptic ulcer disease* frequently occurs and generally is a self-limited process. **Advances in endoscopic therapy have made surgery for this problem uncommon.** Patients usually present with melena, or, if the bleeding is severe enough, hematemesis or hematochezia are present. Bleeding is unpredictable, mandating careful observation of patients suspected of having GI hemorrhage. The treatment team must be prepared to manage severe life-threatening hemorrhage that may occur with little notice. The **routine medical treatment for documented gastroduodenal ulcer disease includes the withdrawal of any exacerbating factors (aspirin or NSAIDs), acid reduction/suppression, and eradication of** *Heliobacter pylori*, if present.

Therapeutic intervention with endoscopic treatment may be indicated in patients with active arterial bleeding at the time of endoscopy or with a visible nonhemorrhaging vessel. The success of endoscopic therapy in controlling peptic ulcer bleeding greatly has reduced the need for surgical intervention. However, surgery must be considered when endoscopic treatment has failed or is impractical. In general, **when patients have required more than six units of blood to be transfused in a 24-hour period, they should be considered for surgery**. An additional indication for surgery exists if a patient stops bleeding clinically and then massively rebleeds. **When surgery is performed, the procedure of choice is oversewing of the bleeding ulcer plus truncal vagotomy and pyloroplasty, truncal vagotomy and antrectomy, or highly selective vagotomy.**

Stress Ulcers: **Stress ulcers** are small, numerous lesions occurring in the superficial mucosa of the gastric fundus. **NSAID ulcers** may appear similar to stress ulcers, but they are distributed primarily in the gastric body and antrum. Their major clinical consequence is the tendency to bleed (but not to perforate). The pathogenesis of these lesions remains unclear. Like most gastric ulcers, the major defect appears to be in the mucosal defense system. However, acid may play a role, the extent of which remains unknown. Because **these lesions are a manifestation of other underlying disease processes**, the mortality associated with a total gastrectomy for stress gastritis is 50% to 80%. If at all possible, **explorations should be avoided in these patients.**

Gastric Ulcers: Bleeding **gastric ulcers that are discrete should be resected**, which easily can be accomplished for greater curvature lesions by performing a wedge resection. Lesser curvature or very large lesions may require a total gastrectomy. Frozen section should be obtained to **identify gastric carcinoma**. Because gastric ulcers cannot be distinguished from gastric carcinoma by gross examination, histologic evaluation is mandated. If carcinoma is found, a formal gastrectomy should be performed: **total gastrectomy for proximal lesions and subtotal for antral lesions**.

Mallory-Weiss Tear: ***Mallory-Weiss tears*** of the esophagus and proximal stomach can occur following emesis. Classically associated with alcoholics, the syndrome is manifested by hematemesis that follows episodes of intense vomiting. More recently, the syndrome has been observed following endoscopy, childbirth, coughing, and CPR. The diagnosis is suggested by a history of vomiting before the onset of hematemesis. Endoscopy reveals linear tears below the gastro-esophageal junction, occasionally extending proximally into the esophagus. Initial management includes **resuscitation and correction of any coagulopathy. Bleeding usually is self-limited. Endoscopic sclerotherapy of a bleeding vessel is effective. Rarely is surgical intervention required.**

Acute Variceal Bleeding: Initial mangement of the patient with ***acute variceal bleeding*** includes **resuscitation** as outlined above. However, **intravascular volume replacement should be performed largely with blood products** because the crystalloid solutions in patients with cirrhosis results in the rapid development of ascites and edema. Patients with active bleeding should be managed in an intensive care unit setting with appropriate hemodynamic monitoring and airway protection. Blood in the GI tract is not well tolerated by cirrhotics, with increased risk of bacterial translocation and sepsis as well as inducing encephalopathy. Lactulose should be given orally or via an NGT or enemas in the comatose patient.

It should be remembered that up to 60% of GI bleeding in alcoholic cirrhotics is of nonvariceal origin. Therefore, **EGD plays a significant role in both the diagnosis and treatment of acute variceal bleeding**. The goal of EGD is to identify active bleeding, detect signs of recent bleeding, and exclude other sources of GI bleeding. Identification of varices as the bleeding site should be accompanied by **initial sclerotherapy or banding**. Acute bleeding can be stopped in 90% of the patients with an endoscopic approach. The use of **octreotide** has supplanted vasopressin as pharmacologic intervention to prevent bleeding. Somatostatin and its synthetic analogue octreotide are potent vasoconstrictors at supraphysiologic doses. Octreotide is given initially as a 50-μg bolus followed by an infusion of 50-μg per hour; this is continued through endoscopic intervention and usually for the subsequent 24 hours.

Patients who have active bleeding that cannot be controlled by pharmacologic and endoscopic management require the **placement of a Sengstaken-Blakemore tube**. The goal is to use the tube to tamponade the bleeding as a temporizing maneuver only, while definitive management is being arranged. Key points of tube insertion include airway protection and correct positioning of the tube under radiologic guidance before the inflation of the balloon.

Definitive management for patients who fail endoscopic management and require balloon placement include **transjugular portasystemic shunts (TIPS) and emergency portocaval shunting**. Since emergency portocaval shunts are associated with a mortality of 50%, there currently is greater enthusiasm for the use of TIPS, an interventional radiologic procedure that creates a communication through the hepatic parenchyma between the hepatic and portal veins. Because the 30-day mortality is significantly better in patients with uncontrolled variceal hemorrhage who receive TIPS, surgical decompression of the portal system in the emergency setting is reserved for those patients in whom TIPS cannot be performed.

Meckel's Diverticulum: **Meckel's diverticulum** represents a true diverticulum composed of a remnant of the duct between the intestinal tract and the yolk sac. Based on autopsy series, Meckel's diverticulum is present in 0.3% to 2.5% of the population. The size and shape can vary, but it usually is between 3 and 5 cm long and is found 10 to 150 cm from the ileocecal valve. Meckel's diverticula contain a mesentery with an independent blood supply from the ileal vessels. Although usually lined by mucosa similar to that seen in the adjacent ileum, approximately 16% to 34% of them can contain heterotopic mucosa, including that of a gastric or duodenal nature.

Meckel's diverticula that contain heterotopic gastric mucosa can produce acid, resulting in ulceration in the adjacent ileal mucosa and subsequent hemorrhage. In fact, hemorrhage is the most common complication associated with Meckel's diverticulum (31%). The passage of blood per rectum in an otherwise healthy child should raise the suspicion of a Meckel's diverticulum. The diagnosis can be made **utilizing a technetium 99 m (Tc-99 m) pertechnetate Meckel's scan** that detects the gastric mucosa within the Meckel's diverticulum and that has been reported to be 90% accurate. Meckel's diverticulum also can be detected **angiographically** in most cases, based primarily on the demonstration of a persistant vitellointestinal artery. When a Meckel's diverticulum causes symptoms or complications, **resection is** indicated.

Lower GI Bleeding

Many pathologic lesions of the colon and rectum can cause lower GI hemorrhage that can be classified as either major (defined as greater than 100 mL) or minor (less than 20 mL). The most common causes of **major lower GI hemorrhage are diverticular disease and arteriovenous malformations (AVM).** Other causes can include **inflammatory bowel disease, neoplasms, ischemic colitis, and a variety of other lesions. Minor bleeding may be related to anal conditions, such as hemorrhoids and anal fissures, or to colonic or rectal lesions, such as neoplasms or mucosal inflammation.** We focus on the management of patients who present with obvious rather than occult blood loss.

Any patient with **significant lower GI bleeding should be admitted to the hospital.** Appropriate **resuscitation** should be initiated as discussed above and as indicated in **Algorithms 20.2 and 20.3.** The patient should be assessed carefully to **determine the rate of bleeding.** If the patient is stable, every attempt should be made **to identify the location** of the hemorrhage site, including the placement of an NGT

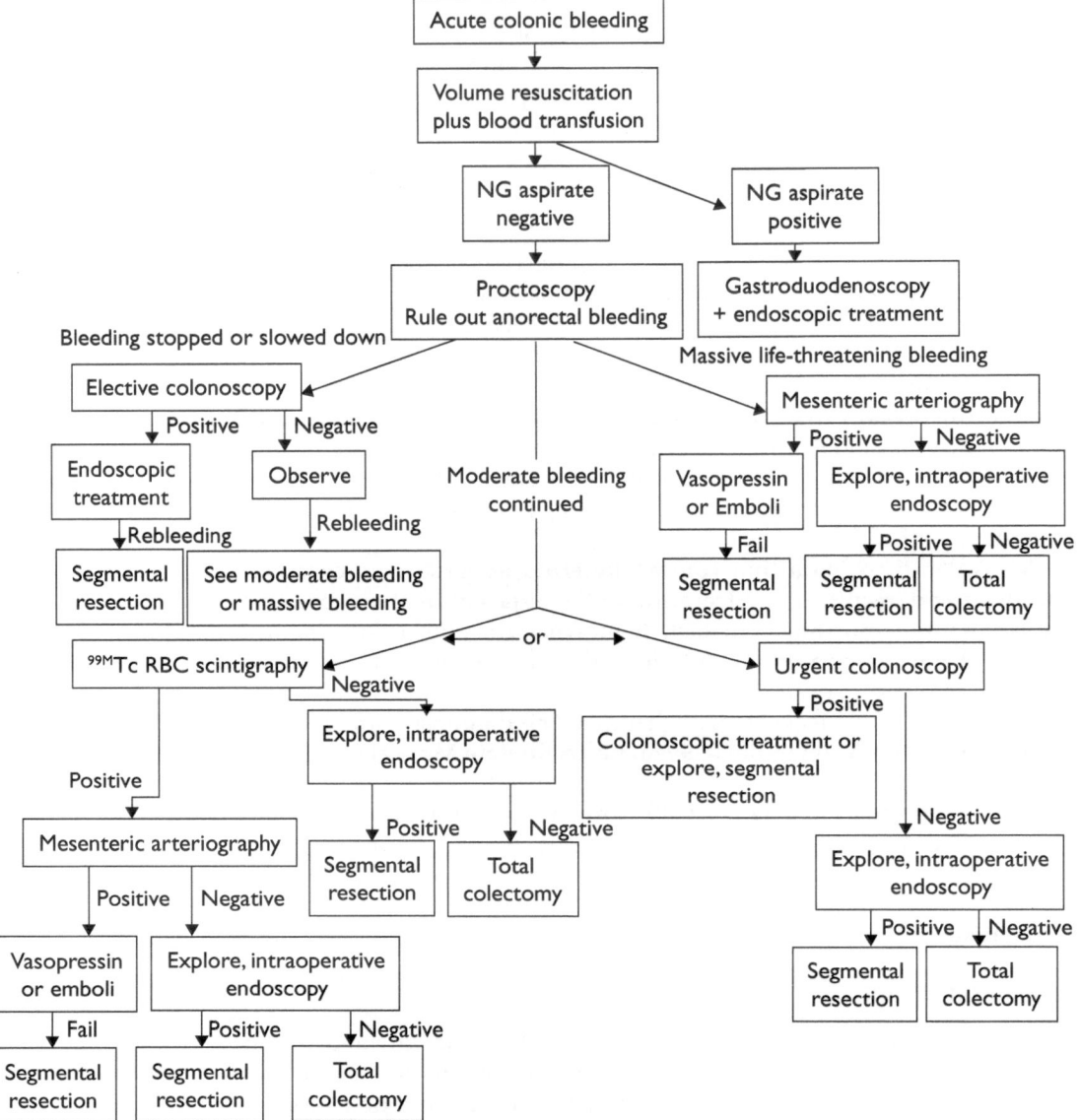

Algorithm 20.3. Algorithm for management and treatment of colonic hemorrhage. (Reprinted from Gordon PH, Nivatvongs S, eds. Principles and Practice of Surgery for the Colon, Rectum, and Anus, 2nd ed. St. Louis: Quality Medical Publishing Inc., 1999, with permission.)

because, as mentioned previously, a significant percentage of lower GI bleeding originates from an upper GI source. Finally, it should be recognized that about 85% of bleeding from lower GI sources stops spontaneously.

Making the Diagnosis

As indicated in **Algorithm 20.3**, the first step in management of patients who present with rectal bleeding, stable or unstable, is a **rigid sigmoi-**

doscopy to exclude rectal lesions as a cause. Information provided by the examination, although it may be limited, can give an indication as to the rate of bleeding and to the appearance of the mucosa. The presence of bleeding internal hemorrhoids can be detected by sigmoidoscopy. However, if an anal source of bleeding is suspected based on the history, then an anoscopy should be performed. These exams still can prove to be unreliable if a large amount of blood remains unevacuated in the rectum. However, it is important to know that this area appears normal in the event that an emergency subtotal or total colectomy may be required.

If the patient is stable but has evidence of ongoing bleeding and the sigmoidoscopy is unrevealing, the following diagnostic studies can be considered: emergency colonoscopy, angiography, and radionuclide scanning, with radionuclide scanning being the preferred first test.

Radionuclide Scanning: If bleeding is thought to be ongoing, radionuclide scanning may prove to be very useful. Technetium 99 m is used because it has a longer half-life and generally less background in the liver and spleen when compared to sulfur colloid. A small aliquot of the patient's blood is withdrawn, the red blood cells are labeled with Tc-99 m, and the blood is returned to the patient. Bleeding at a rate as low as 0.1 mL/min can be detected. If bleeding is brisk, a positive result can occur as quickly as 5 minutes. Success in localization is operator dependent and varies widely between institutions, but sensitivities as high as 97% and specificities of 85% have been reported from multiple centers. Others have had less success, but most centers require this prior to angiography because of the higher sensitivity of the nuclear medicine test compared to angiography: 0.1 mL/min versus 0.5 to 1.0 mL/min.

Angiography: Angiographic localization is attempted in those patients with a positive nuclear medicine scan or in whom bleeding is vigorous or has not stopped spontaneously. However, it is helpful only if the rate of bleeding during the procedure is 2 mL/min or greater. Selective catheterization of all three mesenteric vessels is recommended. This technique allows for confirmation of location and therapeutic intervention with either pitressin infusion (0.1 to 0.4 units per minute) via the catheter positioned in a distal branch or microembolization of a terminal arcade (metal coils or gelatin sponges). Both techniques have a greater than 90% success rate, but pitressin infusion has been associated with a 50% in-hospital rebleed rate. Pitressin infusion has significant cardiac toxicity and requires immobilization in an intensive care unit with a catheter in place, while patients who have had an embolization must be monitored for bowel ischemia, due to a postembolic colon infarction rate that approached 13%.

Urgent Colonoscopy: Emergent colonoscopy after rapid bowel cleansing has been performed successfully as both a diagnostic and a therapeutic technique in select institutions with dedicated teams, but this has not gained widespread acceptance despite excellent results. If the bleeding stops and the pateint is hemodynamically stable, urgent workup is not warranted, but colonoscopy should be performed within 24 hours or as soon as feasible. The patients often will not need to have a bowel prep (this refers to the practice of administering oral agents to "clean out" the colon) because blood in the intestine acts as a cathartic agent. In this instance, administration of enemas achieves adequate preparation of the colon. If the colonoscopy at this time does not identify a bleeding source, such as an AVM or neoplasm, a complete bowel prep should be performed, and the colonoscopy should be repeated electively.

Investigation of Minor Bleeding

Passage of **small amounts of bright red blood per rectum**, either mixed with or on the surface of the stool, can occur. When the bleeding is obvious and bright red, it can be assumed that the blood loss is within or distal to the left colon. If the bleeding is of small volume (i.e., <20 mL) and the patient is stable, further investigation should be performed on an outpatient basis. If there is obviously an anorectal cause in a young healthy patient, no further workup is necessary.

In patients older than 40 years, in patients with a family history of colon cancer, and in patients in whom there is no obvious bleeding source by anoscopy or sigmoidoscopy, an elective colonoscopy following a complete bowel prep is warranted. This is the best test because it is the most sensitive and specific for the detection of mucosal abnormalities or neoplasms. Alternately, **a barium enema and sigmoidoscopy** could be performed if a colonoscopy cannot be performed.

Massive Lower GI Bleeding

In a minority of patients presenting with lower GI bleeding, **the hemorrhage is massive and continuous,** leading to hemodynamic instability. Bleeding is considered massive if transfusions of three to five units of blood are required to maintain hemodynamic stability within the first 24 hours. The most likely source of bleeding in this instance is from **diverticular disease (30–50%), with the remainder being from angiodysplasia (20–30%).** An attempt always should be made to identify the bleeding source prior to surgical intervention. **Rigid sigmoidoscopy should always be performed to exclude an anorectal lesion. If the bleeding is brisk, angiography is more likely to be positive, allowing embolic or vasoconstrictive therapy for definitive management. If localization of the bleeding cannot be performed in an expedient fashion, the patient should be taken to the operating room (OR) without further delay.** The mortality in the group of patients who require emergency surgery without diagnostic information is extremely high, often approaching 30% to 50% because of the requirement for total colectomy. **Hemorrhoids** causing massive bleeding can be managed by banding or suture ligation.

Surgical Management: The indications for surgery and the choice of operation remain controversial and require good clinical judgment. **Efforts to localize the bleeding source are maximized to allow therapeutic intervention as mentioned and to direct a segmental resection if a colectomy is necessary. If the lesion is localized and**

hemorrhage controlled, then elective segmental resection may be carried out based on an assessment of the patient's risks and the risks of rebleeding. An aggressive surgical approach often is advocated by those that argue that these patients often are elderly and tolerate rapid blood loss poorly because of medical comorbidities. However, the natural history of a bleeding source that has been controlled by pitressin or embolization is undefined. **Urgent segmental colectomy is indicated after localization if the bleeding cannot be controlled with the nonoperative measures, if the patient rebleeds during the same hospitalization, if blood products are limited or unavailable while awaiting spontaneous cessation, or if the patient refuses a transfusion (e.g., Jehovah's Witness). "Blind" segmental colectomy is not recommended because of the high recurrence rates and the difficulty in managing patients with postoperative hemorrhage. Blind total colectomy may be necessary when there is massive hemorrhage and when the lesion cannot be localized preoperatively or with intraoperative techniques.** Recurrent bleeding after total colectomy approaches zero, but the morbidity of frequent loose bowel movements, in the elderly in particular, is not insignificant.

Diverticular Bleeding: Bleeding can be expected to occur in 15% to 20% of patients with **diverticulosis**. Of these, 5% experience massive hemorrhage. The source of the bleeding generally is right sided (60%), even though diverticula generally are present on the left, and the source typically is a single diverticulum. The majority of patients (70–82%) stop bleeding, but 12% to 30% continue to bleed and require intervention. The cause of the hemorrhage appears to be erosion into the vasa recta that courses along the diverticula.

Patients with diverticular hemorrhage frequently present with self-limited, minor episodes of bleeding. Patients often describe intermittent passage of bright red or maroon blood per rectum. Often, the patient reports a history of previous GI hemorrhage. Physical examination usually is unremarkable, and evidence of abdominal tenderness is absent. **Treatment for persistent or recurrent bleeding from a known diverticular source traditionally is to remove the affected segment of colon.** Although bleeding generally is considered to be from a single vessel, **endoscopic electrocoagulation has been considered to carry a high risk of perforation of the adjacent diverticulum.**

Angiodysplasia: **Arteriovenous malformations (AVMs)** can occur anywhere in the GI tract and are thought to be responsible for about 6% of all cases of lower GI bleeding. The colon is most commonly involved, usually on the right side. Most of these lesions remain asymptomatic and typically occur in the elderly population, with the average age being 70. When symptomatic, the clinical presentation is one of gross GI bleeding. An AVM is difficult to diagnose via colonoscopy. Therefore, **the best diagnostic tool remains visceral angiography**, which reveals a tortuous knot of blood vessels, sometimes with early filling of a large vein. An AVM is less likely to be controlled by vasopressin infusion because it represents capillary and venous bleeding as opposed to arterial bleeding seen in diverticulosis. The incidence of rebleeding from these lesions is high, with patients often experiencing three to five bleeding episodes before a diagnosis is made. Angiodysplasias can be **managed successfully by colonoscopy and treated by endoscopic electrocoagulation**.

Neoplasms: In recent series, the incidence of massive colonic bleeding from ulcerated carcinomas or polyps ranged from 6% to 32%. **Polyps may be amenable to endoscopic removal, but most carcinomas require resection.**

Inflammatory Bowel Disease: Although **ulcerative colitis and Crohn's disease** both are characterized by bleeding and diarrhea, massive bleeding is quite uncommmon, representing only about 3% to 5% of those presenting with massive hematochezia. When inflammatory bowel disease is the source of a massive lower GI bleed, **it almost always requires surgery**.

Ischemic Colitis: **Ischemic colitis** is the most common form of intestinal ischemia. It is thought to affect "watershed" areas of the colon where two blood supplies may incompletely overlap: the splenic flexure supplied by the left branch of the middle colic artery and the ascending left colon. It may result from a vascular operation or a low flow state. The severity of injury appears to be related to multiple factors including duration of ischemia, vessel caliber, acuity of ischemia onset, collateral circulation, and virulence of intestinal bacteria.

Patients often are elderly and debilitated and in the intensive care unit (ICU) with multiple medical problems. The onset may be insidious, not recognized, or attributed to the medical comorbidities. Onset of acute colonic ischemis is heralded by the sudden onset of crampy abdominal pain. This may be associated with bloody diarrhea, fever, abdominal distention, anorexia, nausea, or vomiting. Physical exam may reveal abdominal distention and tenderness over the involved segment. If the segment is gangrenous, the patient may present in septic shock. **With transient intestinal ischemia, superficial sloughing of the mucosa, submucosal hemorrhage, and edema generally resolve within 1 to 2 weeks without permanent sequelae.** Ischemic strictures can develop in some instances. **If the injury is full thickness, emergency surgery may be required.** Again, massive bleeding is rare with this diagnosis.

Case Investigation of Massive Lower GI Bleeding

The bilious NGT aspirate strongly suggests that the patient is bleeding distal to the ligament of Treitz. His blood pressure remains stable, but his heart rate has risen to 115. A rigid sigmoidoscopy is performed in the emergency room (ER), which reveals no masses and normal rectal mucosa.

The patient passes a third large bloody bowel movement. His systolic blood pressure is now 100. These data suggest that the patient is actively bleeding. It is very important to localize the source of bleeding. To achieve this goal, a bleeding scan is ordered. The bleeding scan is performed and within 15 minutes suggests an area of active hemorrhage in the right colon. Arteriography confirms the location of the bleeding site in the ascending colon, originating from a single vessel.

Gelfoam embolization is performed. Signs and symptoms of active hemorrhage cease.

This patient's history is most consistent with diverticular hemorrhage. The patient spends the next 24 hours in the ICU. He remains stable and is transferred to the floor. The following day, after receiving a gentle bowel prep, a colonoscopy is performed. The procedure demonstrates numerous diverticuli in the descending and sigmoid colon. There are also a few diverticuli located in the right colon. A distinct source for the hemorrhage is not seen. He remains stable and is discharged.

Summary

The first step in managing a patient with a GI hemorrhage is to assess the rate of bleeding and to estimate the blood loss. Patients who have evidence of massive blood loss should be resuscitated immediately. An airway should be established if necessary and supplemental oxygen provided. Two large-bore IVs should be placed and resuscitation should be begun with crystalloid solution. If hematemesis, melena, or hematochezia have not been documented, it is important to establish the site of bleeding by placing an NGT. Remember: 10% to 15% of massive lower GI bleeds are caused by an upper GI source. A careful history and a physical exam may provide clues to the etiology of the hemorrhage.

If the patient is stabilized in the emergency room and hematemesis or bloody nasogastric aspirate has been documented, upper endoscopy is the standard of care for diagnosis and for segregating patients into low- and high-risk groups. Endoscopic treatment of those with major stigmata of ulcer hemorrhage is recommended. Currently, peptic ulcers, acute gastritis, esophageal varices, and Mallory-Weiss tears account for >90% of all upper GI bleeds. Surgical consultation should be obtained and the likelihood for surgical intervention will depend on the etiology of the bleed.

Lower GI hemorrhage stops spontaneously with supportive management alone in up to 90% of cases. The first step in management of patients who present with rectal bleeding, stable or unstable, is a rigid sigmoidoscopy to exclude rectal lesions as a cause. If the patient is stable but has evidence of ongoing bleeding and the sigmoidoscopy is unrevealing, angiography and radionuclide scanning can be considered, with radionuclide scanning being the preferred first test. Recent data suggest an increasing role for colonoscopy in this setting. The most common source of lower GI hemorrhage is diverticulosis. The majority of patients with bleeding diverticula (70–82%) stop bleeding, but 12% to 30% continue to bleed and require intervention.

Selected Readings

Hemming A, Gallinger S, Liver. In: Norton JA, Bollinger RR, Chang AE, et al, eds. Surgery: Basic Science and Clinical Evidence. New York: Springer-Verlag, 2001.

Hodin RA, Matthews JB, Small intestine. In: Norton JA, Bollinger RR, Chang AE, et al, eds. Surgery: Basic Science and Clinical Evidence. New York: Springer-Verlag, 2001.

Jensen DM. Management of severe ulcer rebleeding. N Engl J Med 1999; 340:799–801.

Jensen DM. Where next with endoscopic ulcer hemostasis? Am J Gastroenterol 2002;September:2161–2164.

Jensen DM, Machiacado GA, Jutabha R, Kovacs TO. Urgent colonoscopy for the diagnosis and treatment of severe diverticular hemorrhage. N Engl J Med 2000;342(2):78–82.

Livingston EH. Stomach and duodenum. In: Norton JA, Bollinger RR, Chang AE, et al, eds. Surgery: Basic Science and Clinical Evidence. New York: Springer-Verlag, 2001.

Nathens AB, Maier RV. Shock and resuscitation. In: Norton JA, Bollinger RR, Chang AE, et al, eds. Surgery: Basic Science and Clinical Evidence. New York: Springer-Verlag, 2001.

Savides TJ, Jensen DM. Therapeutic endoscopy for high risk non-variceal gastrointestinal bleeding. Gastrointest Clin North Am 2000;29:465–488.

Vernava AM, Moore BA, Longo WE, Johnson FE. Lower gastrointestinal bleeding. Dis Colon Rectum 1997;40(7):847–858.

Welton ML, Varma MG, Amerhauser A. Colon, rectum, and anus. In: Norton JA, Bollinger RR, Chang AE, et al, eds. Surgery: Basic Science and Clinical Evidence. New York: Springer-Verlag, 2001.

Abdominal Pain

Albert Frankel and Susannah S. Wise

Objectives

1. To understand the etiology of abdominal pain.
2. To understand the difference between visceral and somatic causes of pain.
3. To understand what is important in a directed history of abdominal pain.
4. To understand the relevance of the past medical and past surgical history.
5. To recognize important physical exam findings.
6. To understand the relevance of laboratory and imaging studies.
7. To recognize catastrophic abdominal emergencies.
8. To recognize urgent surgical conditions.
9. To recognize surgical conditions that require further evaluation and eventual operation.
10. To recognize nonsurgical causes of abdominal pain.

Cases

Case 1

A 78-year-old man with a history of myocardial infarction and coronary artery bypass surgery is brought to the hospital by ambulance because of severe abdominal pain that suddenly began 6 hours ago. The patient is confused and disoriented, but he indicates that the pain is excruciating.

The patient's wife reports that he had an urgent desire to defecate when the pain began, but no further stool or flatus has been noted. She provides a list of current medications that includes digoxin, pindolol (a beta-blocker), a baby aspirin, and a nitrate patch.

On examination, he appears gravely ill with cool ashen skin, an irregular pulse of 120, blood pressure of 85/50, and respirations at 28. Rectal temperature is 36.5℃ (97.7°F). The abdomen is minimally distended, and bowel sounds are absent. No abdominal scars are present. There is no muscle guarding, and tenderness is difficult to evaluate. The rectum contains a small smear of liquid stool that is hematest positive.

Case 2

An 18-year-old male college student is awakened with an aching pain in the periumbilical area, anorexia, and nausea. He had shared a pizza and a few beers with friends the previous evening. He skips morning classes and chews a few antacid tablets, but, later in the day, the pain becomes worse, more constant, and moves to the right lower quadrant. Unable to eat, he vomits once and notes that the pain is worse when he tries to walk. At the hospital infirmary, he is found to have lower right quadrant tenderness, involuntary guarding, an oral temperature of 100.9°F, and a white blood count of 12,500 with 80% polymorphonuclear leukocytes.

Case 3

A 59-year-old man is referred to the hospital emergency department by his physician because of lower abdominal pain, fever, and difficulty walking.

The patient has noted intermittent cramps and changing bowel habits over the past 2 months. Recently, he has become constipated, but he also has had occasional episodes of diarrhea. For the past 18 hours, he has had constant, severe pain and soreness in the left lower quadrant. He has no appetite, but he is thirsty.

Physical exam exhibits a blood pressure of 135/85, pulse of 100, and temperature of 39℃ (102°F). He is lying supine, with the left leg flexed at the hip. He does not want to move. There is mild, lower abdominal distention, but no scars or protuberances are noted. Palpation demonstrates involuntary guarding and tenderness in the left lower quadrant. Bowel sounds are almost absent, and percussion is tympanitic. There is fullness and tenderness on the left side of the upper rectum. A small amount of brown stool in the examining glove is negative for occult blood.

Case 4

A 62-year-old African-American woman comes to the hospital emergency department complaining of severe, crampy, midabdominal pain that began approximately 36 hours ago. She simultaneously noted nausea that quickly was followed by multiple episodes of vomiting dark, thick, greenish fluid. The pain and vomiting have persisted, and she feels distended and unable to hold down fluids. She thinks her last bowel movement was 2 days ago and that she has not passed flatus over the past 24 hours. She reports a similar but less severe episode about a week ago; her condition improved when she reduced her oral intake to clear fluids.

On physical examination, she appears uncomfortable and rocks back and forth intermittently. Her blood pressure is 115/70, pulse is 80, respirations are 18, and temperature is 38°C (100.4°F).

Her abdomen is protuberant, symmetrical, and tympanitic, with minimal tenderness. There is a well-healed, lower midline abdominal scar that she explains resulted from a complete hysterectomy performed 20 years ago. Her bowel sounds are hyperactive, with intermittent high-pitched whines and gurgles. Rectal examination demonstrates no masses or tenderness, and the ampulla contains no stool.

Introduction

Abdominal pain is a common clinical symptom. An indicator of either functional or organic pathology of the abdominal wall and the intraabdominal contents, it usually is mild, of short duration, and self-limited. In the overwhelming majority of cases, no cause is ever established. **Persistent, chronic, or recurrent pain** usually can be evaluated safely by systematic observation and diagnostic studies over time and managed electively. On the other hand, **severe abdominal pain** that persists for 6 hours or longer must be diagnosed and treated promptly, as it may portend serious, life-threatening complications.

The so-called acute abdomen has many causes and often requires timely surgical intervention to ensure the best clinical outcome. In most instances, the **acute surgical abdomen** is caused by one of three pathologic processes: **(1) inflammation that has extended beyond or perforated the wall of the organ of origin; (2) acute vascular insufficiency (ischemia) or hemorrhage; (3) acute high-grade obstruction of the alimentary tract and ducts draining secretory or excretory organs**.

The general surgeon has become the specialist of choice for assessing patients with potentially serious abdominal problems. The surgeon's first consideration must be **risk assessment**. How serious is the presenting problem and how quickly must action be taken? Several questions are evident:

1. Is this a catastrophic event that requires immediate recognition, resuscitation, and emergency surgery to avert almost certain death? Severe, persistent abdominal pain associated with hemorrhagic, hypovolemic, or septic shock, severe systemic sepsis unresponsive to antibiotic therapy and fluid replacement, or the "board-like" abdomen of severe generalized peritonitis are typical presentations for these disastrous situations.

2. Is this a noncatastrophic acute surgical abdomen that requires urgent treatment? Most of these cases present with signs of localized peritonitis and a mild to moderate systemic inflammatory reaction. Because the patient is at risk for or already has serious complications, here, too, a prompt and accurate diagnosis must be made. This is followed by a decision for relatively urgent surgery or initial, intensive medical care.

Table 21.1. Examples of disease processes that give rise to abdominal pain.

Catastrophic
  Ruptured abdominal aortic aneurysm
  Intestinal infarction
  Free perforation
    Gastroduodenal ulcer
    Colonic diverticulitis or carcinoma
  Advanced suppurative ascending cholangitis
  Necrotizing infected pancreatitis

Urgent
  Acute appendicitis
  Cholecystitis
  Diverticulitis
  Bowel obstruction
    Incarcerated hernia
    Complete small- or large-bowel obstruction

Elective
  Biliary colic
  Partially obstructing colon carcinoma
  Crohn's disease

Nonsurgical
  Irritable bowel
  Gastroenteritis
  Simple pancreatitis
  Hepatitis
  Pelvic inflammatory disease
  Urinary tract infection/pyelonephritis
  Herpes zoster
  Diabetic ketoacidosis
  Myocardial infarction

3. Is this a transient or recurrent pain caused by a lesion that ultimately requires surgical removal, but that allows an orderly diagnostic workup to be completed safely and an elective date to be set for the procedure?

4. Is this a nonsurgical disorder such as irritable bowel syndrome or a self-limiting and medically treatable organic condition such as viral gastroenteritis or bacterial gastroenteritis? These are the causes of abdominal pain in the majority of patients; these patients are not considered for surgical therapy.

Table 21.1 lists examples of disease processes in each of these above-mentioned categories.

Classification of Abdominal Pain: Is It Visceral or Somatic?

The diagnosis of abdominal pain begins with the acquisition of subjective and objective data. As the clinical history is obtained and the physical examination is performed, it is important to determine if the patient's pain is visceral or somatic in nature. Pain originating from the abdomen is detected and transmitted to the central nervous system via two separate pathways. **Algorithm 21.1** on the **etiology and pathogenesis of abdominal pain** helps elucidate how different processes cause pain.

Visceral receptors are confined to the abdominal organs and their supporting mesenteric structures. These receptors are stimulated by stretching, tension, or ischemia, and their signals are transmitted via the slow C afferent fibers of the regional autonomic nerves. These include vagal and pelvic parasympathetic nerves and the

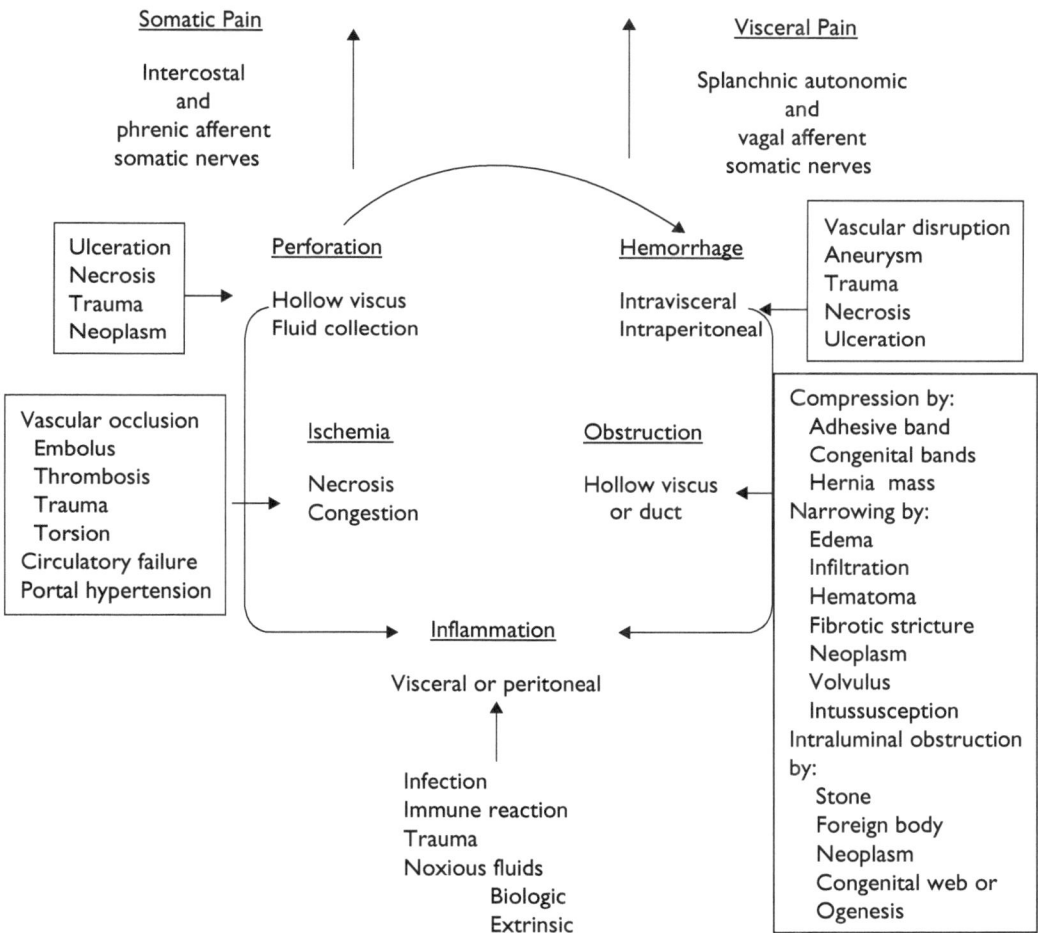

A variety of etiologic factors cause the five pathogenetic processes that produce the disorders that result in abdominal pain.
  Over time, the primary pathology may progress to induce other pathogenic processes. Physiologic responses and pathologic mediators stimulate visceral pain receptors evocative of visceral pain. When mediators extend beyond the organ of origin to pain receptors adjacent to the parietal peritoneum, somatic pain signals are sent to the brain, producing the reflexes and sensations characteristic of peritoneal irritation.

Algorithm 21.1. Etiology and pathogenesis of abdominal pain.

thoracolumbar sympathetic nerves. Within the abdomen, the sympathetic nerves follow the embryonic arterial circulation: the celiac access to the foregut, the superior mesenteric artery to the mid-gut, and the inferior mesenteric artery to the hindgut. Accordingly, pain arising from the foregut structures—stomach, duodenum, liver, biliary tract, pancreas, and spleen—is perceived in the midepigastrium; pain arising from the mid-gut structures—the small intestine distal to the ligament of Treitz to the distal transverse colon, which includes the appendix—is perceived in the periumbilical region; and pain arising from the hindgut—the left colon and rectum—is perceived in the suprapubic area. In all three areas, the pain is central and poorly localized.

Visceral pain is often intermittent, i.e., colicky or crampy in nature with a crescendo/decrescendo tempo. It is characteristic of the response seen in peristaltic muscular conduits that are obstructed. Visceral pain also can be constant and pressing, dull, or lancinating, as seen with gallbladder distention due to outlet obstruction and inappropriately called "biliary colic." Patients suffering visceral pain characteristically move about, seeking a position of relief. A patient doubled over or "climbing the walls" is experiencing visceral pain. Some visceral pain is referred to distant sites, as when gallbladder colic is perceived under the right scapula or urethral colic is referred to the external genital area. A general sense of distress often accompanies visceral pain. "I feel sick to my stomach" means that the patient is experiencing a sense of fullness, anorexia, queasiness, weakness, and malaise. Often, at the outset, the patient experiences an urge to vomit or defecate.

Abdominal somatic pain is transmitted by rapid conducting afferent fiber in the somatic sensory nerves (T7 to L2 anteriorly and L2 to L5 posteriorly). Their receptors lie in the walls of the peritoneal cavity just outside the parietal peritoneum. Somatic abdominal pain, therefore, is sometimes referred to as **parietal pain**, and the signs provoked are referred to as **peritoneal signs**. Somatic pain signals are perceived immediately and with precise localization. Pressure on or motion of the painful area accentuates the pain, and this tenderness provokes a protective reflex spasm of the overlying abdominal wall muscles (involuntary guarding). This is comparable to the somatic pain receptors in a finger touching a hot surface: the burn is recognized rapidly and localized precisely, the finger is withdrawn quickly and reflexively, and the patient avoids further contact with the tender site. Abdominal somatic receptors respond to irritation from inflammatory mediators and physical insults such as cutting, pinching, or burning. The pain usually is sharp, severe, and continuous and is aggravated by pressure, motion, and displacement. Patients suffering somatic pain lie very still, suppress urges to cough or sneeze, and resist being moved or touched in the painful area.

Not infrequently, **the acute abdomen begins with poorly localized visceral pain caused by swelling, distention, or ischemia of the abdominal viscus primarily involved. The pain initially is perceived in the topographic area of the abdomen corresponding to the level of** the gut involved. Subsequent irritation of the parietal peritoneum adjacent to this organ, as the inflammatory process progresses, produces localized pain and tenderness at the exact location of the process.

Diagnosing Abdominal Pain

Diagnosis of the cause of abdominal pain begins with the collection of all relevant clinical information by **history taking, physical examination, and standard diagnostic tests**. Integration of this information allows the physician to reach a preliminary or working diagnosis that may be sufficient for initiating a therapeutic plan or may require further refinement by way of special tests and examinations.

The **history of the present illness** includes a careful characterization of the pain, significant associated symptoms, and **a past history of medical and surgical events** that may be pertinent to the current problem. Because pain syndromes often change over time, the temporal pattern is important. When did the pain start, and was the onset sudden or gradual? What potentially significant events had occurred in the day or hours prior to the onset, and is there anything that makes the pain better or worse? Has the patient had pain like this before, and, if so, how long did it last and what was the final outcome?

The **character of the pain** is equally important. Dull, constant, pressure-like pain often is indicative of an overdistended viscus; colicky pain often is indicative of hyperperistaltic muscular activity; burning and lancinating pain often is neurogenic in origin; and aching or throbbing pain suggests an inflammatory process under pressure. The severity of the pain, described on a scale of 1 to 10, often reflects the seriousness of the underlying process. Pain that is getting better usually means an improvement in the underlying pathology; however, rupture of an abscess or viscus under tension may result in a transient improvement in pain followed by more severe somatic pain.

The **location of the pain**, both at its onset and during the examination, helps in determining the site of the pathology. Is the pain localized, with a point of maximum intensity, or is it diffuse and ill defined? Or, in the worst-case scenario, is the pain constant throughout the abdomen with attendant generalized muscular rigidity?

Pain that radiates to other locations often provides diagnostic clues. Right upper quadrant pain that radiates to the right subscapular area is characteristic of gallbladder disease. Retroperitoneal sources like ureteral colic frequently radiate to the groin and external genital area, while subphrenic irritation often is perceived simultaneously in the upper abdomen and at the root of the ipsilateral neck.

Assumption of a certain body position also has diagnostic significance. Patients with iliopsoas muscle irritation want to keep their hip flexed, while patients with pancreatitis sit, leaning forward, and avoid the supine position. Those with generalized peritonitis lie very still in the supine or fetal position, while those with colicky pain move about seeking a position of comfort to no avail.

Associated Symptoms

Associated symptoms can be useful in assessing the seriousness of the presenting pain syndrome and often help identify the organ system involved.

Hemodynamic instability (shock) is a sign of a life-threatening disorder that requires an urgent diagnostic and therapeutic response. Shock accompanying severe abdominal pain usually is hemorrhagic or hypovolemic, septic, or multifactorial. These patients often are pale, cold, prostrated, and demonstrate global neurologic impairment with confusion, disorientation, or coma.

A coexistent, systemic inflammatory response characterized by high fever and chills, warm flushed skin, and a hyperdynamic cardiovascular response indicates a serious septic process and implies an underlying infectious or necrotizing process.

Organ-specific symptoms help identify primary or secondary involvement of that system. Dyspnea, tachypnea, and hypochondral pain may be due to basilar pneumonia or cardiac infarction referred to the abdomen, or, conversely, severe pancreatitis may produce adult respiratory distress syndrome or cardiac dysfunction.

Abdominal system–specific symptoms may point to the organ affected: anorexia, nausea, and vomiting may point to an upper gastrointestinal (GI) source; middle to lower abdominal cramps, diarrhea, or constipation may point to the lower GI tract; and jaundice may point to the liver and biliary tract.

Lower urinary tract disorders are likely to be associated with frequency, dysuria, nocturia, and hesitancy; however, inflammatory GI disorders in contact with the urinary bladder also may be the cause of these symptoms as well as of microscopic hematuria and pyuria.

Uterine or adnexal disease and pregnancy may produce menstrual irregularities, dysmenorrhea, or vaginal discharge. In males, **urethral discharge or associated prostatic or scrotal tenderness** points to a genitourinary source.

Splenic and other hematologic disorders as a cause of abdominal pain may be reflected in a history of easy bruisability, petechia, or prolonged and excessive bleeding. Other clues may be found in the hemogram, in the form of thrombocyte, erythrocyte, and leukocyte abnormalities.

Past Medical and Surgical History

A relevant past and a current medical history is essential not only for uncovering potential causes for the pain but also for assessing comorbidity. If the current disorder has been going on for some time, **previous medical consultations, diagnostic tests, and procedures** require review.

Itemization of current medications and other treatments helps in recognizing previously diagnosed disorders and in influencing further clinical management. Some medications, such as analgesics, antibiotics, chemotherapeutic agents, and corticosteroids, may be playing a role in the cause of the pain. Previously performed surgical operations and other invasive procedures may be contributing directly to the current pain syndrome or may provide other useful diagnostic information. Allergies and other adverse reactions to previous therapeutic interventions must be identified to prevent repetition of misadventures in the course of diagnosis and treatment of the current illness. Notable are reactions to antibiotics and intravenous radiographic contrast materials. Food-based sensitivities such as gluten sensitivity in patients with celiac disease or milk intolerance in the face of lactase deficiency rarely may explain pain based on maldigestion.

Physical Examination

The **physical examination** provides critical information for reaching a diagnosis and is a simple, low-cost opportunity to assess important findings repeatedly over time. Changing signs are characteristic of certain clinical scenarios and help in ascertaining whether the patient is improving, stabilized, or getting worse. **Impressions reached by the general observation of the patient are invaluable.** Extremely ill individuals often can be identified by their appearance and behavior. What is their state of consciousness and verbal ability? How are they reacting to the pain? These findings, coupled with the **vital signs** (pulse, blood pressure, respirations, and temperature), provide immediate clues to the patient's hemodynamic status and whether or not there is a systemic inflammatory response syndrome.

It is self-evident that **careful examination of the abdomen is of paramount importance but attention also must be paid to the chest, groin, external genitalia, rectal, and pelvic areas**. Observation of the anterior abdominal wall should assess distention, asymmetry, focal protrusions, scars, and other significant skin lesions.

Auscultation of the abdomen is performed primarily to characterize bowel sounds. When bowel sounds are loud and frequent, with high-pitched gurgling and tinkling components, intestinal hyperperistalsis is confirmed. When the peristaltic rushes coincide with crampy pain in the presence of distention and abdominal tympani, the typical picture of mechanical small bowel obstruction is present. A quiet abdomen, on the other hand, is more difficult to assess, since normal bowel sounds may be infrequent. The absence of bowel sounds, however, in the presence of distention suggests paralytic ileus.

The **presence of tenderness** induced by palpation and percussion often is the most informative part of the physical examination. Patients should be made as comfortable as possible, with their knees and head slightly raised, and they should be reassured that every effort will be made to avoid hurting them. The examiner's hand should be warm and dry and should be applied gently to an area as distant as possible from the painful site. Special attention should be paid to eliciting direct and rebound tenderness and involuntary guarding. **Involuntary guarding** and rigidity of the abdominal musculature is a reflex response to parietal irritation. **Voluntary guarding**, on the other hand, is an attempt by the patient to protect the abdomen by consciously tensing the anterior abdominal wall muscles. Many maneuvers have been advocated to distract the patient in order to prevent voluntary guarding and facilitate palpation. One of the most effective is to direct the patient to breathe deeply but slowly through an open mouth without interruption during the examination. This distracts the patient by giving him/her a task to complete and, more importantly, prevents closing of the glottis and the inadvertent Valsalva maneuver required to consciously tense the abdomen. The patient should not breathe rapidly, since hyperventilation produces respiratory alkalosis and possible tentany. **Tenderness and involuntary guarding are hallmarks of parietal peritoneal irritation and a key indicator of an acute surgical abdomen.**

Deep palpation of all quadrants serves to identify organomegaly or abnormal masses. Masses include neoplastic tumors, cysts, hematomas, and inflammatory lesions. Inflammatory masses may be a swollen, distended organ or a composite of inflamed, edematous soft tissues, such as omentum and mesentery surrounding such a primary process, with or without abscess formation. Special attention should be directed to the subcostal areas bilaterally, feeling for an enlarged liver or gallbladder on the right or an enlarged spleen on the left during deep inspiration. A distended urinary bladder or an unexpected gravid uterus may mimic a suprapubic tumor.

Percussion of the abdomen is useful in determining the distribution of tympanitic gas and nontympanitic solid or liquid containing structures. Tympany over the usually dull liver area may be indicative of free air in the peritoneal cavity and requires radiologic verification. Hyperresonance over the central abdomen is indicative of intestinal ileus or obstruction. Midline organomegaly includes pulsatile abdominal aneurysm superiorly, an obstructed closed loop of bowel centrally, and an overfilled urinary bladder inferiorly.

It is important to expose and examine the **inguinal, pubic, and perineal areas**, especially for those with lower abdominal pain. Inflammatory or ulcerative genital lesions associated with sexually transmitted diseases, testicular torsion, epididymo-orchitis, or small cryptic incarcerated inguinal and femoral hernias may not be apparent immediately. Rectal examination should be directed at detection of the pelvic tenderness or masses, the status of the anorectal tissues, and, in males, the prostate gland. Pelvic examination is basic to the evaluation of the lower abdominal pain in females. The examiner looks for cervical discharge or motion tenderness, adnexal masses, and signs of pregnancy and its complications. This requires a bimanual and speculum examination of the vagina and cervix, at which time important smears and cultures of exudates can be obtained.

In either gender, **inspection and analysis of the stool** for gross or occult blood, enteric pathogens, toxins (*Clostridium difficile*), and leukocytes may be indicated.

Basic Laboratory and Imaging Tests

Standard laboratory blood tests, urine analysis, and imaging studies complete the initial assessment of significant abdominal pain.

An abnormal leukocyte count and differential may suggest infection, other forms of inflammation, or hematologic neoplasia, while anemia may signal acute or chronic blood loss or an underlying chronic disease. Platelet abnormalities, together with other coagulation studies, may reflect coagulopathic states and the underlying conditions that produce them. The routine blood or serum multichannel chemical analyses provide a broad spectrum of useful information, and, in particular, they may point to hepatobiliary or renal disease. A serum amylase and lipase are key to diagnosing acute pancreatitis. In women of childbearing age, a β-human chorionic gonadotropin level is a useful screening test for pregnancy and its complications. A clean caught or catheter-obtained urine specimen showing proteinuria, leukocytes, erythrocytes, or bacteria implies primary urinary tract disease.

Traditionally obtained radiographs include a flat and upright plain abdominal film and posteroanterior (PA) and lateral chest films. The abdominal films are most useful for demonstrating abnormal gas patterns and calcifications. Dilated bowel containing air-fluid levels is characteristic of mechanical obstruction or paralytic ileus. The upright chest and abdominal x-rays usually can identify free air within the peritoneal cavity, implying perforation of a gas-containing viscus. Free air is seen most easily between the right hemidiaphragm and the liver on upright films. In patients who cannot assume the upright position, a left lateral decubitis film shows free air between the lateral liver and right abdominal wall. Rarely, gas may be seen in the biliary tree, within the bowel wall, and in the portal vein. The latter two findings are indicative of a gas-producing infection of the intestinal wall with extension to the draining portal veins. Biliary tract gas occurs as a result of enteral-biliary fistula, although gas-producing infection of the gallbladder is another possibility. Strategically located abnormal calcifications are diagnostically helpful. A right lower quadrant appendicolith often is associated with appendicitis, a stone in the course of the ureters with renal colic, calcifications in the pancreas with chronic pancreatitis, and radiopaque gallstones with cholecystitis. "Gallstone ileus" usually occurs in elderly women who present with the classic radiographic picture of small bowel obstruction, air in the biliary tract, and, occasionally, the lightly calcified outline of a large stone lodged in the distal ileum.

Last, an electrocardiogram should be performed on most patients over the age of 50 or younger patients with a history of heart disease or symptoms that may occur with both intraabdominal disorders and myocardial ischemia.

The basic laboratory studies not only are useful for establishing a working diagnosis, but they also are useful for detecting comorbid conditions that would affect management decisions and for establishing a baseline against which further events can be compared.

Synthesis of an Initial Diagnosis

Developing a **reasonable initial diagnosis** requires answers to the clinical questions posed by the unique patient being considered:

1. In what organ or organ system did the pain arise?
2. Is the pain visceral or somatic?
3. What is the primary pathogenic process, and has it progressed to a secondary process?
4. What is the underlying etiology?

In what ways is the patient unique? Certainly, age and gender are important. Certain conditions occur, in the main, at the extremes of age. Infancy and early childhood is the haven for congenital and, to a lesser degree, infectious diseases, while, in the aged, neoplastic and degenerative cardiovascular diseases predominate. Young and middle-aged adults are more likely to exhibit the consequences of substance abuse, alcoholism, sexually transmitted diseases, and trauma. Women of childbearing age may manifest the complications of pregnancy. Preexisting chronic diseases and medications used for their management may predispose the patient to certain disorders, as do certain occupational, dietary, and behavioral practices.

The subjective (S) and objective (O) data obtained from the history, physical examination, and laboratory studies are integrated to reach an initial assessment (A) of the clinical problem. This is the working or initial diagnosis from which a reasoned management plan (P) can be formulated. This so-called **SOAP approach** is a useful tool for addressing and documenting most clinical problems.

The management plan (see **Algorithm 21.2**) may run the gamut from further observation without treatment through performing more advanced problem-focused tests to refine and finalize the diagnosis for medical treatment or surgery. If the initial assessment is that a surgically treatable, catastrophic, life-threatening emergency is present, an immediate surgical intervention is indicated.

Catastrophic Surgical Abdominal Emergencies

Major Intraabdominal Bleeding

Aneurysmal disease of major arteries is the most common etiology for nontraumatic severe intraabdominal bleeding. To avoid the high mortality of aortic aneurysm rupture associated with shock no matter how treated, a prompt diagnosis based on a high level of suspicion is required. The temptation to transport the patient to the radiology department for confirmatory imaging studies or attempts at prolonged preoperative resuscitation should be avoided. Recognition and treatment of a worrisome aneurysm before it ruptures is clearly the best course.

Other potential sources of intraabdominal bleeding are **iliac and visceral aneurysms**, notably of the hepatic and splenic arteries, the latter often rupturing during pregnancy. Still other sources of intraabdominal apoplexy are **ruptured ectopic pregnancy; spontaneous rupture of the spleen; hemorrhage into and from necrosing neoplastic lesions of the liver, kidneys, and adrenal glands; and hemorrhagic pancreatitis.** Spontaneous intra- and retroperitoneal bleeding also may occur after minimal, often unrecognized, trauma in patients with coagulopathies.

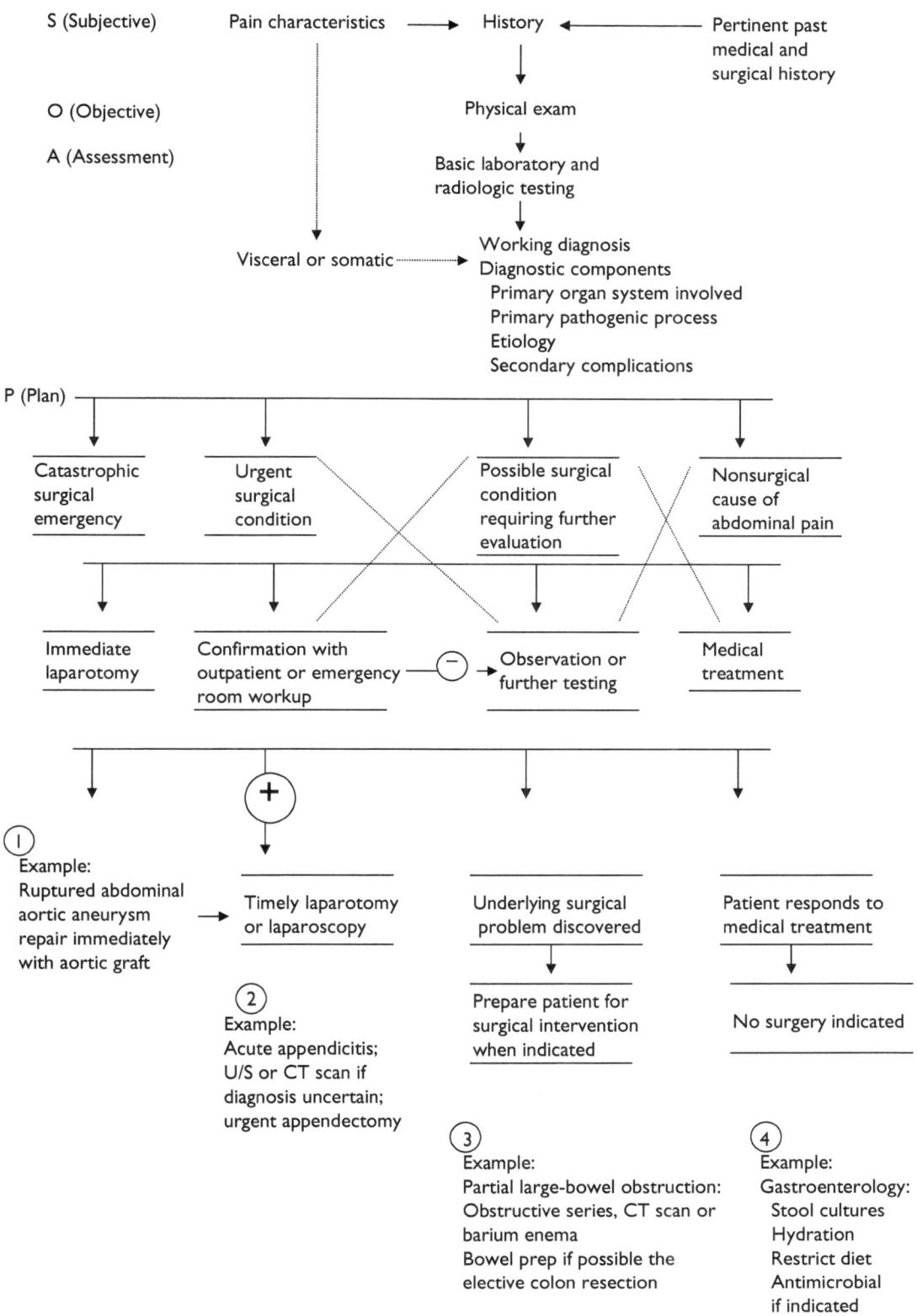

Algorithm 21.2. Evaluation and management of abdominal pain.

Acute thromboembolic occlusion of major mesenteric arteries with intestinal infarction is a dramatic event with rapidly progressive life-threatening consequences. Most common is an occlusive embolus to the superior mesenteric artery. The initial abdominal pain is sudden, severe, and diffuse, with an associated transient hyperperistaltic response. Typically, the pain remains constant and quite severe, in contrast to the few, if any, abdominal physical findings. Peristaltic activity soon ceases, and the abdomen is quiet. This acute embolic syndrome requires prompt diagnosis, laparotomy, and, where indicated, embolectomy and/or resection of necrotic bowel. Thrombotic occlusion of mesenteric arteries and veins also can be associated with heart failure, hypoperfusion, or shock.

Case Discussion

The patient in **Case 1** requires resuscitation and, most likely, operative treatment. He has the classic risk factors for intestinal ischemia from an embolus. His irregular heart rate and medication list lead one to believe that he has an atrial fibrillation. In addition, his recent myocardial infarction and coronary artery bypass procedure highlight underlying cardiac disease. Performing an angiogram and thrombolitic therapy is an option if he does not develop peritonitis and his overall clinical picture improves with fluid resuscitation; however, he is at great risk for transmural ischemia that will require resection in the operating room.

Gastrointestinal Perforation and Generalized Peritonitis

Another disastrous scenario is **generalized peritonitis due to a free perforation of a hollow viscus containing noxious or infectious material. Duodenal and gastric ulcers** are the most common cause of perforation of the gastrointestinal tract in adults. Although many of these patients have a history of ulcer or at least have experienced several days of epigastric discomfort prior to a perforation, it is not unusual for acute perforation to occur unexpectedly.

The perforation is heralded by the sudden onset of severe generalized abdominal pain and anterior wall muscle guarding. The widespread spill produces inflammation of all of the peritoneal surfaces, sequestration of fluid, cessation of intestinal motor activity, and dramatic incapacitation of the patient. See **Figure 21.1** for the classic radiographic picture of free intraabdominal air.

Colonic perforation may occur at the site of diverticular disease, severe transmural inflammation as in toxic dilatation of ulcerative colitis, or transmural cancer. The consequences of colonic rupture usually are more serious because of the large inoculum of fecal bacteria. **Small-bowel perforation** is relatively rare, but it may be encountered as a complication of small-bowel obstruction or severe necrotizing enterocolitis in infants. Insertion of objects into the colorectum and iatrogenic instrumentation, e.g., endoscopy, may lead to accidental perforation.

With rare exceptions, surgical management is required in cases of free perforation. Brisk fluid and electrolyte resuscitation and systemic

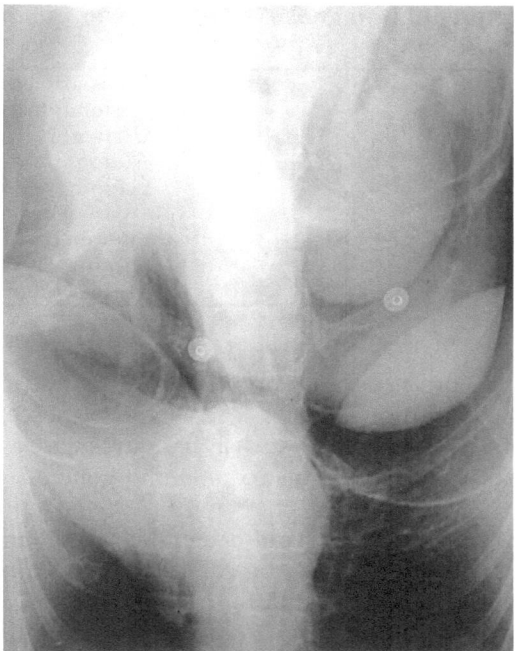

Figure 21.1. X-ray of a massive pneumoperitoneum. A 47-year-old woman developed abdominal pain following a colonoscopy. Erect abdominal radiograph demonstrates air under the diaphragm. Air around the right kidney suggests air in the retroperitoneum also.

antibiotic therapy complement the laparotomy, closure, or resection of the perforated segment and the vigorous peritoneal toilet.

The Acute Surgical Abdomen

Intraabdominal conditions producing localized or regional peritoneal signs often are accompanied by a systemic inflammatory response that characterizes the **acute surgical abdomen**. The majority of these conditions arise from **infections of obstructed ducts or diverticular outpouchings of the gastrointestinal tract and, less often, the genitourinary tract**.

Appendicitis

Appendicitis is the most common of the intraabdominal inflammatory disorders, occurring in both genders and in all age groups. It is most common in older children and young adults, but it does occur in the extremes of age when it is more difficult to diagnose and treat.

In the early stages of the process, the inflammatory edema and distention are confined to the appendix, and the patient perceives visceral pain in the periumbilical area. With time, the diffuse phlegmonous

Table 21.2. Differential diagnosis of right lower quadrant abdominal pain.

Appendicitis	Psoas abscess
Bowel obstruction	Pyelonephritis
Inflammatory bowel disease	Ureteral calculi
Mesenteric adenitis	Abdominal wall hematoma
Cholecystitis	Ectopic pregnancy
Diverticulitis	Ovarian cyst or torsion
Leaking aneurysm	Endometriosis
Perforated ulcer	Salpingitis
Hernia	Mittelschmerz

inflammation can proceed to suppuration and, finally, to gangrene of the appendix. Perforation usually leads to local abscess formation; however, in some circumstances, such as in infants with a poorly developed omentum, walling off is inadequate and generalized peritonitis may occur.

Signs and symptoms may be confusing when an inflamed appendix is in an atypical location. A retrocecal location may mask anterior abdominal signs and produce pain in the back or flank. A high-riding cecum, with the appendix in the subhepatic area, can mimic acute cholecystitis, while a pelvic location mimics acute salpingitis and produces signs most prominent on rectal and pelvic examination.

Other conditions to consider in the differential diagnosis of **right lower quadrant pain** include **mesenteric adenitis in children, cecal or Meckel's diverticulitis, sigmoid diverticulitis when a redundant sigmoid falls toward the right lower quadrant, acute regional ileitis, and a partially contained duodenal ulcer perforation with contents tracking down the right gutter to the right lower quadrant**. In the older age group, **cecal carcinoma** may cause appendicitis by blocking the appendiceal orifice or may mimic appendicitis when it penetrates the full thickness of the cecal wall. Extraintestinal conditions in the differential diagnosis are any of the **many inflammatory and hemorrhagic conditions of the internal female genital tract and urinary tract disorders,** such as ureteral colic, pyelonephritis, perinephric abscess, and renal carcinoma (tumors that outgrow their blood supply necrose centrally and bleed). See **Table 21.2** for a broad differential diagnosis of right lower quadrant pain and **Table 21.3** for a broad differential diagnosis of left lower quadrant pain.

Table 21.3. Differential diagnosis of left lower quadrant abdominal pain.

Diverticulitis	Ureteral calculi
Bowel obstruction	Abdominal wall hematoma
Inflammatory bowel disease	Ectopic pregnancy
Appendicitis	Ovarian cyst or torsion
Leaking aneurysm	Endometriosis
Hernia	Salpingitis
Psoas abscess	Mittelschmerz
Pyelonephritis	

Case Discussion

The young man portrayed in **Case 2** presented to the infirmary with typical signs and symptoms of appendicitis. After evaluation, an operation is scheduled for later in the afternoon. After waiting long enough to ensure an empty stomach and after the infusion of intravenous electrolyte solution and antibiotics, an appendectomy is performed through a small, lower right muscle-splitting incision. An edematous and hyperemic appendix is found and removed, and there is no evidence of perforation or pus in the area. The patient makes an uneventful recovery and is discharged from the hospital on the second postoperative day. The pathology report is acute appendicitis. This is a classic example of the progression of a visceral, pathologic process and its associated pain to a process affecting the parietal peritoneal surfaces and changing into somatic pain. In patients with an uncertain diagnosis, a computed tomography (CT) scan may be warranted (**Fig. 21.2**). The operative approach may be either laparoscopic or open (**Table 21.4**).

Diverticulitis

Diverticular outpouchings from the tubular GI tract are relatively common. Most older adults in the United States have some colonic diverticula, and diverticulitis of the descending and sigmoid colon is not unusual. The severity of inflammation in colonic diverticulitis can be quite variable. The gamut runs from mild attacks treated in the ambulatory setting with bowel rest and oral antibiotics to severe transmural and pericolonic infection. Free perforations and fecal peritonitis may occur occasionally, but most perforations are localized and

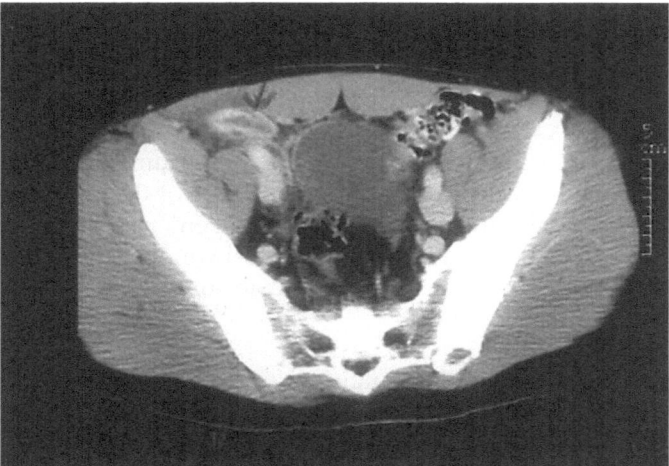

Figure 21.2. Computed tomography (CT) scan of an acute appendicitis. A 14-year-old boy is brought to the emergency department by anxious parents because he has been vomiting and has abdominal pain. CT scan through the midpelvis shows an abnormally enhancing tubular structure that indicates an abnormally inflamed appendix consistent with acute appendicitis.

Table 21.4. Advantages of laparotomy versus laparoscopy approaches to appendectomy.

Laparotomy	Laparoscopy
Shorter time in operating room	Diagnosis of other conditions
Lesser cost of operation	Decreased wound infection
Overall lesser cost of hospital stay	Minimal decrease in hospital stay
Possibly less risk of intraabdominal abscess in perforated cases	Possible decrease in time for convalescence and return to work or normal activity

Source: Based on meta-analysis and reviews of prior prospective controlled randomized trials (level I evidence), including Br J Surg 1997;84:1045–1050, Dis Colon Rectum 1998;41:398–403, J Am Coll Surg 1998;186:545–553. Reprinted from Soybel DI. Appendix. In: Norton JA, Bollinger RR, Chang AE, et al, eds. Surgery: Basic Science and Clinical Evidence. New York: Springer-Verlag, 2001.

produce pericolonic and mesenteric abscesses or penetrate an adjacent organ, producing a fistula. The length of colon involved is variable in extent, but usually it is regional. Chronicity and relapsing attacks can result in obstructive stenosis.

Small intestinal diverticuli are less common, but these do occur in the distal duodenum and the periampullary region. Of special interest, particularly in younger individuals, is the **congenital Meckel's diverticulum of the distal ileum**. This diverticulum is capable of developing inflammatory diverticulitis, may invaginate, and may lead to an intussusception, or, because it often contains ectopic gastric mucosa, it may cause peptic ulceration at its base with bleeding or perforation.

Case Discussion

The man in **Case 3** needs to undergo further evaluation. A CT scan of the abdomen and pelvis would be appropriate to document inflammation of the sigmoid colon, as his presentation seems to indicate that he has a colonic abnormality. Diverticulitis or a perforated sigmoid cancer have similar presentations and may have similar CT scan findings (**Fig. 21.3**). This man will be treated with IV antibiotics initially. If he improves, colonoscopy or barium enema (**Fig. 21.4**) will be done in 6 weeks to determine the cause of the problem definitively. If he does not improve, further management may be required, such as abscess drainage done percutaneously or operative resection of the diseased colon with a temporary colostomy if there is ongoing infection.

Acute Cholecystitis and Cholangitis

The most common pain syndrome associated with **gallbladder dysfunction** occurs as a result of transient mechanical outlet obstruction or dyskinetic motor activity. Typically, the patient develops a pressure-like pain in the right upper quadrant or epigastric area that may radiate to the right subscapular area. This pain is visceral in nature and often is associated with nausea or vomiting. It often occurs after eating and,

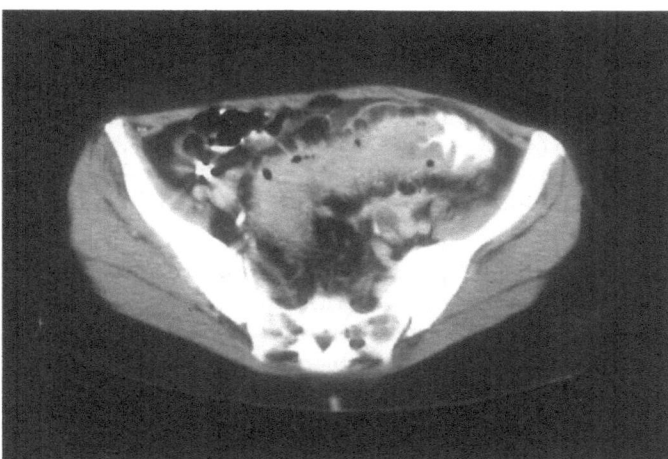

Figure 21.3. CT scan of a sigmoid diverticulitis. A 77-year-old woman is brought to the office with severe left lower quadrant pain, tenderness, and fever. The following findings are consistent with acute sigmoid diverticulitis: CT scan shows an irregularly thickened sigmoid bowel with infiltration of the pericolic fat; air bubbles may indicate diverticula or intramural abscess; the intraluminal contrast is constrained by the edematous wall.

not infrequently, awakes the patient from sleep. This syndrome often is called "gallbladder or biliary colic" and can be variable in duration and intensity and intermittent or constant in nature. Severe or frequently recurring episodes usually initiate ultrasonic examination of the biliary tree; demonstration of gallstones is the most common indication for elective cholecystectomy.

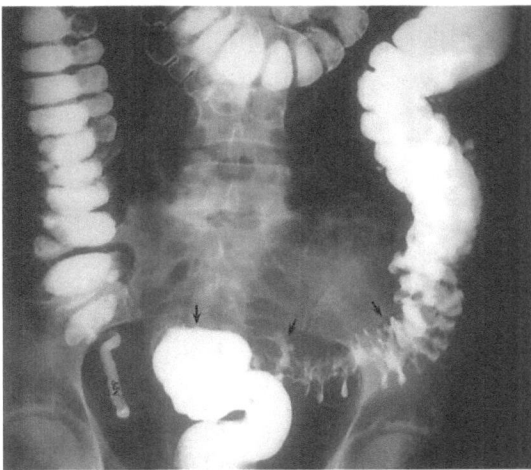

Figure 21.4. Barium enema of a sigmoid diverticulitis. A 77-year-old woman is brought to the office with severe left lower quadrant pain, tenderness, and fever. Contrast enema shows numerous diverticula, spasm, and intramural perforation, findings that are consistent with acute sigmoid diverticulitis.

When the obstructive process is not self-limiting and invasive infection of the gallbladder wall occurs, the pathologic process has advanced to **acute cholecystitis**. The gallbladder wall is thickened by the edema of the inflammatory process, and pus may accumulate within the lumen (empyema of the gallbladder) or gas may be detected within the lumen or wall as a result of gas-producing bacteria (emphysema or the gallbladder). The severity of this infectious process is variable, but it may advance to necrosis of the gallbladder.

Clinically, the patient develops fever, tachycardia, malaise, and polymorphonuclear leukocytosis. Abdominal examination demonstrates right upper quadrant tenderness and involuntary muscle guarding. A sense of fullness or a clearly palpable mass may be present. Murphy's sign, the abrupt cessation of inspiratory effort during palpation in the right subcostal area, occurs when the inflamed gallbladder descends to encounter pressure from the examiner's fingers. Acute cholecystitis is commonly evaluated by ultrasound and sometimes is found on CT scan (**Figs. 21.5 and 21.6**). Treatment may be immediate cholecystectomy or a period of "cooling off" and interval cholecystectomy (**Table 21.5**).

Although **jaundice** may occur with acute cholecystitis, in the absence of obstruction the bilirubin levels usually are not elevated greatly. Migration of stones from the gallbladder into the bile ducts with varying degrees of obstruction is more likely to account for significant jaundice. Obstruction of the bile ducts that occurs acutely usually produces a pain syndrome not unlike that produced by cardiac ischemia. The pain may be severe, is relatively constant and pressing in nature, and is located high in the epigastrium or the lower substernal area. Obstruction of the bile ducts that occurs gradually, as is characteristic

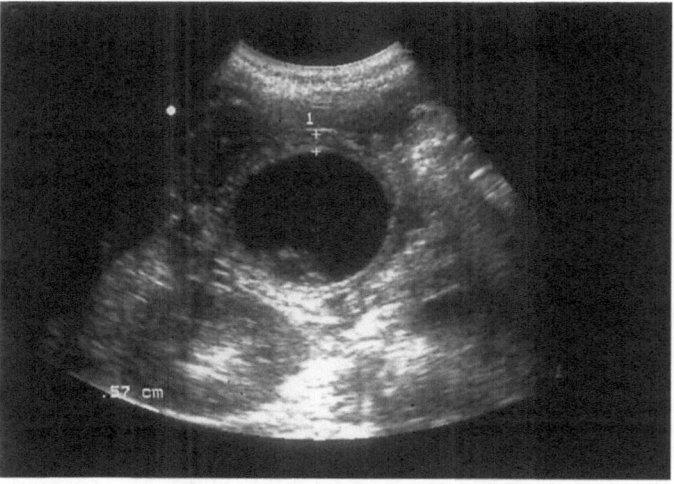

Figure 21.5. Ultrasound of an acute cholecystitis. A 52-year-old woman presents with acute right upper quadrant pain, tenderness, and fever. Ultrasound shows a thickened gallbladder wall and gallstones, findings that are consistent with acute cholecystitis and cholelithiasis.

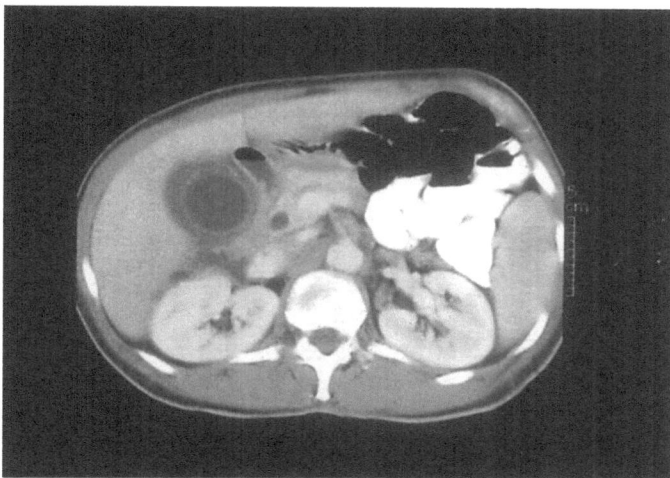

Figure 21.6. CT scan of an acute cholecystitis. A 52-year-old woman presents with acute right upper quadrant pain, tenderness, and fever. CT scan shows the thick gallbladder wall, but the gallstones are not visualized. These findings are consistent with acute cholecystitis and cholelithiasis.

of ductal, periampullary, and pancreatic head neoplasms, may or may not produce pain. Painless or silent jaundice, as it often is referred to, traditionally is attributed to a malignant extrahepatic obstruction, but this clearly is not always the case.

Ascending cholangitis, a serious infection of the bile ducts, almost always is associated with the presence of obstructing foreign bodies, such as stones, sludge, or parasites. These bacteremic patients often exhibit Charcot's triad: upper abdominal pain, chills and fever, and jaundice. In the most severe cases, patients exhibit circulatory insufficiency and impaired mental function as a result of septic shock. All five clinical features are referred to as Reynolds' pentad. Because of its high mortality, ascending cholangitis requires rapid intervention with intravenous antibiotics and drainage of the biliary tract. Drainage is performed best by endoscopic sphincterotomy and placement of a ductal drain, but when this is not possible, open surgical choledochotomy and T-tube drainage is indicated. See **Table 21.6** for a broad differential diagnosis of right upper quadrant pain.

Pancreatitis

Probably the most protean of intraabdominal inflammatory conditions productive of severe abdominal pain is **acute pancreatitis**. Usually abrupt in onset, an attack of pancreatitis may be mild and self-limiting or rapidly may progress to a catastrophic local and systemic life-threatening event. In the severest of cases, **necrotizing hemorrhagic pancreatitis**, the initial visceral inflammation rapidly progresses to widespread retroperitoneal and intraperitoneal inflammation, tissue destruction, and bleeding. In some cases, secondary

Table 21.5. Clinical trials comparing early versus delayed surgery for acute cholecystitis.

Reference	n	Study design	Level of evidence	Complications	Mortality	Findings/comments
Linden and Sunzel 1970,[a] Sweden	140	Randomized, controlled trial	I	Early: 14.3% Delayed: 3.4%	Early: 0% Delayed: 0%	More than two thirds of patients randomized to early surgery underwent operation within 10 days of diagnosis Low mortality, in part the result of excluding 3 high-risk, elderly patients Noted that 17% of patients randomized to delayed surgery ultimately refused operation once acute symptoms resolved No difference in technical difficulty between early and delayed operations when the surgeon was experienced Early surgery (paradoxically) resulted in a 2-day-longer average length of stay, but fewer extended hospitalizations Concluded that early surgery avoids the hazards of diagnostic error, symptom recurrence during the waiting period, and shortened the convalescence period after early surgery
McArthur et al 1975[b] England	35	Randomized, controlled trial	I	Early: 40.0% Delayed: 29.4%	Early: 0% Delayed: 0%	Early surgery defined as immediately following confirmation of the diagnosis Reported no overall difference in the technical difficulty of early versus delayed cholecystectomy, but recommended that early surgery take place within 5 days of diagnosis Most complications were minor infections Concluded that the major benefits of early surgery are the shortened hospitalization and the avoidance of the serious complications of conservative management, including gallbladder perforation and empyema
Lahtinen et al 1978,[c] Finland	100	Randomized, controlled trial	I	Early: 29.7% Delayed: 47.7%	Early: 0% Delayed: 9%	Noted a technically easier operation, shorter OR time (70 vs. 79 min), reduced wound infection rate (6% vs. 18%), and shorter postoperative hospital LOS (12 vs. 15 days) for early vs. delayed surgery High complication rates in both groups predominantly related to localized or systemic infection Authors recommend early surgery

Study	No.	Study design	Level	Mortality	Morbidity/complications	Comments
Norrby et al 1983,[d] Sweden	192	Randomized, controlled, multicenter, trial	I	Early: 0% Delayed: 1.1%	Early: 14.9% Delayed: 15.4%	Early surgery defined as operation within 7 days of symptoms. Studied patients ≤75 years old, randomized by odd vs. even birthdays. Complications were similar between the two groups, but early surgery reduced hospital length of stay by >6 days
Sianesi et al. 1984,[e] Italy	471	Retrospective (1970–77) and prospective (1977–82) data	III	Early: 0% Delayed: 1.6%	Early: 18.5% Delayed: 15%	Study combined retrospective and prospective data, collected over 12 years, during which time patient management evolved. Reported low incidence of biliary infection, low morbidity and mortality, and shorter hospitalization period. Authors recommend early surgery, within 48–72 h of diagnosis
Ajao et al. 1991, Nigeria	81	Retrospective	III	Early: 2.6% Delayed: 0%	Early: 41% Delayed: 12.5%	Retrospective review over 12 months, compared early (≤48 h) versus delayed (7–14 days) surgery. Prohibitive rate of complications reported early surgery including 7 (18%) common bile duct injuries; only complications reported were wound infections (23%) and duct injuries. Authors recommend delayed surgery, recommendations seemingly specific to the practice environment and level of surgical experience
Summary/totals	1019	—	—	Early: 0.2% Delayed: 1.8%	Early: 21.0% Delayed: 16.5%	Early surgery was technically more challenging with a higher complication rate, but shorter hospital stay and convalescence, more rapid return to work, and lower overall mortality than delayed surgery for acute cholecystitis

[a] Linden Wvd, Sunzel H. Early versus delayed operation for acute cholecystitis. A controlled trial. Am J Surg 1970;120:7–13.

[b] McArthur P, Cuschieri A, Sells RA, Shields R. Controlled clinical trial comparing early with interval cholecystectomy for acute cholecystitis. Br J Surg 1975;62:850–852.

[c] Lahtinen J, Alhava EM, Aukee S. Acute cholecystitis treated by early and delayed surgery. A controlled clinical trial. Scand J Gastroenterol 1978;13:673–678.

[d] Norrby S, Herlin P, Holmin T, Sjödahl R, Tagesson C. Early or delayed cholecystectomy in acute cholecystitis? A clinical trial. Br J Surg 1983;70:163–165.

[e] Sianesi M, Ghirarduzzi A, Percudani M, Dell'Anna B. Cholecystectomy for acute cholecystitis: timing of operation, bacteriologic aspects, and postoperative course. Am J Surg 1984;148:609–612.

Source: Reprinted from Harris HW. Biliary system. In: Norton JA, Bollinger RR, Chang AE, et al, eds. Surgery: Basic Science and Clinical Evidence. New York: Springer-Verlag, 2001, with permission.

Table 21.6. Differential diagnosis of right upper quadrant abdominal pain.

Cholecystitis	Herpes zoster
Choledocholithiasis	Myocardial ischemia
Hepatitis	Pericarditis
Hepatic abscess	Pneumonia
Hepatomegaly from congestive heart failure	Empyema
Peptic ulcer	Gastritis
Pancreatitis	Duodenitis
Retrocecal appendicitis	Intestinal obstruction
Pyelonephritis	Inflammatory bowel disease
Nephrolithiasis	

bacterial infection occurs due to loss of alimentary tract and lymphatic integrity.

The etiology of pancreatitis is quite variable, but the majority of cases are due to either transient gallstone obstruction of the common pancreaticobiliary ampulla or destructive effects of alcohol abuse. Initially, the patient experiences severe upper abdominal band-like pain that radiates to the back, is aggravated by recumbency, and partially relieved by sitting or leaning forward. Elevations of serum amylase and lipase are highly diagnostic for acute pancreatitis, and these levels most likely are elevated when drawn shortly after the onset of symptoms. The extent of the elevation, however, is not related directly to the severity of the process. Other blood laboratory tests do correlate with severity and include the degree of acute leukocytosis, anemia, hyperglycemia, hypocalcemia, and elevation of serum lactic dehydrogenase (LDH) and aspartate aminotransferase (AST) concentration. Evidence of hypoxia, cardiac and renal dysfunction, and systemic acidosis, particularly lactic acidosis, has negative prognostic implications. Serial CT scans of the abdomen are useful for confirmation of the diagnosis and the evaluation of the extent, severity, and evolution of the pathologic process (**Fig. 21.7**). Diminished perfusion of the pancreas and peripancreatic areas implies hemorrhage or necrosis, while gas in the soft tissues suggests secondary bacterial infection.

Gallstone-induced pancreatitis rarely requires emergency surgery for removal of a stone impacted at the distal end of the bile duct. There is evidence that, unless increasing jaundice supervenes, the gallstone probably has passed on into the duodenum. Most cases are mild, and treatment with supportive care and observation usually results in clinical improvement within a few days, at which time cholecystectomy, intraoperative cholangiography, and the occasional choledocholithotomy, when indicated, complete the treatment.

Seriously ill patients with multiple risk factors should be treated in an intensive care unit where monitoring and treatment of multisystem organ failure can be performed. Early surgery is generally contraindicated, but it may be required where there is evidence of continued intraabdominal hemorrhage or the cause of the intraabdominal catastrophe is not clear.

Persistent sepsis due to infected pancreatic necrosis is a serious complication that often requires extensive surgical debridement for cure. Patients who go on to develop chronic pancreatitis often have severe nonremitting pain and malabsorption problems that lead to malnutrition and narcotic addiction. Internal surgical duct drainage may help some of these patients.

Gynecologic Pelvic Disorders

Especially during the reproductive years, a woman's pelvic organs are a common site for disorders that produce abdominal and pelvic pain. Two of the **pelvic inflammatory diseases, acute salpingitis and tubo-ovarian abscess**, irritate the pelvic parietal peritoneum, producing a pain syndrome not unlike appendicitis and other inflammatory conditions of the pelvic organs. A comprehensive gynecologic history and thorough pelvic examination, including speculum exposure of the cervix, are mandatory in these patients. A history of prior attacks of pelvic inflammatory disease (PID) and unprotected sexual activity with multiple partners would support this diagnosis. Cervical motion tenderness and a tender adnexal mass are significant findings. A purulent cervical discharge should be cultured. Other adnexal causes of pelvic pain include an **ovarian cyst that has ruptured, an ovary that has undergone torsion and infarction, and an ovary that is the site of a midcycle ovulatory follicle leak ("Mittleschmerz")**. Endometriosis causes pain during menses when hemorrhage occurs into pelvic implants. A serum pregnancy test, β-human chorionic gonadotropin, is

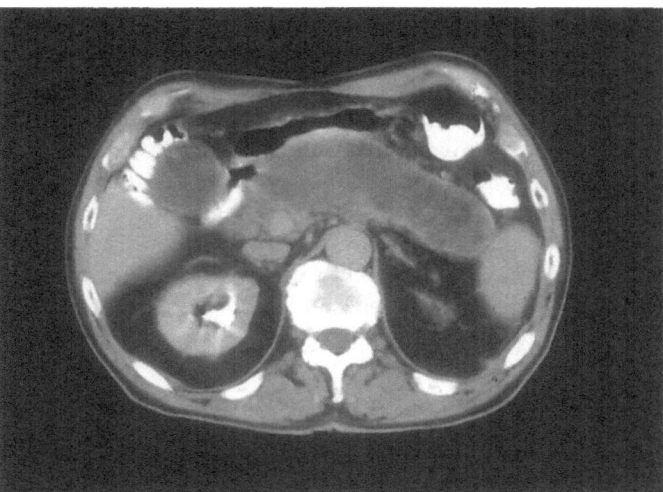

Figure 21.7. CT scan of pancreatitis. A 41-year-old man with a long history of alcoholism has had chronic upper abdominal pain with a recent acute exacerbation. CT scan through the upper abdomen at the level of the gallbladder shows an abnormally enlarged pancreas without any normal pancreatic parenchymal architecture. The low-density material is suggestive of a fluid collection known as a pancreatic pseudocyst.

useful in ruling in a **complication of pregnancy, such as early sponta-neous abortion or ectopic pregnancy**.

Gastrointestinal Obstruction

Although gastrointestinal obstruction conventionally is not character-ized as an acute surgical abdomen, its symptoms mimic the prodrome of an acute abdomen, and its complications merit the same manage-ment urgency.

Gastric outlet obstruction most commonly occurs as a result of **peptic ulcerative disease or neoplasm** in the parapyloric regions. The pain of gastric outlet obstruction results from visceral distention and usually is relatively mild, with a significant sense of fullness and dis-tress in the epigastrium. In the early stages, nausea and vomiting are prominent features. The vomitus usually is free of bile, but it may contain recently ingested food or be stained by blood. Penetrating lesions, such as peptic duodenal ulcer, often induce a variable period of gnawing or burning pain prior to the obstructive symptomatology. This may lead to left upper quadrant pain. See **Table 21.7** for a broad differential diagnosis of left upper quadrant pain.

Acute gastric dilatation, a functional response to major thoracic and upper abdominal surgery or trauma, produces a clinical picture much like mechanical obstruction. Both entities appear as a large, left upper quadrant air-fluid level that outlines the distended stomach on a plain upright abdominal radiograph.

In most cases of gastric dilatation or obstruction, relief can be obtained by decompression of the stomach with a nasogastric tube. Subsequent management depends on etiologic factors that can be assessed with esophagogastric endoscopy. Surgical resection or bypass of the obstructed area is required to relieve most cases of neoplastic or postinflammatory fixed fibrotic stenosis.

The intraperitoneal small intestine distal to the duodenum is the most common site for obstruction of the alimentary tract. The most common causes are bowel entrapment by extravisceral pathology, e.g., adhesions, hernias, or secondary intraperitoneal neoplasms. Most often, a loop of bowel is ensnared within a narrow aperture created by a strategically positioned fibrotic adhesive or congenital band. Similarly, it may be trapped in the neck of an abdominal wall or intraperitoneal hernia. This often creates obstruction at two points: at

Table 21.7. Differential diagnosis of left upper quadrant abdominal pain.

Gastritis	Herpes zoster
Pancreatitis	Myocardial ischemia
Splenic enlargement	Pneumonia
Splenic rupture	Empyema
Splenic infarct	Diverticulitis
Splenic aneurysm	Intestinal obstruction
Pyelonephritis	Inflammatory bowel disease
Nephrolithiasis	

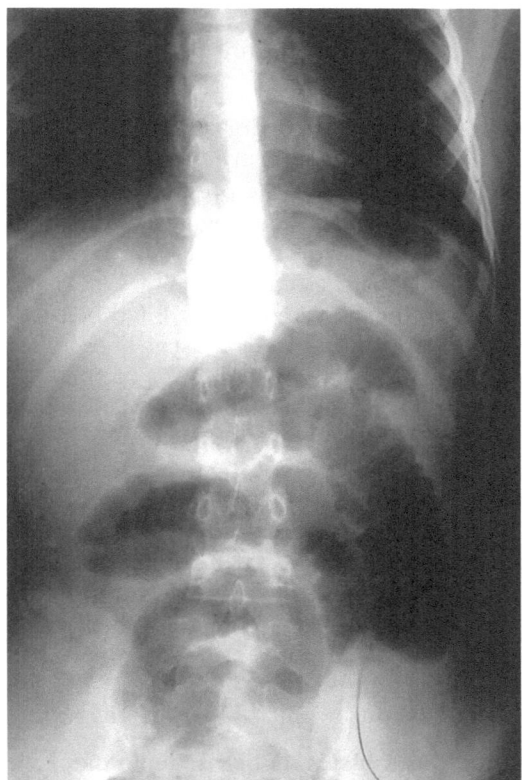

Figure 21.8. X-ray of a small bowel obstruction. A 67-year-old woman presented with vomiting, abdominal pain, and distention. She had a previous appendectomy and hysterectomy. Erect abdominal radiograph shows dilated small bowel with air-fluid levels. There is no air in the colon. These findings are consistent with a small-bowel obstruction.

the entrance and exit sites of the obstructed loop. Unable to empty in either direction, the "closed loop" and its compressed mesentery experience vascular compromise, first venous with resultant congestion and edema, and finally, if unrelieved, arterial with ischemia and necrosis. Air-fluid levels are typically seen on abdominal radiographs (**Fig. 21.8**).

Clinically, **intestinal obstruction** is characterized by the onset of colicky midabdominal pain and vomiting. Vomiting may precede the pain, especially if the site of obstruction is high. The abdomen becomes distended, and the patient is unable to eat. Cessation of bowel movements and flatus usually follow. The abdomen usually is firm if there is significant bowel distention, but initially there is little or no direct tenderness or true abdominal wall guarding. Firm pressure on distended loops of bowel, however, creates a sense of discomfort not to be confused with real tenderness. Bowel sounds are hyperactive, high pitched, and interlaced with gurgling, rumbling, and tinklings.

In the presence of obstruction, an abdominal surgical scar suggests a possible obstructing adhesive band. A tender, irreducible abdominal wall hernia or palpable intraabdominal mass may represent an incarceration, possibly ischemic closed loop of bowel, while ascites or a non-tender firm umbilical or deep mass implies a malignant etiology.

Case Discussion

The woman in **Case 4** has had a prior abdominal operation and now presents with evidence of bowel obstruction. Small-bowel obstruction as a result of adhesions caused by a previous operation is likely. She needs to have fluid resuscitation, a nasogastric tube for decompression of the stomach, and further workup to help determine if she requires an operation. After an obstructive series or CT scan, some pertinent questions that need to be answered are outlined below.

A radiographic obstructive series or CT scan should be obtained, and it usually demonstrates dilated erectile loops of small bowel with air-fluid levels. Air-fluid levels are absent in a small percentage of cases when the bowel contains fluid but little gas or when the obstruction is high in the small bowel and most of the intestine distal to the obstruction is collapsed. If gas is seen in the colon, it suggests an incomplete mechanical obstruction, a functional ileus, or that air has been introduced into the rectum during rectal examination or enema. Partial obstruction may be treated with intestinal decompression and IV fluid. See **Table 21.8** for the success rates of using a short versus a long tube for decompression. Associated free intraabdominal air is an ominous sign, usually indicative of bowel perforation.

The key clinical questions in this setting are the following:

1. Is this mechanical intestinal obstruction a paralytic ileus or gastroenteritis masquerading as obstruction? With ileus, there usually is an identifiable inciting event that has initiated the ileus, and bowel sounds are diminished markedly or absent from the onset. With gastroenteritis, the irritative hyperperistalsis usually produces diarrhea as opposed to the obstipation seen with mechanical obstruction.

Table 21.8. Success rates for standard (short) versus long intestinal tubes in patients with small-bowel obstruction.

| Author | Randomized | Required surgery | | *p* value |
		Short tube	Long tube	
Fleshner[a]	Yes	38/28 (46%)	8/27 (30%)	NS
Brolin[b]	No	80/184 (43%)	83/145 (57%)	NS
Bizer[c]	No	48/91 (53%)	76/154 (49%)	NS

[a] Fleshner P, Siegman M, Slater G, Brolin R, Chandler J, Autses AJ. A prospective randomized trial of short versus long tubes in adhesive small bowel obstruction. Am J Surg 1995;170:366–370.
[b] Brolin R, Krasna M, Mast B. Use of tubes and radiographs in the management of small bowel obstruction. Ann Surg 1987;206:126–133.
[c] Bizer L, Leibling R, Delaney H, Gliedman M. Small bowel obstruction: the role of nonoperative treatment in simple intestinal obstruction and predictive criteria for strangulation obstruction. Surgery (St. Louis) 1981;89:407–413.
Source: Reprinted from Hodin RA, Matthews JB. Small intestine. In: Norton JA, Bollinger RR, Chang AE, et al, eds. Surgery: Basic Science and Clinical Evidence. New York: Springer-Verlag, 2001, with permission.

2. If the obstruction is mechanical, is it complete or incomplete? If complete, the patient is not passing flatus, and gas is not seen within the colon radiographically. A first-time presentation of complete small-bowel obstruction in a previously healthy patient generally requires prompt surgical intervention to achieve the best outcome. Incomplete obstruction, especially when recurrent or presenting as an early complication of abdominal surgery, often responds to nonoperative management using nasogastric decompression. Uncertainty as to whether one is dealing with a complete mechanical obstruction can be answered with an upper gastrointestinal x-ray study using contrast material. With incomplete obstruction, ileus, or gastroenteritis, the contrast material ultimately reaches the colon.

3. At what level is the site of obstruction: is it in the large bowel or the small bowel? Primary carcinoma is the cause of approximately 80% of cases of large-bowel obstruction. The ileocecal valve is competent in most, and gaseous distention is confined between the ileocecal valve and the distal point of colonic obstruction. This produces a nonventable closed loop obstruction of sorts, with a propensity for ischemic necrosis at the widest portion, the tense cecal wall. Large-bowel obstruction in the presence of an incompetent ileocecal valve presents with gas in the small bowel, as well as with a distended gas-filled colon. Conversely, an obstructing lesion of the cecum at the ileocecal valve radiographically appears like a distal small-bowel obstruction. Pain is irregularly colicky or constant and intensifies as wall tension increases. Less common causes of large-bowel obstruction are cecal and sigmoid volvulus, postinflammatory stricture, and fecal impaction. Colorectal obstruction produces the most dramatic degree of gaseous bowel distention. When incomplete, the patient experiences cramps, constipation, or diarrhea and may note a narrowing of stool caliber. Complete obstruction then may develop suddenly, with rapid onset of obstipation and massive dilatation of the colon.

4. Is there vascular compromise of the obstructed bowel? Paramount in the management of an intestinal obstruction is avoidance of ischemic necrosis. Early signs of compromise either are absent or vague and nonspecific. Late signs are the transformation of hyperactive bowel sounds into a quiet abdomen, the transformation of colicky pain into severe constant pain sometimes radiating to the back, and palpation of a tender mass or abdominal wall tenderness and guarding. The systemic findings of significant fever, tachycardia, leukocytosis, and an increasing metabolic acidosis warn that ischemia already is well advanced and surgical intervention may be too late to avoid serious complications. **The admonition "the sun should never be allowed to rise or set on an untreated intestinal obstruction," although overstated, arises from the fact that impending necrosis is difficult to diagnose and delay may be fatal.** By comparison, early surgical intervention, where only the cutting of adhesions or release of an incarcerated hernia may be necessary, is considerably less risky and to the patient's advantage.

Abdominal Pain of Uncertain Cause

In the main, **transient, mild abdominal pain** is self-limited or managed by the patient with over-the-counter remedies. **When the pain is severe or prolonged enough for the patient to seek the care of a physician, the physician must decide whether to observe and treat the patient in an ambulatory setting or refer the patient to a specialist or hospital emergency staff for further management.** The absence of signs of peritonitis, sepsis, or hemodynamic instability in a reliable patient with bearable or controllable pain would allow for the former as long as the home situation is secure.

If these criteria are not met or an acute surgical abdomen is suspected, a hospital setting is essential. This allows for continuous monitoring by medical professionals, advanced diagnostic testing, and, if required, surgical or critical care management.

When **infection** is suspected, **empiric antibiotics** based on the presumed pathogens are the first step in treatment. Second-, third-, and fourth-generation cephalosporins, quinolones, and extended spectrum semisynthetic penicillins in combination with β-lactamase inhibitors are directed at gram-negative rods. Many of these agents provide anaerobic coverage as well. For those that do not, e.g., aminoglycosides, specific antianaerobic antibiotics such as metronidazole and clindamycin may be added.

Because of the rapid and pervasive development of resistance to commonly used antibiotics by extended spectrum β-lactamase–producing gram-negative organisms and many gram-positive pathogens (*Staphylococcus* and *Enterococcus*) and fungal overgrowth, antibiotic selection should be guided by the susceptibility experience of the specific medical institution's microbiology department. This is particularly important for hospital-acquired nosocomial infections. As bacterial resistance renders more of current antibiotics ineffective and new classes of antibiotics are developed, the spectrum of usable, effective agents will continue to change.

Nonsurgical Causes of Abdominal Pain

After clinical assessment, most causes of abdominal pain prove not to require surgery, although some mimic surgical problems and pose a diagnostic dilemma.

The most prevalent causes of abdominal pain are transient functional visceral episodes due to dietary indiscretions, minor undiagnosed infections, and psychosomatic factors. Many patients experience **poorly understood chronic conditions,** such as the irritable bowel syndrome with recurrent episodes of bowel dysmotility and pain. They rarely are considered for surgery.

Abdominal pain as a result of primary peritonitis is relatively rare. Caused by direct blood-borne bacterial infection of the peritoneum, it is seen primarily in children or cirrhotic patients with ascites. **Tuberculous peritonitis** is seen occasionally in this country in patients who are recent immigrants from endemic areas. **Patients receiving peritoneal dialysis develop peritonitis** due to lapses in sterile technique and may require temporary suspension of this treatment and removal of their percutaneous intraabdominal catheter. These patients usually respond to microbiologic examination of aspirated intraperitoneal fluid and culture-directed antibiotic therapy.

Acquired viral infections that affect intraabdominal organs are the multiple forms of viral hepatitis and gastroenteritis. Intercurrent viral infections in children and young adults often also induce **mesenteric lymphadenitis**, which can simulate appendicitis. Bacterial causes of **acquired enterocolitis** are most commonly toxigenic *Escherichia coli, Campylobacter, Salmonella*, and *Shigella*, which cause severe diarrhea as well as crampy pain. Similar symptomatology occurs in **nosocomial antibiotic-related *C. difficile* colitis and the opportunistic infections seen in immunocompromised AIDS patients**. With international travel commonplace today, **endemic agents from around the world**, such as *Entamoeba histolytica, Echinococcus*, protozoa, helminths, and other uncommon organisms, may be encountered as causes of abdominal pain.

Etiologically, **multifactorial erosive and inflammatory disease of the alimentary tract such as gastritis and gastroduodenal ulcer disease, Crohn's enteritis, and ulcerative colitis** require surgery only when intractable or complicated.

Ingestible causes of pain include staphylococcal toxin and other forms of food poisoning; the toxic heavy metals lead, mercury, and arsenic; excessive amount of alcohol; certain medicinal and illicit drugs, and food allergens. **Venomous snake or spider bites** also can cause abdominal pain.

Painful maldigestive syndromes are produced by pancreatic insufficiency, sprue, gluten intolerance, and lactase deficiency.

There are a number of **systemic metabolic disorders** that may include diagnostically ambiguous abdominal pain in their symptomatology. Among these are glutocorticoid deficiency induced by Addison's disease or iatrogenic acute steroid withdrawal, severe hypercalcemia, uremia, and diabetic ketoacidosis.

Autoimmune collagen vascular diseases and other forms of vasculitis may affect adversely the perfusion and ultimately the function of intraabdominal organs. Classically, periarteritis nodosa produces focal ischemic changes, systemic sclerosis, and peristaltic dysfunction. In children, Henoch-Schölein purpura produces a purpuric skin rash as well as abdominal and joint pain.

Sickle cell anemia is the most frequent of the several genetic disorders that can produce diagnostically confusing abdominal pain. Because pigmented gallstones are frequent in these patients, the differential diagnosis often is between acute cholecystitis and a nonsurgical ischemic crisis. The character of repetitive attacks is specific for individual patients, which is a useful diagnostic feature of sickle cell crisis.

Hematologic and infectious disorders, which cause splenomegaly, splenic softening, infarction, and rupture, also may be the etiology for upper abdominal pain. Among the most common are mononucleosis, malaria, hemolytic anemia, leukemia, and other myeloproliferative disorders.

Porphyria is an autosomal-dominant disorder causing defective heme synthesis productive of neurotoxic porphyrins. These patients experience abdominal pain, ileus, muscle weakness, photosensitivity, and psychiatric disturbances. The diagnosis is made by identifying the offending porphyrins in the blood and urine.

Familial Mediterranean fever is a rarely encountered autosomal-recessive disorder. It is characterized by recurrent attacks of abdominal pain, fever, and signs of peritoneal inflammation indistinguishable from an acute surgical abdomen. A strong family history is a clue to the diagnosis.

Rectus sheath hematoma presents as a painful, tender mass in the caudal region of the rectus muscles. It often occurs after minimal trauma, especially in anticoagulated patients. To ascertain whether the mass is intraabdominal or within the abdominal wall, the recumbent patient is asked to tense the abdominal wall musculature by raising the head. If the mass remains palpable, it probably is within the abdominal wall. Computed tomography scan of the area confirms the diagnosis. Although many rectus sheath hematomas are self-limiting and absorb spontaneously, those that are very large or expanding require surgical evacuation and hemostasis. Abdominal wall tumors and hernias usually require surgical treatment as well.

Neurogenic pain can arise from radiculopathy affecting the anterior abdominal wall dermatomes, T7 to L1, due to compression of nerve roots by a disk tumor, infection, or hematoma. Herpes zoster, varicellar viral nerve infection, occurs frequently in older adults and immunosuppressed patients, producing severe burning pain in a dermatomal distribution. It is difficult to diagnose before the typical pox-like eruption appears. Painful peripheral nerve entrapment can complicate abdominal hernias and surgical scars. The diagnosis is made by extinguishing the typical burning pain by injection of a local anesthetic into the trigger zone. Abdominal epilepsy and syphilitic tabes dorsalis are rare central nervous system causes of abdominal pain.

Anatomic structures adjacent to the abdominal cavity may refer pain that is misinterpreted as intraabdominal in origin. Thoracic pain from basilar pleuritis or pericarditis due to pneumonia, pulmonary, or myocardial infarction may mimic subdiaphragmatic pathology. Conversely, subdiaphragmatic pathology, such as gastroesophageal reflux and choledochal disease, may suggest myocardial ischemia and other intrathoracic disorders. A classic example of distal referral from an abdominal pain source is pain felt at the root of the ipsilateral neck due to diaphragmatic irritation. This occurs because the phrenic nerve contains nerve fibers from the cervical 3 and 4 roots that also innervate the neck.

In the lower abdomen, **extraperitoneal pelvic and perineal pathology** may masquerade as intraperitoneal disease.

Clinical awareness of these diagnostic pitfalls and appropriate imaging studies usually lead to the correct diagnostic conclusions and avoidance of nonindicated surgery.

Summary

The list of disease processes that cause abdominal pain is extensive. Most of these maladies never require surgery; however, recognizing when emergent, urgent, or elective operative intervention is required is a necessary skill for general surgeons and most physicians. Starting with a directed history of the nature of the pain and the associated symptoms, one can begin to formulate a differential diagnosis. The past medical and surgical history often provides additional clues as well as a picture of the patient's overall condition. The physical exam is critical. Understanding that the rigid abdomen seen with free air and the involuntary guarding seen with peritoneal irritation are signs of surgical emergencies is the first step. Further refinement of diagnostic skills comes with the number of abdominal exams one performs. The history and physical combined with laboratory and imaging studies usually provide enough information to determine if the patient has a catastrophic abdominal emergency, an urgent surgical condition, an elective surgical condition, or a nonsurgical condition.

Selected Readings

Balthazar EJ. Imaging of the acute abdomen. Radiol Clin North Am 2003;41(6).

Burns BJ. Intestinal ischemia. Gastroenterol Clin 2003;32(4).

Cohn DE, Rader JS. Gynecology. In: Norton JA, Bollinger RR, Chang AE, et al, eds. Surgery: Basic Science and Clinical Evidence. New York: Springer-Verlag, 2001.

Harris HW. Biliary system. In: Norton JA, Bollinger RR, Chang AE, et al, eds. Surgery: Basic Science and Clinical Evidence. New York: Springer-Verlag, 2001.

Hemming A, Gallinger S. Liver. In: Norton JA, Bollinger RR, Chang AE, et al, eds. Surgery: Basic Science and Clinical Evidence. New York: Springer-Verlag, 2001.

Hodin RA, Matthews JB. Small intestine. In: Norton JA, Bollinger RR, Chang AE, et al, eds. Surgery: Basic Science and Clinical Evidence. New York: Springer-Verlag, 2001.

Lefor AT, Phillips EH. Spleen. In: Norton JA, Bollinger RR, Chang AE, et al, eds. Surgery: Basic Science and Clinical Evidence. New York: Springer-Verlag, 2001.

Livingston EH. Stomach and duodenum. In: Norton JA, Bollinger RR, Chang AE, et al, eds. Surgery: Basic Science and Clinical Evidence. New York: Springer-Verlag, 2001.

Mulvihill SJ. Pancreas. In: Norton JA, Bollinger RR, Chang AE, et al, eds. Surgery: Basic Science and Clinical Evidence. New York: Springer-Verlag, 2001.

Schecter WP. Peritoneum and acute abdomen. In: Norton JA, Bollinger RR, Chang AE, et al, eds. Surgery: Basic Science and Clinical Evidence. New York: Springer-Verlag, 2001.

Scott DJ, Jones DB. Hernia and abdominal wall defects. In: Norton JA, Bollinger RR, Chang AE, et al, eds. Surgery: Basic Science and Clinical Evidence. New York: Springer-Verlag, 2001.

Silen W. Copes' Early Diagnosis of the Acute Abdomen, 19th ed. New York: Oxford University Press, 1995.

Soybel DI. Appendix. In: Norton JA, Bollinger RR, Chang AE, et al, eds. Surgery: Basic Science and Clinical Evidence. New York: Springer-Verlag, 2001.

Welton ML, Varma MG, Amerhauser A. Colon, rectum, and anus. In: Norton JA, Bollinger RR, Chang AE, et al, eds. Surgery: Basic Science and Clinical Evidence. New York: Springer-Verlag, 2001.

Abdominal Masses: Solid Organs and Gastrointestinal

Thomas J. Kearney

Objectives

1. To describe the causes of hepatomegaly; to discuss the role of imaging and liver biopsy; to discuss the most frequently encountered benign and malignant liver masses and their management.
2. To describe the differential diagnosis of a pancreatic mass; to discuss the most useful imaging studies and the role of biopsy.
3. To understand the relationship of the pancreatic duct to the common bile duct and how this may affect the diagnosis and treatment of a pancreatic mass; to discuss the management of cysts of the pancreas.
4. To describe the causes of hypersplenism; to discuss the common signs and symptoms of hypersplenism and contrast with splenomegaly; to discuss the role and consequences of splenectomy in the treatment of splenic disease.
5. To discuss the most frequently encountered retroperitoneal masses; to contrast the management of lymphomas and sarcomas.

Cases

Case 1

A 46-year-old male police officer noticed mild pressure in his abdomen when he bent to tie his shoes. His colleagues teased him that he was getting fat. However, he had not gained any weight. Further questioning revealed early satiety, and physical examination revealed a large epigastric mass that was firm but not hard. It was not tender. A computed tomography (CT) scan was ordered.

Case 2

A 72-year-old woman presented to the hospital with hematemesis. She had noticed a 10-pound weight loss and early satiety over the past month. She denied changes in her bowel habits or jaundice. Physical examination revealed a midline epigastric mass along with an enlarged spleen. Neither was tender. A CT scan was ordered.

Case 3

A 22-year-old man complained of bleeding gums and epistaxis. Examination was otherwise unremarkable. He did not have a left upper quadrant mass. Platelet count was 15,000/μL.

Case 4

A 48-year-old man presented with increasing abdominal girth and decreased appetite. Examination revealed a large left-sided mass. A CT scan revealed a large mass in the retroperitoneum with fat density.

Case 5

A 45-year-old man presented with intermittent nausea and blood in his stools. Examination revealed a mass in the midabdomen. A CT scan suggested a colon cancer that was locally advanced. Colonoscopy revealed a cancer.

Introduction

Abdominal masses may be caused by a large variety of pathologic conditions. All abdominal masses need to be thoroughly and expeditiously evaluated, sometimes with significant urgency. A detailed history and physical examination, combined with knowledge of normal anatomy, allow the physician to generate a reasonable differential diagnosis. Additional diagnostic tests then can be obtained. **In certain situations, notably rupturing abdominal aortic aneurysms, the physician must take the patient directly to the operating room without further testing to avoid exsanguination.**

Several classification systems are available to help guide evaluation of a patient with an abdominal mass (**Table 22.1**). Surgeons often use

Table 22.1. Classification systems for abdominal masses.

Anatomic
  Organ based
  Location
Etiology
Clinical course
  Acute
  Chronic
  Urgent

Table 22.2. Anatomic classification.

Organ based
Liver
Pancreas
Spleen
Renal
Vascular
Gastrointestinal
Connective tissue
Location based
Abdominal wall
Intraperitoneal
Pelvic
Right lower quadrant
Left lower quadrant
Mid-pelvis
Retroperitoneal
Flank
Epigastric
Right upper quadrant
Left upper quadrant

anatomic systems (**Table 22.2**). These systems can be divided into an organ-based system or a location-based system. In addition, an etiologic system (**Table 22.3**) is equally valuable and may be preferred by some. As always, **the physician must be sure the patient does not have an emergency situation requiring immediate operation**.

General Evaluation

A **detailed history** must include information about the onset of the mass (sudden vs. chronic). Incidentally discovered masses often represent neoplasms. Symptomatic and acute masses imply an infectious or inflammatory cause. Abdominal aneurysm rupture usually is sudden and acute. (See Chapter 23 for vascular abdominal masses.) Changes in size over time and symptoms associated with the gastrointestinal, hepatobiliary, urinary, or gynecologic systems can provide clues to the

Table 22.3. Etiologic classification.

Neoplastic
Benign
Malignant
Primary
Metastatic
Infectious
Bacterial
Parasitic
Fungal
Traumatic
Inflammatory
Congenital
Degenerative

nature of the mass. These symptoms could include nausea, vomiting, diarrhea, melena, jaundice, vaginal bleeding, and hematuria. The physician should ask about the presence of pain along with details about pain quality, location, radiation, timing, severity, and factors that alleviate or exacerbate the pain. Details about preexisting or chronic conditions are required.

Physical examination should include an evaluation of the patient's general status, including vital signs and any evidence of impending cardiac or respiratory collapse. Try to identify the general location of the mass. Contour and texture (hard, fluctuant) provide clues to the diagnosis. Evidence of bowel perforation, such as diffuse abdominal tenderness or tympany from free air, should be sought. Examination of the chest as well as rectal and pelvic examination are essential. Masses that are tender and associated with signs of sepsis (fever, hypotension) or masses associated with perforation require urgent evaluation.

Upon completion of the history and physical examination, the physician usually knows if urgent evaluation and treatment are needed or if more leisurely evaluation is safe. In nonurgent situations, radiologic evaluation plays a key role. Plain radiographs of the chest and abdomen combined with **basic laboratory evaluation** (complete blood count with differential, electrolytes, renal and liver function, urinalysis, pregnancy test) are the first steps in further evaluation. The plain radiographs should include a flat and upright abdominal film along with posteroanterior and lateral chest radiographs. These films detect signs of perforation or obstruction as well as mass effect.

After initial evaluation, **the probable site of abnormality guides further workup**. Findings suggestive of gastric or colonic disease would lead to endoscopic evaluation or possibly gastrointestinal (GI) contrast studies. If a CT scan is contemplated, it must be performed prior to GI contrast studies. Masses of the uterus and ovaries usually are evaluated initially with ultrasound, either transabdominal or transvaginal. Ultrasound also is useful for suspected biliary disease as well as for evaluation of nonurgent abdominal aortic aneurysms. Masses of the solid organs (liver, spleen, and pancreas) or the retroperitoneum require CT scan, almost always with oral and intravenous contrast. Magnetic resonance imaging (MRI) is useful for further characterization of some solid organ masses. Intravenous pyelography (IVP) is useful for evaluation of the urinary system. Cystoscopy is useful for bladder evaluation and should be included in any evaluation of hematuria. Radionuclide imaging is less used than previously due to the excellent anatomic detail available from modern CT scanning. Angiography occasionally is used in the evaluation of operative approaches for abdominal masses. Magnetic resonance angiography is an evolving technique that may provide similar information less invasively than angiography.

Liver Masses

Liver masses may present with symptoms or may be discovered incidentally on scans done for other reasons. Multiple causes are possible (**Table 22.4**). Pain usually is dull, aching, and fairly constant. Fever and

Table 22.4. Liver masses.

Tumors	Cysts	Abscesses
Benign	Acquired	Pyogenic
Hemangioma	Parasitic (hydatid)	
Adenoma	Traumatic	
Focal nodular hyperplasia		
Malignant: primary	Congenital	Amebic
Hepatoma	Single	
Cholangiocarcinoma	Multiple	
Angiosarcoma		
Malignant: metastatic		Fungal
Unresectable		
Resectable		

tenderness could represent an infectious etiology, such as abscess. A personal history of cancer, particularly colon and rectal cancer, could be a clue to hepatic metastases. Patients with a history of alcoholism or hepatitis leading to cirrhosis are at risk for hepatocellular cancer. The patient in **Case 1** had none of these. His occupation as a police officer may have exposed him to blunt abdominal trauma while arresting a suspect. This could lead to a hematoma, but he could not recall any particular incident. A CT scan revealed a large 12-cm hemangioma of the left lobe of the liver. The patient's symptoms were managed with mild analgesics, and the decision was made to avoid surgical resection in this patient. On follow-up the next year, size and symptoms had increased. A left hepatectomy was performed. A scheme for management of liver tumors is presented in **Algorithm 22.1**.

Tumors

Tumors of the liver can be classified as **benign or malignant. Hemangioma** is the most common benign tumor of the liver, occurring in up to 20% of patients in some autopsy series. They usually are asymptomatic and require removal only if disabling symptoms are present. The risk of rupture is quite low, even in large hemangiomas. The diagnosis can be confirmed with near certainty by an MRI or nuclear imaging studies. Other benign tumors include **hepatic adenomas** associated with oral contraceptive use in young women. Hepatic adenomas that are symptomatic or larger than 5 cm usually are removed due to the 10% to 20% chance of subsequent rupture. **Focal nodular hyperplasia (FNH)** of the liver also usually is asymptomatic. It is not associated with oral contraceptives, and the etiology is not clear. Resection rarely is needed.

    Malignant tumors of the liver can be either primary or secondary. In the United States, metastatic liver tumors are 20 times as common as primary tumors. **Almost every cancer site can metastasize to the liver, and liver metastases represent systemic disease. Only in the specific setting of colon and rectal cancer can liver metastases potentially represent regional disease without systemic spread.** Patients with one or several metastases technically amenable to resection and no sign of systemic disease can expect a 25% to 35% 5-year survival

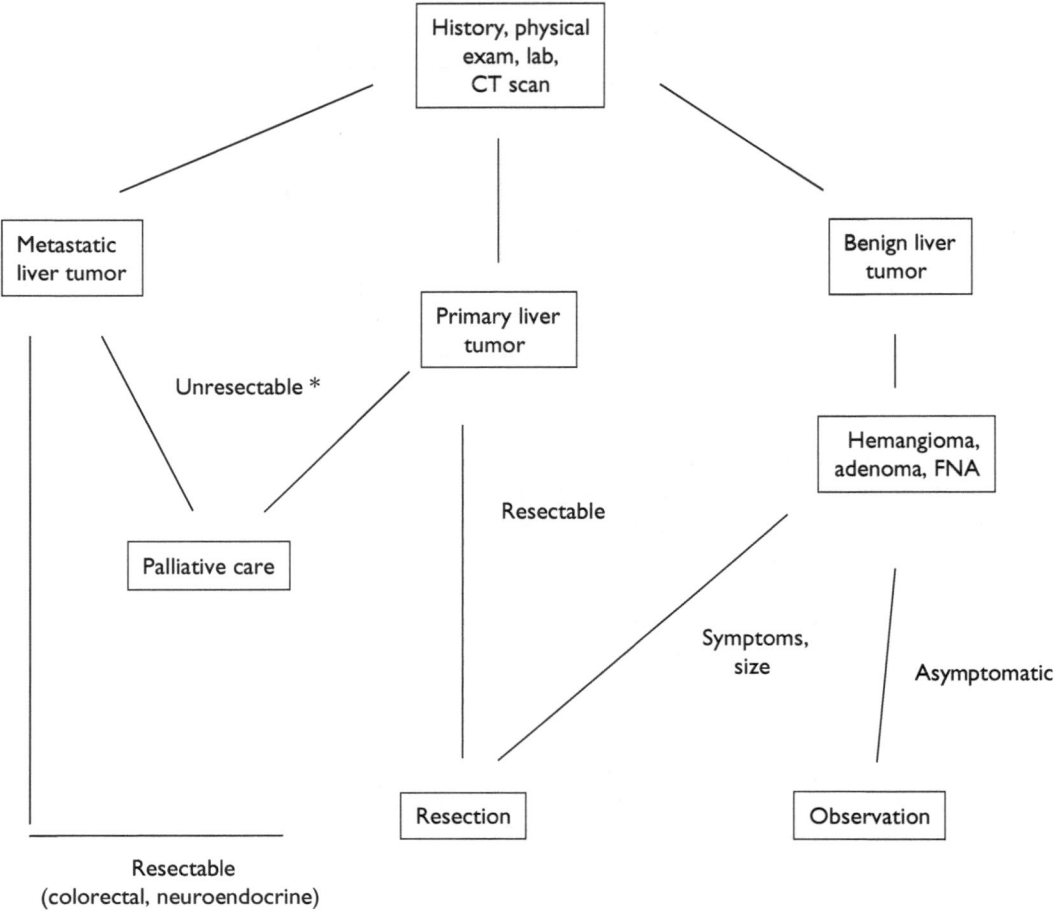

* Consider ablation (thermal, cryo) in selected cases

Algorithm 22.1. Algorithm for evaluation and treatment of liver tumors. FNA, fine-needle aspiration.

(**Table 22.5**). Most patients' metastases are not resectable. Patients with symptomatic liver metastases from neuroendocrine tumors also benefit from liver resection even if this is not curative.

Primary malignant liver tumors are rare in the United States, but worldwide these represent a significant cancer burden. **Hepatocellular carcinoma** (also known as hepatoma) usually arises in patients with cirrhosis. Patients present with abdominal pain, weight loss, and jaundice. The underlying parenchymal liver disease severely limits the ability to safely perform liver resection in most patients. Patients able to have resection can have 5-year survival exceeding 25%. Patients undergoing liver transplantation for end-stage liver disease sometimes have incidentally discovered small hepatomas. The prognosis for these patients is much better. Other forms of primary liver tumors include **intrahepatic cholangiocarcinoma and angiosarcoma.** Patients with unresectable and incurable liver tumors do not benefit from surgery. The diagnosis usually can be obtained with core needle biopsy or fine-needle aspiration. Occasionally, biopsy requires laparoscopic or open surgical techniques, but this situation is rare.

Cysts

Hepatic cysts can be classified as acquired or congenital. Acquired cysts usually are either parasitic or posttraumatic. In South American or Mediterranean countries and Australia, echinococcal (hydatid) cysts are prevalent. Patients present with symptoms of abdominal pain.

Table 22.5. Five-year survival following liver resection for colorectal cancer metastases.

Number of cases	5-Year survival (%)	Comments	Reference (year, location)
56	25		Cobourn et al[a] (1987, Toronto)
859	33	Summary data from 24 institutions	Hughes et al[b] (1988, Sacramento)
100	30		Doci et al[c] (1991, Milan)
266	31		Scheele et al[d] (1991, Erlangen)
280	25		Rosen et al[e] (1992, Rochester)
204	32		Gayowski et al[f] (1994, Pittsburgh)
81	32		Yasui et al[g] (1997, Nagoya)
456	38	6-year consecutive series	Fong et al[h] (1997, New York)
123	34		Taylor et al[i] (1997, Toronto)
94	30	Only include 94 of 231 reported cases with definite negative margins	Ambiru et al[j] (1998, Chiba)
111	25	25-year consecutive series	Ohlsson et al[k] (1998, Lund)

[a] Cobourn CS, Makowka L, Langer B, et al. Examination of patient selection and outcome for hepatic resection for metastatic disease. Surg Gynecol Obstet 1987;165:239–246.

[b] Hughes KS, Simon R, Songhorabodi S, et al. Resection of the liver of colorectal carcinoma metastases: a multi-institutional study of indications for resection. Surgery (St. Louis) 1988;103:278–288.

[c] Doci R, Gennari L, Bignami P, et al. One hundred patients with hepatic metastases from colorectal cancer treated by resection: analysis of prognostic determinants. Br J Surg 1991;78:797–801.

[d] Scheele J, Stangl R, Altendorf-Hofman A, et al. Indicators of prognosis after hepatic resection for colorectal secondaries. Surgery (St. Louis) 1991;110:13–29.

[e] Rosen CB, Nagorney DM, Taswell HF, et al. Perioperative blood transfusion and determinants of survival after liver resection for metastatic colorectal carcinoma. Ann Surg 1992;216:493–505.

[f] Gayowski TJ, Iwastsuki S, Madariaga JR, et al. Experience in hepatic resection for metastatic colorectal cancer: analysis of clinical and pathologic risk factors. Surgery (St. Louis) 1994;116:703–711.

[g] Yasui K, Hirai T, Kato T, et al. A new macroscopic classification predicts prognosis for patient with liver metastases from colorectal cancer. Ann Surg 1997;226:582–586.

[h] Fong Y, Kemeny N, Paty P, et al. Treatment of colorectal cancer: hepatic metastasis. Semin Surg Oncol 1996;12:219–252.

[i] Taylor M, Forster J, Langer B, et al. A study of prognostic factors for hepatic resection for colorectal metastases. Am J Surg 1997;173:467–471.

[j] Ambiru S, Miyazaki M, Ito H, et al. Resection of hepatic and pulmonary metastases in patients with colorectal carcinoma. Cancer (Phila) 1998;82:274–278.

[k] Ohlsson B, Stenram U, Tranberg K-G. Resection of colorectal liver metastases: 25-year experience. World J Surg 1998;22:268–277.

Source: Reprinted from Hemming A, Gallinger S. Liver. In: Norton JA, Bollinger RR, Chang AE, et al, eds. Surgery: Basic Science and Clinical Evidence. New York: Springer-Verlag, 2001, with permission.

Eosinophilia is common. A calcified cyst often can be seen on plain radiography. Treatment requires excision of the cyst, with special care taken to avoid spillage of the parasitic contents. Traumatic cysts lack an epithelial lining, and thus they are not true cysts. They represent hemorrhage into the liver parenchyma following significant trauma. Management is conservative observation.

Congenital cysts usually are single, but they may be multiple. They usually are asymptomatic. Patients with multiple cysts often have polycystic kidneys as well. Treatment rarely is required. Rare cases of cystic neoplasms of the liver have been reported.

Abscess

The final category of liver mass is the **hepatic abscess**. **Pyogenic bacterial abscess** usually follows an episode of biliary or gastrointestinal tract sepsis. Patients have fever and rigors. Treatment requires percutaneous drainage and antibiotics. **Amebic abscess** presents with similar findings. Treatment with metronidazole is effective, and drainage is required only in complicated cases. **Fungal abscess** usually is associated with immunosuppression.

Pancreatic Masses

In **Case 2**, the patient's history and examination immediately do not suggest the cause of her problem. A CT scan revealed an enlarged spleen along with a heterogeneous mass posterior to the stomach. The head and body of the pancreas were well visualized, but the tail seemed to blend into the mass. The mass did not appear to invade surrounding structures and radiographically appeared resectable. To further evaluate the pancreatic mass, endoscopic retrograde cholangiopancreatography (ERCP) was performed. The bile duct was normal, as was most of the pancreatic duct. The pancreatic duct in the tail of the pancreas did not communicate with the mass, but it was displaced caudally. The patient underwent a distal pancreatectomy. Pathology revealed a cystadenoma of the pancreas.

The **presentation of a pancreatic mass is dependent on the location and nature of the mass**. Masses in the head of the pancreas (usually neoplasms) obstruct the common bile duct due to proximity. These patients present with obstructive jaundice, and the masses tend to be only a few centimeters in diameter. Neoplasms in the body or tail of the pancreas grow larger and cause symptoms by impinging on surrounding structures. In this case, the mass had caused splenic vein thrombosis, leading to bleeding gastric varices from left-sided portal hypertension. The mass effect on the posterior stomach led to early satiety and weight loss. Pancreatic enlargement associated with pancreatitis usually involves signs of systemic inflammation. Patients with pancreatic pseudocysts usually have a past history of pancreatitis. An algorithm for the evaluation and treatment of pancreatic masses is presented in **Algorithm 22.2**.

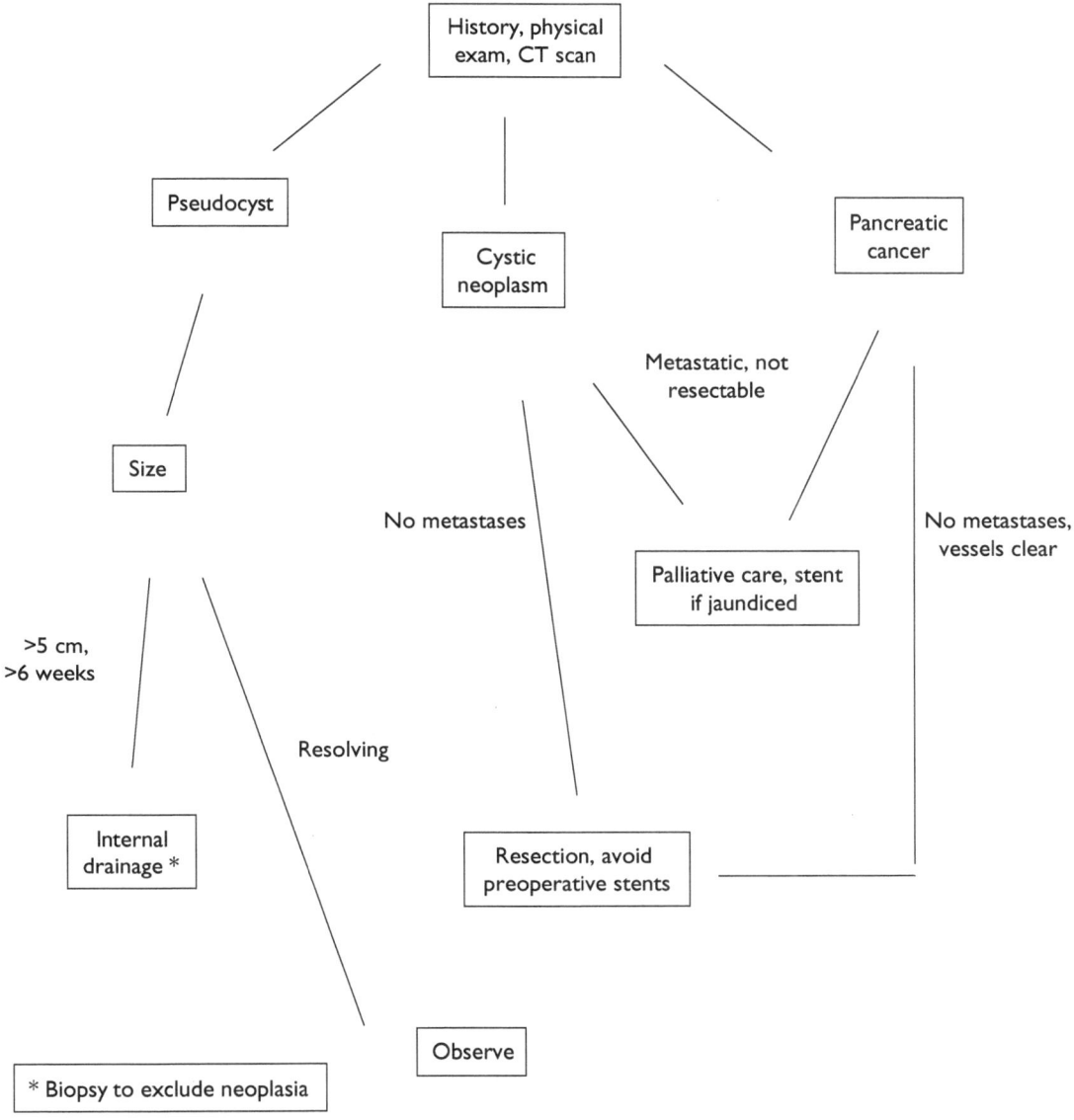

Algorithm 22.2. Algorithm for evaluation and treatment of pancreatic tumors.

Tumors

Solid pancreatic masses almost always represent neoplasia. Almost all pancreatic tumors are malignant. Classically, tumors of the body and tail of the pancreas grow silently and eventually produce symptoms by invasion of surrounding organs. They almost never are resectable. **Confirmation of the diagnosis can be made with percutaneous fine-needle aspiration guided by ultrasound or CT.**

Tumors of the head of the pancreas occasionally come to attention earlier due to the development of obstructive jaundice. The proximity of the common bile duct to the head of the pancreas allows small pancreatic tumors the opportunity to obstruct the bile duct. This causes symptoms when the pancreatic tumor is still small. **A patient with painless obstructive jaundice should be assumed to have pancreatic cancer until proven otherwise.** A small proportion of such patients (15%) have no evidence of systemic disease on imaging. These patients are candidates for curative pancreaticoduodenectomy (Whipple procedure). **Patients with potentially resectable cancers of the head of the pancreas should not undergo percutaneous needle biopsy.** This procedure may risk seeding the abdominal cavity and eliminating a chance of cure. The techniques of pancreatic surgery are advanced enough that mortality rates should be under 3% at specialized centers.

Occasionally, an intraoperative diagnosis of pancreatic cancer cannot be made. If the tumor is technically resectable, the surgeon must be prepared to perform definitive resection without a tissue diagnosis. Five-year survival may be as high as 20% with truly localized disease resected with a negative margin and combined with adjuvant therapy.

Pseudocysts and Cystic Tumors

Some pancreatic masses are cystic in nature. The differential diagnosis is between a true cystic neoplasm and a pancreatic pseudocyst. **Cystic neoplasms can be benign cystadenomas or malignant cystadenocarcinomas. Pancreatic pseudocysts arise in the setting of pancreatitis.**

Persistent pain and the development of an abdominal mass following a bout of acute pancreatitis should raise suspicion about a pseudocyst. **About one third to one half of acute pseudocysts resolve spontaneously within about 6 weeks.** Pseudocysts that are present longer than 6 weeks are termed chronic pseudocysts. Those that become chronic can be observed if small and asymptomatic. Chronic pseudocysts with symptoms of pain, obstruction, and infection usually require treatment. **Various treatment options exist, including external percutaneous drainage, internal endoscopic drainage (cystogastrostomy), and internal surgical drainage (cystogastrostomy or cystojejunostomy).** Percutaneous drainage works well for some patients, but, when the technique fails, the patient often has a complicated course. Endoscopic drainage is relatively new. Surgical drainage is the gold standard with recurrence rates less than 10%. Surgical drainage allows for biopsy of the pseudocyst wall to exclude cystic malignancy.

Cystic neoplasms can be either benign or malignant. They account for about 20% of cystic masses of the pancreas. **The treatment for malignant cystic tumors of the pancreas is resection.** These malignant tumors have much higher cure rates with surgical resection compared to noncystic tumors. Some series report 5-year survival rates greater than 50%.

Splenomegaly

In **Case 3**, the patient has thrombocytopenia. Further testing included a bone marrow aspirate revealing an increased number of megakaryocytes. Platelet-associated immunoglobulin G (IgG) antibodies were

Table 22.6. Primary and secondary hypersplenism.

Primary	Secondary
Hereditary spherocytosis	Cirrhosis
Hemoglobinopathies (sickle cell)	Splenic vein thrombosis
Hemolytic anemia	Myeloid metaplasia
Idiopathic thrombocytopenic purpura	Chronic myelogenous leukemia
Thrombotic thrombocytopenic purpura	

present in serum. The diagnosis of idiopathic thrombocytopenic purpura (ITP) was made. The patient was treated with prednisone. Unlike 80% of patients, he did not respond. He was vaccinated against encapsulated organisms, and a laparoscopic splenectomy was performed, revealing a mildly enlarged spleen. His platelet count returned to normal.

Hypersplenism and Splenomegaly

The patient in **Case 3** had signs of **hypersplenism (increased function of the spleen)**. Although it was not appreciated on physical examination, he had mild splenomegaly. **Hypersplenism and splenomegaly are separate findings related to function and size of the spleen.** Due to the spleen's location under the left rib cage, mild enlargement often can be missed on physical examination. One of the normal functions of the spleen is to clear abnormal and aged cellular elements from the blood. **If an increased number of abnormal cells are presented to the spleen with increased destruction, the patient has primary hypersplenism. Alternatively, a patient may develop splenic enlargement due to intrinsic splenic disease that leads to secondary hypersplenism (Table 22.6).** In the case presented, the patient's spleen is inherently normal, but it has enlarged as a consequence of increased clearance of abnormal platelets.

A **variety of illnesses can lead to splenomegaly (Table 22.7)**. Malaria probably is the most common cause of splenomegaly throughout the world. A variety of bacterial, parasitic, and viral infections can lead to increased proliferation of immune system cells (e.g., mononucleosis). Sarcoidosis can lead to granulomatous enlargement of the spleen.

Table 22.7. Causes of splenomegaly.

Malaria
Granulomatous disease
Rheumatoid disease
Hematologic disorders
Cirrhosis
Lymphoma
Splenic abscess
Storage disease
Leukemia
Splenic cysts
Viral infection

Metabolic abnormalities, such as Gaucher's disease, can lead to accumulation of unmetabolized products in the spleen. A variety of hematologic disorders, such as ITP, thrombotic thrombocytopenic purpura, hereditary spherocytosis, and β-thalassemia, lead to some splenic enlargement as a consequence of primary hypersplenism. In primary hypersplenism, the spleen inherently is normal, but it enlarges in size and increases function in response to an increased work load. Disorders such as cirrhosis, portal vein obstruction, and congestive heart failure can lead to splenomegaly due to restricted venous outflow. Myeloid metaplasia (also known as myelofibrosis) leads to bone marrow failure. The spleen compensates and becomes a major site of erythropoiesis. In chronic myelogenous leukemia, massive splenomegaly can develop and lead to difficult problems with anemia. **Cysts and abscesses are rare, but they can produce splenic enlargement.** All of these situations reflect secondary hypersplenism: increased function resulting from abnormally increased size.

Splenectomy

The most common reason for splenectomy in the United States today **is splenic trauma**. The spleen is the organ most commonly injured in blunt trauma. The diagnosis is made based on the mechanism of injury and left upper quadrant pain and tenderness. Splenic injury also may be relatively asymptomatic and discovered on CT scan following blunt trauma.

The management of splenic trauma can involve observation in the stable patient. In the unstable patient, splenectomy and occasionally splenorrhaphy are used. The degree of splenic injury and the presence of associated injuries guide the surgeon to either removal or repair. The presence of splenomegaly is not an indication for elective splenectomy by itself. Rather, the underlying condition must be one that responds to splenectomy. Elective splenectomy most commonly is performed for hematologic disorders, with ITP being the most common reason in most series (**Table 22.8**). Surgical staging of Hodgkin's disease was performed in the past to help decide on treatment modalities. This technique is used less today due to the increasing use of systemic chemotherapy even in early-stage patients. In the past, open splenectomy was performed through a left upper quadrant incision. Increasingly, **laparoscopic techniques** are used to remove the spleen (**Table 22.9**). During laparoscopic splenectomy, the spleen is morcellated into fragments and removed. The size of the spleen is the primary determinant of the decision to use laparoscopic or open techniques. Laparoscopic removal is preferred if an experienced team is available.

Whether performed electively or emergently, there are some **complications** common to all splenectomies. Injury to the greater curvature of the stomach during ligation of the short gastric vessels can lead to perforation. Hemorrhage is seen in 5% of splenectomies. Atelectasis is more common following open splenectomy. Accessory splenic tissue is present in over 10% of patients and can cause relapse in some of the hematologic conditions. Overwhelming postsplenectomy infection

Table 22.8. Indications for elective splenectomy.

ITP (idiopathic thrombocytopenia purpura)
Hereditary spherocytosis
Autoimmune hemolytic anemia
Staging for Hodgkin's disease
Lymphoma
Thrombocytopenic thrombotic purpura
AIDS-related thrombocytopenia
Leukemia
Splenic abscess
Gaucher's disease
Myelofibrosis
Splenic infarct

Source: Reprinted from Lefor AT, Phillips EH. Spleen. In: Norton JA, Bollinger RR, Chang AE, et al, eds. Surgery: Basic Science and Clinical Evidence. New York: Springer-Verlag, 2001, with permission.

(OPSI) is a unique complication that can occur in about 4% of patients. Patients without spleens are particularly susceptible to infection with *Streptococcus pneumoniae, Haemophilus influenzae,* and *Neisseria meningitidis.* This complication is life threatening. **Early institution of antibiotics is needed for postsplenectomy patients who present with nonspecific flu-like symptoms to prevent progression of OPSI.** Prior to elective splenectomy and following emergent splenectomy, all patients should be vaccinated with pneumococcal vaccine to prevent OPSI.

Retroperitoneal Masses

The patient in **Case 4** had further evaluation, including a chest CT that revealed no sign of disease outside of the retroperitoneum. He underwent exploratory laparotomy with en bloc resection of the mass including the left colon, the left kidney, and the adrenal gland. Pathology review showed an intermediate-grade liposarcoma. The retroperitoneal margin was involved focally. It is common to have microscopically involved margins, even with en bloc resection of retroperitoneal sarcoma. Most patients have a recurrence. Repeat resection is indicated, since recurrences can remain low grade. Eventually, many of these low-grade sarcomas become high-grade with an increased chance of systemic (usually pulmonary) metastases.

Tumors

The differential diagnosis of retroperitoneal masses is fairly limited. **Retroperitoneal sarcomas usually are liposarcomas or leiomyosarcomas.** A CT scan and MRI can be used to assess the nature and potential resectability of retroperitoneal masses. Other potential diagnoses include **testicular tumors in men and primary germ cell tumors in both sexes**. Evaluation should include serum markers for germ cell

Table 22.9. Adult matched retrospective studies of laparoscopic versus open splenectomy for disease (level II evidence).

Reference	Procedure	n	Operating room time (min)	EBL (mL)	Spleen size (cm)	Major morbidity	Postoperative stay (days)	Total cost ($)	Operating room cost ($)
Delaitre (1997)[a]	Lap	28	183			3	5.1		
	Open	28	127			8	8.6		
	Conversion	3 (%)							
Diaz (1997)[b]	Lap	15	196 ± 71	385 ± 168		1	2.3 ± 1.5	18,015 ± 2,550	12,827 ± 2,253
	Open	15	116 ± 64	359 ± 318		2	8.8 ± 6.8	16,362 ± 8,752	4,372 ± 2,038
Smith (1996)[c]	Lap	10	261 ± 31		17	0	3.0 ± 0.5	17,071 ± 1,849	8,400 ± 720
	Open	10	131 ± 12		14.5	2	5.8 ± 0.2	13,196 ± 1,418	3,627 ± 270
	Conversion	1 (%)							

Lap: laparoscopy.

Data are mean ± SD.

Clinical studies are classified according to the design of the study and the quality of the resulting data. Class I, prospective randomized studies; class II, prospective nonrandomized studies or case-controlled retrospective studies; class III, retrospective analyses without case controls.

[a] Delaitre B, Pitre J. Laparoscopic splenectomy versus open splenectomy: a comparative study. Hepatogastroenterology 1997;44:45–49.

[b] Diaz J, Eisenstat M, Chung R. A case-controlled study of laparoscopic splenectomy. Am J Surg 1997;173:348–350.

[c] Smith CD, Meyer TA, Goretsky MJ, et al. Laparoscopic splenectomy by the lateral approach. Surgery (St. Louis) 1996;120:789–794.

Source: Reprinted from Lefor AT, Phillips EH. Spleen. In: Norton JA, Bollinger RR, Chang AE, et al, eds. Surgery: Basic Surgery and Clinical Evidence. New York: Springer-Verlag, 2001, with permission.

tumors such as β-human chorionic gonadotropin (β-HCG) and α-fetoprotein. The treatment of germ cell tumors requires systemic
chemotherapy, and surgery is not needed. **Retroperitoneal lymphoma**
also can present as an abdominal mass, although patients usually have
lymphadenopathy elsewhere. Finally, **intraabdominal spread from
other more common gastrointestinal tumors** can cause retroperitoneal
masses. An algorithm for the evaluation and treatment of retroperitoneal tumors is presented in **Algorithm 22.3**.

When retroperitoneal tumors appear unresectable or when the suspicion of lymphoma or germ cell tumor is high, **percutaneous needle
biopsy** is appropriate. **In the setting of a potentially resectable
retroperitoneal sarcoma, percutaneous biopsy can lead to tumor
seeding of the abdomen, preventing a curative resection.** Patients
with potentially resectable retroperitoneal masses should be prepared

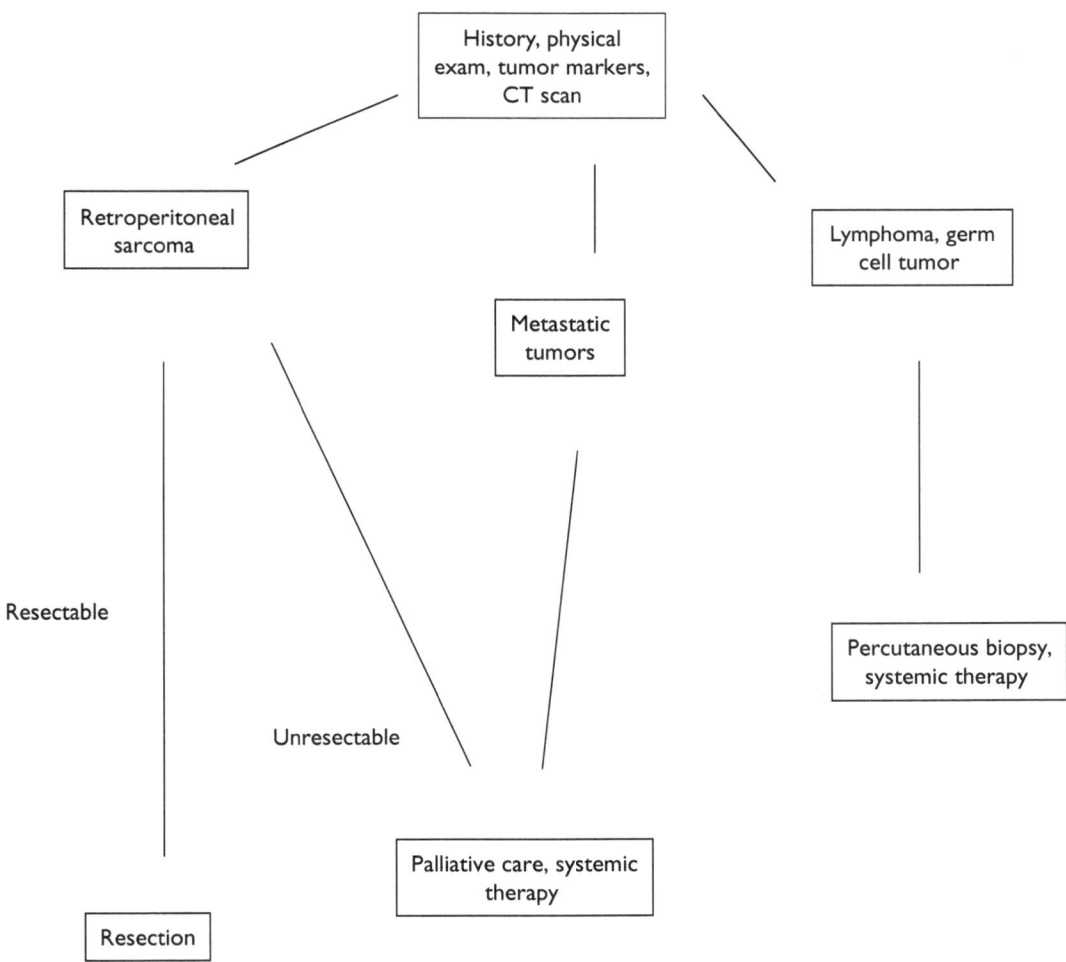

Algorithm 22.3. Algorithm for evaluation and treatment of retroperitoneal masses.

for **en bloc resection** of the mass with attached organs as needed. Partial resection does not appear to aid survival. The most common reasons for unresectability include involvement of the aorta or cava along with intraoperative discovery of distant spread of disease. Neither radiotherapy nor adjuvant chemotherapy has demonstrated usefulness in the postoperative treatment of patients undergoing complete resection. Selected series reveal resectability rates ranging from 25% to about 75%.

Other Abdominal Masses

The patient in **Case 5** was taken to the operating room and underwent a resection of the right and transverse colon together with a portion of the stomach and small bowel. Negative margins were achieved. He received postoperative adjuvant chemotherapy. Although this patient had an abdominal mass, careful questioning revealed that his primary symptoms were related to partial obstruction of the GI tract along with GI bleeding.

Tumors of the stomach, small bowel, and colon can present as abdominal masses. However, the symptom complex usually is related to bleeding and obstruction. These symptoms and their evaluation are covered in Chapters 20 and 21. Abdominal and pelvic masses also can present from **tumors of the ovaries**. A large variety of ovarian tumors, both malignant and benign, can produce tumors of enormous size. All female patients with an abdominal mass should have a pelvic exam performed with imaging studies ordered as needed. The details of the management of ovarian masses are best addressed in the student's obstetrics and gynecology rotation. Finally, **large renal masses** can present with an abdominal mass. The triad of flank mass, flank pain, and hematuria raise suspicion of a renal cell cancer. The discussion of this topic is covered in Chapter 37.

Summary

A patient who presents with a palpable abdominal mass, without signs or symptoms of obstruction or bleeding, probably has a mass arising from the liver, pancreas, spleen, or retroperitoneum. In certain circumstances, gynecologic, gastrointestinal, or renal masses can be responsible. A focused history and physical exam, combined with appropriate imaging studies, can help the student identify the anatomic origin of the mass. In addition, a general classification of the mass as neoplastic, infectious, or inflammatory usually can be made. Malignant neoplastic masses usually require surgical resection for cure. Some benign neoplasms also require resection, while others safely can be observed. Infectious masses most often are treated with antibiotics, although undrained purulent collections usually require percutaneous drainage. In all cases, the physician should bear in mind that vascular masses, such as an abdominal aortic aneurysm, may require emergency repair rather than extended workup.

Selected Readings

Flowers JL, Lefor AT. Laparoscopic splenectomy in patients with hematologic diseases. Ann Surg 1996;1996:19–28.

Fong Y, Cohen AM, Fortner JG, et al. Liver resection for colorectal metastases. J Clin Oncol 1997;15:938–946.

Fong Y, Sun RL. An analysis of 412 cases of hepatocellular carcinoma at a western center. Ann Surg 1999;229:790–800.

Friedman RL, Hiatt JR. Laparoscopic or open splenectomy for hematologic disease; which approach is superior? J Am Coll Surg 1997;185:49–54.

Hemming A, Gallinger S. Liver. In: Norton JA, Bollinger RR, Chang AE, et al, eds. Surgery: Basic Science and Clinical Evidence. New York: Springer-Verlag, 2001.

Karakousis CP, Gerstenbluth R. Retroperitoneal sarcomas and their management. Arch Surg 1995;130:1104–1109.

Karpoff HM, Klimstra DS. Results of total pancreatectomy for adenocarcinoma of the pancreas. Arch Surg 2001;136:44–47.

Lefor A, Phillips E. Spleen. In: Norton JA, Bollinger RR, Chang AE, et al, eds. Surgery: Basic Science and Clinical Evidence. New York: Springer-Verlag, 2001.

Lewis JJ, Leung D. Retroperitoneal soft-tissue sarcoma; analysis of 500 patients treated and followed at a single institution. Ann Surg 1998;228:355–365.

Lieberman MD, Kilburn H. Relation of perioperative deaths to hospital volume among patients undergoing pancreatic resection for malignancy. Ann Surg 1995;222:638–645.

Mulvihill S. Pancreas. In: Norton JA, Bollinger RR, Chang AE, et al, eds. Surgery: Basic Science and Clinical Evidence. New York: Springer-Verlag, 2001.

Yeo CJ, Cameron JL. Pancreaticoduodenectomy for cancer of the head of the pancreas. Ann Surg 1995;221:721–733.

23

Abdominal Masses: Vascular

Rocco G. Ciocca

Objectives

1. To describe the evaluation and management of abdominal aortic aneurysms.
2. To discuss appropriate imaging studies for aneurysms.
3. To discuss which patients need angiograms.
4. To discuss the relationship of aortic aneurysms to other vascular aneurysms.
5. To discuss how to determine which patients need surgical repair of the aneurysm.
6. To discuss the risks of surgical treatment and the risks of the aneurysm left untreated.

Case

A 65-year-old man is undergoing a prophylactic colonoscopy, and, during the procedure, the gastroenterologist notices some prominent pulsation along the medial border of the left colon. The colonoscopy is negative other than for the presence of some diverticular disease. Upon completion of the study, the doctor examines the patient's abdomen and finds that he indeed does have a significant pulsatile abdominal mass at the level of the umbilicus. The gastroenterologist orders a STAT computed tomography (CT) scan and places an urgent call to a vascular surgeon.

Introduction

The primary vascular mass of clinical significance is an abdominal aortic aneurysm (AAA). Approximately 200,000 new cases of AAA are diagnosed each year, and 50,000 to 60,000 surgical AAA repairs are performed annually. Ruptured AAAs are responsible for approximately

15,000 deaths in the United States each year, making AAA the 14th leading cause of death in this country, similar in magnitude to emphysema, renal disease, and homicide.

Note that Chapter 22 covers abdominal masses that are not vascular.

Presentation

The most common presentation of an AAA is that of a painless pulsatile abdominal mass. The primary clinical concern regarding an AAA is that of **rupture**. Rupture of an AAA is associated with a mortality rate of between 50% and 90%. **It therefore is incumbent upon the clinician to recognize an asymptomatic AAA and to refer the patient with the aneurysm for appropriate management.**

Pathophysiology and Etiology

The **pathophysiology and the etiology of AAA** remain somewhat controversial. Abdominal aortic aneurysms long have been considered to be **atherosclerotic in nature**, and several of the major risk factors for atherosclerotic occlusive disease, such as smoking, hypertension, and elevated cholesterol, may be additive to the patient's inherent risk of AAA development. The question then is: Why do some patients with the above-mentioned risk factors develop occlusive disease, while other patients have dilated vessels with or without associated occlusive disease? Patients who have AAA may be **congenitally predisposed** to the development of AAA. This may explain the approximately 5:1 predominance of males to females with this condition.

Relationship to Other Vascular Aneurysms

Patients with AAA also may be predisposed to peripheral aneurysms. It therefore is incumbent upon the examining physician to examine the patient closely for the presence of other aneurysms. Fortunately, most peripheral aneurysms can be diagnosed by physical exam. The popliteal artery is the most common site for peripheral aneurismal disease. **The danger of popliteal artery aneurysms is their propensity to thrombosis, embolization, and, rarely, rupture, making them similar to femoral artery aneurysms and all peripheral aneurysms.** A patient with unilateral popliteal artery aneurysms has an approximately 50% chance of a contralateral aneurysm and a greater than 30% chance of having an AAA. The complications of acute thrombosis or distal embolization of a peripheral aneurysm can be severe and can be associated with amputation rates as high as 20% to 50%. It is best to treat these and all aneurysms electively and prior to the development of symptoms. **Surgical exclusion and bypass** usually are the preferred therapy, with very acceptable long-term results. **Thrombolytic therapy** can be very helpful in opening distal outflow in acutely thrombosed peripheral aneurysms.

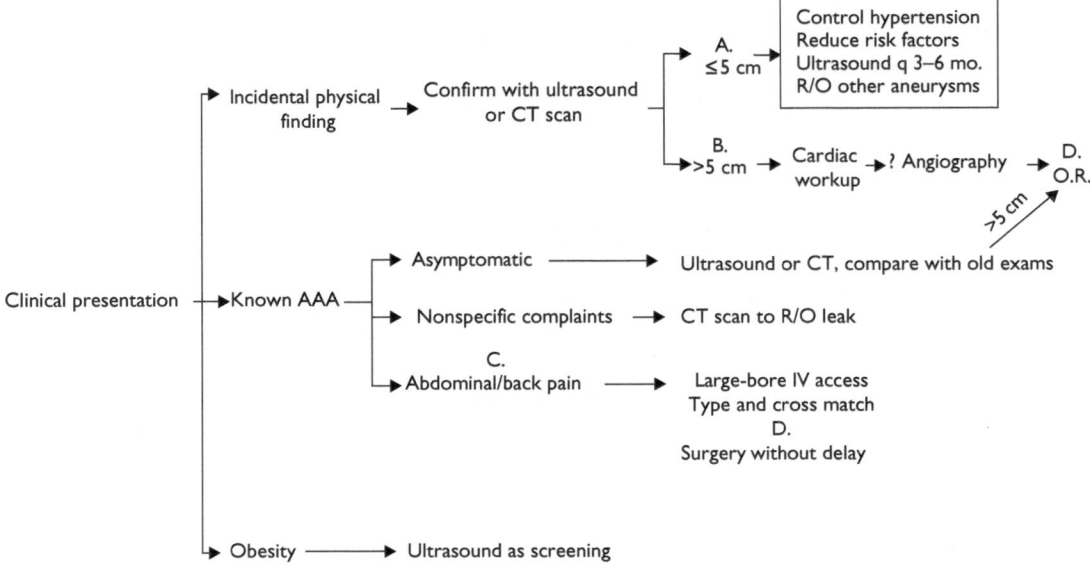

CT scan:
1. rules out leaking or inflammatory abdominal aneurysm
2. determines suprarenal involvement
3. assesses quality of aneurysm wall (blebs)
4. rules out iliac aneurysms

Aortography:
1. assesses renal arteries (number, location, involvement)
2. assesses inferior mesenteric artery patency
3. assesses iliac disease and distal runoff

Algorithm 23.1. Algorithm for the evaluation and treatment of abdominal aortic aneurysms. (Reprinted from March, RJ. Abdominal aortic aneurysm. In: Millikan KW, Saclarides TJ, eds. Common Surgical Diseases. New York: Springer-Verlag, 1998.)

Appropriate Imaging Studies for Aneurysms

Abdominal aortic aneurysms tend to be a condition that presents late in life. See **Algorithm 23.1** for the evaluation and treatment of abdominal aortic aneurysms. The diagnosis of a ruptured AAA must be suspected in an elderly man who presents with abdominal pain and hypotension. The pain frequently radiates to the back, but it may manifest itself as almost any type of abdominal pain. A patient with a contained rupture of an AAA may present with stable vital signs.

A thorough abdominal exam with special attention to a pulsatile mass is the most important initial diagnostic evaluation. Other diagnostic modalities include **abdominal ultrasonography,** which is sensitive and specific for the presence of an AAA, but it is not anatomically detailed enough to provide a surgeon with the information necessary for surgical repair. It also is not a very good study for evaluating the presence or absence of a leak. A **CT scan with oral and IV contrast** can provide excellent anatomic detail and frequently is more than adequate for operative intervention. A CT scan also may be helpful in the diagnosis of a ruptured AAA, but **a hemodynamically unstable**

patient must *never* be sent to the CT scanner. Stable patients in whom a possible leaking or symptomatic AAA is suspected but whose diagnosis is uncertain should have a CT scan only if escorted by a physician, only with continuous blood pressure (BP) monitoring, and only with a large-bore (16-gauge or larger catheters) IV access in place. The patient should have had a vial of blood sent to the blood bank for type and crossmatch as well. It is highly recommended that the hospital's operating room (OR) staff be notified that a possible leaking or ruptured AAA is being evaluated so that the OR can be ready for an expeditious transfer for operative repair. In short, a CT scan for the evaluation of a possible ruptured AAA is a useful and proactive study.

The role of **angiography** in preoperative assessment has evolved from an absolute necessity to one selectively employed for those patients for whom a specific indication exists (e.g., renal vascular disease or severe peripheral vascular disease). A high-quality CT scan with IV contrast generally is felt to be the preoperative test of choice for most vascular surgeons. With the advent of **endovascular stent graft repair of AAA**, many surgeons now again are using angiography routinely for precise measurement and planning of stent graphs.

How to Determine Which Patients Need Surgical Repair of an Aneurysm

The primary concern with AAA is that there is **increased tension on the arterial wall as the AAA expands. Remember Laplace's law: the larger the aneurysm, the greater the likelihood of rupture and the resultant catastrophic consequences (Tables 23.1 and 23.2).** It there-

Table 23.1. Estimates of annual growth rates based on initial aneurysm size (cm/yr).

Study	n	3.0–3.9	4.0–4.9	5.0–5.9	Total
Bernstein[a]	49	0.31	0.61	—	0.46
Bernstein and Chan[b]	110	0.47	0.42	0.51	0.44
Nevitt[c]	103	0.31	0.55	—	0.38
Limet[d]	114	0.63	0.83	—	
Kremer[e]	35	0.23	0.22	—	0.20
Delin[f]	35	0.65	0.56	0.56	0.62
Brown[g]	460	0.37	0.63	—	0.50
Total	906	0.42	0.55	0.54	0.43

Source: Modified from Wilson K, et al. Expansion rates of abdominal aortic aneurysms. Eur J Endovasc Surg 1997;13:521–526, with permission. Copyright 1997 Elsevier LTD. With permission from Elsevier. Reprinted from Winterstein BA, Baxter BT. Diseases of the Abdominal Aorta and Its Branches. In: Norton JA, Bollinger RR, Chang AE, et al, eds. Surgery: Basic Science and Clinical Evidence. New York: Springer-Verlag, 2001, with permission.
[a] Bernstein EF, et al. Surgery 1976;80(6):765–773.
[b] Bernstein EF, et al. Ann Surg 1984;200(3):255–263.
[c] Nevitt MP, et al. N Engl J Med 1989;321(15):1009–1014.
[d] Limet R, et al. J Vasc Surg 1991;14(4):540–548.
[e] Kremer H, et al. Klin Wochenschr 1984;62(23):1120–1125.
[f] Delin A. Br J Surg 1985;72(7):530–532.
[g] Brown P, et al. J Vasc Surg 1996;23(2):213–220.

Table 23.2. Risk factors associated with aneurysm expansion and rupture.

Initial size of aneurysm
Hypertension
Cigarette smoking
Chronic obstructive pulmonary disease
Severe cardiac disease
Advanced age
Previous stroke
Family history of abdominal aortic aneurysm

Source: Reprinted from Winterstein BA, Baxter BT. Diseases of the abdominal aorta and its branches. In: Norton JA, Bollinger RR, Chang AE, et al, eds. Surgery: Basic Science and Clinical Evidence. New York: Springer-Verlag, 2001, with permission.

fore is necessary to define the risk/benefit ratio of AAA rupture versus operative risk.

Such analysis has been done, and, while there is evidence to support operative intervention of "small" aneurysms (those between 4 and 5 cm in size) in selected cases, **most surgeons feel that 5 cm is the size for which the risk of rupture is high enough to accept the operative risk of intervention**. This surgical threshold may change with the evolution of endovascular stent grafting.

Preoperative Risk Assessment and Surgical Approach

Preoperative evaluation of patients with AAA includes a **thorough history and physical exam, with particular attention to the patient's medical comorbidities**. A great deal has been written about preoperative risk assessment (see Chapter 1), and, intuitively, it would make sense to evaluate the patient for significant coronary artery disease (CAD) and intervene if significant CAD was unmasked. There is very little evidence, however, that aggressive preoperative cardiac risk assessment significantly has lowered operative mortality. The primary improvements in surgical outcome more likely can be attributed to improved surgical and anesthetic techniques.

Operative repair of AAA is performed best electively on asymptomatic patients with AAAs greater than 5 cm in transverse diameter. The patients should be medically stable. Standard open surgical repair remains a significant operative intervention, with an operative mortality rate of between 3% and 5% at the best surgical centers.

Operative intervention carries significant morbidity, including myocardial infarction (MI), stroke, renal insufficiency, blood loss, colonic ischemia, distal ischemia, and, very infrequently, spinal ischemia. The majority of these complications can be avoided with proper preoperative planning, proper intraoperative technique, and superb postoperative care.

Standard open operative repair remains the gold standard of care for patients with AAA. Endovascular stent grafts increasingly are being employed successfully on selected patients with AAA and have resulted in promising short- and medium-term results. The obvious appeal of an endovascular approach is that it is minimally invasive and obviates the significant incisional discomfort and recovery of the standard operation. The overall cost-effectiveness and utility of this procedure await further testing and development.

Case Discussion

With regard to the case presented at the beginning of this chapter, several important points can be made. The diagnosis of an AAA is made ideally and most cost-effectively by a thorough physical exam, and such an exam ideally is done prior to an intervention and not after the fact. Frequently, very large aneurysms cannot be palpated readily on physical exam due to the significant girth of many patients, and the "incidental" finding of an AAA is becoming more and more the norm rather than the exception. The ordering of the CT scan in this case is appropriate, although it probably does not need to be done on an emergent basis. Obviously, if the patient were having severe abdominal pain after the procedure, then a more urgent radiologic exam, if not emergent surgery, would be indicated. The concern about an emergent CT scan is that it frequently is performed hastily and frequently does not employ IV contrast, which greatly helps the surgeon understand the vascular anatomy. Such hastily performed CT scans are adequate for revealing the presence or absence of an aneurysm, something that the physician already knows based on his physical exam; however, frequently these scans lack the anatomic detail that is clinically helpful. In this case, it would be better to evaluate the patient electively with a high-quality CT scan of the abdomen and pelvis with 3-mm cuts. This allows the vascular surgeon to evaluate optimally the extent of an aneurysm and to make an accurate assessment as to the best and safest way to repair the aneurysm. If the aneurysm is greater than 5 cm in transverse diameter, it should be repaired electively, assuming that the patient is a reasonable operative risk.

Summary

The diagnosis, workup, and treatment of vascular abdominal masses have been presented in this chapter. A basic understanding of abdominal anatomy and physiology greatly assists in the evaluation of a patient with a vascular abdominal mass. Classifying the mass anatomically, based on etiology and clinical course, greatly helps in the understanding of the problem and type of intervention necessary to facilitate proper therapy. The diagnosis and treatment of vascular abdominal masses frequently requires input from several medical and surgical specialists. In addition to primary care specialists, gastroenterologists, oncologists, general surgeons, surgical oncologists, gynecologists, radiologists, infectious disease specialists, urologists, and vascular surgeons often contribute in the management of a patient with a vascular abdominal mass. The overall prognosis of a patient with a vascular abdominal mass depends on the nature of the mass, the timing of the diagnosis, and the overall condition of the patient. Elective intervention, whether medical or surgical, generally is better than delayed or emergent intervention.

Selected Readings

Busuttil R, Abou-Zamzam AM, Machleder HI. Collagenase activity of the human aorta: a comparison of patients with and without abdominal aneurysms. Arch Surg 1980;115:1373–1378.

Carpenter JP, Barker CF, Roberts B, Berkowitz HD, Lusk EJ, Perloff LJ. Popliteal artery aneurysms: current management and outcome (see comments). J Vasc Surg 1994;19:65–72; discussion 72–73.

Golden MH, Whittemore AD, Donaldson MC, et al. Selective evaluation and management of coronary artery disease in patients undergoing repair of abdominal aortic aneurysms: a 16-year experience. Ann Surg 1990;212: 415–423.

Johnston K, Rutherford RB, Tilson MD, et al. Suggested standards for reporting on arterial aneurysms. J Vasc Surg 1991;3:452–458.

March RJ. Abdominal aortic aneurysm. In: Millikan KW, Saclarides TJ, eds. Common Surgical Diseases. New York: Springer-Verlag, 1998.

Moore W, Rutherford R. Transfemoral endovascular repair of abdominal aortic aneurysm: results of the North American EVT phase 1 trial. J Vasc Surg 1996;23:543–553.

Shortell C, DeWeese JA, Ouriel K, Green RM. Popliteal artery aneurysms: a 25-year surgical experience. J Vasc Surg 1991;14:771–776; discussion 776–779.

Winterstein BA, Baxter BT. Diseases of the abdominal aorta and its branches. In: Norton JA, Bollinger RR, Chang AE, et al, eds. Surgery: Basic Science and Clinical Evidence. New York: Springer-Verlag, 2001.

Zarins C, Harris EJ. Operative repair for aortic aneurysms: the gold standard. J Endovasc Surg 1997;4:232–241.

24

Jaundice

Thomas J. Kearney

Objectives

1. To understand bilirubin metabolism and classify jaundice as nonobstructive or obstructive.
2. To describe common benign and malignant causes of obstructive jaundice.
3. To understand common symptoms and physical signs associated with jaundice.
4. To describe the usefulness and limitations of blood tests and hepatobiliary imaging in the evaluation of a jaundiced patient.
5. To discuss the management of common conditions associated with jaundice.

Cases

Case 1

A 43-year-old woman has had intermittent episodes of right upper quadrant pain, usually associated with eating fatty foods. That pain radiates to her right shoulder, but it spontaneously resolves after several hours. She now presents to the emergency room with a deeper, more persistent pain in the right upper quadrant. She noticed yellowing of her eyes and darkening of her urine for the past 36 hours. Her last bowel movement was light gray. Physical exam reveals tenderness in the right upper abdomen but no mass. She is clinically jaundiced. She has a fever of 101.8F and is mildly tachycardic.

Case 2

A 63-year-old man complains to his physician about yellow discoloration of his eyes. He had lost weight recently and had noticed a decreased appetite. Examination reveals a nontender mass in the right upper quadrant, indicating an enlarged gallbladder (Courvoisier's sign). The patient's urine is dark and his stools gray, sometimes with silver streaks.

Case 3

A 23-year-old man presents to the emergency room with fatigue and jaundice. The patient is an intravenous drug user. Examination reveals an enlarged, tender liver. The urine is dark, but his stools are brown. The bilirubin level is mildly elevated, but alkaline phosphatase is normal. Serum transaminases are very high. A hepatitis panel is obtained.

Introduction

The appearance of jaundice in a patient is a visually dramatic event. It invariably is associated with significant illness, although long-term outcome is dependent on the underlying cause of the jaundice. **Jaundice is a physical finding associated with a disturbance of bilirubin metabolism.** It often is accompanied by other abnormal physical findings and usually is associated with specific symptoms. **The student should be able to classify jaundice broadly as obstructive or nonobstructive based on history and physical examination. The appropriate use of blood tests and imaging allows further refinement of the differential diagnosis.**

In general, nonobstructive jaundice does not require surgical intervention, whereas obstructive jaundice usually requires a surgical or other interventional procedure for treatment. Greater emphasis is placed on surgical jaundice than on medical jaundice in this chapter.

Bilirubin Metabolism and the Classification of Jaundice

Bilirubin is a normal body product that results from the breakdown of heme primarily from red blood cells but also from other body constituents. This bilirubin, known as unconjugated or indirect bilirubin, is bound to albumin and is not water-soluble. Indirect bilirubin is transported into hepatocytes. There it is conjugated with glucuronic acid to form conjugated bilirubin. Conjugated bilirubin is soluble in water and also is referred to as direct bilirubin. The conjugated bilirubin then is released into the biliary tree and from there into the intestinal tract. In the colon, the bilirubin undergoes further conversion into several products, including urobilinogen. A portion of the urobilinogen is reabsorbed, while the remainder passes in the stools. The brown color of normal stool is due to these breakdown products of bilirubin metabolism.

An interruption in any portion of the metabolic pathway can result in an excess of bilirubin and the clinical syndrome of jaundice. Patients with jaundice have yellow skin, usually with itching. The sclerae usually are the first site of color abnormality, typically becoming yellow with a bilirubin level of about 2.5 mg/dL. Skin yellowing is evident at levels of 4 to 5 mg/dL, depending on skin pigmentation.

The urine usually is dark, since the kidneys excrete the excess bilirubin. Stools may be gray if no bilirubin is excreted into the intestinal tract as in obstructive jaundice. Gray stool usually is a sign of complete lack of bilirubin excretion into the intestinal tract. In medical or nonobstructive jaundice, bilirubin does pass into the intestinal tract and the stools remain brown. These signs and symptoms are common to all patients with jaundice. Additional signs and symptoms may be present depending on the cause of the jaundice. These accompanying findings often contain the key to proper classification of the jaundice.

It is clear that multiple mechanisms can produce jaundice. Overproduction of bilirubin from hemolysis can overwhelm the liver's ability to excrete. Hemolysis may be secondary to a congenital hemolytic syndrome or may be acquired in transfusion reactions, trauma, or sepsis. Deficiencies of unconjugated bilirubin uptake into the hepatocytes can produce jaundice. The most common reason for this is Gilbert's syndrome, a congenital reduction in the enzyme bilirubin glucuronyl transferase. This condition affects about 5% to 7% of the general population. Sepsis and certain drugs (e.g., rifampin) also can impair uptake. In neonates, immaturity of the conjugating and transport system can cause jaundice. These conditions are considered **prehepatic jaundice**.

Hepatic jaundice, most commonly from viral hepatitis, results from hepatocyte dysfunction. Other acquired or congenital conditions, including alcoholic hepatitis, Wilson's disease, hepatic cirrhosis, drug reactions, primary biliary cirrhosis, and exposure to hepatotoxins (carbon tetrachloride, acetaminophen), may cause hepatic jaundice. Patients may progress to complete hepatic failure. Genetic defects, such as Dubin-Johnson and Rotor's syndrome, may be responsible for impaired excretion of conjugated bilirubin.

Finally, **posthepatocyte obstruction** to bile flow can produce jaundice. This final cause often is called **surgical or obstructive jaundice** due to the requirement for an intervention in most cases in order to relieve the obstruction. **Obstructive jaundice can be divided further into benign and malignant obstruction.**

Algorithm 24.1 lists a schema for a general classification of jaundice: prehepatic, hepatic, and posthepatic. **Obstructive jaundice often is referred to as posthepatic since the defect lies in the pathway of bilirubin metabolism past the hepatocytes. The other forms of jaundice are referred to as nonobstructive jaundice. These forms are due to a hepatocyte defect (hepatic jaundice) or a prehepatic condition.** **Table 24.1** lists some common and uncommon causes of the three major categories of jaundice: prehepatic, hepatic, and posthepatic.

Obstructive Jaundice

Benign Stone Disease

In **Case 1** the patient is acutely ill with jaundice. The previous right upper quadrant pain suggests biliary colic from gallstones. Tenderness in the right upper quadrant (Murphy's sign) suggests cholecystitis. The patient also is exhibiting the clinical syndrome of Charcot's triad—fever, right upper quadrant pain, and jaundice. This symptom complex suggests cholangitisbiliary infection combined with obstruction. This condition requires intervention with antibiotics and biliary drainage to prevent serious septic complications. Patients with Charcot's triad who exhibit mental confusion and shock (Reynolds' pentad) have advanced

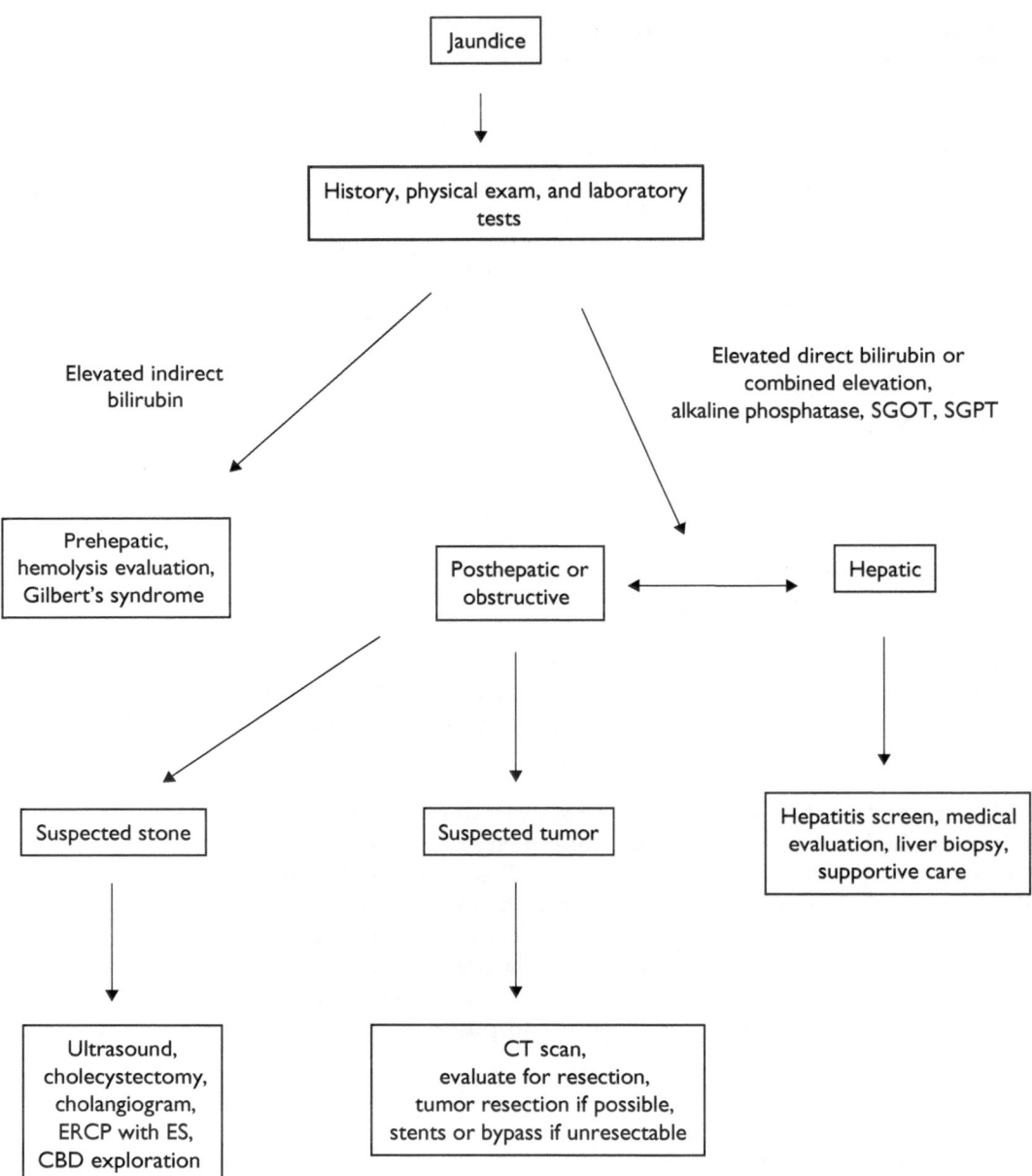

Algorithm 24.1 Evaluation of the jaundiced patient. CBD, common bile duct; ERCP, endoscopic retrograde cholangiopancreatography; ES, endoscopic sphincterotomy; SGOT, serum glutamic-oxaloacetic transaminase; SGPT, serum glutamic-pyruvic transaminase.

Table 24.1. Classification and causes of jaundice.

Prehepatic	Hepatic	Posthepatic (obstructive)
Hemolytic anemia	Viral hepatitis	Choledocholithiasis
Hereditary spherocytosis	Alcoholic hepatitis	Periampullary cancer
Acute hemolysis	Hepatic cirrhosis	Bile duct cancer
Gilbert's syndrome	Dubin-Johnson syndrome	Sclerosing cholangitis
Drugs	Rotor's syndrome	Pancreatitis
Crigler-Najjar syndrome	Mononucleosis	Choledochal cyst
	Hepatotoxins	Biliary atresia
	Primary biliary cirrhosis	Mirizzi's syndrome
	Acetaminophen	Iatrogenic injury
	Autoimmune hepatitis	Gallbladder cancer
	Storage diseases	Biliary parasites
	Idiopathic hepatitis	Cytic fibrosis
		Duodenal diverticula
		Peribiliary adenopathy

biliary sepsis and require urgent intervention to decompress the biliary system.

The patient in **Case 1** was placed on intravenous antibiotics to cover the most common biliary pathogens: *Klebsiella, Escherichia coli,* and *Enterococcus*. Blood tests for bilirubin revealed elevated direct and indirect bilirubin. The combined bilirubin level was 7.3 mg/dL. The presence of elevated direct bilirubin implies that this is not just prehepatic jaundice. Prehepatic jaundice from hemolysis rarely causes a bilirubin level above 5.0 mg/dL in the absence of other hepatic dysfunction. The alkaline phosphatase level was elevated markedly, but the transaminases were normal. This pattern suggests biliary obstruction without any inherent abnormality of the hepatocytes. Other useful markers of hepatocyte function include prothrombin time and albumin. The proteins required for the coagulation pathway as well as albumin are synthesized in the liver. Abnormalities suggest hepatocyte dysfunction. Elevated prothrombin time usually responds to vitamin K administration in obstructive jaundice but not in hepatic jaundice. These levels were normal in this patient. Amylase and lipase levels also should be evaluated due to the association between choledocholithiasis and pancreatitis (gallstone pancreatitis). This patient had mildly elevated amylase. This pattern of abnormalities suggests **biliary obstruction with normal hepatocytes (Table 24.2).** The history is suggestive of **benign biliary obstruction.**

An ultrasound was ordered; it revealed stones in the gallbladder with gallbladder wall thickening and a dilated common bile duct. A stone could be seen in the distal common bile duct. The normal common bile duct should be under 10 mm in diameter. **Ultrasound is the procedure of choice for patients with suspected benign obstructive jaundice from gallstone disease (see Algorithm 24.1).** The main limitation of ultrasound is its inability in many cases to visualize the most distal portion of the common bile duct due to duodenal or colonic gas.

Table 24.2. Evaluation of liver function tests in jaundice.

Test	Source	Pattern in gallstone obstruction of the biliary tree	Pattern in malignant obstruction of the biliary tree	Pattern in acute hepatitis
Total bilirubin	Red blood cell destruction, hepatocyte processing	Elevated, but typically less than 10 mg/dL	Elevated, commonly more than 10 mg/dL	Elevated
Direct bilirubin	Conjugation by hepatocytes	Elevated	Markedly elevated	Mildly elevated
Indirect bilirubin	Red blood cell turnover, hepatocyte processing	Minimally elevated	Elevated	Elevated
Alkaline phosphatase	Biliary epithelial cells and bone	Elevated	Markedly elevated	Minimally elevated
Transaminases	Hepatocytes	Minimally elevated	Minimally elevated	Markedly elevated
Gamma-glutamyl transferase	Biliary epithelial cells	Elevated	Markedly elevated	Minimally elevated

Source: Reprinted from Mulvihill SJ. Pancreas. In: Norton JA, Bollinger RR, Chang AE, et al, eds. Surgery: Basic Science and Clinical Evidence. New York: Springer-Verlag, 2001, with permission.

This patient needs two interventions for two problems. The impacted stone needs to be removed from the common bile duct. The gallbladder needs to be removed to prevent future episodes of common duct stones and to relieve the cholecystitis. In previous decades, the patient would have undergone open cholecystectomy with open cholangiography and common bile duct exploration (CBDE). **With the advent of laparoscopic and endoscopic techniques in the 1990s, the management plan becomes more complex.** Individual hospital and physician abilities may influence the choice and timing of procedures.

Patients with cholelithiasis are quite common. In general, **asymptomatic cholelithiasis** does not require treatment. The condition results from an imbalance among levels of bile acid, lecithin, and cholesterol in the gallbladder. There are several scenarios in which patients with asymptomatic cholelithiasis should consider prophylactic cholecystectomy. These include patients with hematologic disorders, such as sickle cell disease or hereditary spherocytosis. Immunocompromised patients and patients requiring immunosuppression (e.g., renal transplant) with cholelithiasis should undergo cholecystectomy. The signs of acute cholecystitis can be masked by the immunosuppressive state. Cholecystectomy in diabetic patients formerly was thought to require prophylactic surgery due to the high rate of gangrenous cholecystitis. This recommendation is controversial, however. Patients with a porcelain gallbladder have a high rate of harboring gallbladder cancer and should have surgery. The majority of otherwise normal patients with asymptomatic cholelithiasis will not suffer an episode of cholecystitis. Prophylactic surgery is not recommended.

Patients with **mildly symptomatic cholecystitis** can be managed safely in most cases with laparoscopic cholecystectomy. Although shock-wave lithotripsy, bile acids, and gallbladder perfusion with solvents all have been tried to dissolve gallstones, surgery remains the main form of therapy. In elective cases, the rate of conversion to open cholecystectomy is under 5%, and the rate of bile duct injury (a rare but extremely serious complication) is about 3 per 1000 cases. Patients undergoing elective laparoscopic cholecystectomy with normal liver function tests rarely have common bile duct (CBD) stones and do not require an intraoperative cholangiogram, provided the anatomy is delineated clearly. Mildly elevated bilirubin or alkaline phosphatase levels or a history of jaundice or pancreatitis make CBD stones more likely. An intraoperative cholangiogram would be prudent in such circumstances. The discovery of CBD stones would require laparoscopic or open CBD exploration or postcholecystectomy endoscopic retrograde cholangiopancreatography (ERCP) with stone extraction. The gallbladder always should be inspected at the time of removal to evaluate for the rare case of unsuspected gallbladder cancer.

Gallbladder cancer is seen in about 1 of 200 cholecystectomy specimens and is the fifth most common gastrointestinal tract cancer in the United States. Stage I gallbladder cancer (confined to the mucosa) is treated with simple cholecystectomy. Advanced gallbladder cancer (stages III and IV) rarely is curable. The treatment of stage II gallbladder cancer (no extension beyond the serosa or into the liver) is controversial, but most experts would recommend radical cholecystectomy, which includes removal of the gallbladder and a wedge of the hepatic gallbladder bed along with a biliary node dissection.

Patients with suspected **acute cholecystitis** are managed best with intravenous hydration, antibiotics, and cholecystectomy within 24 to 48 hours. The diagnosis is made by history and physical exam and confirmed with ultrasound or occasionally by biliary scintigraphy using technetium 99 m (^{99m}Tc)-labeled hepatic 2,6-dimethyl-iminodiacetic acid (HIDA) compounds scan. The practice of "cooling down" the patient and scheduling elective cholecystectomy at a later date is less desirable than early cholecystectomy. This approach has been validated by clinical trials (**Table 24.3**). Originally, acute cholecystitis was felt to be a contraindication to laparoscopic cholecystectomy. The majority of patients today can undergo laparoscopic cholecystectomy in the setting of acute cholecystitis if an experienced surgeon is available.

Cholecystectomy, whether laparoscopic or open, does not address the management of patients presenting with **CBD stones (choledocholithiasis)**. At many institutions, this patient would undergo ERCP with endoscopic sphincterotomy (ES). A CBD stone would be found in the majority of patients, and the stone could be extracted in greater than 90% of patients. The patient then would undergo laparoscopic cholecystectomy. If the ERCP with ES was unsuccessful, CBD exploration would be needed; CBD exploration could be either open or laparoscopic. Another option would be laparoscopic cholecystectomy with planned laparoscopic common bile duct exploration, skipping the preoperative ERCP. Laparoscopic CBDE can be accomplished with a

Table 24.3. Clinical trials comparing early versus delayed surgery for acute cholecystitis.

Reference	n	Study design	Level of evidence	Complications	Mortality	Findings/comments
Linden and Sunzel 1970,[a] Sweden	140	Randomized, controlled trial	I	Early: 14.3% Delayed: 3.4%	Early: 0% Delayed: 0%	More than two thirds of patients randomized to early surgery underwent operation within 10 days of diagnosis Low mortality, in part the result of excluding 3 high-risk, elderly patients Noted that 17% of patients randomized to delayed surgery ultimately refused operation once acute symptoms resolved No difference in technical difficulty between early and delayed operations when the surgeon was experienced Early surgery (paradoxically) resulted in a 2-day-longer average length of stay, but fewer extended hospitalizations Concluded that early surgery avoids the hazards of diagnostic error, symptom recurrence during the waiting period, and shortened the convalescence period after early surgery
McArthur et al. 1975[b] England	35	Randomized, controlled trial	I	Early: 40.0% Delayed: 29.4%	Early: 0% Delayed: 0%	Early surgery defined as immediately following confirmation of the diagnosis Reported no overall difference in the technical difficulty of early versus delayed cholecystectomy, but recommended that early surgery take place within 5 days of diagnosis Most complications were minor infections Concluded that the major benefits of early surgery are the shortened hospitalization and the avoidance of the serious complications of conservative management, including gallbladder perforation and empyema
Lahtinen et al. 1978,[c] Finland	100	Randomized, controlled trial	I	Early: 29.7% Delayed: 47.7%	Early: 0% Delayed: 9%	Noted a technically easier operation, shorter OR time (70 vs. 79 min), reduced wound infection rate (6% vs. 18%), and shorter postoperative hospital LOS (12 vs. 15 days) for early vs. delayed surgery High complication rates in both groups predominantly related to localized or systemic infection Authors recommend early surgery

Study	N	Study type		Outcome	Comments
Norby et al. 1983,[d] Sweden	192	Randomized, controlled, multicenter, trial	I	Early: 0% Delayed: 1.1%	Early surgery defined as operation within 7 days of symptoms Studied patients ≤75 years old, randomized by odd vs. even birthdays Complications were similar between the two groups, but early surgery reduced hospital length of stay by >6 days
Sianesi et al. 1984,[e] Italy	471	Retrospective (1970–77) and prospective (1977–82) data	III	Early: 0% Delayed: 1.6%	Study combined retrospective and prospective data, collected over 12 years, during which time patient management evolved Reported low incidence of biliary infection, low morbidity and mortality, and shorter hospitalization period Authors recommend early surgery, within 48–72h of diagnosis
Ajao et al. 1991, Nigeria	81	Retrospective	III	Early: 2.6% Delayed: 0%	Retrospective review over 12 months, compared early (≤48h) versus delayed (7–14 days) surgery Prohibitive rate of complications reported early surgery, including 7 (18%) common bile duct injuries; only complications reported were wound infections (23%) and duct injuries Authors recommend delayed surgery, recommendations seemingly specific to the practice environment and level of surgical experience
Summary/totals	1019	—	—	Early: 0.2% Delayed: 1.8%	Early surgery was technically more challenging with a higher complication rate, but shorter hospital stay and convalescence, more rapid return to work, and lower overall mortality than delayed surgery for acute cholecystitis

Note: Additional outcome columns shown: Early: 14.9% / Delayed: 15.4% (Norby); Early: 18.5% / Delayed: 15% (Sianesi); Early: 41% / Delayed: 12.5% (Ajao); Early: 21.0% / Delayed: 16.5% (Summary/totals).

[a] Linden Wvd, Sunzel H. Early versus delayed operation for acute cholecystitis. A controlled trial. Am J Surg 1970;120;7–13.

[b] McArthur P, Cuschieri A, Sells RA, Shields R. Controlled clinical trial comparing early with interval cholecystectomy for acute cholecystitis. Br J Surg 1975;62:850–852.

[c] Lahtinen J, Alhava EM, Aukee S. Acute cholecystitis treated by early and delayed surgery. A controlled clinical trial. Scand J Gastroenterol 1978;13:673–678.

[d] Norby S, Herlin P, Holmin T, Sjodahl R, Tagesson C. Early or delayed cholecystectomy in acute cholecystitis? A clinical trial. Br J Surg 1983;70:163–165.

[e] Sianesi M, Ghirarduzzi A, Percudani M, Dell'Anna B. Cholecystectomy for acute cholecystitis: timing of operation, bacteriologic aspects, and postoperative course. Am J Surg 1984;148:609–612.

Source: Reprinted from Harris HW. Biliary system. In: Norton JA, Bollinger RR, Chang AE, et al, eds. Surgery: Basic Science and Clinical Evidence. New York: Springer-Verlag, 2001, with permission.

Table 24.4. Periampullary cancer.

Pancreatic adenocarcinoma
Cholangiocarcinoma of distal common bile duct
Ampullary cancer
Duodenal cancer

transcystic duct approach or via a choledochotomy. This procedure requires advanced laparoscopic skills. The patient also could be managed primarily with an open cholecystectomy with intraoperative cholangiogram. Open common bile duct exploration then could be performed. Finally, ERCP and ES could follow laparoscopic cholecystectomy. However, this last scenario might require further intervention if common duct stones were seen but could not be extracted via ERCP with ES. Ultimately, the experience of the surgical team and gastroenterologist and the availability of specialized equipment influence the exact management algorithm at a particular institution.

Malignancy

Case 2 also presents a patient who is quite ill. The history of insidious onset of jaundice with weight loss strongly suggests a malignancy. The dilated gallbladder locates the patient's obstruction at a point distal to the junction of the common hepatic duct with the cystic duct. His laboratory profile, with elevated bilirubin and alkaline phosphatase, would be similar to that of the first patient. His albumin might be low due to poor nutrition. Although ultrasound could be used as an initial screening test, computed tomography (CT) of the abdomen would be a better choice (see **Algorithm 24.1**). This patient almost certainly has cancer. An evaluation of the periampullary area is accomplished better with fine-cut CT. In addition, metastases can be identified and surgical resectability often can be predicted based on local involvement of the superior mesenteric artery and vein.

Periampullary cancer usually occurs from one of the four causes listed in **Table 24.4**. This patient has an **ampullary cancer**, one of the rarer causes of periampullary obstruction. The silver streaks in the gray stools represent intermittent bleeding into the lumen of the duodenum. The blood coats the gray stools, causing a silver discoloration. Usually, **pancreatic adenocarcinoma** is the cause of malignant periampullary obstruction. Patients without signs of distant metastases and without signs of local unresectability are candidates for pancreaticoduodenectomya Whipple procedure. The cure rate (survival at 5 years) is about 20%. Survival from bile duct, ampullary, and **duodenal cancers** is slightly better then for pancreatic adenocarcinoma.

Most experienced pancreatic surgeons prefer direct referral without any other interventional studies. There is no convincing evidence that preoperative biliary decompression provides any advantage to patients with resectable lesions, and it may be harmful. Patients with distant metastases or local unresectability almost always should undergo ERCP with placement of a biliary stent. This relieves obstruction. Brush biopsy often can provide a diagnosis, and the patient can receive palliative systemic therapy without requiring an operation. In some cases, local resectability is not clear after CT imaging. Angiography can be used to assess potential involvement of unresectable vessels. Newer technologies, such as endoscopic ultrasound (EUS), magnetic resonance cholangiopancreatography (MRCP), and magnetic resonance angiography (MRA), can provide additional anatomic information.

Another cause of malignant biliary obstruction is **cholangiocarcinoma**. This rare tumor occurs much less frequently then pancreatic cancer. When obstruction occurs in the distal common bile duct, the patient is managed as a patient with periampullary cancer. Intrahepatic cholangiocarcinoma usually does not cause jaundice, since a portion of the liver remains unobstructed. Cholangiocarcinoma in the common hepatic duct or at the bifurcation of the right and left hepatic duct (Klatskin's tumor) represents the most common site of extrahepatic cholangiocarcinoma. Patients present with obstructive jaundice, but they typically do not have a dilated gallbladder. Ultrasound reveals dilated intrahepatic ducts, but it also reveals a collapsed extrahepatic system and gallbladder. Percutaneous transhepatic cholangiography (PTC) is preferred to ERCP for upper bile duct tumors due to better delineation of the proximal extent of the tumor. Stents can be placed percutaneously for palliation in unresectable cases. If the tumor is localized and there are no distant metastases, resection is indicated. The entire extrahepatic biliary system is removed, and biliary drainage is reestablished with a Roux-en-Y hepaticojejunostomy. Occasionally a partial hepatectomy is required to provide a negative margin of resection. Aggressive surgical resection of hilar bile duct cancer can produce cure (5-year survival) in about 20% of patients.

Uncommon Causes

There are other rare causes of biliary obstruction that are not related to cancer but that are not secondary to gallstone disease either (**Table 24.5**). They are mentioned here for completeness. **Benign bile duct strictures** can result from operative injury. The rate of bile duct injury from laparoscopic cholecystectomy is estimated at 0.3%, higher than the 0.1% estimate from the open cholecystectomy era. Patients often are managed initially with endoscopic balloon dilation and stent placement. Long-term success usually requires definitive surgical excision, with reconstruction similar to malignant biliary strictures. The other cause of benign biliary stricture that must be mentioned is **sclerosing cholangitis**: an inflammatory narrowing of the biliary ducts usually

Table 24.5. Uncommon causes of biliary obstruction.

Benign biliary stricture (iatrogenic)
Sclerosing cholangitis
Biliary atresia
Choledochal cyst

associated with inflammatory bowel disease. The rise in bilirubin is more gradual. The disease ultimately results in cirrhosis of the liver. Patients with isolated strictures are rare and can be treated with resection. Usually, liver transplantation is required once end-stage liver disease occurs. A congenital cause of biliary obstruction is **biliary atresia**. These pediatric patients require decompressive hepatic portoenterostomy (Kasai procedure). Many of these patients progress to further biliary obstruction, cirrhosis, and eventual liver transplantation. Finally, **choledochal cysts**, an entity with unknown etiology that can be congenital or acquired, can require resection and bilioenteric reconstruction.

Hepatic Jaundice

Viral Hepatitis

The patient's presentation in **Case 3** suggests **nonobstructive jaundice**. This patient is at high risk of **viral hepatitis** due to his IV drug usage. He also should be tested for **HIV infection**. Other conditions also can result in hepatocyte injury. These include **alcoholic hepatitis, cirrhosis, and drug or toxin induced hepatocellular injury. Patients with such illnesses have a clinical picture consistent with liver malfunction and failure, and the jaundice is merely a representation of this underlying liver failure.** Often, liver biopsy is required to confirm a diagnosis in equivocal situations (see **Algorithm 24.1**). There usually is no requirement for surgical intervention, except for cases of fulminant hepatic failure or end-stage liver disease requiring liver transplantation.

Medical management of viral hepatitis is generally supportive. Treatment for chronic hepatitis B includes the use of interferon or lamivudine. Both hepatitis A and B can be prevented through preexposure vaccination. Hepatitis immune globulin can be used for postexposure prophylaxis. Medical management of alcohol- and toxin-induced liver damage also is primarily supportive in nature. Acetaminophin poisoning can be treated with acetylcysteine, but most hepatic toxins do not have a specific antidote.

Summary

Jaundice is a manifestation of an abnormality with bilirubin metabolism. The abnormality may be prehepatic, hepatic, or posthepatic. There are certain signs and symptoms common to all jaundiced patients (yellow skin, itching). Specific items from the history and physical examination along with blood work can help the clinician classify jaundice into obstructive and nonobstructive jaundice. Surgical or other mechanical intervention almost exclusively is restricted to cases of obstructive (posthepatic) jaundice. Imaging evaluation of the gallbladder and biliary system plays an important role in the evaluation of obstructive jaundice by locating the site and disclosing the nature of the obstruction. Ultrasound imaging usually is the first step for suspected biliary stone disease. The physician's level of suspicion about benign versus malignant causes of obstructive jaundice will lead to different radiologic tests and interventions.

Stone disease usually is managed with laparoscopic gallbladder removal. Stones in the biliary system may pass spontaneously if small. More often, an endoscopic procedure is required to clear the bile ducts. Laparoscopic techniques also are available. Patients with malignant causes of obstructive jaundice are seriously ill. Major surgical resections are required for cure, and only a minority of patients are cured of their malignancy. Excellent palliation can be achieved, however, either with surgical bypass or stents. Surgical bypass tends to be more durable, but immediate morbidity is higher. **Algorithm 24.1** summarizes the management of the jaundiced patient, with an emphasis on surgical therapy of obstructive jaundice.

Selected Readings

Barkun AN, Barkun JS. Useful predictors of bile duct stones in patients undergoing laparoscopic cholecystectomy. Ann Surg 1994;220(7):32–39.

Bauer TW, Morris JB. The consequences of major bile duct injury during laparoscopic cholecystectomy. J Gastrointest Surg 1998;2(1):61–66.

Harris HW. Biliary system. In: Norton JA, Bollinger RR, Chang AE, et al, eds. Surgery: Basic Science and Clinical Evidence. New York: Springer-Verlag, 2001.

Houdart R, Pernicieni T. Predicting common bile duct lithiasis: determination and prospective validation of a model predicting low risk. Am J Surg 1995;170(7):38–43.

Klempnauer J, Ridder GJ, Waisielewski R, Werner M, Weimann A, Pichlmayr R. Resectional surgery of hilar cholangiocarcinoma: a multivariate analysis of prognostic factors. J Clin Oncol 1997;15(3):947–954.

Newman L, Newman C. An institutional review of the management of choledocholithiasis in 1616 patients undergoing laparoscopic cholecystectomy. Am Surg 1994;60(4):273–277.

Yeo CJ, Sohn TA, Cameron J. Periampullary adenocarcinoma: analysis of 5-year survivors. Ann Surg 1998;227(6):821–831.

25

Colon and Rectum

Stephen F. Lowry and Theodore E. Eisenstat

Objectives

1. To describe the presentation and potential complications of ulcerative colitis and Crohn's disease.
2. To contrast the pathology, anatomic location and pattern, cancer risk, and diagnostic evaluation of ulcerative colitis and Crohn's disease.
3. To discuss the role of surgery in the treatment of patients with ulcerative colitis and Crohn's disease.
4. To outline the diagnosis and management of colonic volvulus and diverticular disease.
5. To outline the treatment of carcinoma located at different levels of the colon and rectum.

Cases

Case 1

A 35-year-old Caucasian man presents with a 48-hour history of bloody diarrhea, diffuse abdominal pain, and feverishness. He experienced some blood in his stools 6 months previously, but he did not seek medical attention. His temperature is 102F and his white blood count (WBC) is 20,000 cm². Rectal exam shows gross blood and mucus in the stool. Physical exam reveals abdominal distention, slight rebound tenderness diffusely, and hyperactive bowel sounds. Aside from evidence of dehydration, there are no other significant findings. An abdominal series reveals diffusely dilated large bowel with no evidence of obstruction.

Case 2

A 60-year-old man presents with a 12-hour history of persistent bright red blood per rectum. Aside from a weight loss of 5 pounds over the prior 2 months, he has been healthy with no significant medical history. His blood pressure is 100/50 (supine), and his pulse is 100 beats per minute. A hematocrit reading is 28%. Abdominal exam reveals no masses or tenderness. Radiographs of the chest and abdomen are unrevealing.

Anatomy and Physiology of the Colon and Rectum

The colon is one structural unit with two embryologic origins. The cecum, right colon, and midtransverse colon are of midgut origin and as such are supplied by the superior mesenteric artery. The distal transverse colon, splenic flexure, descending colon, and sigmoid colon are of hindgut origin and receive blood from the inferior mesenteric artery. The transverse and sigmoid colons are completely covered with peritoneum and are attached by long mesenteries, allowing for great variation in the location of these structures (**Fig. 25.1**).

The blood supply to the colon is quite variable, but general patterns exist (**Fig. 25.2**). The venous drainage (**Fig. 25.3**) of the colon is through veins that bear the same name as the arteries with which they run except for the inferior mesenteric vein.

Small numbers of lymphatics actually exist in the lamina propria, but, for practical purposes, lymphatic drainage and therefore, the

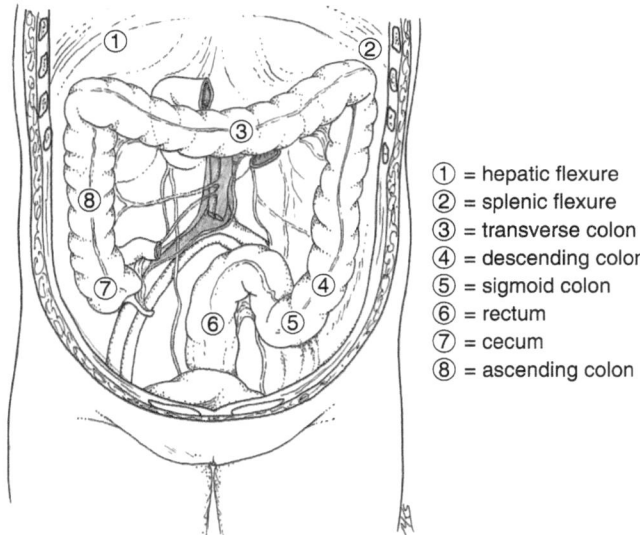

① = hepatic flexure
② = splenic flexure
③ = transverse colon
④ = descending colon
⑤ = sigmoid colon
⑥ = rectum
⑦ = cecum
⑧ = ascending colon

Figure 25.1. The posterior aspects of the ascending and descending colon are "extraperitoneal," as those surfaces are not covered with peritoneum, whereas the transverse and sigmoid colon are completely intraperitoneal, as these segments are completely peritonealized and on mesenteries. (Reprinted from Schecter WP. Peritoneum and Acute Abdomen. In: Norton JA, Bollinger RR, Chang AE, et al, eds. Surgery: Basic Science and Clinical Evidence. New York: Springer-Verlag, 2001, with permission.)

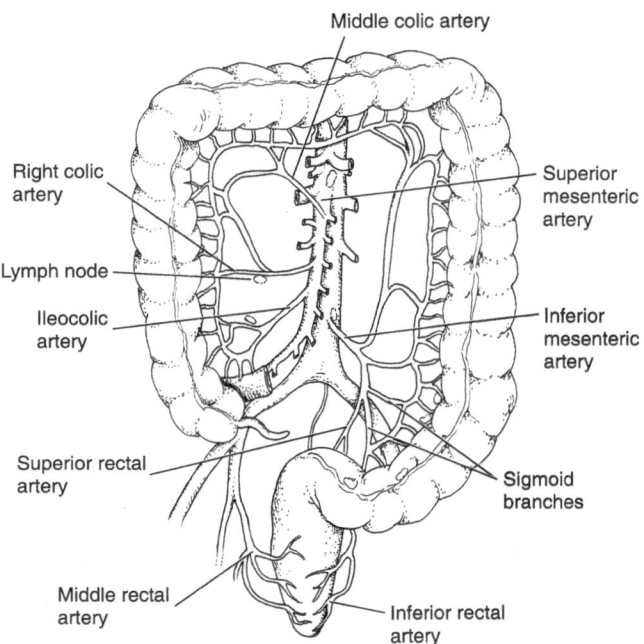

Figure 25.2. The arterial supply to the colon and rectum. The lymphatic drainage parallels the arterial supply. (Reprinted from Schecter WP. Peritoneum and Acute Abdomen. In: Norton JA, Bollinger RR, Chang AE, et al, eds. Surgery: Basic Science and Clinical Evidence. New York: Springer-Verlag, 2001, with permission.)

ability of malignancies to metastasize, begin once the tumor has invaded through the muscularis mucosa. The extramural lymphatic vessels and nodes follow along the arteries to their origins at the superior and inferior mesenteric vessels. The colon is innervated via the sympathetic and parasympathetic nervous systems. Sympathetic stimulation inhibits peristalsis, whereas it is promoted by the parasympathetic system.

The major functions of the colon are absorption, storage, propulsion, and digestion of the output of the proximal intestinal tract. Absorption of the salts and water of the ileal output is critical in the maintenance of normal fluid and electrolyte balance. It is regulated through a complex, integrated, neurohormonal pathway in normal individuals; the ileum expels approximately 1500 mL of fluid per day, of which 1350 mL is absorbed by the colon.

The rectum is approximately 12 to 15 cm long. It extends from the rectosigmoid junction, marked by the fusion of the taenia, to the anal canal, marked by the passage of the bowel into the pelvic floor musculature. The rectum lies in the hollow of the sacrum and forms three distinct curves, creating folds that, when visualized endoscopically, are known as the valves of Houston.

See **Algorithm 25.1** for the initial workup of large-bowel disease.

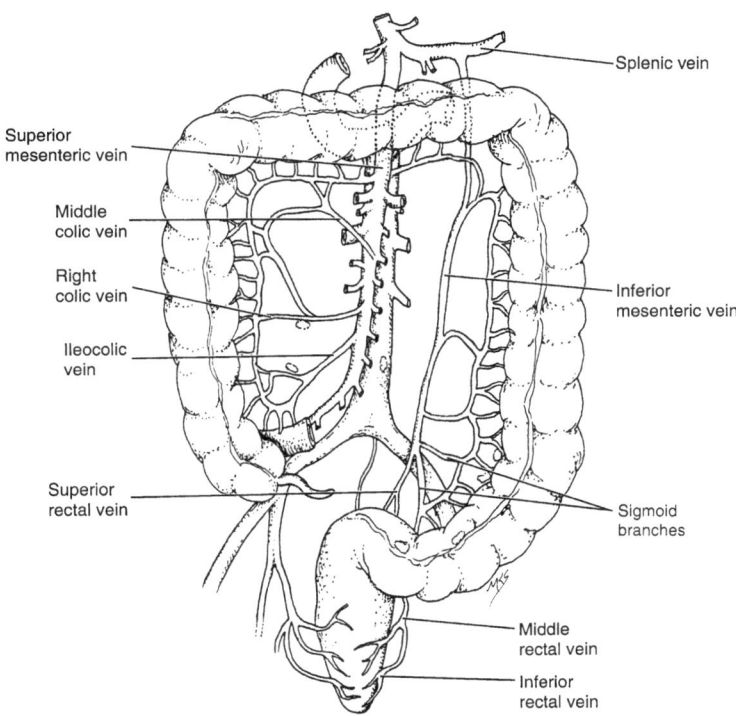

Figure 25.3. The venous drainage of the colon and rectum. (Reprinted from Schecter WP. Peritoneum and Acute Abdomen. In: Norton JA, Bollinger RR, Chang AE, et al, eds. Surgery: Basic Science and Clinical Evidence. New York: Springer-Verlag, 2001, with permission.)

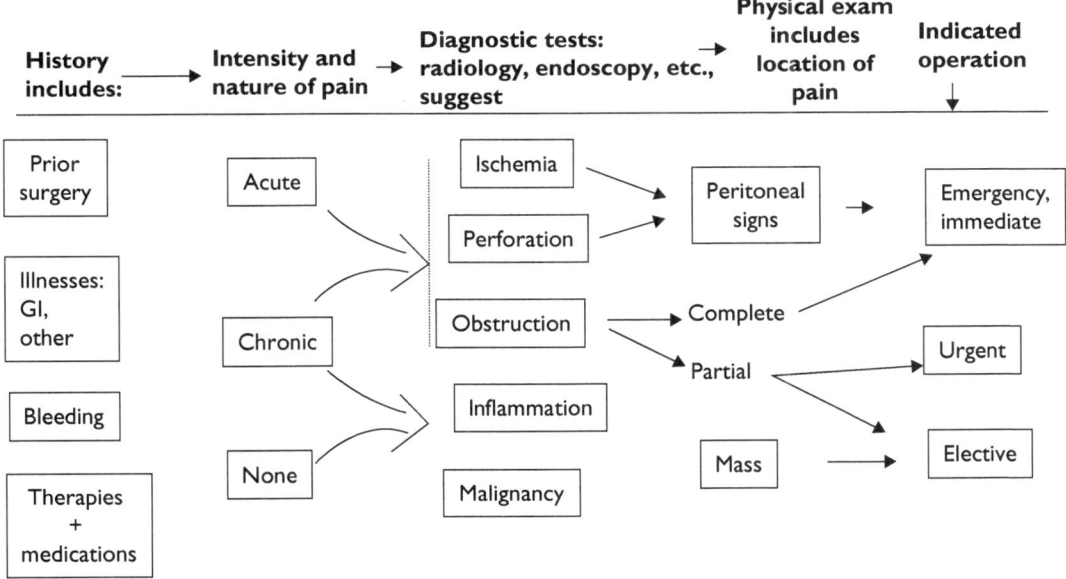

Algorithm 25.1. Algorithm for the initial workup of large-bowel disease.

Benign Diseases

Inflammatory Bowel Disease

Crohn's Disease

The etiology of Crohn's disease remains elusive, as does the etiology of ulcerative colitis with which it shares many similarities. **The presentation of Crohn's disease can be difficult to appreciate**. Patients have a variety of symptoms that are directly related to the extent, character, and location of the inflammation. **The classic symptoms are abdominal pain, diarrhea (which can be bloody), and weight loss**. Other signs and symptoms include fever, nausea, vomiting, anorexia, palpable abdominal mass, aphthous ulcerations of the mouth, cholelithiasis, and renal calculi.

The nature of Crohn's disease can be divided into three categories: inflammatory, stricturing, and fistulizing. Patients with stricturing Crohn's disease may have only symptoms of obstruction, whereas those with a fistula or abscess may have a more septic presentation. Patients with an inflammatory presentation may have symptoms of malabsorption with its sequelae.

The evaluation for Crohn's disease verifies the diagnosis and assesses the severity and extent of the disease. **Upper and lower endoscopy** with directed and random biopsies and radiographic imaging help to elucidate the diagnosis. **Stool cultures** may find evidence of infectious enterocolitis that may mimic Crohn's disease. **Colonoscopy** is the most sensitive test for identifying a patchy distribution of inflammation, terminal ileal involvement, and rectal sparing that are highly suggestive of Crohn's. **Endoscopic findings** include mucosal edema and erythema, aphthous or linear ulcerations, and fibrotic strictures.

Many patients with colonic disease also have **small-bowel findings**, which distinguishes Crohn's from ulcerative colitis. To evaluate the extent of the disease, an upper gastrointestinal (GI) examination with small-bowel follow-through is imperative to find lesions of the stomach, duodenum, or small intestine such as strictures or fistulas.

The most common **symptoms found outside the GI tract** involve the skin, eyes, and joints. Multiple subcutaneous nodules that are tender, red, raised, and microscopically composed of lymphocytes and histiocytes characterize erythematous lesions that may form a tender necrotizing ulcer. Most of these occur in the pretibial area, but they also can occur anywhere on the body. Ocular manifestations include uveitis, iritis, episcleritis, vasculitis, and conjunctivitis. These findings are associated more commonly with colonic disease and infrequently precede any intestinal symptoms.

The incidence of carcinoma is increased in the setting of Crohn's disease and should be suspected in patients with a severe or chronic stricture.

Medical Therapy: **The primary treatment of Crohn's disease is medical. Surgery is indicated for complications of the disease process.**

Sulfasalazine and mesalamine are the two aminosalicylates used for Crohn's disease. For patients with exacerbations leading to moderate or severe Crohn's disease, steroids are the primary therapy.

As increasing evidence points to an immunologic etiology of inflammatory bowel disease, efforts have been made to utilize various **immunotherapies**. The drugs most commonly used are azathioprine and its metabolite, 6-mercaptopurine (6-MP). Methotrexate is a folate analogue that inhibits purine and pyrimidine synthesis and has been shown in a number of trials to be effective in treating Crohn's disease. However, this drug has significant side effects including hepatotoxicity and bone marrow suppression and thus is reserved for patients with severe Crohn's that is refractory to other therapies. Recently, anti–α-tumor necrosis factor (α-TNF) monoclonal antibody has been proven to be useful in the management of Crohn's disease.

Surgical Therapy: As previously noted, **the primary treatment of Crohn's disease is medical, and surgery is considered for patients with specific complications of the disease.** See **Algorithm 25.2.** Crohn's disease cannot be cured by an operation, but surgery can help ameliorate certain situations (**Table 25.1**).

Small intestinal or ileocolic stenotic disease is treated by resection with primary anastomosis. Only grossly involved intestine should be resected, because wide resection or microscopically negative margins of resection have no impact on the recurrence rate of the

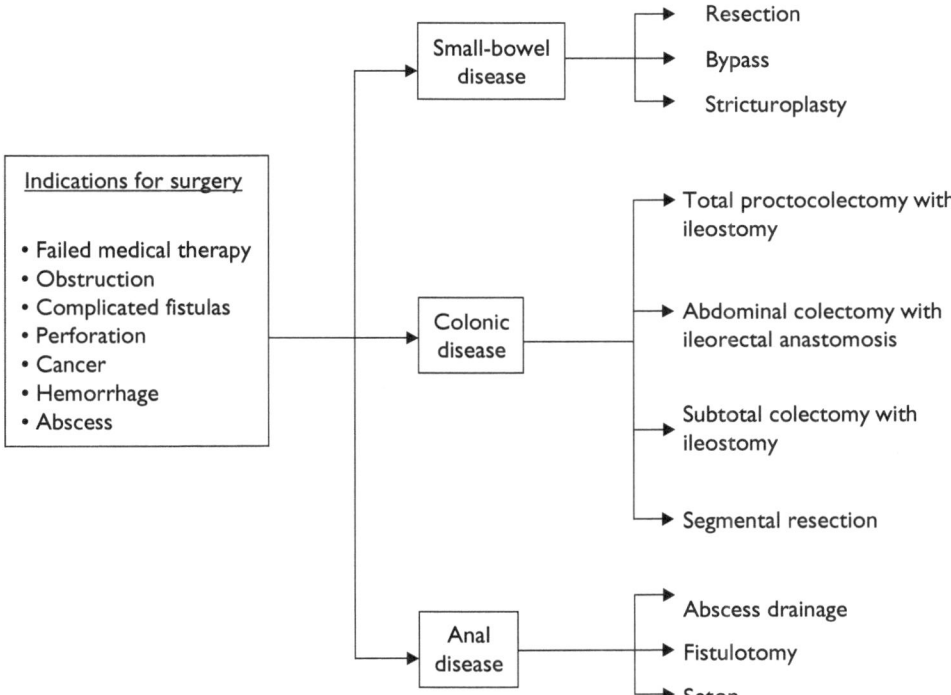

Algorithm 25.2. Algorithm for the management of Crohn's disease.

Table 25.1. Indications for surgical treatment of Crohn's disease.

Failure of medical treatment
  Persistence of symptoms despite corticosteroid therapy for longer than 6 months
  Recurrence of symptoms when high-dose corticosteroids tapered
  Worsening symptoms or new onset of complications with maximal medical therapy
  Occurrence of steroid-induced complications (cushingoid features, cataracts, glaucoma, systemic hypertension, aseptic necrosis of the head of the femur, myopathy, or vertebral body fractures)
Obstruction
Intestinal obstruction (partial or complete)
Septic complications
  Inflammatory mass or abscess (intraabdominal, pelvic, perineal)
  Fistula if
    Drainage causes personal embarrassment (e.g., enterocutaneous, enterovaginal fistula, fistula in ano)
    Fistula communicates with the genitourinary system (e.g., entero- or colovesical fistula)
    Fistula produces functional or anatomic bypass of a major segment of intestine with consequent malabsorption and/or profuse diarrhea (e.g., duodenocolic or enterorectosigmoid fistula)
    Free perforation
Hemorrhage
Carcinoma
Growth retardation
Fulminant colitis with or without toxic megacolon

Source: Reprinted from Michelassi F, Milsom J. Operative Strategies in Inflammatory Bowel Disease. New York: Springer-Verlag, 1999.

disease. It may lead to additional complications, such as short bowel syndrome.

Patients who present with fistulizing disease with either established fistulas or undrained sepsis require the greatest amount of judgment and caution. The surgical inclination is to operate urgently. However, percutaneous drainage, parenteral nutrition, and bowel rest usually control sepsis and allow the inflammation of the uninvolved bowel and surrounding structures to resolve.

For isolated Crohn's colitis, a total proctocolectomy with ileostomy or total abdominal colectomy with ileorectal anastomosis or ileostomy and rectal stump are the primary therapies.

The manifestations of **perianal Crohn's disease** are multiple, including abscesses, fistulas, fissures, ulcers, strictures, and incontinence. Perianal disease is the first presentation of Crohn's disease in 8% of cases. Estimates of the number of Crohn's patients who develop perianal manifestations at some time range from 10% to 80%. As with Crohn's disease proximally, palliation of symptoms and preservation of functional bowel are the priorities guiding surgical intervention. Likewise, the aim of therapy is the treatment of complications of disease rather than the disease itself. Two mandates clarify these **principles with respect to perianal disease: (1) the management of a septic focus is an indication for surgery, and (2) the sphincter should be preserved as long as the patient is coping well.** As painful as Crohn's perineal lesions often appear, they surprisingly are well tolerated. In fact, the complaint of pain is indicative of an abscess, and surgical consultation should be arranged promptly.

Ulcerative Colitis

Ulcerative colitis (UC) is a mucosal inflammatory condition of the GI tract confined to the colon and rectum. Like Crohn's, it is considered a manifestation of inflammatory bowel disease (IBD), as discussed in **Case 1. Although the medical therapy is similar for Crohn's disease and ulcerative colitis, the surgical therapies for each differ greatly, and it is imperative that a clear diagnosis is made whenever possible.**

The clinical manifestations of ulcerative colitis vary with the severity of the disease. Patients may have active disease with intervening periods of quiescence. The most common symptom of ulcerative colitis is **bloody diarrhea**. Patients with mild disease may have occasional blood and mucus and a moderate number of stools. Frequent, explosive diarrhea with significant bleeding or discharge of mucus and pus manifests more severe disease. Massive hemorrhage from ulcerative colitis is rare. Severe disease also may be associated with fever, abdominal pain, tenesmus, malaise, anemia, or weight loss. Some may have fecal incontinence with severe disease activity.

Most patients present with mild to moderate disease involving the rectum and a contiguous segment of the distal colon. About 20% of patients present with pancolitis. The so-called **toxic "megacolon" is a presentation of fulminant colitis** with fever, abdominal pain, and leukocytosis that may or may not be associated with radiographic evidence of colonic dilatation. As presented **in Case 1, patients may require emergent operation for perforation or resistance to medical therapy**.

The diagnosis of ulcerative colitis is made endoscopically. **A sigmoidoscopy may be diagnostic, and colonoscopy is hazardous (perforation) when active disease is present. Enemas should not be given before the exam for the same reasons. Surveillance by colonoscopy in ulcerative colitis is important because of the increased risk of colorectal dysplasia and carcinoma.** Patients at higher risk are those with colitis proximal to the splenic flexure and those with long-standing disease, at least 8 to 10 years.

The **extraintestinal manifestations** of ulcerative colitis are similar to those of Crohn's disease, with the exception of hepatobiliary complications, which are more common and can be quite severe. Primary sclerosing cholangitis (PSC) is uncommon with Crohn's disease and occurs in 7.5% of patients with UC. The only cure for this disease is liver transplant.

Medical Therapy: **The medical therapy for ulcerative colitis overlaps significantly with those therapies used for Crohn's disease**, discussed earlier. Sulfasalazine, as well as preparations that delay the release of the active ingredient [5-acetylsalicylic acid (5-ASA)], are more useful in treating ulcerative colitis. Drugs to treat the presumed immune basis for UC also may be useful.

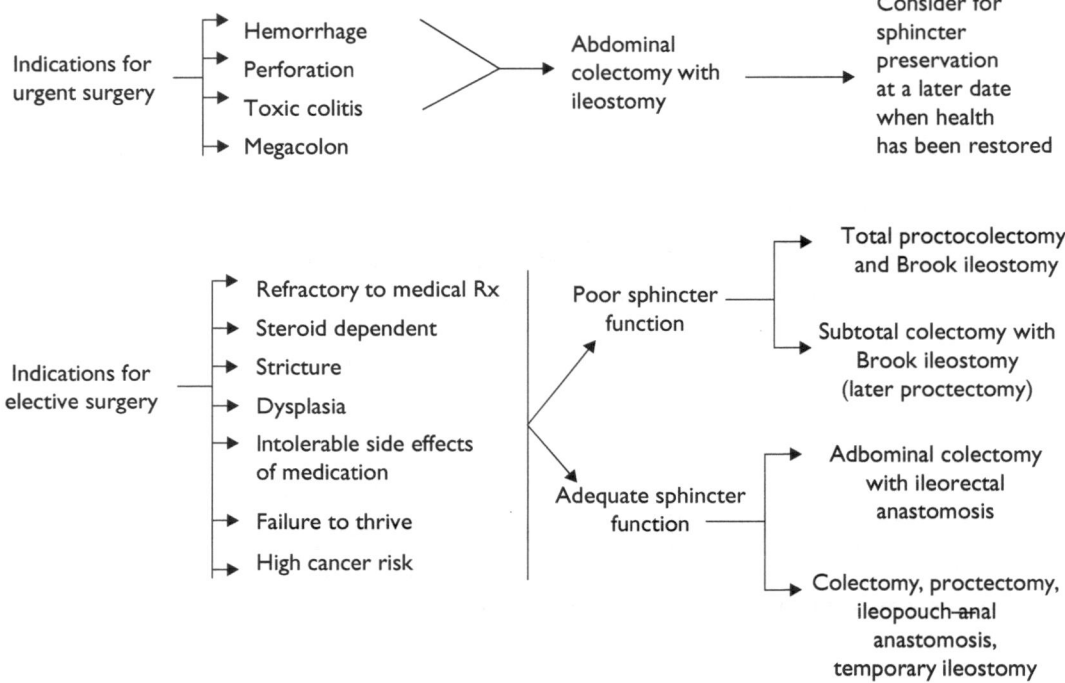

Algorithm 25.3. Algorithm for the management of ulcerative colitis.

Surgical Therapy: Approximately 30% of all patients with ulcerative colitis ultimately have surgery. (See **Algorithm 25.3.**) The surgical therapy employed most often involves removing the colon and, in most cases, the rectum. For patients with chronic active or quiescent disease, the indications for surgery include an inability to wean from steroids, extracolonic manifestations that may respond to colectomy, and the presence of dysplasia or carcinoma on colonoscopy screening. Children with UC may require surgery to treat delayed growth and maturation secondary to medical therapy or malnutrition.

The **ileal pouch–anal anastomosis** has become the standard operation for ulcerative colitis. The advantage of the procedure is that it allows the patient to void per anus, thus avoiding a stoma. The disadvantages are that the procedure is associated with significant morbidity and that the risk of cancer is not completely eliminated, as it is when a **standard proctocolectomy** is performed.

Diverticular Disease

Diverticulosis: **Diverticulosis** is common. As the incidence of diverticulosis increases with age, the risk of complications, other than bleeding, does not increase. In fact, the risk of complications related to perforation may be higher in the younger age groups. Medical treatment is less effective for recurrent attacks, and complications associated with an acute attack increase from 23% for the first attack to 58% after more than one attack. Complications requiring surgery occur only in approximately 1% of patients with the disease, whereas nearly one third of symptomatic patients may require surgery at some point.

Colonoscopy is preferred over barium enema in the initial workup of suspected diverticular disease because of its superior sensitivity and specificity. However, colonoscopy is less rewarding and more dangerous in the evaluation of acute complications of perforated diverticular disease.

Fiber is the mainstay of the medical management of uncomplicated diverticulosis or mild diverticulitis. A high-fiber diet is believed to reduce intracolonic pressures, presumably eliminating the "cause" of diverticular disease.

Complications of colonic diverticula that may require surgical consultation or intervention are hemorrhage and the complications of perforation of a diverticulum, which include chronic left lower quadrant pain, phlegm, abscess, peritonitis, fistula, and stricture. Hemorrhage occurs in up to 20% of patients with diverticulosis. In 5%, the hemorrhage is massive. The source of the bleeding is generally right sided, even though the diverticula predominantly are present on the left. The majority of patients (70–82%) stop bleeding; up to one third continue to bleed and require intervention.

Once resuscitation is under way, attention is directed toward localization of the source. If the nasogastric tube and proctosigmoidoscopic evaluation suggest a distal source, a nuclear medicine test is the preferred first step. Angiographic localization is attempted in those with a positive nuclear medicine scan. Embolization or Pitressin infusion following angiography may control bleeding.

Diverticulitis: Diverticulitis develops when a diverticulum ruptures. In most cases, the perforation is microscopic, causing localized inflammation in the colonic wall or paracolic tissues. In more severe cases, an abscess may form or the diverticulum freely may rupture into the peritoneal cavity, causing generalized peritonitis. The average age at presentation is the early 60s; more than 90% of cases occur after 50 years of age.

Patients with acute diverticulitis typically present with the gradual onset of left lower quadrant pain and low-grade fever. The pain is constant and does not radiate. On physical examination, tenderness to palpation usually is present in the left lower quadrant or suprapubic region. A mass suggestive of a peridiverticular abscess or phlegmon also may be palpable. Rectal examination may reveal a boggy mass anteriorly if a pelvic abscess is present. Unlike diverticulosis, acute diverticulitis usually is not associated with hemorrhage, but 30% to 40% of cases have guaiac-positive stool.

Plain-film abdominal series including an upright chest x-ray should be obtained to rule out free intraperitoneal air or lower lobe pneumonia. These studies may be normal or may demonstrate a distal large-bowel obstruction, localized ileus, or extracolonic air. **Computed tomography** with IV, oral, and rectal contrast is the study of choice (**Fig. 25.4**). Endoscopy generally is contraindicated in the setting of acute diverticulitis.

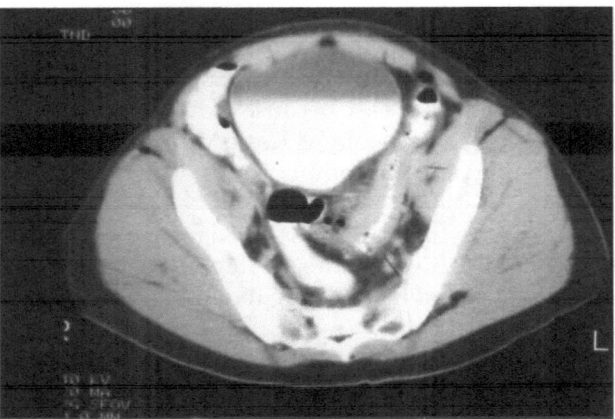

Figure 25.4. Computed tomography (CT) scan of a patient with acute diverticulitis. Note the "streaking" of the fat characteristic of inflammation and the thickening of the sigmoid colon bowel wall. (Reprinted from Schecter WP. Peritoneum and Acute Abdomen. In: Norton JA, Bollinger RR, Chang AE, et al, eds. Surgery: Basic Science and Clinical Evidence. New York: Springer-Verlag, 2001, with permission.)

Mild cases of acute diverticulitis in immunocompetent patients can be managed on an outpatient basis with clear liquids and oral antibiotics. Ideal patients for outpatient management are those who are able to tolerate a diet, have no systemic symptoms or peritoneal signs, and are reliable. Immunocompromise, steroid therapy, and advanced age are contraindications to outpatient therapy (see **Algorithm 25.4**).

Purulent or fecal peritonitis may develop secondary to rupture of a contained abscess or free perforation of a diverticulum. Most present with an acute abdomen and some degree of septic shock. **Aggressive intravenous resuscitation, antibiotics, and surgery are required for patients who present in this fashion.** The presentation in the immunosuppressed population may not be as clear, and abdominal films and a computed tomography (CT) scan may be necessary to make the diagnosis. Nonetheless, the treatment is the same. They are explored urgently, and a resection with descending colostomy and oversewing of the rectal stump is performed in all but the sickest patients.

Fistulas develop in only 2% of patients with diverticulitis, but fistula is the indication for surgery in 20% of those undergoing surgery for diverticulitis and its associated complications (**Fig. 25.5**). The bladder is affected most commonly, with nearly two thirds of all patients in one series having colovesical fistulas. Such patients may present with pneumaturia, fecaluria, abdominal pain, urinary symptoms (frequency, urgency, dysuria), hematuria, and fever and chills. Colovaginal fistulas, the next most common diverticular fistula, present with vaginal discharge, air, or stool per vagina.

The indications for surgery for diverticulitis are recurrent attacks, a severe attack, age less than 50 years, immunocompromised patients, or a severe complication of perforation such as significant

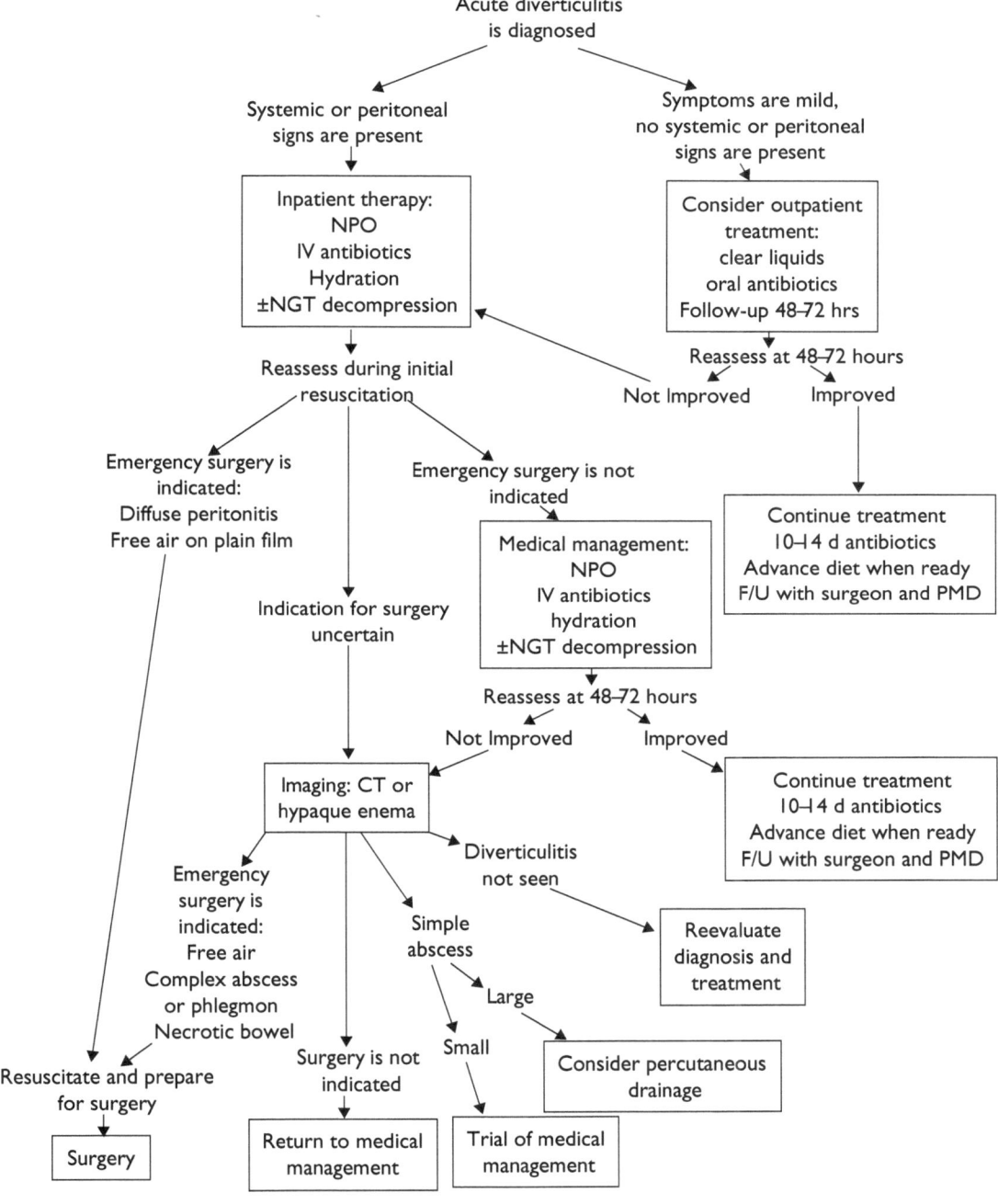

Algorithm 25.4. Algorithm for the management of acute diverticulitis. NGT, nasogastric tube; PMD, primary medical doctor. (Reprinted from Schecter WP. Peritoneum and Acute Abdomen. In: Norton JA, Bollinger RR, Chang AE, et al, eds. Surgery: Basic Science and Clinical Evidence. New York: Springer-Verlag, 2001, with permission.)

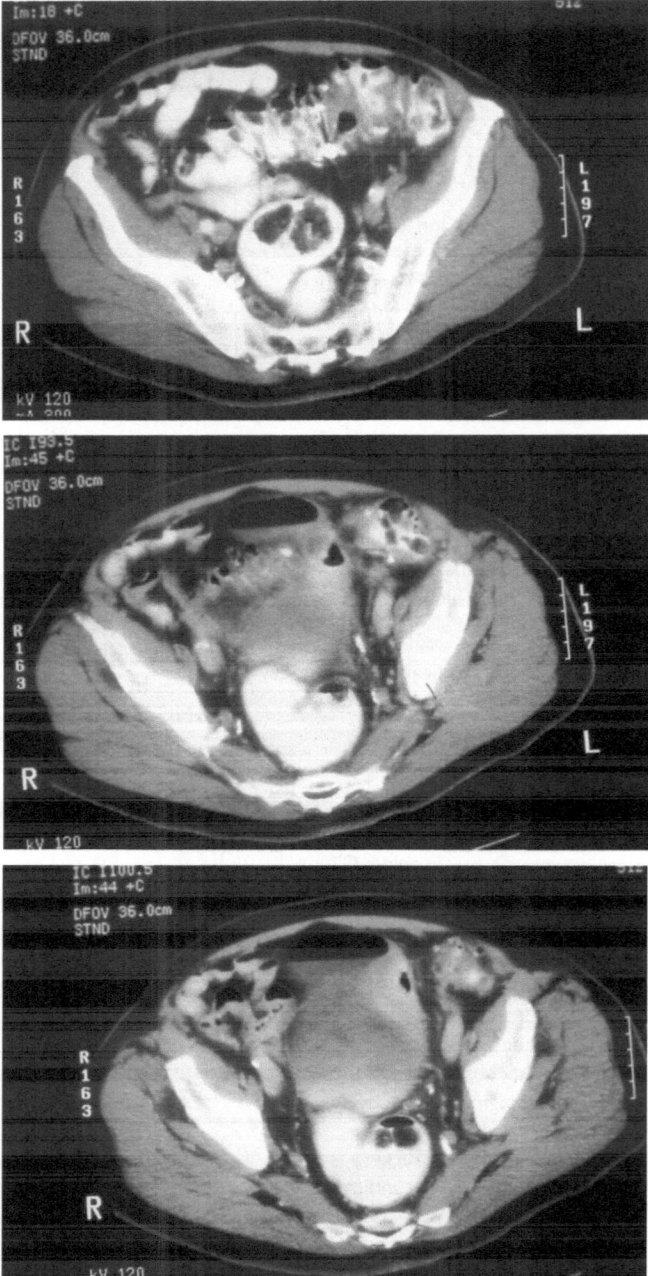

Figure 25.5. CT scan of a patient with a fistula to the bladder. Note the air collection outside the colon that can be traced down to the bladder on serial images. Air in the bladder without a history of recent catheterization is diagnostic of a communication with the gastrointestinal tract. (Reprinted from Schecter WP. Peritoneum and Acute Abdomen. In: Norton JA, Bollinger RR, Chang AE, et al, eds. Surgery: Basic Science and Clinical Evidence. New York: Springer-Verlag, 2001, with permission.)

phlegmon/abscess, peritonitis, fistula, or stricture. The goals of surgical therapy are to minimize morbidity and mortality, remove the septic focus and diseased colon, avoid or at least minimize the risks of a second operation, and convert an emergent situation to an urgent or elective operation.

Infectious Colitides

Infections of the large bowel usually cause diarrhea and can produce fever or abdominal pain. **Infectious colitis must be differentiated from other etiologies of colitis.** It is critical to elicit a complete history from the patient, including recent travel, unusual ingestions suspect for food poisoning, similar illnesses among family members, recent hospitalizations, treatment with antibiotics, sexual history, immunosuppression, and evidence of systemic disease.

Diarrhea that develops during antibiotic administration may be related to a change in the bacterial flora of the colon. This resolves spontaneously after cessation of therapy. However, a minority of patients on antibiotics have a proliferation of the toxin-producing strains of *Clostridium difficile*, a gram-positive, anaerobic organism. It is now known that any antibiotic can produce this colitis. Patients present with watery diarrhea, fever, and leukocytosis. Abdominal pain and tenderness also are common. Some patients develop toxic megacolon. Symptoms can occur both during antibiotic administration and weeks to months after cessation of treatment. The diagnosis is made by rapid immunoassays that test for antigens or toxins in the stool. On endoscopic exam, the mucosa can look inflamed or develop plaque-like membranes, which is why it has been called "pseudomembranous" colitis.

Volvulus

Intestinal volvulus is a closed-loop obstruction of the bowel resulting from an axial twist of the intestine upon its mesentery of at least 180 degrees; this results in luminal obstruction and progressive strangulation of the blood supply. **The early diagnosis and treatment of volvulus are important in avoiding intestinal ischemia or gangrene that can lead to a high morbidity and mortality.**

The more common **sigmoid volvulus** usually presents with the triad of abdominal pain, distention, and obstipation. Upon questioning, one often elicits a history of previous attacks. On exam, the abdomen is distended dramatically, with high-pitched bowel sounds and tympany to percussion. The diagnosis may be confirmed with an abdominal radiograph (**Fig. 25.6**). Minimal tenderness may be elicited in spite of this presentation.

When patients do not show signs of intestinal strangulation, the initial treatment of choice is **endoscopic decompression**; this allows the volvulus to reduce so that surgical treatment can be performed electively, after a full mechanical bowel preparation, with lower morbidity and mortality. **Rigid sigmoidoscopy** can reduce and decompress the bowel, evaluate the rectal and colonic mucosa, and allow for the passage of a rectal tube to keep the bowel decompressed. Endoscopic decompression is successful about 85% of the time.

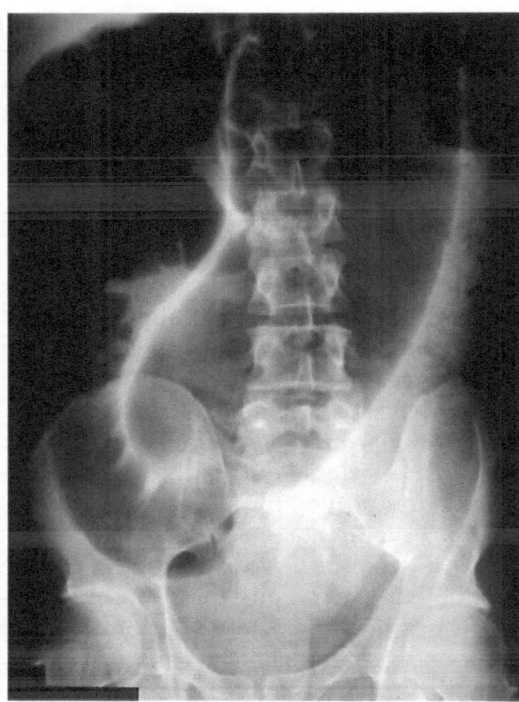

Figure 25.6. Classic sigmoid volvulus. Note that pelvis of kidney bean–shaped volvulus points to origin of volvulus. (Reprinted from Schecter WP. Peritoneum and Acute Abdomen. In: Norton JA, Bollinger RR, Chang AE, et al, eds. Surgery: Basic Science and Clinical Evidence. New York: Springer-Verlag, 2001, with permission.)

Patients with gangrene may present with a more fulminating picture of systemic illness and an acute abdomen. The goals of treatment are to untwist and decompress the bowel before strangulation and to prevent recurrences. **Those patients admitted with signs of sepsis indicative of gangrenous bowel must be resuscitated aggressively and taken emergently to the operating room.**

Cecal volvulus is the second most common type of volvulus, although it is the cause of only 1% of all intestinal obstructions. Most patients present with symptoms of a small-bowel obstruction: nausea, vomiting, cramping, abdominal pain, and distention. Two types of volvulus can occur: an ileocolic twisting, generally in a clockwise direction; or a cecal bascule, which is an anterior and superior folding of the cecum over the ascending colon. The latter is much less common, occurring 10% of the time.

These patients cannot be reduced endoscopically and require operation for definitive treatment. If the bowel is gangrenous, right hemicolectomy with ileostomy is the standard treatment. The mortality of this procedure ranges from 22% to 40%. However, if no perforation is present and the patient is hemodynamically stable, then an ileocolectomy and primary anastomosis may be performed safely.

Malignant Diseases

Incidence

Colorectal cancer is the second leading cause of death by cancer in the United States (estimated at 15% of all malignancies). Approximately 30% are located in the rectum, 28% in the sigmoid, 9% in the descending colon, 11% in the transverse colon, 9% in the ascending colon, and 13% in the cecum.

Screening and Surveillance

Cancer screening refers to the testing of a population of apparently asymptomatic individuals to determine the risk of developing colorectal cancer. Various screening and surveillance modalities are available to detect colorectal cancers and adenomatous polyps (**Table 25.2**). Surveillance refers to the ongoing monitoring of individuals who have an increased risk for the development of a disease. **For colorectal cancer, surveillance is reserved for patients with inflammatory bowel disease, family cancer syndromes, APC disorders, and a previous history of colorectal cancer or colorectal adenomas.**

Signs and Symptoms

The presentation of large-bowel malignancy generally falls into three categories: insidious onset of chronic symptoms, acute onset of intestinal obstruction, and acute perforation. The most common presentation is that of an insidious onset of chronic symptoms (77–92%), followed by obstruction (6–16%), and perforation with local or diffuse peritonitis (2–7%).

   As in Case 2, **bleeding is the most common symptom of colorectal malignancy. Unfortunately, patient and physician alike often attribute the bleeding to hemorrhoids. Change in bowel habits is the second most common complaint, with patients noting either diarrhea or constipation. Perforation is the third general class of presentation of colorectal malignancy.** It may result in localized peritonitis or gen-

Table 25.2. Patients who should be screened or in surveillance programs.

Screen				Surveillance
Average risk and symptoms	Average risk and age >50	Average risk and request screen	Increased risk	Personal history
Change in bowel habits, per anal bleeding, unclear abdominal pain, unclear anemia			Family history of CRC, adenomas in 1st-degree relatives <60 years old, genetic family syndrome (HNPCC, FAP)	IBD, previous adenomas, previous CRC, genetic syndromes

CRC, colorectal carcinoma; FAP, familial adenomatous polyposis; HNPCC, hereditary nonpolyposis coli syndrome; IBD, inflammatory bowel disease.
Source: Reprinted from Welton ML, Varma MG, Amerhauser A. Colon, rectum, and anus. In: Norton JA, Bollinger RR, Chang AE, et al, eds. Surgery: Basic Science and Clinical Evidence. New York: Springer-Verlag, 2001, with permission.

eralized peritonitis, or, if walled off, it may present with obstruction or fistula to an adjacent structure, such as the bladder.

Staging

Staging systems are important for predicting outcomes, selecting patients for various therapies, and comparing therapies for like patients across institutions. **For a tumor to be considered as an invasive cancer and staged, it must penetrate through the muscularis mucosa.** Several classification systems are utilized, including the Dukes, which is based on the extent of direct extension, along with the presence or absence of regional lymphatic metastases for the staging of rectal cancer. Dukes' A lesions are those in which the depth of penetration of the primary tumor is confined to the bowel wall. Dukes' B lesions have primary tumor penetration through the full thickness of the bowel to include serosa or fat. Dukes' C lesions have local (C_1) or regional (C_2) nodal involvement. Although not initially described, it became accepted by common practice to add a fourth category for distant spread (D) outside the resected specimen.

The TNM (tumor/node/metastasis) classification was proposed by the American College of Surgeons' Commission on Cancer to incorporate findings at laparotomy. The stages of the TNM system roughly correlate to the stages of Dukes' C; stage 4 is the equivalent of Dukes' D (**Tables 25.3 and 25.4**).

The American Joint Committee on Cancer (AJCC) has settled on two classifications: low grade (well and moderately differentiated) and high grade (poorly and undifferentiated). DNA ploidy assessment is the

Table 25.3. TNM staging system.

Stage	Depth	Nodal status	Distant metastasis
Stage 1	T1, T2	N0	M0
Stage 2	T3, T4	N0	M0
Stage 3	Any T	Any N (except N0)	M0
Stage 4	Any T	Any N	M1

TX	Primary tumor cannot be assessed
T0	No evidence of primary tumor
Tis	Carcinoma in situ
T1	Tumor invades into submucosa
T2	Tumor invades into muscularis propria
T3	Tumor invades through muscularis propria
T4a	Tumor perforates visceral peritoneum
T4b	Tumor directly invades other structures
NX	Regional lymph nodes cannot be assessed
N0	No regional lymph nodes
N1	1–3 regional lymph nodes
N2	More than 4 regional lymph nodes
N3	Regional lymph nodes along a named vascular trunk
MX	Presence of distant metastasis cannot be assessed
M0	No distant metastases
M1	Distant metastases

Source: Reprinted from Welton ML, Varma MG, Amerhauser A. Colon, rectum, and anus. In: Norton JA, Bollinger RR, Chang AE, et al, eds. Surgery: Basic Science and Clinical Evidence. New York: Springer-Verlag, 2001, with permission.

Table 25.4. Comparison of TNM system to Dukes' classification.

	Tumor	Nodes	Distant disease
A	Tis, T1, T2 T3	N0	M0
B	T4	N0	M0
C1	T1, T2, T3	Any N (except N0)	M0
C2	T4	Any N (except N0)	M0
D	ANY T	ANY N	M1

Source: Reprinted from Welton ML, Varma MG, Amerhauser A. Colon, rectum, and anus. In: Norton JA, Bollinger RR, Chang AE, et al, eds. Surgery: Basic Science and Clinical Evidence. New York: Springer-Verlag, 2001, with permission.

measurement of the quantum amount of DNA in cells. Diploidy is correlated with good prognoses; aneuploidy is correlated with poor prognoses. Bowel perforation and elevated preoperative carcinoembryonic antigen (CEA) are associated with poorer prognosis.

Preoperative Staging for Colorectal Cancer

The general physical examination remains a cornerstone in assessing a patient preoperatively to determine the extent of the local disease, disclosing distant metastases, and appraising the general operative risk. Special attention should be paid to weight loss, pallor as a sign of anemia, and signs of portal hypertension. In addition, a complete workup should include the investigations listed in **Table 25.5.**

Cancer of the Colon

Natural History

Surgery remains the cornerstone of treatment for colorectal cancer, but it has inherent limitations imposed by the biology and stage of the tumor as well as its location. Ultimately, 50% of patients who undergo curative resection develop local, regional, or widespread recurrence. Operative management is discussed briefly below, and additional therapies, based on pathologic findings, are outlined in **Algorithm 25.5.**

Table 25.5. Preoperative evaluation for colorectal malignancy.

Routine blood work
Colonoscopy
Radiographs
Ultrasound
CBC, LFT, CEA
Tissue diagnosis, synchronous disease
CXR, seleced CT abdomen/pelvis
Transrectal ultrasound

CBC, complete blood count; CEA, carcinoembryonic antigen; CT, computed tomography; CXR, chest x-ray; LET, liver function test.
Source: Reprinted from Welton ML, Varma MG, Amerhauser A. Colon, rectum, and anus. In: Norton JA, Bollinger RR, Chang AE, et al, eds. Surgery: Basic Science and Clinical Evidence. New York: Springer-Verlag, 2001, with permission.

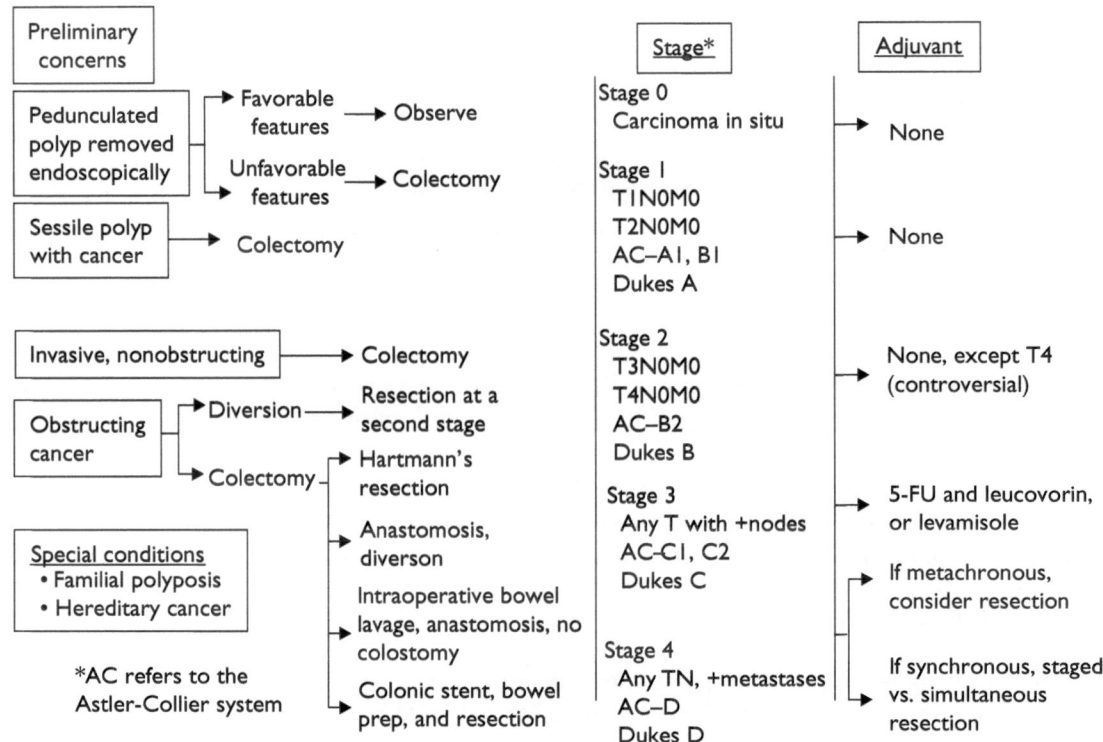

Algorithm 25.5. Algorithm for the management of colon cancer. 5-FU, 5-fluorouracil.

Cancer of the Cecum, Ascending Colon, or Hepatic Flexure

For lesions located in the cecum or ascending colon, **a right hemi-colectomy** to encompass the bowel served by the ilii-colic, right colic, and right branch of the middle colic vessels is recommended. For lesions involving the hepatic flexure, **a more extended resection** is indicated, including the right colon and proximal and midtransverse colon, including both branches of the middle colic artery. This often is referred to as "an extended right hemicolectomy."

Cancer of the Transverse Colon

Depending on the exact location of the tumor, the **transverse colon often is resected,** including either the hepatic or splenic flexure.

Cancer of the Splenic Flexure

Splenic flexure lesions require **removal of the distal half of the transverse colon** and the descending colon.

Cancer of the Sigmoid Colon

Sigmoid lesions are treated by **removal of the sigmoid colon**. The exact boundaries of resection depend on the level of the tumor. Resections of higher sigmoid lesions include the descending sigmoid junction.

Subtotal colectomy is the treatment of choice for patients with synchronous lesions at different sites. If synchronous lesions are located in the same anatomic region, a conventional resection may be performed.

Cancer of the Rectum

Rectal cancer has traditionally been treated with **abdominal perineal resection**, which removes the whole rectum and anus. More recently, the **low anterior resection and local excision with and without radiation** have gained popularity. Both preserve continence and can result in equal 5-year survival rates in properly selected patients.

Cancer Arising in a Colon Polyp

A colorectal polyp is defined as a mass that protrudes into the lumen of the colon. These masses may be either sessile or pedunculated (**Fig. 25.7**).

Adenomas are benign neoplasms with dysplasia. Nonneoplastic polyps are without dysplastic features and include mucosal, hyperplastic, inflammatory, and hamartomatous (including juvenile) polyps. Approximately 70% of colonoscopically removed polyps are adenomas.

There is now a general consensus that **most colon cancers arise from preexisting polyps**. The lifetime risk of an adenoma transforming into a malignancy is estimated to be 5% to 10%, and the time for transforming is estimated to be 5 to 15 years. Less than 2% of adenomas smaller than 1 cm harbor a carcinoma, whereas the percentage increases to about 10% in adenomas between 1 and 2 cm and 50% in adenomas larger than 2 cm. **Colonoscopy and complete polypectomy are curative in patients with carcinoma in situ**, as these lesions appear to have no potential for metastases.

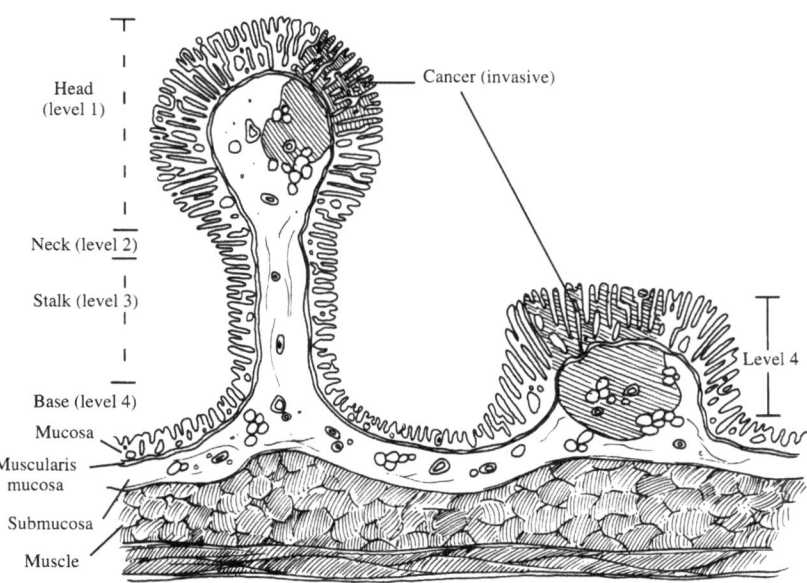

Figure 25.7. Sessile and pedunculated polyps illustrating Haggitt's classification of levels of invasion. (Reprinted from Bailey HR, Snyder MJ, eds. Ambulatory Anorectal Surgery. New York: Springer-Verlag, 2000, with permission.)

Therapy for Metastatic Colorectal Cancer

Of 100 patients with colorectal cancer, roughly 50 are cured by surgery, 15 develop local recurrence, and 35 develop blood-borne distant metastases. The organs most frequently involved with metastases are the liver, the lung, the bone, and the brain. Up to 15% of patients present with liver metastases at their initial operation, and 30% of patients undergoing apparently curative resection already have hepatic metastases that are not evident to the surgeon at the time of operation. **Patients with disseminated disease beyond the scope of surgical resection are eligible for chemotherapy.**

Therapy for Local Recurrent Colorectal Cancer

Of all colorectal cancer recurrences, 70% occur within 2 years of operation. Local recurrences vary between 1% and 20% for colon cancer and between 3% and 32% for rectal cancer. Many patients are eligible for **surgical therapy of localized recurrence, but this should always be considered in conjunction with options for chemotherapy.**

Polyposis Coli Syndromes

Familial Adenomatous Polyposis

Familial adenomatous polyposis (FAP) is an inherited, non–sex-linked, dominant disease characterized by the progressive development of hundreds of polyps. The mutated gene is found on the long arm of chromosome 5 and is called the *APC* gene. Genetic testing to detect FAP and its variants is available.

The condition is characterized by the development of hundreds to thousands of colonic adenomatous polyps and an extreme risk of colon cancer. Polyps occur at a mean age of 16 years, and almost all affected persons exhibit adenomas by age 35 years. Seven percent of untreated individuals have cancer by age 21, 50% by age 39, and 90% by the age of 45 years.

Hereditary Nonpolyposis Coli Syndromes I and II (HNPCC)

Hereditary nonpolyposis coli syndrome is an autosomal-dominant inherited disease with a high risk of colon cancer. The average age of colon cancer diagnosis is 45 years, and the lifetime risk of colon cancer is 80% in gene carriers.

All patients with HNPCC need to be entered in a surveillance program by the age of 20 to 25 years. Screening not only should be directed at the colon but also at the pancreas, breast, cervix, ovary, and bladder. Colonoscopic surveillance should be performed every other year until 30 years of age and annually thereafter.

Summary

Complaints related to large bowel and rectal disease are frequent. The physician must be attentive to acute conditions that require active resuscitation and expeditious diagnosis. While many inflammatory bowel conditions may not require acute surgical interventions, surgery may represent an appropriate therapy for acute toxicity or intractable chronic symptoms. Surgical resection is the only option for potential cure of large bowel and rectal cancers.

Selected Readings

Bartlett JG, Chang TW, Gurwith M, Gorbach SL, Onderdonk AB. Antibiotic-associated pseudomembranous colitis due to toxin-producing clostridia. N Engl J Med 1978;(10):531–534.

Beart RW, Melton LJd, Maruta M, Dockerty MB, Frydenberg HB, O'Fallon WM. Trends in right- and left-sided colon cancer. Dis Colon Rectum 1983; 26(6):393–398.

Bokhari M, Vernava AM, Ure T, Longo WE. Diverticular hemorrhage in the elderly is-it well tolerated? Dis Colon Rectum 1996;39(2):292–295.

Casarella WJ, Galloway SJ, Taxin RN, Follett DA, Pollock EJ, Seaman WB. "Lower" gastrointestinal tract hemorrhage: new concepts based on arteriography. AJR 1974;121:357–368.

Gunderson LL, Sosin H, Levitt S. Extrapelvic colon areas of failure in a re-operation series: implications for adjuvant therapy. Int J Radiat Oncol Biol Phys 1985;11(4):731–741.

Hachigian MP, Honickman S, Eisenstat TE, Rubin RJ, Salvati EP. Computed tomography in the initial management of acute left-sided diverticulitis [published erratum appears in Dis Colon Rectum 1993;36(2):193] [see comments]. Dis Colon Rectum 1992;35(12):1123–1129.

Kelly CP, Pothoulakis C, LaMont JT. Clostridium difficile colitis [see comments]. N Engl J Med 1994;330(4):257–262.

McGuire HH Jr. Bleeding colonic diverticula. A reappraisal of natural history and management. Ann Surg 1994;220(5):653–656.

McGuire HH Jr, Haynes BW Jr. Massive hemorrhage for diverticulosis of the colon: guidelines for therapy based on bleeding patterns observed in fifty cases. Ann Surg 1972;175(6):847–855.

Morson BC, Dawson IMP. Gastrointestinal Pathology. London: Blackwell, 1972.

Muto T, Bussey HJ, Morson BC. The evolution of cancer of the colon and rectum. Cancer (Phila) 1975;36(6):2251–2270.

Pontari MA, McMillen MA, Garvey RH, Ballantyne GH. Diagnosis and treatment of enterovesical fistulae. Am Surg 1992;58(4):258–263.

Rothenberger DA, Wiltz O. Surgery for complicated diverticulitis. Surg Clin North Am 1993;73(5):975–992.

Russell AH, Tong D, Dawson LE, Wisbeck W. Adenocarcinoma of the proximal colon. Sites of initial dissemination and patterns of recurrence following surgery alone. Cancer (Phila) 1984;53(2):360–367.

Sagar PM, Pemberton JH. Surgical management of locally recurrent rectal cancer. Br J Surg 1996;83(3):297–304.

Smirniotis V, Tsoutsos D, Fotopoulos A, Pissiotis AC. Perforated diverticulitis: a surgical dilemma. Int Surg 1992;77(1):44–47.

Welton ML, Varma MG, Amerhauser A. Colon, rectum, and anus. In: Norton JA, Bollinger RR, Chang AE, et al, eds. Surgery: Basic Science and Clinical Evidence. New York: Springer-Verlag, 2001.

26

Perianal Complaints

Stephen F. Lowry and Theodore E. Eisenstat

Objectives

1. To understand the etiologies of and therapeutic approaches to diarrheal diseases.
2. To develop a differential diagnosis for a patient with common perianal disorders (including benign, malignant, and inflammatory causes).
3. To discuss the characteristic history and findings for common perianal problems.
4. To discuss a treatment plan for each diagnosis covered by Objective 1, including nonoperative interventions and the role and timing of surgical interventions.

Cases

Case 1

A 48-year-old diabetic man presents with a 2-day history of throbbing perianal pain that is worsened with bowel movement. His temperature is 102℉; his pulse is 108; his blood pressure is 94/50. He has dizziness on standing. Rectal examination reveals a painful, indurated perianal mass. There are no external sinus tracts.

Case 2

A 60-year-old woman presents with a remote history of blood coating her stool. She now has had 12 hours of severe, constant perianal pain. Examination reveals a tender, purplish subcutaneous mass below the dentate line.

Anatomy of the Anus

The anatomic anal canal starts at the dentate line and ends at the anal verge. However, a practical definition is the surgical anal canal, which extends from the termination of the muscular diaphragm of the pelvic floor to the anal verge. The anal canal is "supported" by the surrounding anal sphincter mechanism, composed of the internal and external sphincters. The internal sphincter is a specialized continuation of the circular muscle of the rectum. The external sphincter is composed of voluntary striated muscle.

Hemorrhoids are found in the subepithelial tissue above and below the dentate line. These are cushions composed of vascular and connective tissues and supportive muscle fibers. The middle rectal veins drain the lower rectum and upper anal canal into the systemic system via the internal iliac veins. The inferior rectal veins drain the lower anal canal, communicating with the pudendal veins and draining into the internal iliac veins.

Sensations of noxious stimuli above the dentate line are conducted through afferent fibers of these parasympathetic nerves and are experienced as an ill-defined dull sensation. Below the dentate line, the epithelium is exquisitely sensitive and richly innervated by somatic nerves. The internal sphincter, composed of smooth muscle, generates 85% of the resting tone. It is innervated with sympathetic and parasympathetic fibers.

Hemorrhoids are important participants in maintaining continence and minimizing trauma during defecation. They function as protective pillows that engorge with blood during the act of defecation, protecting the anal canal from direct trauma due to passage of stool.

See **Algorithm 26.1** for the initial workup of perianal conditions.

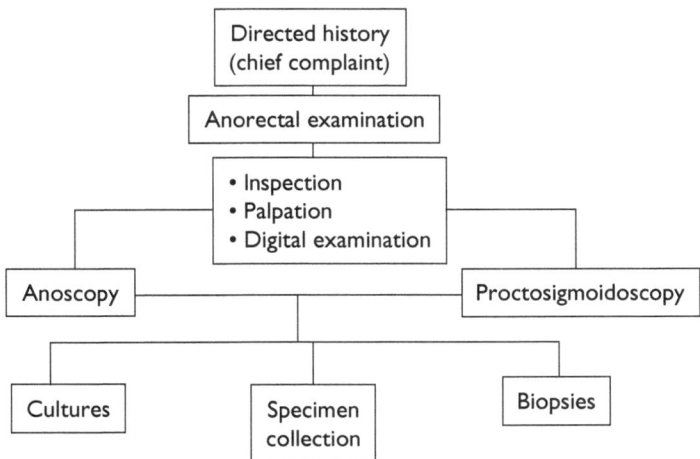

Algorithm 26.1. Algorithm for the initial workup of perianal conditions.

Diarrhea: Diagnosis and Management

Diarrhea is defined as liquid stool, rather than soft or formed stool, which has a daily weight exceeding 250 g and is accompanied by excess fluid loss and a number of bowel movements. Four general mechanics are responsible for diarrhea: morphologic alterations of intestinal mucosa, osmotic malabsorption, secretory derangement, and aberrant intestinal motility.

The **management of diarrhea** begins with a history and physical examination, including a thorough drug, dietary, and travel history as well as questions regarding food ingestion, recent medication changes, exposure to others with diarrhea, and family history. Chronic diarrhea lasts at least 3 to 6 weeks.

All patients with diarrhea should have stool samples tested for fecal leukocytes, occult blood, excess fat, and bacterial cultures. The presence of white blood cells (WBCs) implies an exudative or inflammatory process, usually as a result of an infectious enteritis or inflammatory bowel disease. The presence of blood in the stool without WBCs should arouse suspicion for neoplasm or colonic ischemia. Evaluations for ova and parasites, fecal qualitative fat, or mucosal biopsy are indicated in select cases.

Inflammatory diarrhea is characterized by the presence of fecal leukocytes and persistent diarrhea despite fasting. **Infections** are the most common cause. Etiologies include viral gastroenteritis (rotavirus), AIDS-related enteritis (giardia, salmonella, cryptosporidium), and pseudomembranous colitis (*Clostridium difficile*). Assays for *C. difficile* toxin and visual identification of organisms (giardia) on stain or culture can be diagnostic; antibiotic therapy should be directed against the causative agent. If negative, endoscopy should be performed to directly visualize the mucosa.

Examination of the stool for qualitative fecal fat can help diagnose **malabsorption**. A 24-hour fecal fat measurement should be ordered; greater than 10 g of fat per 24-hour period is indicative of malabsorptive or maldigestive steatorrhea.

Exogenous agents that may produce an osmotic diarrhea include laxatives (magnesium sulfate); magnesium-based antacids; dietetic foods with sorbitol, mannitol, or xylitol; and certain drugs used chronically (cholestyramine, colchicines, neomycin, and lactulose).

Endogenous sources are caused by congenital conditions including disaccharidase deficiencies or generalized malabsorptive/maldigestive processes (cystic fibrosis, congenital lymphangiectasia).

Acquired causes include pancreatic exocrine deficiency, bacterial overgrowth, celiac sprue, bile salt diarrhea, thyrotoxicosis, and adrenal insufficiency. Bacterial overgrowth syndromes can be confirmed by a hydrogen breath test that detects fermentation of carbohydrates by direct measure of hydrogen in the breath. Patients with small-bowel bacterial overgrowth have hydrogen peaks within 3 hours; those with colonic fermentation peak later, thereby identifying the site of the problem.

Secretory diarrhea is characterized by watery stools with volumes greater than 1 L per day. Etiologies include enterotoxin-induced secretion (cholera and enterotoxigenic *Escherichia coli*, diagnosed by toxin identification or organism culture), carcinoid syndrome (serotonin and substance P), pancreatic islet cell tumor syndrome [vasoactive intestinal polypeptide (VIP) induced], medullary thyroid carcinoma syndrome (calcitonin), and Zollinger-Ellison syndrome (gastrin).

Treatment of diarrhea should be directed to the underlying specific cause whenever possible. **Treatment of volume depletion is the first step in the management of diarrhea**; this can be accomplished in mild cases by avoiding solid foodstuffs and ingesting clear liquids. More severe volume depletion requires intravenous resuscitation.

Benign Diseases

Anorectal Abscess and Fistula

The anal canal has 6 to 14 glands that lie in or near the intersphincteric plane between the internal and external sphincters. Projections from the glands pass through the internal sphincters and drain into the crypts at the dentate line. Glands may become infected when a crypt is occluded, trapping stool and bacteria within the gland. If the crypt does not decompress into the anal canal, an abscess may develop in the intersphincteric plane. The abscess may track within or across the intersphincteric plane. Abscesses are classified by the space they invade (**Fig. 26.1**). Regardless of abscess location, **the extent of disease often is difficult to determine without examination under anesthesia.**

Antibiotics given while allowing the abscess to "mature" are not helpful. Early surgical consultation and operative drainage are the

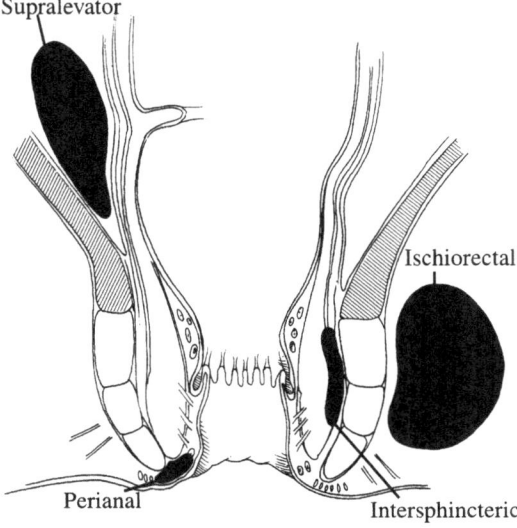

Figure 26.1. Abscesses are classified by location. (Reprinted from Vasilevsky CA. Fistula-in-ano and abscess. In: Beck DE, Wexner SD, eds. Fundamentals of Anorectal and Colonic Diseases, 2nd ed. New York: McGraw-Hill, 1992, with permission.)

best measures to use to avoid the disastrous complications associated with undrained perineal sepsis. When drained either surgically or spontaneously, 50% of abscesses have persistent communication with the crypt, creating a fistula from the anus to the perianal skin or fistula in ano. A fistula in ano is not a surgical emergency because the septic focus has drained.

As in **Case 1**, an abscess typically causes severe, continuous, throbbing anal pain that may worsen with ambulation and straining. Occasionally, patients present with fever, urinary retention, and life-threatening sepsis, which especially is true in diabetics and the immunocompromised host.

Physical examination of the patient with an abscess reveals a tender perianal or perirectal mass. No imaging studies are necessary in uncomplicated abscess fistulous disease, but imaging studies such as sinograms, transrectal ultrasound, computed tomography (CT), and magnetic resonance imaging (MRI) may be useful in the evaluation of complex or recurrent disease. An approach to surgical management of perianal abscesses/fistulas is shown in **Algorithm 26.2**.

Abscess fistula disease of cryptoglandular origin must be differentiated from complications of Crohn's disease, pilonidal disease, hidradenitis suppurativa, tuberculosis, actinomycosis, trauma, fissures, carcinoma, radiation, chlamydia, local dermal processes, retrorectal tumors, diverticulitis, and ureteral injuries. Five percent to 10% of patients with Crohn's disease initially present with anorectal abscess or fistulous disease. A colonic source may be suspected in a patient with known inflammatory bowel disease or diverticular disease.

The complications of an undrained anorectal abscess may be severe. If the abscess is not drained surgically or spontaneously, the infection may spread rapidly, which may result in extensive tissue loss, sphincter injury, and even death. **Abscesses should be drained surgically.** Patients often require drainage in the operating room, where anesthesia allows for adequate evaluation of the extent of the disease.

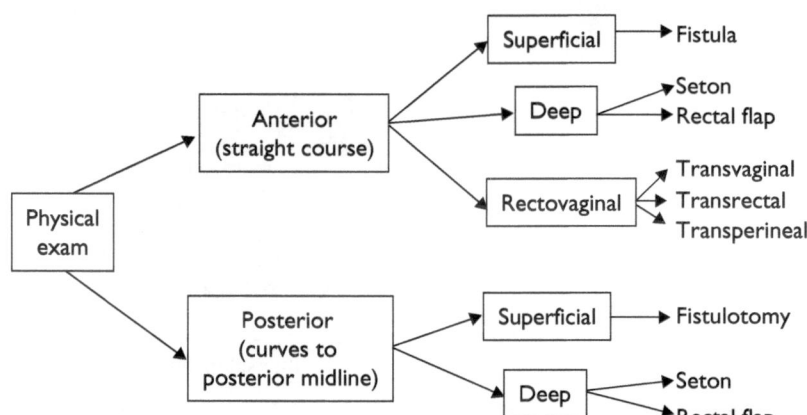

Algorithm 26.2. Algorithm for an approach to the surgical management of perianal abscesses/fistulas.

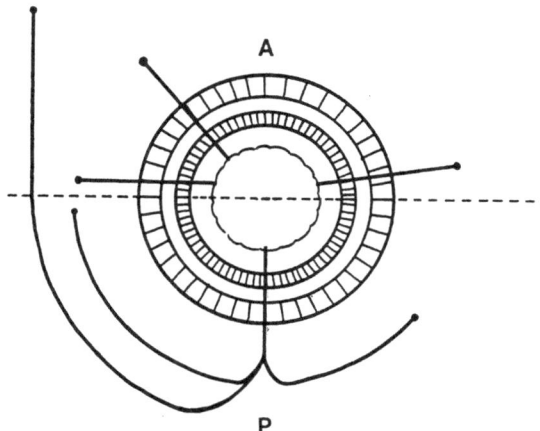

Figure 26.2. Goodsall's rule: External openings anterior to a line drawn between the 3 and 9 o'clock positions communicate with an internal opening along a straight line drawn toward the dentate line. Posterior external openings communicate with the posterior midline in a nonlinear fashion. The exception may be an interior opening that is greater than 3 cm from the dentate line. (Reprinted from Marti M-C, Givel J-C, eds. Surgical Management of Anorectal and Colonic Diseases, 2nd ed. Heidelberg: Springer-Verlag, 1999, with permission.)

Patients with a chronic or recurring abscess after apparent adequate surgical drainage often have an undrained, deep, postanal space abscess that communicates with the ischiorectal fossa via a "horseshoe fistula." Immunocompromised patients are a particular challenge, as seen in **Case 1**. These patients are more prone to necrotizing anorectal infections.

The **treatment of fistulas** is dictated by the course of the fistula. Goodsall's rule is of particular assistance in identifying the direction of the tract (**Fig. 26.2**) in fistulas with posterior external openings, but reliability is decreased anteriorly and in particular as the distance from the verge is increased.

Anal Fissure/Ulcer

An anal fissure is a split in the anoderm. An ulcer is a chronic fissure. Fissures most frequently occur in the midline just distal to the dentate line. Fissures result from forceful dilation of the anal canal, most commonly during defecation. Classically, the initial insult is believed to be a firm bowel movement. The pain associated with the initial bowel movement is great, and the patient therefore ignores the urge to defecate for fear of experiencing the pain again. A self-perpetuating cycle of pain, poor relaxation, and reinjury results.

Fissures cause pain and bleeding with defecation. The pain is often tearing or burning, worse during defecation, and subsides over a few hours. Anoscopy and proctosigmoidoscopy should be deferred until healing occurs or the procedure can be performed under anesthesia. **Although anoscopy and rigid sigmoidoscopy may not be performed** in the initial evaluation of a patient with a fissure, they must be performed during a subsequent visit because the presence of associated anorectal malignancy or inflammatory bowel disease must be excluded.

Ulcers occurring off the midline or away from the mucocutaneous junction are suspect. Crohn's disease, anal TB, anal malignancy, abscess/fistula disease, cytomegalovirus (CMV), herpes, chlamydia, syphilis, AIDS, and some blood dyscrasias all may mimic certain aspects of fissures/ulcer disease.

Treatment using stool softeners, bulk agents, and sitz baths is successful in healing 90% of anal fissures. Patients are instructed to soak in a hot bath and contract the sphincters to identify the muscle in spasm and then focus on relaxing that muscle. Botox infiltration into the internal sphincters may be effective in the treatment of anal fissures. Lateral internal sphincterotomy is the procedure of choice for many surgeons after conservative measures have failed.

Hemorrhoids

Patients with perianal pathology often present or are referred with a chief complaint of "hemorrhoids." A thorough history frequently suggests the diagnosis. **Those individuals with painless bleeding due to hemorrhoids must be distinguished from those with bleeding from colorectal malignancy, inflammatory bowel disease, diverticular disease, and adenomatous polyps.** Rectal prolapse must be distinguished from hemorrhoids because it is safe to band a hemorrhoid but not a prolapsed rectum.

Hemorrhoidal tissues are part of the normal anatomy of the distal rectum and anal canal. The disease state of "hemorrhoids" exists when the internal complex becomes chronically engorged or the tissue prolapses into the anal canal as the result of laxity of the surrounding connective tissue and dilatation of the veins. External hemorrhoids may thrombose, leading to acute onset of severe perianal pain. An approach to the management of hemorrhoid disease is shown in **Algorithm 26.3**.

Internal hemorrhoids may have two main pathophysiologic mechanisms seen in two distinct but not exclusive groups: **older women and younger men**. Internal hemorrhoids originate above the dentate line and are lined with insensate rectal columnar and transitional mucosa. In older women, the pathophysiologic mechanism may be related to earlier pregnancy or chronic straining, which leads to vascular engorgement and dilatation, resulting in stretching and disruption of the supporting connective tissue surrounding the vascular channels. Another suggested pathologic mechanism, and the one that may be more important in younger men, is that of increased resting pressures within the anal canal, leading to decreased venous return. Internal hemorrhoids typically do **not** cause pain but rather bright-red bleeding per rectum, mucous discharge, and a sense of rectal fullness or discomfort.

External hemorrhoids may develop an acute intravascular thrombus, which is associated with acute onset of extreme perianal pain. The pain

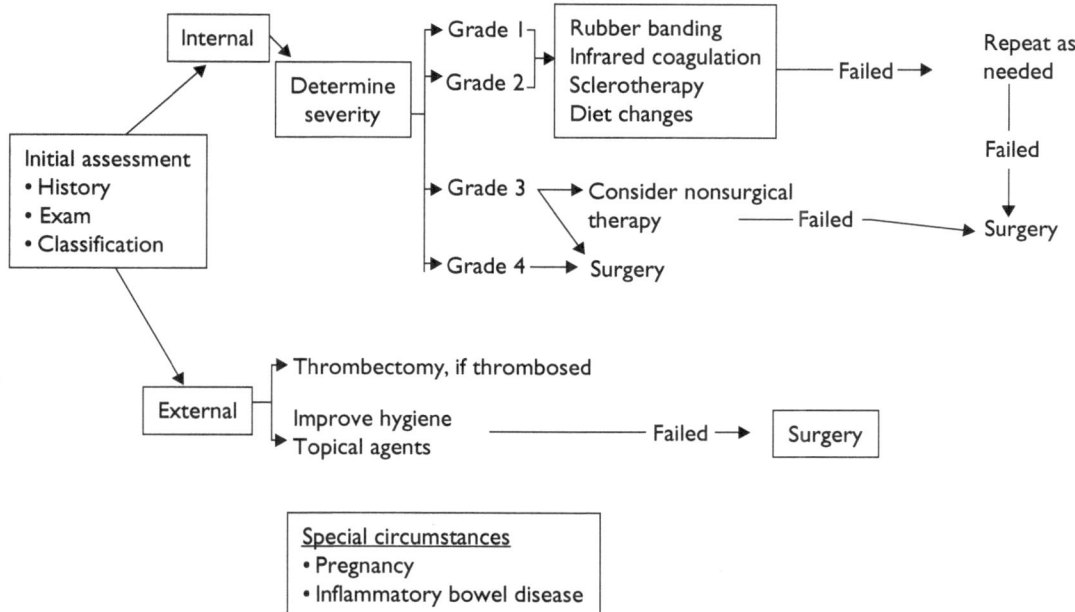

Algorithm 26.3. Algorithm for an approach to the management of hemorrhoid disease.

usually peaks within 48 hours. Repeated episodes of dilatation and thrombosis may lead to enlargement of the overlying skin, which is seen as a skin tag on physical exam. As in **Case 2**, the acutely thrombosed external hemorrhoid is seen as a purplish, edematous, tense subcutaneous perianal mass that is quite tender.

The complications of internal or external hemorrhoids are the indications for medical or surgical intervention: bleeding, pain, necrosis, mucous discharge, moisture, and, rarely, perianal sepsis. Initial medical management for all but the most advanced cases is recommended. Dietary alterations, including elimination of constipating foods (e.g., cheeses), addition of bulking agents, stool softeners, and increased intake of liquids are advised. Internal hemorrhoids that fail to respond to medical management may be treated with elastic band ligation, sclerosis, photocoagulation, cryosurgery, excisional hemorrhoidectomy, and many other local techniques that induce scarring and fixation of the hemorrhoids to the underlying tissues. The acutely thrombosed external hemorrhoid may be treated with excision of the hemorrhoid or clot evacuation if the patient presents within 48 hours of onset of symptoms. If the patient presents more than 48 hours after onset of symptoms, conservation management with warm sitz baths, high-fiber diet, stool softeners, and reassurance is advised.

Pilonidal Disease

Patients with pilonidal disease may present with small midline pits or an abscess(es) off the midline near the coccyx or sacrum. The workup is limited to a physical exam unless one suspects Crohn's disease; then a more extensive evaluation may be necessary. The differential diagnosis includes abscess/fistulous disease of the anus, hidradenitis suppurativa, furuncle, and actinomycosis.

Pilonidal abscesses may be drained under local anesthesia. For those who fail to heal after 3 months or develop a chronic draining sinus, **definitive therapy** is recommended. The preferred method is **to excise the pilonidal disease and primarily close the defect with rotational flaps over closed suction drainage. Simple primary closure has an unacceptably high dehiscence rate.**

Neoplasms

Historically, the anal canal has been defined as the region above the dentate line, and the anal margin has been defined as the area below the dentate line. Squamous cell tumors of the anal margin are well differentiated, keratinizing tumors that behave similarly to squamous cell tumors of the skin elsewhere. Tumors of the anal canal are aggressive, high-grade tumors with significant risk for metastasis. The staging system for anal tumors is shown in **Table 26.1**.

Tumors of the Anal Margin

Squamous Cell Carcinoma
Patients frequently complain of a lump, bleeding, itching, pain, or tenesmus (complaints common to most lesions of this region). Typically, the lesions are large, are centrally ulcerated with rolled everted

Table 26.1. Staging for anal cancer.

Anal Canal			
T1	≤2 cm		
T2	>2 to 5 cm		
T3	>5 cm		
T4	Adjacent organ(s)		
N1	Perirectal		
N2	Unilateral internal iliac/inguinal		
N3	Perirectal and inguinal, bilateral internal iliac/inguinal		
Stage Grouping			
Stage 0	Tis	N0	M0
Stage I	T1	N0	M0
Stage II	T2	N0	M0
	T3	N0	M0
Stage IIIA	T1	N1	M0
	T2	N1	M0
	T3	N1	M0
	T4	N0	M0
Stage IIIB	T4	N1	M0
	Any T	N2, N3	M0
Stage IV	Any T	Any N	M1

Source: Reprinted from Welton ML, Varma MG, Amerhauser A. Colon, rectum, and anus. In: Norton JA, Bollinger RR, Chang AE, et al, eds. Surgery: Basic Science and Clinical Evidence. New York: Springer-Verlag, 2001, with permission.

edges, and have been present for more than 2 years before detection. **All chronic or nonhealing ulcers of the perineum should be biopsied to rule out squamous cell carcinoma.**

Tumors of the Anal Canal

Epidermoid Carcinoma
Generally, there is a long history of minor perianal complaints such as bleeding, itching, or perianal discomfort. **Early lesions that are small, mobile, confined to the submucosa, and well differentiated may be treated with local excision. Radiation therapy or chemoradiotherapy is the preferred treatment option for larger lesions of the anal canal.**

Summary

Patients with perianal problems often are referred with a diagnosis of hemorrhoids. The sometimes life-threatening causes of perianal complaints require attention to history and a thorough physical examination. While hemorrhoidal disease often can be treated expectantly or by local therapies, improperly treated infectious and malignant causes of such complaints often result in devastating consequences.

Selected Readings

Allal A, Kurtz JM, Pipard G, et al. Chemoradiotherapy versus radiotherapy alone for anal cancer: a retrospective comparison. Int J Radiat Oncol Biol Phys 1993;27(1):59–66.

Beahrs OH, Wilson SM. Carcinoma of the anus. Ann Surg 1976;184(4):422–428.

Bernstein WC. What are hemorrhoids and what is their relationship to the portal venous system? Dis Colon Rectum 1983;25(12):825–834.

Cirocco WC. Lateral internal sphincterotomy remains the treatment of choice for anal fissures that fail conservative therapy [letter; comment]. Gastrointest Endosc 1998;47(2):212–214.

Duthie HL, Gairns FW. Sensory nerve-endings and sensation in the anal region of man. Br J Surg 1960;47:585–594.

Haas PA, Fox TA Jr, Haas GP. The pathogenesis of hemorrhoids. Dis Colon Rectum 1984;27(7):442–450.

Hiltunen KM, Matakainen M. Anal manometric findings in symptomatic hemorrhoids. Dis Colon Rectum 1985;28(11):807–809.

Lin JK. Anal manometric studies in hemorrhoids and anal fissures. Dis Colon Rectum 1989;32(10):839–842.

Milligan ETC, Morgan CN. Surgical anatomy of the anal canal. Lancet 1933;2:1150–1156.

Mĺler C, Saksela E. Cancer of the anus and anal canal. Acta Chir Scand 1970;136(4):340–348.

Papillon J, Montbarron JF. Epidermoid carcinoma of the anal canal. Dis Colon Rectum 1987;30(5):324–333.

Thomson WH. The nature of haemorrhoids. Br J Surg 1975;62(7):542–552.

Vasilevsky C-A. Results of treatment of fistula-in-ano. Dis Colon Rectum 1984;28:225–231.

Welton ML, Varma MG, Amerhauser A. Colon, rectum, and anus. In: Norton JA, Bollinger RR, Chang AE, et al, eds. Surgery: Basic Science and Clinical Evidence. New York: Springer-Verlag, 2001.

Groin Hernias and Masses, and Abdominal Hernias

James J. Chandler

Objectives

1. To be able to discuss the differential diagnosis of inguinal pain and the diagnosis and management of groin masses and hernias.
2. To develop an understanding of the anatomy, location, and treatment of different types of hernias; this includes the frequency, indications, surgical options, and normal postoperative course for inguinal, femoral, and umbilical hernia repairs.
3. To understand the definition and clarification of the clinical significance of incarcerated, strangulated, reducible, and Richter's hernias.
4. To develop an awareness of the urgency of surgical referral, the urgency of treating some hernias.
5. To develop an understanding of the differential diagnosis of an abdominal wall apparent hernia or mass, including adenopathy, desmoid tumors, rectus sheath hematoma, true hernia, and neoplasm.

Cases

Case 1

A 74-year-old woman has noted an intermittent small lump in the right groin for 8 months. This has seemed to go away when she lies down, but it is present when she showers in the morning. Two nights ago, she could feel the lump when supine. It was slightly tender. Yesterday, she began feeling a steady ache in the groin and had poor appetite. The discomfort became worse, and she slept fitfully last night. This morning she felt awful, had a lemon-sized tender right groin mass, and had nausea and some diarrhea. You found her moaning, holding her distended abdomen, and trying to vomit. On examination, there were intermittent gurgles heard in the abdomen, and a slightly pink, skin-covered, very tender lump was present in the right groin. Abdominal x-ray: dilated intestinal loops with air-fluid levels. Laboratory studies: hemoglobin, 14.6; BUN, 24; electrolytes normal; urine specific gravity, 1.028.

Case 2

A male college student, age 20, presents with a 4-year history of inter-mittent soft mass in his groin and a large lump in the right side of the scrotum, which is now uncomfortable. He does not notice any groin mass on awakening, but he becomes aware of the groin and scrotal masses later in the morning, toward noon.

Definitions

A **hernia** is present when an object goes through an opening and is now in any unexpected location. There may be a covering of the object; this covering, called the **sac**, usually is the peritoneum. An organ, a portion of omentum, or part of the intestine, bladder, or stomach may herniate through an opening in the abdominal wall or diaphragm. This has occurred in both **Case 1** and **Case 2**.

A **femoral hernia**, much more common in women, presents through the femoral canal, and an **indirect inguinal hernia** protrudes through the abdominal wall in the spermatic cord or alongside the round liga-ment. **Pediatric inguinal hernias** are **indirect. Direct inguinal hernias** are rare in females and in males younger than 35 years of age.

An **internal hernia** occurs when the intestine goes through an opening inside the abdominal cavity. In a **Richter's hernia (Case 1)**, only a **part of the intestinal wall**, covered by a sac formed by the overlying peritoneum, protrudes through an opening (usually in the femoral canal), and the intestinal lumen remains open. **In Case 1, the woman has both a lump in the groin and not complete intestinal obstruction, meaning that she could have a knuckle of bowel wall caught in an opening but with an open lumen, as in a Richter's hernia. This patient is dehydrated and seriously ill! (See Algorithms 27.1 and 27.2.)**

If an organ or a portion of the intestine **uncovered by peritoneum protrudes through and forms part of the hernia sac**, this is called a **sliding hernia**. When an intestinal loop comes out through an opening and this hernia does not go back by itself or cannot be gently pushed back, the hernia cannot be **reduced. The hernia is incarcerated.** When part of the intestine (or stomach) is incarcerated, there can be a shut-ting off of the venous drainage and/or the arterial circulation; this is now a **strangulated** hernia. **Gangrenous changes develop, leading to possible perforation and possible death.**

Groin Masses: Differential Diagnosis

These are the differential diagnoses for groin masses.

- **Inguinal hernia:** Protrudes through the internal ring, at the level of the public tubercle; exits via the external ring (see **Algorithm 27.1**).

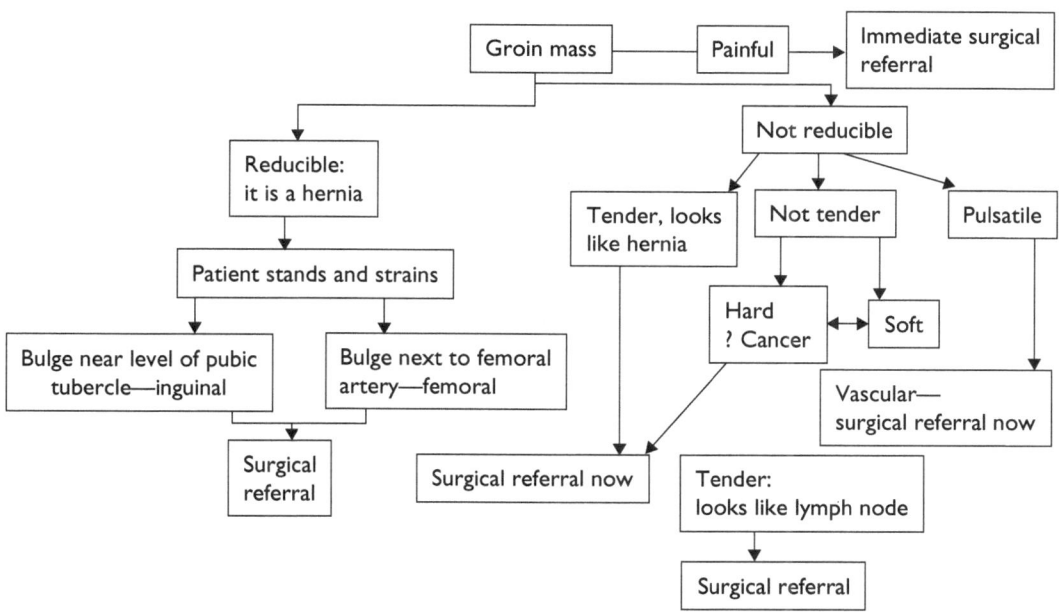

Algorithm 27.1. Algorithm for the evaluation of groin masses.

There may be a sausage-shaped mass going all the way down into the scrotum, as in **Case 2**.

- **Femoral hernia:** Bulge/mass appears medial to the femoral vein (see **Algorithm 27.1**), can rise higher, and can be difficult to distinguish from an inguinal hernia.
- **Lymph node mass:** This does not disappear with pressure on it. This usually is a nontender mass that is firm, overlying the femoral artery. Lymph nodes **may** be inflamed and tender from infection or enlarged and firm because of cancer, a lymphoma, or metastatic cancer (see **Algorithm 27.1**).

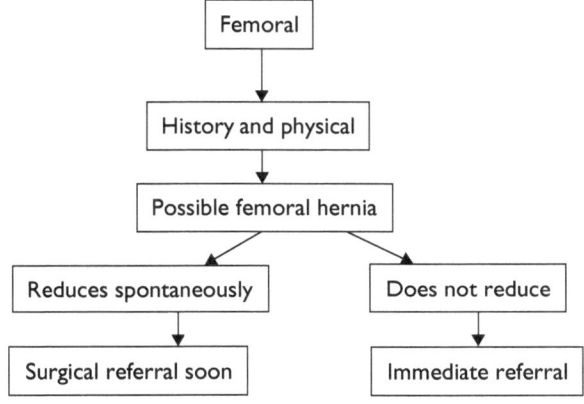

Algorithm 27.2. Algorithm for the evaluation of likely femoral hernia.

- **Varicocele:** Irregular, nontender type lump palpable in the spermatic cord superior to the left testicle. If diagnosis is uncertain, order duplex color-coded ultrasonography.
- **Hydrocele:** "Water sac." A fluid-filled membrane, around or above the testicle, which may extend up into the inguinal canal and may communicate with a hernia sac. A hydrocele can be transilluminated by holding a flashlight behind it.
- **Femoral artery aneurysm:** Pulsatile, expansile mass. **Refer for vascular surgery, now!**
- **Psoas muscle abscess:** Rare. Formerly more common when due to tuberculosis. Pus in the muscle sheath dissects inferiorly and bulges into the groin. If due to staphylococcus, patient is very ill and febrile, and the mass is acutely tender.
- **Tumor (benign) of spermatic cord:** A fibroma is firm, nontender, and can be moved a little to the side, in the inguinal canal.
- **Seroma:** Collection of serum in the groin. Edges are poorly defined. These generally follow a groin-area surgical procedure, such as groin dissection or arterial surgery. Hematomas are fairly common after hernia repair, but large ones are rare.
- **Abscess:** This would be unlikely unless following a surgical procedure. Tender, warm skin overlying.
- **Cryptorchid:** An undescended testicle. Duplex ultrasonography diagnosis it.

See **Algorithm 27.3** for a general workup for an abdominal or groin lump/mass.

Anatomy of the Groin

The layers of tissue found in the lower abdomen are the external oblique muscle, internal oblique, transversus abdomen, transversalis fascia, preperitoneal fat, and peritoneum (**Fig. 27.1**).

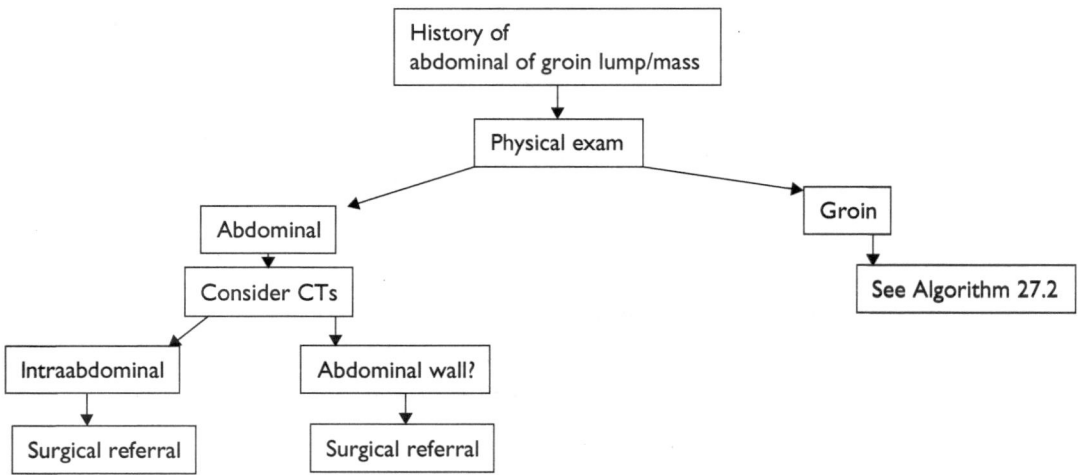

Algorithm 27.3. Algorithm for general workup for abdominal or groin lump/mass.

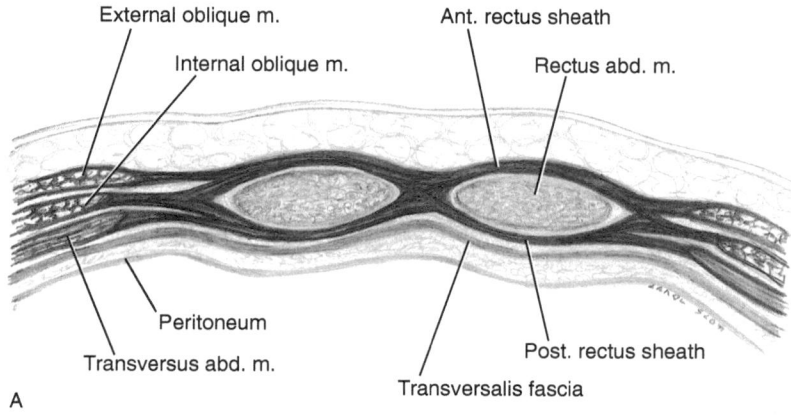

External oblique m.

Internal oblique m.

Ant. rectus sheath

Rectus abd. m.

Peritoneum

Transversus abd. m.

Post. rectus sheath

Transversalis fascia

A

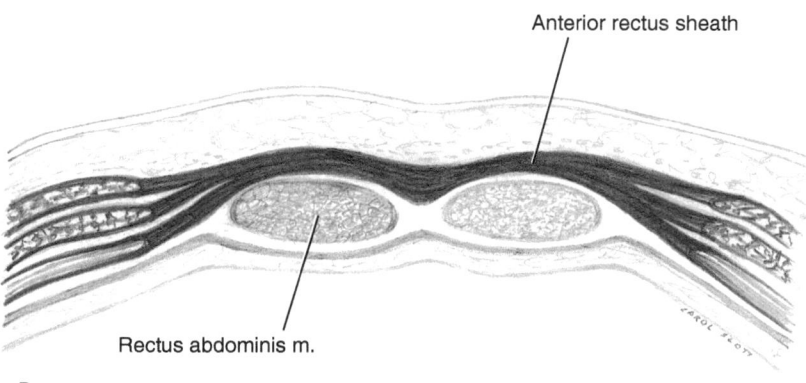

Anterior rectus sheath

Rectus abdominis m.

B

Figure 27.1. Abdominal wall layers: (A) above the semilunar line of Douglas; (B) below the semilunar line. (Reprinted from Scott DJ, Jones DB. Hernias and abdominal wall defects. In: Norton JA, Bollinger RR, Chang AE, et al, eds. Surgery: Basic Science and Clinical Evidence. New York: Springer-Verlag, 2001, with permission.)

The **inguinal canal** courses obliquely from the **internal ring** opening in the transversalis fascia to the pubic bone and the **external ring** opening in the external oblique. The spermatic cord in the male comes through the internal ring; the external ring is where the spermatic cord exits to head down into the scrotum. Included in this "cord" are superficial and external spermatic fascial layers, cremaster muscle, external spermatic artery (in the cremaster), internal spermatic fascia, vas deferens, testicular artery, pampiniform plexus of little veins, and some sympathetic fibers. The genital branch of the genital femoral nerve, often said to be **in the spermatic cord**, actually courses through the internal ring in the edge of posterior cremaster fibers and easily is separated from the cord. This nerve lies posterior to the cord with its accompanying vessels in the inguinal canal. The boundaries of the inguinal canal are the transversalis fascia posterior, external oblique anterior, internal oblique muscle and rectus sheath superior, inguinal ligament inferior, pubic bone medial, and internal ring lateral. See **Figure 27.2** for the relationships of the inguinal canal.

A hernia going through the internal ring, outside the inferior epigastric artery, and inside the spermatic cord courses obliquely with the cord and is termed an **indirect inguinal hernia (Case 2)**. A protrusion through thinned-out transversalis fascia comes straight out through the abdominal wall and is called a **direct inguinal hernia**, which is medial to the inferior epigastric artery. These hernias bulge through Hesselbach's triangle, which is bounded by the rectus sheath, inguinal ligament, pubis, and inferior epigastric artery (**Fig. 27.3**). A hernia presenting through both the internal ring and Hesselbach's triangle is termed a **pantaloon hernia**, with a "leg" of the hernia coming out on both sides of the inferior epigastric artery.

Groin Hernias

Femoral Hernia

Unknown in children and relatively rare in males, this is a hernia presenting in the femoral sheath, through the femoral canal, medial to the nerve, artery, and vein there. The femoral ring has firm, unyielding

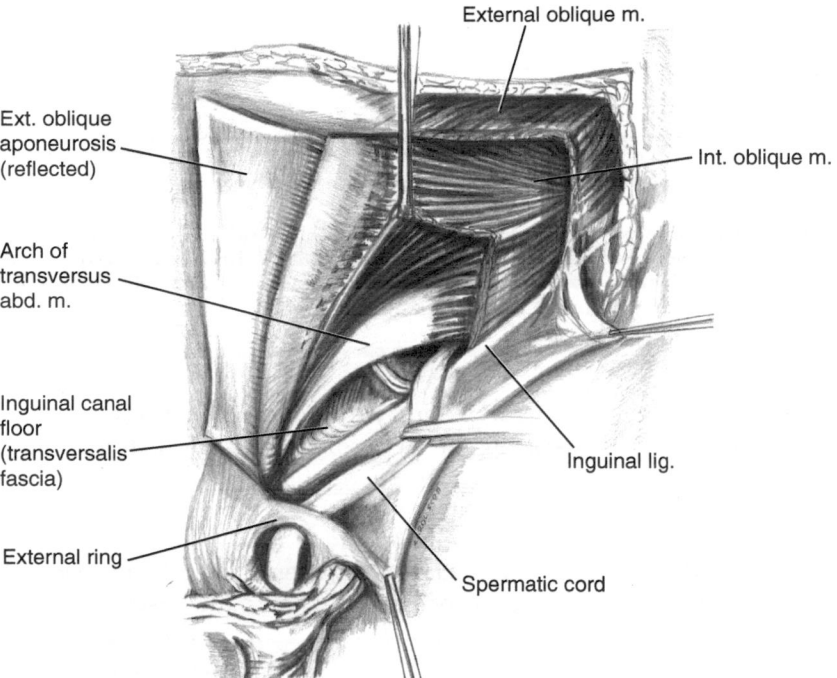

Figure 27.2. The left inguinal canal with external oblique aponeurosis incised and reflected. (Reprinted from Scott DJ, Jones DB. Hernias and abdominal wall defects. In: Norton JA, Bollinger RR, Chang AE, et al, eds. Surgery: Basic Science and Clinical Evidence. New York: Springer-Verlag, 2001, with permission.)

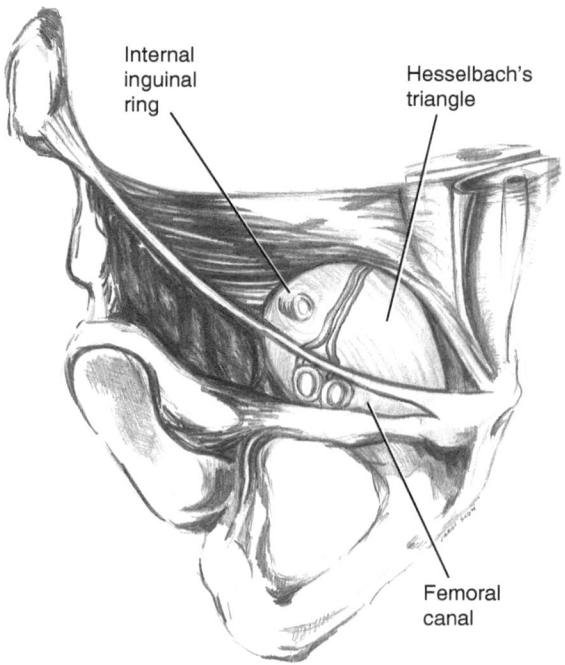

Figure 27.3. Indirect hernias occur through the internal ring. Direct inguinal hernias occur through Hesselbach's triangle, which lies between the inguinal ligament, the rectus sheath, and the inferior epigastric vessels. Femoral hernias occur through the femoral canal, which lies between the inguinal ligament, the lacunar ligament, Cooper's ligament, and the femoral vein. Fruchaud's myopectineal orifice refers to the entire musculoaponeurotic area through which inguinal and femoral hernias can occur. (Reprinted from Scott DJ, Jones DB. Hernias and abdominal wall defects. In: Norton JA, Bollinger RR, Chang AE, et al, eds. Surgery: Basic Science and Clinical Evidence. New York: Springer-Verlag, 2001, with permission.)

borders: the superior inguinal ligament, the inferior Cooper's ligament, and the medial half-moon–shaped **lacunar ligament**. Because of this, **these hernias frequently are incarcerated and are prone to develop strangulation, with intestinal wall gangrene**, as in **Case 1**.

Diagnosis
Diagnosis can be difficult because of the short distance between the inguinal canal and the medial groin presentation site of the femoral hernia. The usual **history** includes the awareness of a lump in the groin, but it is in the leg crease where the pelvis meets the thigh medially. Direct pain or tenderness, vague groin or lower abdominal discomfort, nausea, and discomfort on prolonged standing or while walking are frequent findings. **Examination** is most helpful with the patient standing. If, when she strains and increases intraabdominal pressure, a lump is seen or felt, the base of the femoral hernia will be below the level of the top of the pubic bone, as noted in **Algorithm 27.1**. Also, if the examiner's forefinger is in the femoral canal when the patient strains, the fingertip can be backed away slowly, allowing the

hernia to pop out of the canal. With an incarcerated hernia in a woman, there is some tissue swelling, and it can be difficult to differentiate between femoral or inguinal hernia. The **gentlest pressure can be tried** with the patient supine to see whether an inguinal hernia will reduce. **Caution is required because an incarcerated femoral hernia usually should be diagnosed in the operating room; no significant pressure should be applied to attempt reduction (see Algorithm 27.2)!**

Surgical Treatment of Femoral Hernia

The surgeon must know several operative methods and be able to choose the best method for the particular patient and situation. In the **open, preperitoneal approach**, the surgeon opens the inguinal canal and then may enter the preperitoneal space through Hesselbach's triangle or by going above the canal and entering through the posterior rectus sheath. A piece of nonabsorbable mesh may be used for repair. **In approaching the femoral hernia from below**, one incises over the femoral canal, dissects through the fat and lymphatic tissue, reduces a sac found, and occludes the canal with rolled mesh or with stitched tissue adjacent. The sac is opened to check for evidence of ischemic intestine (bloody fluid). **Normal postoperative course** includes the following. The individual has moderate pain after the effects of local anesthetic have cleared. She/he can resume a light diet, returning to normal in 24 hours; constipation may be a problem. With return home within a few hours after the operation, the patient is up and around but requires more rest for the next week. Patients return to work from within a few days to 2 weeks after surgery.

Inguinal Hernias

Diagnosis

In **Case 2**, we are presented with a man who has had a long history of groin and associated scrotal mass. **Diagnosis** of an inguinal hernia is a simple matter when given a **history** of an inguinal bulge felt or seen, especially if it is a new discovery and if it disappears when supine, as in **Case 2**. This young man should be **examined** while he is standing, with unclothed lower body. Seat yourself before him, ask him to strain or cough, and watch the hernia roll down the inguinal ligament and into the upper scrotum. Then see if gentle upward pressure with your or the patient's fingers can reduce the hernia; if not, have him lie down, and try again. When examining a standing male patient without an obvious bulge, the examiner's finger pushes up through the upper scrotal skin and is placed against the external inguinal ring. As the patient strains and coughs, a soft mass coming out through the ring and pushing your finger away gives you the diagnosis of a hernia. If the hernia is continuously bulging and will not reduce with position change or gentle upward pressure, **surgical referral is indicated without delay** (see **Algorithm 27.4**).

Examination of females also is best done with the patient standing, but invagination of labial skin is next to impossible. One also desires to assess whether this is an inguinal or femoral hernia, which can be difficult (see **Algorithm 27.1**). Whether a hernia is even present also

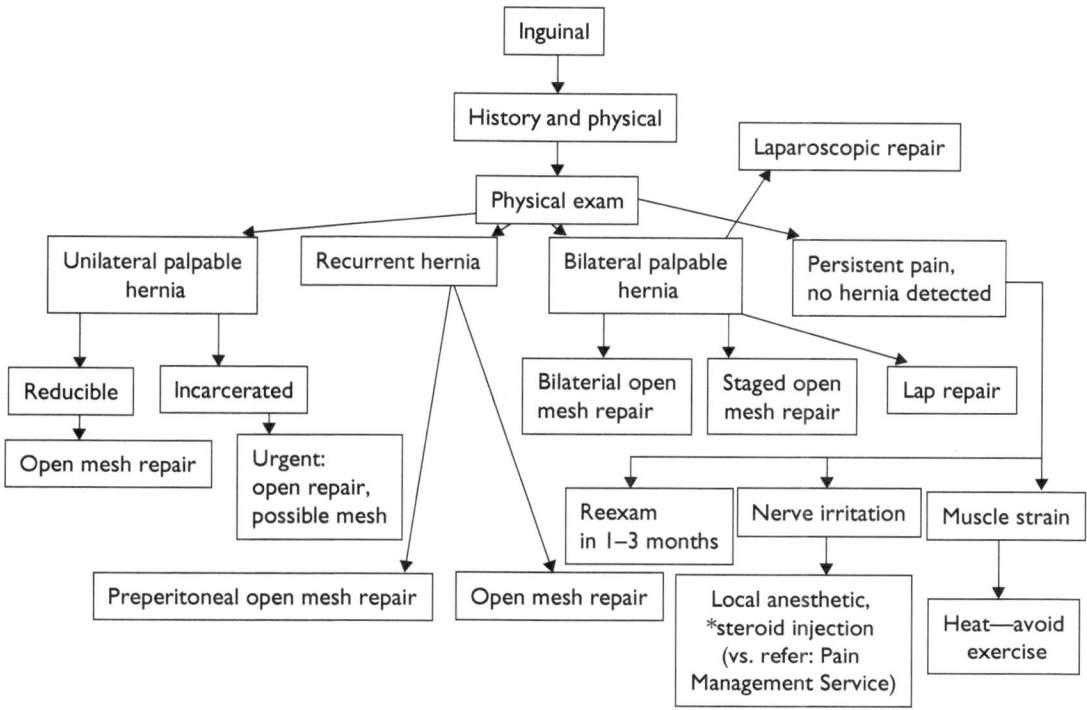

Algorithm 27.4. Decision tree for inguinal hernia and inguinal pain.

may be especially difficult to decide in females and in any obese male. On occasion, the examiner will admit uncertainty and recommend follow-up exam or examination by another physician (see **Algorithm 27.4**). Operating and finding no hernia to repair is to be avoided.

Pain upon straining or lifting but with no appreciable bulge can be the first evidence of inguinal hernia. The groin lump may appear some days later after discomfort from muscle disruption and after inflammation in the muscle have subsided. Pain from inguinal hernia can be poorly or well localized by the patient. Discomfort usually is intermittent and related to prolonged standing or walking or increased intraabdominal pressure. "Burning," "dragging feeling," and "ache" all have been used as descriptions. **Persistent pain and groin mass suggest incarceration, which requires urgent surgical treatment. Fever, nausea and vomiting, rapid heart rate, marked tenderness over the mass, and abdominal distention must bring to mind likely bowel ischemia, "strangulation," and the required emergency treatment.**

Surgical Treatment of Inguinal Hernia

Open Repair: **Open repair** is the term used to differentiate from a **laparoscopic technique.** The open repair can be via an **anterior approach** or via an **approach from behind the inguinal canal, through the preperitoneal space, termed "preperitoneal approach."** Many hernia repair techniques have been described. General surgeons know multiple methods. The Italian surgical genius Bassini developed an elaborate anterior open and successful operation using layers of native tissue.[1] The modern, currently most popular and successful open anterior technique with native tissue is the **Canadian Repair** developed at the Shouldice Clinic.[2] This features **local anesthesia** and very early ambulation, after a repair utilizing running stitches in several layers of tissue. Nyhus[3] is given credit both for promoting an understanding of the surgical anatomy above the pelvis and for demonstrating advantages in hernia repair with a preperitoneal approach. Lichtenstein[4] opened the **mesh repair** floodgates with his introduction of a highly successful open, anterior technique using inert mesh laid onto the posterior inguinal canal, repairing a hernia without the tension caused by bringing tissues together with stitches. Repairs then were developed that featured mesh placed in the preperitoneal space and repairs in which mesh is used both in that space and over the floor of the inguinal canal. Laparoscopic repairs also have evolved.

The young man in **Case 2** had his hernia diagnosed through the history and the exam method described earlier. Many repair techniques could be used. With the expected small opening at the internal ring and the congenital-type indirect inguinal hernia, the sac could be ligated high or stitched, with redundant sac tissue excised, or the sac could be dissected high and inverted. A few stitches taken medially to tighten the internal ring (the Marcy repair) might suffice in a case with firm layer of transversalis fascia in Hesselbach's triangle. A mesh plug could be used in the internal ring. After an internal ring plug is placed, onlay of mesh covering the inguinal canal provides some insurance against recurrence. The **normal postoperative course** is similar to the course after femoral hernia repair. However, lifting more than 35 pounds and heavy work are to be avoided for 6 postoperative weeks.

Pitfalls and Perils of Open Inguinal Hernia Repair: **Complication** rates vary from minimal to 20%. Nerve entrapment or neuroma with virtually constant pain, bleeding and large hematoma, ischemic orchitis, vas deferens injury, intestinal injury, or failure to recognize pregangrene all are known and relatively unusual, but feared. Pain after surgery has been reduced markedly by using a tension-free procedure combined with local anesthesia. Mesh sheets shrink 20% in size. Mesh plugs shrink up to 70% in volume, harden, and may allow a hernia to develop adjacent to the plug. Patient-related complications are ileus, nausea, cardiac, and respiratory. Other complications that can follow hernia

[1] Wright AJ, Gardner GC, Fitzgibbons RJ Jr. The Bassini repair and its variants. In: Fitzgibbons RJ, Greenberg AG, eds. *Nyhus and Condon's Hernia*, 5th ed. Philadelphia: Lippincott, 2002:105–114.

[2] Bendavid R. The Shouldice repair. In: Fitzgibbons RJ, Greenberg AG, eds. *Nyhus and Condon's hernia*, 5th ed. Philadelphia: Lippincott, 2002:129–138.

[3] Nyhus LM, Condon RE, Harkins HW. Clinical experiences with preperitoneal hernia repair for all types of hernia in the groin: with particular reference to the importance of tranversalis fascia analogs. Am J Surg 1960;100:234–244.

[4] Lichtenstein IL, Shulman AG. Ambulatory outpatient hernia surgery, including a new concept, introducing tension-free repair. Int Surg 1986;71:1–4.

repair include chronic pain, testicular atrophy or ejaculation abnormality, wound seroma or infection, hydrocele, and scrotal or retroperitoneal hematoma. **Recurrence of hernias after surgical repair is of major concern to surgeons and patients alike.** Many patients are not closely followed, and many with a recurrence seek aid elsewhere, making recurrence rates difficult to establish. In summary, all of the open approaches now in popular usage have acceptable rates of long-term hernia cure when the reports of centers with large numbers of repairs are reviewed.

Laparoscopic Inguinal Hernia Repair: **Laparoscopic repair** requires general anesthesia, has been controversial, and is not widely used. However, recent reports of highly acceptable recurrence rates, lessened postoperative pain, and rapid return to regular work have caused genuine increasing interest, demonstrated in a recent compilation of prospective, randomized trials comparing open and laparoscopic repairs (**Table 27.1**).

Pitfalls and Perils of Laparoscopic Repair of Inguinal Hernias: While some surgeons have excellent reported results, laparoscopic repair has had numerous **complications** related to this technique, in addition to the usual list of potential complications of open hernia surgery. These include bleeding in the retroperitoneal space, in the abdominal wall, or inside the abdomen; intraabdominal intestinal or artery injury; bladder perforation; trocar-site hernia; stapling a nerve; and small-bowel obstruction. Recurrences have resulted from inadequate mesh fixation, too small a mesh, missed hernia, and mesh displacement. Cost of repairing a hernia with a laparoscopic method is greater than the costs associated with other methods.

Watchful Waiting

Whether watchful waiting is ever indicated is controversial, and the conventional approach is to plan repair when a hernia is diagnosed. The conventional approach is being questioned, however, in asymptomatic hernias. Somewhere between one-half and three-quarter million hernias are operated upon yearly in the United States. It is estimated that an even larger number are not operated upon because individuals are not choosing to have them repaired. Most surgeons recommend repair in order to avoid the higher complication rate and the greater difficulty of repair in cases of incarceration or strangulation, and because of the belief that incarceration/strangulation are likely to occur, when in fact this may be unlikely. Also, long-term complications, including chronic pain, may follow surgical repair. Data are insufficient now to develop clear indications for watchful waiting. **An inguinal hernia that is asymptomatic, has a large defect or almost no bulge at all, and that reduces quickly with the patient supine should be able to be observed for some period of time. Also, with a patient who presents with possible incarceration of a hernia that you find to be easily reduced with very gentle pressure, surgical intervention can be delayed for a few hours and, in some cases, for 1 or 2 days.**

Table 27.1. Prospective randomized trials comparing laparoscopic and open repairs (level I evidence).

Reference	Study design	Average follow-up (months)	No. of repairs	Complications (not including recurrences)	Recurrences
Paganini et al 1998, Italy[a]	TAPP vs. Lichtenstein	28	TAPP: 52	14 (26.9%) total complications 4 (7.7%) hematoma 1 (1.9%) hydrocele 5 (9.6%) paresthesia 4 (7.7%) seroma*	2 (3.8%)
			Licht.: 56	15 (26.8%) total complications 8 (14.3%) hematoma 2 (3.6%) hydrocele 5 (8.9%) paresthesia 0 seroma*	0
Zieren et al 1998, Germany[b]	TAPP vs. Plug & Patch vs. Shouldice	25	TAPP: 80	2 (3%) intraop bleeding* 15 (19%) postop complications	0
			Plug: 80	12 (15%) postop complications	0
			Shouldice: 80	13 (16%) postop complications	0
Liem et al 1997, Netherlands[c]	TEP vs. open (Marcy, Lichtenstein, Bassini, Shouldice, McVay)	20.2	TEP: 487	24 (5%) Conversion to TAPP or open 54 (11%) total postop complications 0 deep wound infection* 10 (2%) chronic pain* 7 (1%) seroma* 3 (1%) pneumoscrotum >1 day	17 (3%)*
			Open: 507	99 (19.5%) total postop complications 6 (1%) deep wound infection* 70 (14%) chronic pain* 0 seroma*	31 (6%)*
Champault et al 1997, France[d]	TEP vs. Stopps	20.2	TEP: 51	4% total complications* 3 (6%) conversions to open	3 (6%)
			Stoppa: 49	20% total complications*	1 (2%)

Table 27.1. *Continued*

Operative time (min)	Cost	Postoperative pain	Return to work (days)	Conclusions/details
66.6 Unilateral primary* 71.1 Unilateral recurrent 85.7 Bilateral	$1249	↓ pain score @ 48 h*	15	95% of Lichtenstein repairs performed under local anesthesia. TAPP had less postop pain. TAPP should not be adopted routinely unless its cost can be reduced.
48.2 Unilateral primary* 41.2 Unilateral recurrent 75.9 Bilateral	$306	↑ discomfort @ 7 d, 3 mon	14	
61*	$1211		16 18	Plug & Patch and TAPP cause less pain and have faster return to work than Shouldice; Plug & Patch cost less than TAPP and can be performed faster and under local anesthesia.
36	$124			
47	$69	↑ pain score *	26*	
45*	—	↓ pain score *	14*	TEP has more rapid recovery and fewer recurrences than open repairs, but takes slightly longer to perform.
40*	—		21*	
"Significantly longer"*	—	↓ pain score * ↓ meds *	17*	45% bilateral, 43% recurrent. Mesh for TEP was not fixed in place; mesh size increased from 6 × 11 cm to 12 × 15 cm due to early recurrences. Single piece of mesh for bilateral hernias believed to reduce recurrence rates.
	—		35*	TEP has the same long-term recurrence rate as the Stoppa procedure, but confers a real advantage in the early postop period.

Continued

Table 27.1. *Continued*

Reference	Study design	Average follow-up (months)	No. of repairs	Complications (not including recurrences)	Recurrences
Kald et al 1997, Sweden[e]	TAPP vs. Shouldice	12	TAPP: 122	8 (6.6%) total complications	0*
			Shouldice: 89	9 (10.1%) total complications	3 (3.4%) *
Bessell et al 1996, Australia[f]	TEP vs. Shouldice	7.3	TEP: 39	6 conversion to open 3 conversion to TAPP 4 (10%) postop complications	2 (5.1%)
			Shouldice: 74	7 (9.5%) postop complications	0
Wright et al 1996, Scotland[g]	TEP vs. open (Lichtenstein or preperitoneal)	—	TEP: 67	6 (9%) conversion to open 15 (22%) postop complications 1 (1%) hematoma* 0 seroma*	—
			Open: 64	46 (72%) postop complications 20 (31%) hematoma* 7 (11%) seroma*	—
Tschudi et al 1996, Switzerland[h]	TAPP vs. Shouldice	6.7	TAPP: 52	6 (12%) total complications	1 (1.9%)
			Shouldice: 56	9 (16%) total complications	2 (3.6%)
Barkun et al 1995, Canada[i]	TAPP or IPOM vs. open (Bassini, McVay, Shouldice, Lichtenstein, Plug & Patch)	14	TAPP: 33 IPOM: 10	10 (22.5%) total complicaions	0
			Open: 49	6 (12.2%) total complications	1 (2%)
Vogt et al 1994, US[j]	IPOM (with meshed PTEE) vs. open (Bassini, McVay)	8	IPOM: 30	5 (17%) total complications 1 (3.3%) bladder perforation	1 (3.3%)
			Open: 31	5 (16%) total complications	2 (6.5%)

Table 27.1. *Continued*

Operative time (min)	Cost	Postoperative pain	Return to work (days)	Conclusions/details
72*	+ $483 direct cost	—	10*	TAPP had faster recovery and return to work with comparable complication rates.
62*	+ $1364 indirect cost	—	23*	TAPP more cost-effective if indirect cost compared, which included income lost by a delay in return to work.
87.5*	—	↓ pain score * ↓ meds	30.5	Study biased because of larger crossover to open group. Substantial conversion rate to open and TAPP repairs. TEP has significant decrease in pain, equivalent return to work, but longer operative time. TEP alleviates the inherent dangers associated with TAPP, but further studies needed.
50*	—		32	
58*	—	↓ pain score * ↓ meds	—	Acute study focusing on early outcome. No data for length of follow-up or recurrences. Significant decrease in pain but increased OR time for TEP. Significant conversion rate. Very high complication rates for both groups. Also looked at pulmonary and metabolic measures; no differences found.
45*	—		—	
87 unilateral* 124 bilateral	—	↓ pain score * ↓ meds *	25	Study biased because patients undergoing open repairs told not to resume activity for 4–6 weeks. Significantly less pain with TAPP, but longer OR time. Long-term follow-up needed for analysis of recurrences.
59 unilateral* 79 bilateral	—		48	
43	$1718	↓ meds *	9.6	Improved quality of life and decreased pain with laparoscopic repairs, but at increased cost. Laparoscopic repairs are feasible and comparable to open repairs.
	$1224		10.9	
62.5	—	↓ med	7.5	Less pain and faster return to work with IPOM, with comparable efficacy and morbidity. Longer follow-up needed.
80.9	—		18.5	Two patients had IPOM under local anesthesia.

Continued

Table 27.1. *Continued*

Reference	Study design	Average follow-up (months)	No. of repairs	Complications (not including recurrences)	Recurrences
Stoker et al 1994, UK[k]	TAPP vs. open (nylon darn plication)	7	TAPP: 83	6 (7%) total complications* 1 deep wound infection 3 persistent pain 1 hematoma	0
			Open: 84	16 (19%) total complications* 5 deep wound infection 6 persistent pain 3 hematoma	0
Payne et al 1994, US[l]	TAPP vs. Lichtenstein	10	TAPP: 48	6 (13%) total complications 0 groin pain >1 mon. 2 (4%) conversions to open 1 (2%) incarcerated omentum in peritoneal flap	0
			Licht: 52	9 (17%) total complications 4 (8%) groin pain >1 mon.	0

TAPP, transabdominal preperitoneal approach; IPOM, intraperitoneal onlay mesh repair; TEP, totally extraperitoneal approach; PTEE, polytetrafluoroethylene.

*, Statistically significant.

[a] Paganini AM, Lezoche E, Carle F, et al. A randomized, controlled, clinical study of laparoscopic vs open tension-free inguinal hernia repair. Surg Endosc 1998;12:979–986.

[b] Zieren J, Zieren H, Jacobe CA, et al. Prospective randomized study comparing laparoscopic and open tension-free inguinal hernia repair with Shouldice's operation. Am J Surg 1998;175:330–333.

[c] Liem MSL, Van Der Graff Y, Van Steensel CJ, et al. Comparison of conventional anterior surgery and laparoscopic surgery for inguinal-hernia repair. N Engl J Med 1997;336:1541–1547.

[d] Champault G, Rizk N, Catheline JM, et al. Inguinal hernia repair: totally pre-peritoneal laparoscopic approach versus Stoppa operation, randomized trial: 100 cases. Hernia 1997;1:31–36.

[e] Kald A, Anderberg B, Carlsson P, Park PO, et al. Surgical outcome and cost-minimization analyses of laparoscopic and open hernia repair: a randomized prospective trial with one year follow-up. Eur J Surg 1997;163:505–510.

[f] Bessell JR, Baxter P, Riddell P, Watkin S, et al. A randomized controlled trial of laparoscopic extraperitoneal hernia repair as a day surgical procedure. Surg Endosc 1996;10:495–500.

Source: Reprinted from Scott DJ, Jones DB. Hernias and abdominal wall defects. In: Norton JA, Bollinger RR, Chang AE, et al, eds. Surgery: Basic Science and Clinical Evidence. New York: Springer-Verlag, 2001, with permission.

Abdominal Wall Hernias

Ventral hernias are those protruding through the anterior wall of the abdomen. **Umbilical hernias** are **ventral**, but they are placed in their own category because etiology and repair techniques are so different from those used for **ventral incisional hernias**. With a weakened area of the wall or with significant increased intraabdominal pressure, hernia develops. At the umbilicus, hernia usually is congenital, but hernia can follow childbirth, increased weight, or be at the upper or

Table 27.1. *Continued*

Operative time (min)	Cost	Postoperative pain	Return to work (days)	Conclusions/details
50 unilateral* 92 bilateral	+£168	↓ pain score * ↓ meds *	14*	TAPP has less pain, faster return to work, and fewer complications, but increased operative time. Substantial economic savings in lost work days.
35 unilateral* 60 bilateral			28*	
68 unilateral 87 bilateral 67 recurrent	$3093 *	—	9 unilat.* 7.5 bilat. 11.4 recurr.	TAPP can be performed with similar operative times and short-term recurrence rates, with faster return to work, but an increased cost. 90% of Lichtenstein's used local anesthesia. Biggest impact on faster return to work and increased ability to perform straight leg raises seen in manual labor population.*
56 unilateral 93 bilateral 73 recurrent	$2494 *	—	17 unilat.* 25 bilat. 26 recurr.	

[g] Wright DM, Kennedy A, Baxter JN, et al. Early outcome after open versus extraperitoneal endoscopic tension-free hernioplasty: a randomized clinical trial. Surgery (St. Louis) 1996;119:552–557.

[h] Tschudi J, Wagner M, Klaiber C, Brugger JJ, et al. Controlled multicenter trial of laparoscopic transabdominal preperitoneal hernioplasty vs Shouldice herniorrhaphy. Surg Endosc 1996;10:845–847.

[i] Barkun JS, Wexler MJ, Hinchey EJ, Thibeault D, et al. Laparoscopic versus open inguinal herniorrhaphy: preliminary results of a randomized controlled trial. Surgery (St. Louis) 1995;118:703–710.

[j] Vogt DM, Curet MJ, Pitcher DE, et al. Preliminary results of a prospective randomized trial of laparoscopic onlay versus conventional inguinal herniorrhaphy. Am J Surg 1995;169:84–90.

[k] Stoker DL, Spiegelhalter DJ, Singh R, Wellwood JM. Laparoscopic versus open inguinal hernia repair: randomized prospective trial. Lancet 1994;343:1243–1245.

[l] Payne JH, Grininger LM, Izawa MT, et al. Laparoscopic or open inguinal herniorrhaphy? A randomized prospective trial. Arch Surg 1994;129:973–981.

Source: Reprinted from Scotl DJ, Jones DB. Hernias and abdominal wall defects. In: Norton JA, Bollinger RR, Chang AE, et al, eds. Surgery: Basic Science and Clinical Evidence. New York: Springer-Verlag, 2001, with permission.

lower end of a healed incision (an **incisional umbilical hernia**). Preperitoneal fat, omentum, or gut may protrude, causing a bulge, symptoms of pain, and nausea. A huge umbilical hernia may allow a large portion of bowel to enter the sac, to become twisted and compromised, and to perforate. Some umbilical hernias can be repaired using local anesthesia, but most require general anesthesia and muscle relaxation. Asymptomatic hernias may be able to be controlled with an abdominal binder. Symptomatic umbilical hernias are repaired by incising halfway around the umbilical skin, dissecting down to the fascia, separating the overlying skin from the hernia sac, separating the fascial ring from the sac, reducing the sac and contents, and closing the fascial defect with permanent suture. A piece of prosthetic mesh often is placed just under the fascial closure, held in place with one or more of the closure stitches.

Epigastric hernias occur in the upper abdomen through a defect in the linea alba and are repaired with simple closure with permanent suture, often buttressed with a piece of mesh in the preperitoneal space. Abdominal wall mass differential diagnosis includes metastatic cancer at the navel ("Sister Mary Joseph" tumor) or dermal metastasis, varicose veins (umbilical, secondary to portal hypertension), lymph node groin mass encroaching onto the abdominal wall, rectus sheath hematoma (usually in an anticoagulated patient: the hard, tender mass is confined to one entire rectus sheath), and desmoid tumor. Desmoids are seen in patients with familial polyposis syndrome and, although benign, can be a problem and difficult to remove surgically. Biopsy is diagnostic, and imaging studies aid in management decision.

Incisional hernias may be small or large and enlarging. Huge symptomatic hernias in an obese patient can be very difficult to repair, carrying the risks of intestinal injury (while freeing adhesions in the abdomen) and of major pulmonary, cardiac, and wound complications postoperatively. Numerous operations have been developed. Almost all repairs used today involve the use of mesh placement somewhere. (For more information, see the chapter "Hernias and Abdominal Wall Defects" by D.J. Scott and D.B. Jones in *Surgery: Basic Science and Clinical Evidence*) edited by J.A. Norton, et al, published by Springer-Verlag, 2001.) Of particular interest for repair of large and complex incisional hernias are techniques using a giant piece of mesh. The newer laparoscopic methods seem promising, with fewer reported complications and less pain postoperatively.

Other Abdominal Hernias

In a **spigelian hernia**, fat or an intestinal loop comes through a weak point in the lateral posterior rectus sheath at the semilunar line (in the lower abdomen). This hernia is in the abdominal wall between muscles and fascia, which makes the hernia difficult to locate. It usually is reducible, but it is intermittently painful. Laparoscopic repair works well for these, as does an incision directly onto the palpable lump or through the midline. When a midline incision is used, the site of the abdominal wall is lifted up so that the opening can be seen from underneath and the hernia defect repaired.

In a **lumbar hernia**, a posterior-lateral bulge is noted, possibly following trauma, through one of the two muscular lumbar triangles. **Pelvic floor hernias** are rare, and a computed tomography (CT) scan is useful for diagnosis and in planning the operative approach. **Parastomal hernias** usually develop alongside a colostomy, but they can occur next to an iliostomy. These are common and may require correction, but the recurrence rate is high.

Congenital and Diaphragmatic Hernias

Infants born with congenital diaphragmatic hernia constitute a pediatric and pediatric surgical emergency. While prenatal diagnosis with ultrasound and prenatal treatment is desirable, when not done, a rapid postnatal diagnosis can be crucial. The child has a huge opening in the posterolateral diaphragm (foramen of Bochdalek), the abdominal contents are up in the chest; the child has a scaphoid abdomen, and may have easily heard bowel sounds in the chest. After an abnormality is noted in the child's breathing and a rapid chest radiograph is ordered, one often can make the diagnosis from seeing gut in the chest and a shift of the mediastinum. **A very small amount of contrast put through a tiny nasogastric tube should help clarify the diagnosis.** With rapid diagnosis and appropriate treatment (neonatal intensive care before and after surgical correction), formerly high mortality rates have been reduced to acceptable levels.

A sliding hiatal hernia (widened esophageal hiatus with part of the stomach in the chest) exists in almost all patients with gastroesophageal reflux disease. Wrapping some upper stomach around the esophagogastric junction and holding it there with stitches **(Nissen repair)** has excellent results in those requiring surgical intervention. This procedure lends itself well to a laparoscopic approach, with rapid return home and to work. Preoperative evaluation includes manometry and endoscopy.

In a **paraesophageal hiatal hernia**, the gastric fundus herniates up through the diaphragm and is superior to the location of the most distal point of the esophagus. Reflux symptoms, possible mild or severe pain, and even gangrenous changes in the herniated portion of the stomach can result. A lateral chest radiography usually is diagnostic; an upper gastrointestinal study always is. If at all symptomatic, a paraesophageal hernia always should be corrected surgically without delay. **Traumatic hernia through the diaphragm always requires repair.**

Summary

Evaluation of a suspected or definite groin mass and evaluation of groin pain can be a challenge to any primary physician. History and physical examination, while keeping the different etiologic possibilities in mind, frequently clarify the diagnosis. The most commonly performed general surgical procedure is groin hernia repair. General surgeons are referred for many patients with groin area pains of all types. Almost all patients with groin mass or groin pain are, sooner or later, referred to a surgeon. The sooner this is done, the better.

The transition in hernia surgery to widespread use of local anesthesia and rapid return to home and normal activities has been aided by shorter operating times and use of some type of inert, nonabsorbable mesh. Outcomes and patient satisfaction have improved. Types of hernia repairs and their pros and cons have been presented, along with discussion of definitions, differential diagnoses, and anatomic and special considerations. Abdominal wall hernias as well as congenital and diaphragmatic hernias have been briefly discussed.

Selected Readings

Bendavid R. Complications of groin hernia surgery. Surg Clin North Am 1998;78(6):1089–1103.

Cunningham J, Fry DE, Richards AT, et al. Part IV: complications of groin hernias. In: Fitzgibbons RJ, Greenburg AG, eds. Nyhus and Condon's Hernia, 5th ed. Philadelphia: Lippincott, 2002:279–324.

Felix E, et al. Causes of recurrence after laparoscopic hernioplasty. A multicenter study. Surg Endosc 1998;123:226–231.

Gilbert AI, Graham MF. Tension-free hernioplasty using a bilayer prosthesis. In: Fitzgibbons RJ, Greenburg AG, eds. Nyhus and Condon's Hernia, 5th ed. Philadelphia: Lippincott, 2002:173–180.

Hair A, et al. What effect does the duration of an inguinal hernia have on patient symptoms? J Am Coll Surg 2001;193:125–129.

Lichtenstein IL, Shulman AG. Ambulatory outpatient hernia surgery, including a new concept, introducing tension-free repair. Int Surg 1986;71:1–4.

Loham AS, et al. Mechanisms of hernia recurrence after preperitoneal mesh repair. Traditional and laparoscopic. Ann Surg 1997;225(4):422–431.

Neuhauser D. Elective inguinal herniorrhapy versus truss in the elderly. In: Bunker JP, Barnes BA, Mosteller F, eds. Costs, Risks and Benefits of Surgery. New York: Oxford University Press, 1977:223–239.

Nyhus LM, Condon RE, Harkins HN. Clinical experiences with preperitoneal hernia repair for all types of hernia in the groin: with particular reference to the importance of tranversalis fascia analogs. Am J Surg 1960;100:234–244.

Payne JH, Grininger LM, Izawa MT, et al. Laparoscopic or open inguinal herniorrhaphy? A randomized prospective trial. Arch Surg 1994;129:973–981.

Scott DJ, Jones BJ. Hernias and abdominal wall defects. In: Norton JA, Bollinger RR, Chang AE, et al, eds. Surgery: Basic Science and Clinical Evidence. New York: Springer-Verlag, 2001:727–823.

Shulman AG, Amid PK, Lichtenstein IL. The safety of mesh repair for primary inguinal hernia: results of 3,019 operations from five diverse surgical sources. Am Surg 1992;58:255–257.

Stassen, et al. Reoperation after recurrent groin repair. Ann Surg 2001;234:122–126.

Stoppa RE. The treatment of complicated groin and incisional hernias. World J Surg 1984;13:545–554.

Wantz GE. The Canadian repair: personal observations. World J Surg 1989;13:516–521; J Am Coll Surg 2000;190:645–650.

28

The Ischemic Lower Extremity

Rocco G. Ciocca

Objectives

1. To describe atherosclerosis, its etiology, prevention, and sites of predilection.
   - To discuss the intimal injury that characterizes the process and how that injury affects therapy and prevention.
2. To describe the differential diagnosis of hip, thigh, buttock, and leg pain associated with exercise.
   - To discuss neurologic versus vascular etiologies of walking-induced leg pain.
   - To discuss musculoskeletal etiologies.
   - To discuss the relationship of impotence to the diagnosis.
3. To describe the pathophysiology of intermittent claudication.
   - To discuss the diagnostic workup of chronic arterial occlusive disease.
   - To discuss the role of segmental Doppler studies and arteriography.
   - To discuss the medical management of arterial occlusive disease.
   - To discuss risk factors associated with arterial occlusive disease.
   - To discuss operative and nonoperative interventions for aortoiliac, femoropopliteal, and distal vascular occlusion.
4. To describe the pathophysiology of ischemic rest pain.
   - To discuss evaluation and management of rest pain.
   - To discuss the role of anticoagulation in peripheral vascular disease.

- To discuss the indications for amputation and choice of amputation level.
5. To describe the etiologies and presentation of acute arterial occlusion.
   - To discuss embolic versus thrombotic occlusion.
   - To discuss the signs and symptoms of acute arterial occlusion (the "Ps").
   - To discuss the medical and surgical management.
   - To discuss the complications associated with prolonged ischemia and revascularization.
   - To discuss the diagnosis and treatment of compartment syndrome.

Case

An 80-year-old woman presents to her primary care physician with a several-hour history of pain in her left foot. The pain was rather sudden in onset and has progressed to the point that she is having difficulty moving and feeling her toes. She states that in the past she has had difficulty walking more than a block or two without severe pain in her calves bilaterally. She also has an extensive past medical history that includes coronary artery bypass surgery, hypertension, smoking, and insulin-dependent diabetes mellitus (IDDM). She is on multiple medications, but, unfortunately, she forgot to bring her list of medications.

Introduction

The most important question to ask when evaluating someone with an ischemic or painful leg is the following: Is the leg ischemic? Put a better way: **Is the pain that the patient is experiencing caused by decreased blood flow?** As we shall discuss in this chapter, determining the adequacy of blood flow is relatively easy using history, physical exam, and simple, noninvasive tests.

As in all physical conditions, the cornerstone of medical therapy begins and sometimes ends with a thorough history and a thorough physical exam.

History

The leading cause of lower extremity ischemia usually is related to **some form of or complication of atherosclerotic disease,** known as "hardening of the arteries" in lay terms. With that in mind, it is helpful to elicit very early in a patient's history the risk factors for atherosclerotic disease. These risk factors include smoking, hypertension, elevation of cholesterol, diabetes, obesity, and a sedentary lifestyle. Finding out about these risk factors early in the evaluation helps to narrow the diagnosis and helps to stratify risk for possible surgical intervention. It has been estimated that the prevalence of intermittent claudication is about 15% for patients older than 50, and about 1% of this population has critical limb ischemia.

Unfortunately, patients, even in this age of information overload, do not always have tremendous insight into their underlying health problems. Despite one's best efforts, patients frequently are unable to provide an accurate listing of their **past medical history and associated comorbidities**. To obtain the proper answers concerning a particular condition, **it is vital for a physician to ask the correct questions**. For example, the question "Do you have high blood pressure?" may be appropriately answered by the patient on hypertensive medications with "No." The more appropriate question is "Are you currently being treated for high blood pressure?" Very often, the knowledgeable physician can piece together accurately the salient points of patients' history based on the medications that they are on. **Always encourage your patients to carry a list of their current medications and the doses.** Along with the information regarding medications, it is helpful to obtain a **history of any adverse drug reactions or allergies**. When dealing with patients who have cardiovascular disease, it also is helpful to obtain a history of "dye" reactions or allergies to iodine. This is due to the fact that the patient with the acutely ischemic extremity may require an angiogram with iodinated intraarterial contrast. A previous contrast reaction does not rule out the use of angiography as a diagnostic or therapeutic tool. It simply means that appropriate precautions need to be taken.

As in all conditions, the **acuity of the problem** also must be taken into account. The reasons for this should be obvious. Patients with chronic ischemia rarely seem to present with acute limb-threatening ischemia. This is not to say that they are not at risk for limb loss or that they will not require aggressive revacularization procedures, but it is rare for these patients to require urgent/immediate surgical intervention. If the onset of the ischemia is **acute and particularly if it is unilateral, then an embolic or thrombotic etiology must be considered**. This is especially true in a patient such as the one in the case presented who has a long-standing history of lower extremity ischemia and who has a sudden change. You must ask: Why? What has happened that has led to the acute change? For patients with chronic symptoms of leg pain, it is important to elicit the nature of the pain. Is it exercise induced? Does it go away at rest? What part of the leg does the pain affect? How far can one walk before the pain starts? Has it been getting better or worse? Does it affect both legs equally? What we are looking for here is a **history of claudication**. We generally refer to intermittent claudication, which is a complex of symptoms characterized by absence of pain or discomfort in a limb when at rest, the commencement of pain, tension, and weakness after walking is begun, intensification of the condition until walking becomes impossible, and the disappearance of the symptoms after a period of rest.

Epidemiologic studies suggest that up to 5% of men and 2.5% of women over 60 years of age have symptoms of claudication.[1,2] The natural history of claudication, fortunately, is that of a generally benign course, with 70% of patients reporting no change in symptoms over 5 to 10 years, with 20% to 30% eventually progressing to require some form of intervention, and with less than 10% eventually requiring amputation. However, it is important to recall that **intermittent claudication reflects systemic vascular disease, with affected patients carrying a threefold increase in cardiovascular mortality.**

Rest pain is not merely claudication while at rest; rather, it is pain, usually in the forefoot, that occurs at rest and often is relieved by dependency of the affected limb. Rest pain indicates reduced perfusion of the extremity even at rest and portends eventual progression to frank tissue loss.

In the case presented, the patient, by her history, has chronic ischemia of her lower extremity, but she has experienced a rather profound and unfortunately negative change. Did she acutely thrombose already diseased but patent lower extremity vessels, or did she embolize a clot from her heart or from another more diseased proximal vessel leading to her current limb that is in a threatened state? A physical exam will give some clues to the etiology of her current state.

Physical Examination

When treating a patient who presents with an ischemic extremity, it is necessary to examine that extremity. But one must not forget to examine the entire patient. By examining a patient in a head-to-toe manner, one is much less likely to miss important physical findings.

The Ps of acute ischemia are pain, pallor, pulselessness, paresthesia, paralysis, and poikilothermy. It is helpful to think in this order because, generally, it is the order in which the patient complains of symptoms. Patients do not come in saying that their leg is poikilothermic, although they may say that it is cold. Generally, patients present because their leg hurts. The pain coincides with the pallor and the pulselessness. Optimally, the patient is seen prior to the onset of paresthesia and paralysis. The extremity that has been paralyzed secondary to ischemia usually predicts a less than optimal outcome, even if expedient revascularization is performed. Patients with acutely ischemic extremities present with painful, cold, and pale extremities. If they do not improve or are revascularized, they become numb and immobile.

The critical and yet frequently missed physical finding is the **presence or absence of pulses.** It is critically important to examine and honestly document the presence or absence of all pulses in both the upper

---

[1] Reunanen A, Takkunen H, Aromaa A. Prevalence of intermittent claudication and its effect on mortality. Acta Med Scand 1982;211:249–256.

[2] Jelnes R, Gaardsting O, Hougaard Jensen K, Baekgaard N, Tonnesen KH, Schroeder T. Fate in intermittent claudication: outcome and risk factors. Br Med J (Clin Res Ed) 1986;293:1137–1140.

and lower extremities. It also is helpful to note whether the pulse is regular or not. The presence of a cardiac rhythm other than sinus may have some critical implications to the understanding of the patient's problem. If pulses are absent to palpation, then it is helpful to employ the aid of a hand-held Doppler. The presence or absence of Doppler signals goes a long way in assessing the degree of limb ischemia. If the leg is absent of both pulses and Doppler signal, it generally is profoundly ischemic and will require revascularization sometime in the near future.

In addition to palpating pulses, it is important **to feel for thrills**, which are a "buzzing" vibratory sensation above the vessel. If there is a thrill, then you can expect to find an **audible bruit**. One must listen for bruits over the areas of major pulsation, most notably the neck, abdomen, groin, and occasionally the popliteal fossa. The presence of a bruit generally implies turbulence within the underlying vessel, and that generally is due to atherosclerotic plaque. Documentation and recognition of an irregular pulse are exceedingly important and frequently help to explain the source of embolization as a case of an acutely ischemic extremity.

The chronically ischemic leg has several other salient physical findings: thickened, brittle toenails; thin, fragile, almost shiny skin; absence of hair on the dorsum of the toes; increased capillary refill times; and frequently, dependent rubor.

Diagnostic Tests

Generally, diagnostic tests should form a logical progression from the history and physical exam. The tests should focus and clarify what the physician has found on the physical exam. If an operation is indicated to treat the problem, the tests frequently define the anatomy in question in a better manner. See **Algorithm 28.1** for management options for claudication.

In general, one should start with a noninvasive and relatively inexpensive test first before proceeding to more expensive and invasive studies. It is important to individualize the approach to a patient. For example, the patient in the case presented at the start of this chapter, based on her presentation, would benefit from an angiogram, providing an emergent operation is not required. **Order the test that the patient needs and that gives the information that is needed to take care of the patient optimally.**

The **most common and frequently the most valuable noninvasive vascular study is the ankle brachial index (ABI)**. This is a simple test to perform and is easy to learn. It simply is the ankle systolic pressure taken by Doppler over either the posterior tibial or dorsalis pedis artery (whichever is highest) divided by the brachial systolic pressure, also taken by Doppler. The ratio should be greater than 1.0. Values less than 1.0 suggest some component of peripheral vascular disease. The lower the value, the greater the degree of ischemia, with the important caveat that patients with very calcified lower extremity vessels (e.g., diabetic

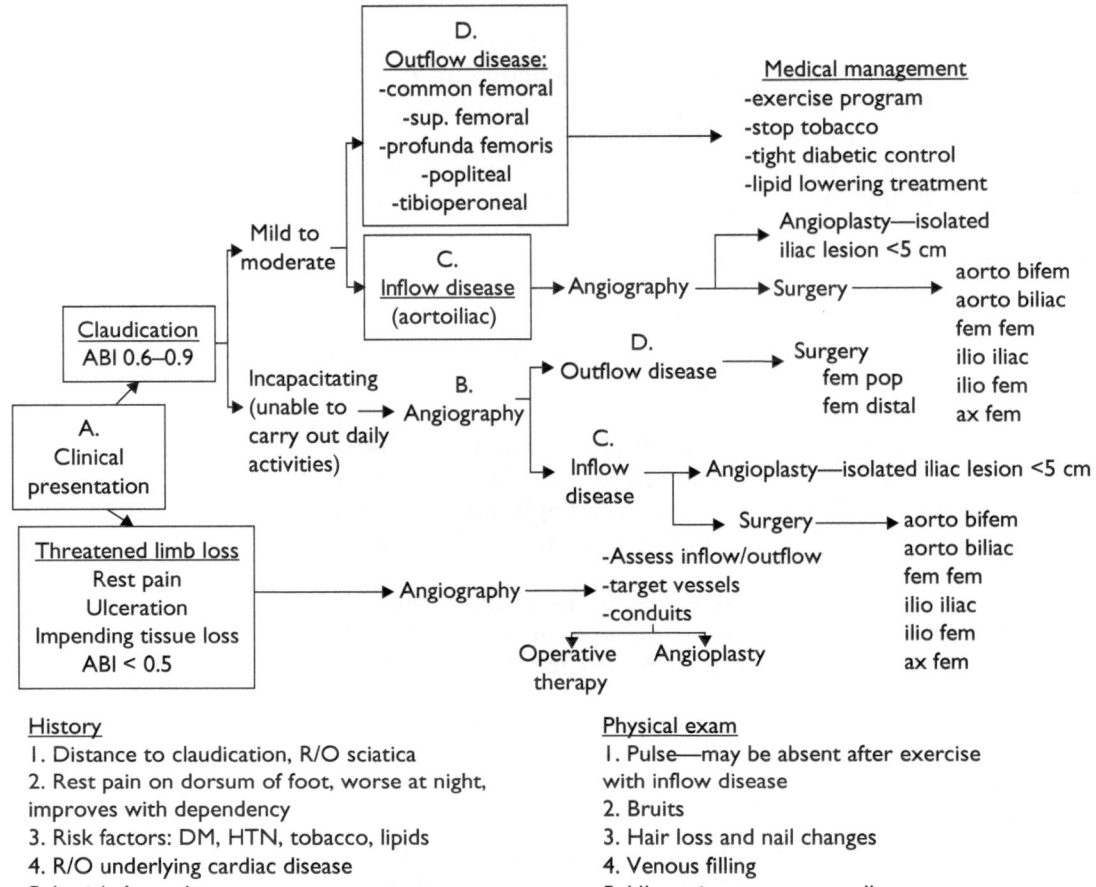

Algorithm 28.1. Algorithm for the management of claudication. ABI, ankle brachial index; DM, diabetes mellitus; HTN, hypertension. (Reprinted from Millikan KW, Saclarides TJ, eds. Common Surgical Diseases: An Algorithmic Approach to Problem Solving. New York: Springer-Verlag, 1998, with permission.)

patients) tend to have noncompressible vessels and, therefore, falsely elevated ABIs.

With the limitations of the ABI in mind, more formal, noninvasive testing frequently is indicated. We prefer to use a combination of **pulse volume recordings (PVRs) and segmental pressure measurement**. These relatively easy-to-perform and inexpensive studies provide very accurate and reproducible information regarding lower extremity ischemia. The PVRs are measurements of the increase in blood volume at a given level of the extremity with each heartbeat. If there is an obstructing lesion or occlusion of a blood vessel proximal to the placement of the PVR cuff, the amount of blood flow to that level will be diminished, and the PVR waveform will be flattened.

It also is important to recognize that the above-mentioned studies also can be performed after the patient has exercised. The normal response to exercise is an increase in heart rate, blood pressure, and arterial vasodilation, with a resultant increase in blood flow to the lower extremity and concomitant rise in the ABI. In patients with vascular occlusive disease, however, one sees a drop in the ABI due to the patients' inability to increase blood flow past the obstructing lesions(s) and distal exercised induced vasodilatation.

Other noninvasive studies worth mentioning are **arterial duplex ultrasound and transcutaneous O$_2$ measurement**. Duplex ultrasound is the combination of B-mode ultrasound with Doppler ultrasound. While it has become the gold standard for noninvasive imaging of the carotid arteries, its usefulness in lower extremity imaging is defined less clearly. It is much more labor intensive than the above-mentioned studies and frequently more time-consuming to perform. Duplex scanning has been reported to detect significant stenoses, with an average 82% sensitivity and 92% specificity depending on the vessels studied.[3] Transcutaneous O$_2$ measurements can be useful in assessing the oxygen saturation at a given level of an extremity. The higher the level of O$_2$, the better the arterial perfusion and generally the more likely a wound is to heal at that level. Transcutaneous O$_2$ levels greater than 50 mm Hg correlate with good perfusion and generally good wound healing. Conversely, transcutaneous O$_2$ levels below 25 mm Hg indicate poor arterial perfusion and low likelihood of wound healing. Transcutaneous O$_2$ measurements can be helpful in assessing the need to reperfuse an extremity prior to amputation or in assessing the proper level of amputation.

Magnetic resonance angiography (MRA) is an additional noninvasive means of obtaining an anatomic assessment of lower extremity ischemia. While safe and particularly helpful for patients who have absolute contraindications for conventional angiography, there are several limitations. Not all MRAs are the same. The best results are obtained when a specific area is being interrogated rather than when a global assessment is being made.

Treatment

Treatment of the ischemic extremity varies over a wide range of options and degrees of intervention. **A large segment of patients who have nondisabling claudication can and should be treated conservatively.** The recommendation for such conservatism is borne out by the fact that only 7% of patients with claudication at 5 years and only 12% at 10 years progress to amputation if left alone. **The cornerstone of conservative therapy is risk management.** This includes a program of exercise, smoking cessation, and control of lipids, glucose, and blood pressure. The addition of antiplatlet and rheologic medications can be helpful. The patient, particularly the diabetic patient, must be educated about how to meticulously care for the lower extremity.

---

[3] Kohler TR, Nance DR, Cramer MM, Vandenburghe N, Strandness DE Jr. Duplex scanning for diagnosis of aortoiliac and femoropopliteal disease: a prospective study. Circulation 1987;76:1074–1080.

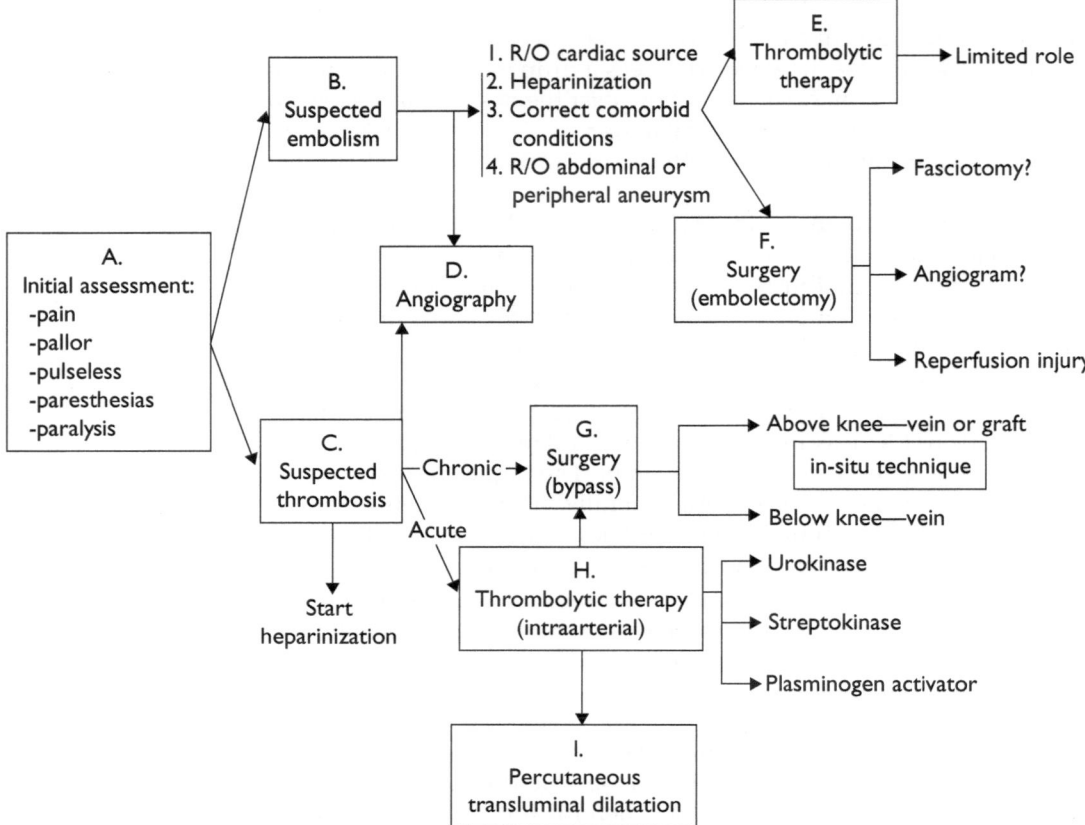

Algorithm 28.2. Algorithm for the management of cold leg. (Reprinted from Millikan KW, Saclarides TJ, eds. Common Surgical Diseases: An Algorithmic Approach to Problem Solving. New York: Springer-Verlag, 1998, with permission.)

Acutely ischemic extremities, such as the one in our case, generally must be treated more aggressively. See **Algorithm 28.2** for management options for the cold leg. **If conservative measures are unsuccessful or if the patient presents with advanced disease, then vascular intervention is indicated.** The guiding principles of vascular reconstruction are **inflow, outflow, and a conduit.** In addition, the reconstructions may be performed anatomically, extraanatomically, and, increasingly, endovascularly (within the artery itself). **Inflow** refers to the source of good blood flow above the occlusive disease. It can be any artery in the body that has unobstructed arterial pressure. It is important to note that, occasionally, patients are in such a low cardiac output state that good inflow cannot be had. These patients generally have a dismal overall prognosis unless their cardiac status can be improved. **Outflow** generally refers to the target vessel below the occlusive disease to which blood will be supplied. Frequent outflow vessels in the ischemic lower extremity include the above-knee popliteal artery, the below-knee popliteal artery, tibial arteries, and, increasingly, particularly in diabetic patients, pedal arteries. Occasionally, patients lack an adequate outflow vessel and succumb to limb loss. The **conduit** refers to the connection between the inflow and outflow vessels. Conduits may be prosthetic, and, in fact, prosthetic conduits (particularly Dacron grafts) are the conduit of choice for large-vessel reconstruction such as the aorta and iliac segments. They may be autologous, such as the greater saphenous vein (GSV). The GSV is the conduit of choice for infrainguinal reconstructions. Alternate veins, such as the lesser saphenous vein and the arm vein, also can be useful alternatives if the GSV is not available or if it is of poor quality. In the absence of an autologous conduit, prosthetic conduits, usually polytetrafluoroethylene (PTFE), may be used. The success of prosthetic conduits for lower extremity conduits generally are inferior to vein conduits. There are various adjunctive procedures that may be employed to enhance the success of these bypass procedures (**Table 28.1**).

Lower extremity reconstructions can be performed safely on properly selected patients with very acceptable morbidity and mortalities. Five-year survival, however, remains low, in the range of 50% to 60%, and this speaks to the advanced age of these patients and to the comorbidities, particularly coronary artery disease, that afflict these patients.

We generally speak in terms of primary and secondary patency and limb salvage when describing the success of lower extremity reconstructions. Increasingly, functional outcome data also are being assessed, which helps to provide a more detailed understanding of the benefits of revascularization.

In general, anatomic reconstructions have better long-term patency than extraanatomic reconstruction (e.g., aortobifemoral bypass versus axillobifemoral bypass). Autologous conduits have better patency than prosthetic bypasses, particularly when the distal anastomosis is to an artery below the knee joint. It is important to remember that veins have valves and that these must be accounted for when a vein is going to be used as an arterial conduit. The vein must be reversed or the valves must be lysed.

Endovascular procedures have been around since the early 1960s, but they have been refined over the past decade. Most of these procedures can be performed percutaneously and therefore obviate the need for an incision and the associated pain, healing, and recovery. Many endovascular procedures, therefore, readily can be done using only local anesthesia or in combination with mild sedation. This is a significant advance over conventional surgery, particularly when one considers the prevalence of significant comorbidities on the part of patients who present with advanced pulmonary vascular disease (PVD). Most of the techniques are preformed with a guidewire technique devised originally by Seldinger.[4] Current interventions include balloon angioplasty, balloon angioplasty plus stenting, and various thrombolytic techniques. These are all in a state of evolution, but there is growing evidence to support their use in properly selected patients (**Table 28.2**).

---

[4] The Seldinger Technique. Reprint from Acta Radiologica. AJR 1984;142(1):5–7.

Table 28.1. Infrapopliteal grafts.

	1 Year	4 Year
Primary patency		
Reverse saphenous vein[t,r,d,o,a,j,s,c,f,p,e,g,h]	76%	62%
In-situ vein bypass[k,i,l,b,s]	81%	68%
Secondary patency		
Reverse saphenous vein[r,s,c,e,h]	83%	76%
In-situ vein bypass[l,b,s]	87%	81%
PTEE[t,o,s,g,h]	47%	21%
Limb salvage		
Reverse saphenous vein[t,j,f,p,e,g,q]	85%	82%
In-situ vein bypass[i,m]	91%	83%
PTFE[t,j,g]	68%	48%

PTFE, polytetrafluoroethylene.

[a] Anonymous. Comparative evaluation of prosthetic, reversed, and in situ vein bypass grafts in distal popliteal and tibialperoneal revascularization. Veterans Administration Cooperative Study Group 141. Arch Surg 1988;123: 434–438.

[b] Bandyk DF, Kaebnick HW, Stewart GW, Towne JB. Durability of the in situ saphenous vein arterial bypass: a comparison of primary and secondary patency. J Vasc Surg 1987;5:256–268.

[c] Barry R, Satiani B, Mohan B, Smead WL, Vaccaro PS. Prognostic indicators in femoropopliteal and distal bypass grafts. Surg Gynecol Obstet 1985;161:129–132.

[d] Bergan JJ, Veith FJ, Bernhard VM, et al. Randomization of autogenous vein and polytetrafluoroethylene grafts in femoral-distal reconstruction. Surgery (St. Louis) 1982;92:921–930.

[e] Berkowitz HD, Greenstein SM. Improved patency in reversed femoral-infrapopliteal autogenous vein grafts by early detection and treatment of the failing graft. J Vasc Surg 1987;5:755–761.

[f] Cantelmo NL, Snow JR, Menzoian JO, LoGerfo FW. Successful vein bypass in patients with an ischemic limb and a palpable popliteal pulse. Arch Surg 1986;121:217–220.

[g] Dalsing MC, White JV, Yao JS, Podrazik R, Flinn WR, Bergan JJ. Infrapopliteal bypass for established gangrene of the forefoot or toes. J Vasc Surg 1985;2:669–677.

[h] Flinn WR, Rohrer MJ, Yao JS, McCarthy WJ III, Fahey VA, Bergan JJ. Improved long-term patency of infragenicular polytetrafluoroethylene grafts. J Vasc Surg 1988;7:685–690.

[i] Harris RW, Andros G, Dulawa LB, Oblath RW, Apyan R, Salles-Cunha S. The transition to "in situ" vein bypass grafts. Surg Gynecol Obstet 1986;163:21–28.

[j] Hobson RW Jr, Lynch TG, Jamil Z, et al. Results of revascularization and amputation in severe lower extremity ischemia: a five-year clinical experience. J Vasc Surg 1985;2:174–185.

[k] Kent KC, Whittemore AD, Mannick JA. Short-term and midterm results of an all-autogenous tissue policy for infrainguinal reconstruction. J Vasc Surg 1989;9:107–114.

[l] Leather RP, Shah DM, Chang BB, Kaufman JL. Resurrection of the in situ saphenous vein bypass. 1000 cases later [see comments]. Ann Surg 1988;208:435–442.

[m] Leather RP, Shan DM, Karmody AM. Infrapopliteal arterial bypass for limb salvage: increased patency and utilization of the saphenous vein used "in situ." Surgery 1981;90:1000–1008.

[n] Rosenbloom MS, Walsh JJ, Schuler JJ, et al. Long-term results of infragenicular bypasses with autogenous vein originating from the distal superficial femoral and popliteal arteries. J Vasc Surg 1988;7:691–696.

[o] Rutherford RB, Jones DN, Bergentz SE, et al. Factors affecting the patency of infrainguinal bypass. J Vasc Surg 1988;8:236–246.

[p] Schuler JJ, Flanigan DP, Williams LR, Ryan TJ, Castronuovo JJ. Early experience with popliteal to infrapopliteal bypass for limb salvage. Arch Surg 1983;118:472–476.

[q] Taylor LM Jr, Edwards JM, Brant B, Phinney ES, Porter JM. Autogenous reversed vein bypass for lower extremity ischemia in patients with absent or inadequate greater saphenous vein. Am J Surg 1987;153:505–510.

[r] Taylor LM Jr, Edwards JM, Porter JM. Present status of reversed vein bypass grafting: five-year results of a modern series. J Vasc Surg 1990;11:193–205.

[s] Varty K, Allen KE, Jones L, Sayers RD, Bell PR, London NJ. Influence of Losartan, an angiotensin receptor antagonist, on neointimal proliferation in cultured human saphenous vein. Br J Surg 1994;81:819–822.

[t] Veith FJ, Gupta SK, Ascer E, et al. Six-year prospective multicenter randomized comparison of autologous saphenous vein and expanded polytetrafluoroethylene grafts in infrainguinal arterial reconstructions. J Vasc Surg 1986;3: 104–114.

Data from McCann RL. Peripheral artery aneurysms. In: Porter JM, Taylor LM Jr, eds. Basic Data Underlying Clinical Decision Making in Vascular Surgery. St. Louis: Quality Medical, 1994:137–140. *Source*: Reprinted from Neschis DG, Golden MA. Arterial disease of the lower extremity. In: Norton JA, Bollinger RR, Chang AE, et al, eds. Surgery: Basic Science and Clinical Evidence. New York: Springer-Verlag, 2001, with permission.

Table 28.2. Percutaneous transluminal angioplasty patency.

	1 Year	4 Year
Aortoiliac[c,a,b,e]	88%	75%
Femoropopliteal[c,a,b,d]	81%	63%

[a] Gallino A, Mahler F, Probst P, Nachbur B. Percutaneous transluminal angioplasty of the arteries of the lower limbs: a 5-year follow-up. Circulation 1984;70:619–623.
[b] Hewes RC, White RI, Jr., Murray RR, et al. Long-term results of superficial femoral artery angioplasty. AJR 1986; 146:1025–1029.
[c] Johnston KW, Rae M, Hogg-Johnston SA, et al. 5-year results of a prospective study of percutaneous transluminal angioplasty. Ann Surg 1987;206:403–413.
[d] Krepel VM, van Andel GJ, van Erp WF, Breslau PJ. Percutaneous transluminal angioplasty of the femoropopliteal artery: initial and long-term results. Radiology 1985;156: 325–328.
[e] Spence RK, Freiman DB, Gatenby R, et al. Long-term results of transluminal angioplasty of the iliac and femoral arteries. Arch Surg 1981;116:1377–1386.
Data from Wilson SE, Sheppard B. Results of percutaneous transluminal angioplasty for peripheral vascular occlusive disease. In: Porter JM, Taylor LM Jr, eds. Basic Data Underlying Clinical Decision Making in Vascular Surgery. St. Louis: Quality Medical, 1994:144–148. *Source*: Reprinted from Neschis DG, Golden MA. Arterial disease of the lower extremity. In: Norton JA, Bollinger RR, Chang AE, et al, eds. Surgery: Basic Science and Clinical Evidence. New York: Springer-Verlag, 2001, with permission.

Case Discussion

The most appropriate first step in dealing with the presented patient would be to anticoagulate her with systemic heparin. If she is a reasonable operative candidate, then one could go to the operating room and, under local anesthesia, perform a diagnostic angiogram. Depending on the findings, a decision could be made as to whether the ischemia could be resolved with either endovascular techniques (e.g., thrombolytic therapy) or limited open surgery. Caution should be taken, however, to avoid lengthy emergent surgical procedures on these very elderly patients with significant comorbidities.

Summary

Lower leg ischemia as a manifestation of peripheral arterial disease is common. Frequently, it can be noninvasively diagnosed and conservatively managed. Patients, like the patient in our case, may present with acute ischemia and warrant more aggressive management. The level of intervention, however, always must be tailored to the overall condition of the patient. Given the presences of significant comorbidities in our patient, significant caution is warranted before embarking on aggressive surgical intervention. Fortunately, with the advent of less invasive endovascular techniques, vascular interventionalists have more and potentially safer options.

Selected Readings

Chew DE, Conte MS, Belkin M, et al. Arterial reconstruction for lower limb ischemia. Acta Chir Belg 2001;101(3):106–115.

Cikrit DF, Dalsing MC. Lower extremity arterial endovascular stenting. Surg Clin North Am 1998;78(4):617–629.

Cronenwett JL, Warner KG, Zelenock GB, et al. Intermittent claudication. Current results of nonoperative management. Arch Surg 1984;119:430–436.

Dalman RL, Taylor LM Jr. Infrainguinal revascularization procedures. In: Porter JM, Taylor LM Jr, eds. Basic Data Underlying Clinical Decision Making in Vascular Surgery. St. Louis: Quality Medical, 1994:141–143.

Kannel WB, Skinner JJ Jr, Schwartz MJ, Shurtleff D. Intermittent claudication. Incidence in the Framingham Study. Circulation 1970;875–883.

Mills JL, Porter JM. Acute limb ischemia. In: Porter JM, Taylor LM Jr, eds. Basic Data Underlying Clinical Decision Making in Vascular Surgery. St. Louis: Quality Medical, 1994:134–136.

Neschis DG, Golden MA. Arterial disease of the lower extremity. In: Norton JA, Bollinger RR, Chang AE, et al., eds. Surgery: Basic Science and Clinical Evidence. New York: Springer-Verlag, 2001.

Ouriel K, Veith FJ, Sasahara AA. A comparison of recombinant urokinase with vascular surgery as initial treatment for acute arterial occlusion of the legs. Thrombolysis or Peripheral Arterial Surgery (TOPAS) Investigators [see comments]. N Engl J Med 1998;338:1105–1111.

29

The Swollen Leg

Rocco G. Ciocca

Objectives

1. To describe the differential diagnosis of the swollen leg.
   - To discuss how to differentiate lymphedema from venous disease.
   - To discuss painful versus nonpainful swelling.
2. To describe the factors that lead to venous thrombosis and embolism.
   - To discuss the usual locations of thrombosis.
   - To discuss differing implications of deep and superficial venous thrombophlebitis.
   - To discuss the common invasive and noninvasive diagnostic tests for deep venous thrombosis (DVT).
   - To discuss methods for DVT prophylaxis and identify high-risk patients.
   - To discuss the risks, benefits, and available options for anticoagulation and thrombolysis.
   - To discuss the signs, symptoms, diagnostic evaluation, and treatment of pulmonary embolism.
3. To describe the diagnosis, workup, and management options for symptomatic varicose veins and venous ulcers.
   - To discuss the physical exam and tests for venous valvular competence.
   - To discuss the role of venography and ultrasound.
   - To discuss medical versus surgical management.
   - To discuss the role of stripping, sclerosis, and laser ablation.

Case

You are asked to see a 43-year-old woman with a "swollen leg." She states that she has had a swollen left leg for several months and that her primary care physician wanted her to see a specialist for this condition. The left leg is somewhat larger on exam than the right leg, but, other than a sensation of "fullness," the patient denies any discomfort.

History and Physical Examination

As in all things that pertain to patient care, **the history and the physical exam** are the cornerstones to getting at the etiology of the swollen leg. Giving the patient adequate time to explain the problem is critical and frequently can save valuable time and useless diagnostic studies. Of critical importance, however, is obtaining a sense of the immediacy of the problem. In other words, is this an **acute or a chronic problem**? Once the timing of the swelling is ascertained, then a relatively simple thought process can be followed. See **Algorithm 29.1** for an algorithm of the management of the swollen leg.

The physical exam is critically important in the evaluation of the swollen leg, and, while not 100% accurate, it helps narrow the differential diagnosis of the problem. In the case presented above, the patient has had swelling for several months. The chronic nature of the situation may alter somewhat the aggressiveness of the workup. Things to focus on include any obvious trauma, evidence of infection, or bony abnormality. The presence of edema and the nature of the edema may be very telling. Ultimately, one must decide if the swelling is **systemic in nature, due to a vascular (venous) abnormality, or secondary to lymphedema. The unilateral nature of the swelling described by the patient in the case presented leads one to think that the etiology of the swelling is not systemic in nature. Systemic conditions like obesity or congestive heart failure generally lead to bilateral lower extremity swelling.**

All physical exams should include a thorough head-to-toe evaluation. **Head and neck evaluation**, with particular attention to the presence or absence of jugular venous distention, is important. Documentation of any masses may be telling when considering the etiology of venous or thromboembolic disease. The **chest exam** is important with regard to the presence or absence of rales or rhonchi. Decreased breath signs and dullness to percussion also are important to identify. A careful **abdominal exam** is critical. The presence of abdominal masses, which may be a source of venous or lymphatic obstruction, must be noted. Abdominal masses also may be indicative of an intraabdominal tumor and therefore a nidus for a hypercoaguable state. Checking the patient's **stool for occult blood** also is important as an indicator of a possible neoplasm but also in planning therapy, particularly if anticoagulation is indicated. **Obesity**, a frequent cause of a "swollen" extremity, frequently is overlooked or disregarded as an etiology.

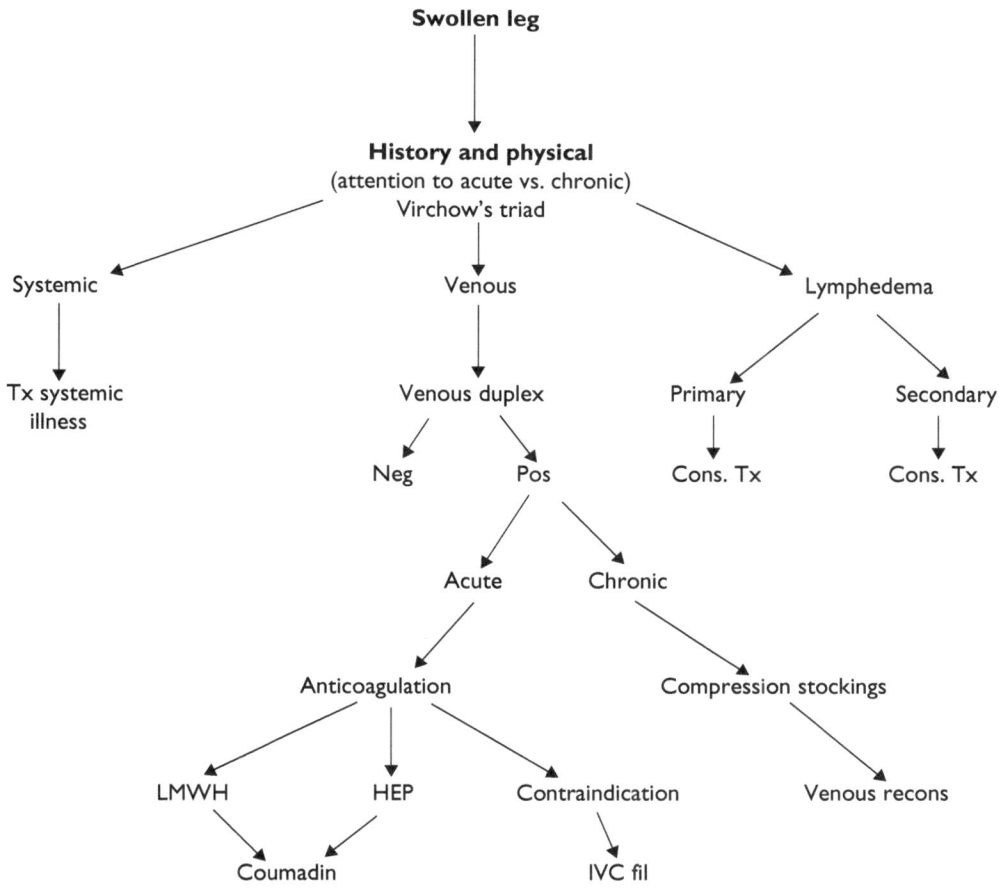

Cons. Tx, conservative treatment
LMWH, low molecular weight heparin
HEP, conventional heparin
IVC-FIL, inferior vena cava filter
Venous Recons., venous reconstruction

Algorithm 29.1. Algorithm for the management of swollen leg.

Unilateral swelling, as in the case patient, certainly could be due to an intrabdominal mass or deep venous thrombosis. It is critically important to examine both legs. Inspection often fails to identify any difference between the extremities. This implies that the swelling is bilateral in nature or that the "swelling" may be due to some other process. Remember the obesity discussion above.

The nature of the swelling, the presence or absence of edema, the nature of the edema, the evidence of trauma, cellulitis, the nature and texture of the skin, the presence of ulcerations, and the locations and nature of the ulcerations all are important to document. The presence of pain, the location of pain, and the presence or absence of varicosi-

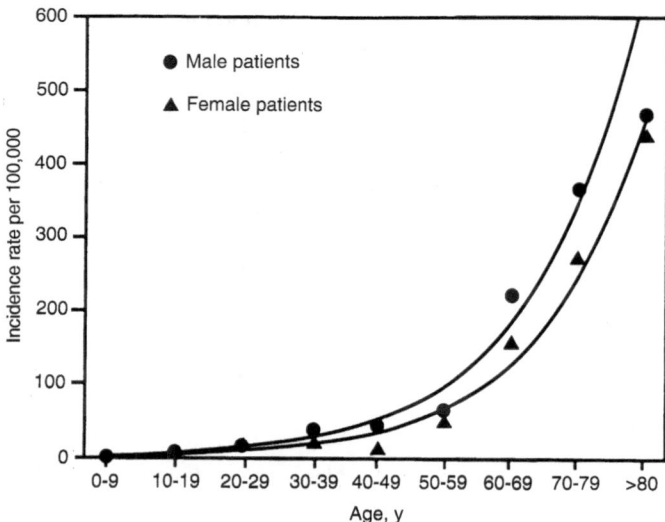

Figure 29.1. Incidence rate of clinically recognized deep vein thrombosis and/or pulmonary embolism per 100,000 population. The increase in rates for both male and female patients is well approximated by an exponential function of age. (Reprinted from Anderson FA Jr., Wheeler HB, Goldberg RJ, et al. A population-based perspective of the hospital incidence and case-fatality rates of deep venous thrombosis and pulmonary embolus. Arch Intern Med 1991;151:933–938, with permission. Copyright © 1991, American Medical Association. All rights reserved.)

ties are important to document. While arterial insufficiency rarely presents as swelling, the presence of peripheral pulses is important to document.

Acute versus Chronic

When the history obtained from the patient indicates that the swelling has occurred acutely, the differential veers toward disease processes that need to be diagnosed quickly and treated aggressively. If the process is chronic, a more leisurely diagnostic workup may follow.

Deep venous thrombosis (DVT) is exceedingly prevalent. The annual incidence is estimated at 48 per 100,000.[1] Deep venous thrombosis is a component of a larger process, **venous thromboembolism (VTE)**. The incidence of VTE is age dependent (**Fig. 29.1**). The diagnosis of DVT is *always* predicated on **Virchow's triad**. Rudolf Virchow, a 19th century pathologist, surmised that three conditions tended toward thrombosis: intimal injury, stasis of blood flow, and a hypercoaguable state. These observations have stood the test of time and are as true today as they were in Virchow's time. Most risk factors for DVT are related in some way to Virchow's triad (**Table 29.1**). In the case pre-

---

[1] Anderson FA Jr, Wheeler HB, Goldberg RJ, et al. A population-based perspective of the hospital incidence and case-fatality rates of deep venous thrombosis and pulmonary embolus. Arch Intern Med 1991;151:933–938.

Table 29.1. Risk factors for venous thromboembolism (VTE).

History of VTE
Age
Major surgery
Malignancy
Obesity
Trauma
Varicose veins/superficial thrombophlebitis
Cardiac disease
Hormones
Prolonged immobilization/paralysis
Pregnancy
Central venous catheterization
Hypercoaguable states

Source: Reprinted from Foley MI, Moneta GL. Venous disease
and pulmonary embolism. In: Norton JA, Bollinger RR,
Chang AE, et al, eds. Surgery: Basic Science and Clinical Evidence. New York: Springer-Verlag, 2001, with permission.

sented, the patient may have had a DVT for the past several months
that simply had not been diagnosed. Therefore, the presence of a DVT
needs to be ruled out.

Trauma is without question a risk factor for DVT (**Table 29.2**). Stasis
frequently follows trauma or surgery and frequently is contributory to
the development of DVT and pulmonary embolus (PE) (**Table 29.3**).

It can, at times, be difficult to **differentiate an acute DVT from a
chronic DVT**. Obviously, the patient's history is critical in helping to
do this. If the patient had a normal extremity and suddenly developed
a painful swollen extremity, the diagnosis is straightforward. Unfortunately, patients frequently present in a less than straightforward
manner. In those cases, it is best to err on the side of caution and treat
the patient as if he/she has an acute problem. A duplex scan, as discussed in the next section, may help in the diagnosis of an acute versus
chronic DVT.

Diagnosis

As with many disease processes in medicine, the diagnosis of DVT has
evolved. A thorough history and a thorough physical exam remain

Table 29.2. Risk factors for venous thromboembolism in 349 trauma
patients.[a]

Risk factor	Odds ratio (95% confidence interval)
Age (each 1-year increment)	1.05 (1.03–1.06)
Blood transfusion	1.74 (1.03–2.93)
Surgery	2.30 (1.08–4.89)
Fracture of femur or tibia	4.82 (2.79–8.33)
Spinal cord injury	8.59 (2.92–25.28)

[a] Determined by multivariate logistic regression.
Source: Reprinted from Geerts WH, Code KI, Jay RM, et al. A prospective study of venous
thromboembolism after major trauma. N Engl J Med 1994;331:1601–1606. Copyright ©
1994 Massachusetts Medical Society. All rights reserved.

Table 29.3. Pattern of injury analysis: pulmonary embolus (PE) vs. control.

Injury pattern	Number	Number (%) of pulmonary emboli	Odds ratio
Head + spinal cord injury	195	3 (1.5)	4.5*
Head + long bone fracture	471	11 (2.3)	8.8%
Severe pelvis + long bone fracture	106	4 (3.8)	12*
Mutliple long bone fracture	275	8 (2.9)	10*

*$p < .05$ compared with control group.
Source: Reprinted from Winchell RJ, Hoyt DB, Walsh JC, et al. Risk factors associated with pulmonary embolism despite routine prophylaxis: implications for improved protection. J Trauma 1994;37(4):600–606. With permission from Lippincott Williams and Wilkins.

the primary initial diagnostic modalities, but they suffer from a lack of sensitivity.

Venography had been considered the "gold standard" in the diagnosis of DVT. It currently is performed rarely. Venography or **phlebography** involves the cannulation of a peripheral hand or foot vein, application of a tourniquet to occlude the superficial venous system and to direct blood flow into the deep system, and injection of radiopaque contrast medium. Clot is outlined by the contrast material, thereby confirming the diagnosis. The procedure is painful for the patient, technically difficult to perform, and not always easy to interpret.

Duplex ultrasongraphy has surpassed venography as the diagnostic test of choice for DVT. It is a combination of B-mode ultrasonograpy and Doppler. The study allows determination of vein compressibility as well as flow characteristics. Veins generally are thin-walled and easily compressed. Veins that are incompressible with firm pressure applied by the ultrasound probe are considered thrombosed. Flow within the veins also can be assessed easily. Normal venous flow should be phasic, decreasing with inspiration. Flow can be increased by distal compression and decreased by increasing intraabdominal pressure. With experience, duplex ultrasonography can achieve greater than 90% sensitivity and greater than 95% specificity in the diagnosis of DVT.[2] A venous duplex scan would be an appropriate diagnostic study for the patient in the case presented in this chapter.

Clinicians frequently ask the vascular lab to help differentiate between an acute and a chronic DVT. There are no strict criteria to achieve the differentiation; however, there are some "soft" signs that can be helpful. If the thrombus is acute, it generally is not echogenic on duplex and is relatively soft on compression. The veins distal to the thrombus frequently are dilated. The clot may appear free floating

---

[2] Heijboer H, Buller HR, Lensing AWA, et al. A randomized comparison of the clinical utility of real time compression ultra-sonography versus impedance plethysmography in the diagnosis of deep-vein thrombosis in symptomatic outpatiens. N Engl J Med 1993;329:1365–1369.

and not completely adherent to the vein wall. Chronic DVTs are more commonly echogenic. There may be evidence of recanalization of the vein, and the veins distal to DVT are not as dilated as in an acute DVT. Comparison to a previous study, if available, can be very helpful.

A less specific but occasionally useful test for the diagnosis of DVT is the **D-dimer assay**. A new rapid assay currently is available to detect D-dimer, which is a specific derivative of cross-linked fibrin that is released when fibrin is lysed by plasmin. It is a useful screening test for patients suspected of DVT, with sensitivity approaching 93%. Its utility is questionable, however, if duplex ultrasonography is available readily.

Pulmonary Embolus

Embolization of DVT into the pulmonary artery is the most dreaded complication of DVT. **Pulmonary embolus (PE)** is estimated to be responsible for the deaths of 50,000 to 100,000 persons per year in U.S. hospitals who would otherwise not be expected to die of their underlying disease process.[3]

One should be suspicious of PE when a patient at risk develops signs and symptoms of dyspnea, tachypnea, chest pain, tachycardia, cyanosis, hemoptysis, hypotension, syncope, evidence of right-sided heart failure, and a pleural rub or rales.

The diagnosis of PE usually is not easy, but significant prospective data have been collected by the Prospective Investigation of Pulmonary Embolism Diagnosis (PIOPED).[4] There are multiple nonspecific tests that are helpful and usually are ordered when a patient presents with the above-mentioned symptoms. The tests include **arterial blood gas, chest x-ray (CXR), and electrocardiogram (ECG)**. The arterial blood gas characteristically reveals a respiratory alkalosis, decreased CO_2, and decreased O_2, which results in an increased alveolar-arterial (A-a) gradient. Suggestive findings on CXR include prominent central pulmonary artery, decreased pulmonary vascularity (Westermark's sign), and a pleural-based, wedge-shaped pulmonary density. These findings, while strongly suggestive of PE, rarely are seen. The most common ECG findings are nonspecific ST segment or T-wave changes. The importance of these nonspecific tests is to rule out other pathologic processes with similar signs and symptoms to PE.

Pulmonary angiography (PA) is the "gold standard" diagnostic study for PE. It is performed by placing a catheter into the pulmonary artery, usually via a femoral vein puncture, and injecting contrast into both lungs. The diagnosis of PE is confirmed by evidence of either com-

---

[3] Dismuke SE, Wagner EH. Pulmonary embolism as a cause of death; the changing mortality in hospitalized patients. JAMA 1986;255(15):2039–2042.

[4] The PIOPED Investigators. Value of the ventilation/perfusion scan in acute pulmonary embolism; results of the prospective investigation of pulmonary embolism diagnosis (PIOPED). JAMA 1990;263:2753–2759.

plete obstruction of, or filling defects within, the pulmonary vessels. The study is invasive and has a significant list of complications, including cardiac arrthymias, contrast reaction, and bleeding. It is both sensitive and specific, and a negative PA effectively rules out PE.

The noninvasive test of choice for the diagnosis of PE is a **ventilation/perfusion scan (V/Q)**. Perfusion scans involve the injection of radiolabeled colloid into a peripheral vein, followed by scanning of the lung in several positions. This is followed by inhalation of a radiolabeled aerosol for the ventilation portion of the study. The diagnosis of PE is confirmed by a perfusion defect without a corresponding ventilation defect. The scans are graded as normal, very low probability, low probability, intermediate probability, and high probability (**Table 29.4**).

When the V/Q scan is intermediate probability, many physicians also obtain a **lower extremity venous duplex scan**. If that is positive, then the patient should be anticoagulated, if there are no contraindications and no further testing is necessary. Additional diagnostic studies for PE currently being developed are **helical computed tomography (CT) and magnetic resonance angiography (MRA)**.

Table 29.4. PIOPED[a] central scan interpretation categories and criteria.

High probability
≥2 large (>75% of a segment) segmental perfusion defects without corresponding ventilation or roentgenographic abnormalities or substantially larger than either matching ventilation or chest roentgenogram abnormalities
≥2 moderate segmental (≥25% and ≤75% of a segment) perfusion defects without matching ventilation or chest roentgenogram abnormalities and 1 large mismatched segmental defect
≥4 moderate segmental perfusion defects without ventilation or chest roentgenogram abnormalities
Intermediate probability (indeterminate)
Not falling into normal, very low, low-, or high-probability categories
Borderline high or borderline low
Difficult to categorize as high or low
Low probability
Nonsegmental perfusion defects (e.g., very small effusion causing blunting of the costophrenic angle, cardiomegaly, enlarged aorta, hila and mediastinum, and elevated diaphragm)
Single moderate mismatched segmental perfusion defect with normal chest roentgenogram
Any perfusion defect with a substantially larger chest roentgenogram abnormality
Large or moderated segmental perfusion defects involving no more than 4 segments in 1 lung and no more than 3 segments in 1 lung region with matching ventilation defects either equal to or larger in size and chest roentgenogram either normal or with abnormalities substantially smaller than perfusion defects
>3 small segmental perfusion defects (<25% of a segment) with a normal chest roentgenogram
Very low probability
≤3 small segmental perfusion defects with a normal chest roentgenogram
Normal
No perfusion defects seen
Perfusion outlines exactly the shape of the lungs as seen on the chest roentgenogram (hilar and aortic impressions may be seen, chest roentgenogram and/or ventilation study may be abnormal)

[a] Prospective Investigation of Pulmonary Embolism Diagnosis.
Source: Reprinted from The PIOPED Investigators. Value of the ventilation/perfusion scan in acute pulmonary embolism; results of the prospective investigation of pulmonary embolism diagnosis (PIOPED). JAMA 1990;263: 2753–2759, with permission. Copyright © 1990 American Medical Association. All rights reserved.

Treatment

Once the diagnosis of a venous thromboembolic event has been confirmed and, occasionally, before it has been confirmed and, if the index of suspicion is high, the patient should be **anticoagulated**. In addition to conventional anticoagulation, a small subset of patients may benefit from **thrombolytic therapy**. There is a role for the use of thrombolytic therapy in the treatment of VTE in highly selected patients. Many patients have contraindications or relative contraindications to the use of thrombolysis that obviate their use.

Patients with VTE usually are treated with a bolus dose of **unfractionated heparin** (UFH), which functions as an anticoagulant via two mechanisms: (1) it binds to antithrombin III (ATIII) and amplifies the inhibition of thrombin and activated factor X by ATIII, and (2) it catalyzes the inhibition of thrombin by heparin cofactor II. The half-life of UFH is 90 minutes. The adequacy of anticoagulation is monitored by the activated prothrombin time (aPTT), which usually is monitored at 6-hour intervals until the level has achieved a steady state. One generally attempts to increase the aPTT to 1.5 to 2.5 times above control.

Evidence indicates that it is best to dose UFH according to a nomogram.[5] Treatment with UFH generally is continued until the patient is fully anticoagulated with oral agents, namely **warfarin**. Complications of UFH use include bleeding and heparin-induced thrombocytopenia (HIT). HIT is estimated to occur in approximately 2% to 5% of patients receiving heparin. It is believed to be due to antibodies directed against platelet complexes with heparin. Due to the possibility of HIT, it is important that patients treated with UFH have a platelet count at some point after the initiation of therapy. Consequences of HIT include problems with both bleeding and thrombosis. All forms of heparin should be withheld once the diagnosis is considered.

Warfarin, the oral anticoagulant of choice, acts by interfering with the production of both the procoagulant (II, VII, IX, X) and anticoagulant (proteins C and S) vitamin K–dependent cofactors. Response to warfarin is variable depending on the patient's liver function, diet, age, and concomitant medications. The levels of anticoagulation produced by warfarin are monitored by following the prothrombin time (PT). Secondary to a wide variability of thromboplastin reagents used, the international normalized ratio (INR) was created. An INR of 2.0 to 3.0 generally is accepted to be therapeutic in most patients with VTE.

It initially was thought that several days of UFH were necessary before initiating warfarin therapy. Multiple studies have shown that starting warfarin therapy in addition to heparin is safe and effective. Warfarin has a long half-life, variable depending on the patient, and must be withheld for several days prior to any significant intervention. It generally is felt that a patient with VTE should be continued on

---

[5] Raske RA, Reilly BM, Guidry JR, et al. The weight-based heparin dosing nomogram compared with a "standard care" nomogram: a randomized controlled trial. Ann Intern Med 1993;119:874–881.

Table 29.5. Randomized trials of LMWH[a] versus UFH[b] for treatment of deep venous thrombosis (DVT) (level I evidence).

Agent	Dose	Recurrent DVT (%); LMWH vs. UFH	Major bleeding (%); LMWH vs. UFH
Fraxiparine[d]	<55 kg 12,500 XaIU[c] >55 kg <80 kg 15,000 XaIU >80 kg 17,500 XaIU (Q 12 h)	7 vs. 14 ($p = ns$)	1 vs. 4 ($p = ns$)
Dalteparin[e]	200 XaIU/kg (Q 24 h)	5 vs. 3 ($p = ns$)	None, either group
Enoxaparin[f]	100 XaIU/kg (Q 12 h)	1 vs. 10 ($p < .02$)	None, either group
Logiparin[g]	175 XaIU/kg (Q 24 h)	3 vs. 7 ($p = .07$)	0.5 vs. 5 ($p = 0.06$)

[a] Low molecular weight heparin.
[b] Adjusted dose unfractionated heparin.
[c] Factor Xa inhibitory units.
[d] Prandoni P, Lensing AWA, Buller HR, et al. Comparison of subcutaneous low-molecular-weight heparin with intravenous standard heparin in proximal deep-vein thrombosis. Lancet 1992;339:441–445.
[e] Lindmarker P, Holstrom M, Granqvist S, et al. Comparison of once-daily subcutaneous fragmin with continuous intravenous unfractionated heparin in the treatment of deep vein thrombosis. Thromb Haemostasis 1994;72(2):186–190.
[f] Simmonneau G, Charbonnier B, Decousus H, et al. Subcutaneous low-molecular-weight heparin compared with continuous intravenous unfractionated heparin in the treatment of proximal deep vein thrombosis. Arch Intern Med 1993;153:1541–1546.
[g] Hull RD, Raskob GE, Pineo GF, et al. Subcutaneous low-molecular-weight heparin compared with continuous intravenous heparin in the treatment of proximal-vein thrombosis. N Engl J Med 1992;326:975–982.
Source: Reprinted from Foley MI, Moneta GL. Venous disease and pulmonary embolism. In: Norton JA, Bollinger RR, Chang AE, et al, eds. Surgery: Basic Science and Clinical Evidence. New York: Springer-Verlag, 2001, with permission.

warfarin therapy for at least 3 to 6 months depending on their risk factors. Patients with a recurrence should be treated indefinitely.[6,7]

The most exciting new development in the treatment of VTE is the use of **low molecular weight heparins (LMWHs) (Table 29.5)**. They have longer half-lives and better bioavailability than UFH and allow for once or twice daily subcutaneous dosing. They have a predictable anticoagulant effect based on body weight, so that laboratory monitoring is unnecessary. It is important to note that different LMWHs differ in their anti-Xa and anti-IIa activity and therefore do not perform in the same manner. Multiple randomized trials have been performed comparing various LMWHs to UFH in the initial treatment of VTE. [8–10]

[6] Schulman S, Rhedin AS, Lindmarker P, et al. A comparison of six weeks with six months of oral anticoagulant therapy after a first episode of venous thromboembolism. N Engl J Med 1995;332:1661–1665.
[7] Schulman S, Granqvist S, Holmstrom M, et al. The duration of oral anticoagulant therapy after a second episode of venous thromboembolism. N Engl J Med 1997;336: 393–398.
[8] Lindmarker P, Holstrom M, Granqvist S, et al. Comparison of once-daily subcutaneous fragmin with continuous intravenous unfractionated heparin in the treatment of deep vein thrombosis. Thromb Haemostasis 1994;72(2):186–190.
[9] Simmonneau G, Charbonnier B, Decousus H, et al. Subcutaneous low-molecular-weight heparin compared with continuous intravenous unfractionated heparin in the treatment of proximal deep vein thrombosis. Arch Intern Med 1993;153:1541–1546.
[10] Hull RD, Raskob GE, Pineo GF, et al. Subcutaneous low-molecular-weight heparin compared with continuous intravenous heparin in the treatment of proximal-vein thrombosis. N Engl J Med 1992;326:975–982.

The advantages of LMWH have allowed patients with VTE to be successfully treated as outpatients. [11]

The role for **surgical intervention** in the treatment of VTE is limited. The most commonly performed surgical intervention is the placement of an inferior cava filtration device. The indications for cava filter placement are the presence of VTE in the presence of an absolute contraindication to anticoagulation or the failure of anticoagulation. These are rare. Most commonly, cava filters are placed for relative contraindications to anticoagulation or, increasingly, for pulmonary embolus prophylaxis for patients who cannot be anticoagulated safely. While inferior cava filters are safe and effective, they do not treat VTE; rather, they prevent the most dreaded complication: pulmonary embolus.

Other more aggressive surgical interventions for VTE have been described, but they rarely are indicated. Simple procedures, such as high ligation of the greater saphenous vein at the saphenofemoral junction, are reasonable for superficial thrombosis of the greater saphenous vein. More significant operations, such as iliofemoral venous thrombectomy or surgical pulmonary embolectomy, have a role, but fortunately they only rarely need to be employed.

Referring back to the patient who presented with a swollen leg, one might surmise that she may have had a left lower extremity DVT that was missed. While the likelihood of this being the case is low in the absence of injury, stasis, or history of a hypercoagulable state, it would be reasonable to interrogate her venous anatomy with a venous duplex scan. If the duplex scan is positive for DVT, then the clinician may be left with a bit of a dilemma: Should the patient be treated with anticoagulants or not? One of the limitations of duplex ultrasonogaphy is differentiating acute versus chronic DVTs. Particularly with the development of safe and effective outpatient therapies for DVT, a physician probably should treat a duplex proven DVT with anticoagulation.

Chronic Venous Insufficiency

One of the most common causes of a swollen leg is **chronic venous insufficiency (CVI)**. It has been estimated that 27% of the U.S. population has some form of detectable lower-extremity venous abnormality.[12]

Patients with CVI frequently complain of leg fatigue, discomfort, and heaviness. Signs include venous telangiectasias, swelling, and varicose veins, as well as lipodermatosclerosis and venous ulceration. **Lipodermatosclerosis** represents a constellation of skin changes, including thickening of the skin, hemosiderin deposition of the skin, and a dry scaly dermatitis of the skin. These changes most commonly affect the

---

[11] Koopman MMW, Prandoni P, Piovella F, et al. Treatment of venous thrombosis with intravenous unfractionated heparin in the hospital as compared with subcutaneous low-molecular-weight heparin administered at home. N Engl J Med 1996;334:682–687.

[12] Band FN, Dannenberg AL, Abbott RD, Kannel WB. The epidemiology of varicose veins: the Framingham study. Am J Prev Med 1988;4:96.

medial aspect of the calf, the so-called gator region of the leg. Risk factors associated with varicose veins may include prolonged standing, heredity, female sex, parity, and history of phlebitis. Venous ulcerations particularly are problematic. In addition to the previously mentioned risk factors, patients with venous ulceration tend to be older, have a history of previous DVT, and have a history of lower extremity trauma; they tend to be male, and are obese.

The diagnosis of deep venous insufficiency generally is made clinically based on **history and clinical exam**. It can be confirmed by noninvasive studies, such as **air plethysmography (APG)** and, most commonly, via **duplex ultrasound evaluation**. The APG is performed by placing a polyvinyl chloride bladder on the lower leg. Various volumes of the leg are then calculated with the patient in several positions (**Fig. 29.2**). The information gathered from the APG may assess calf muscle pump function, venous reflux, and overall lower-extremity venous function. The duplex ultrasound, in addition to ruling out the presence of DVT, can be used to evaluate venous reflux in individual segments of the lower extremity. Particular attention currently is being paid to communicating veins, those that connect the deep and superficial venous systems. Incompetence of the perforating veins has been implicated in the development of venous stasis ulcers.

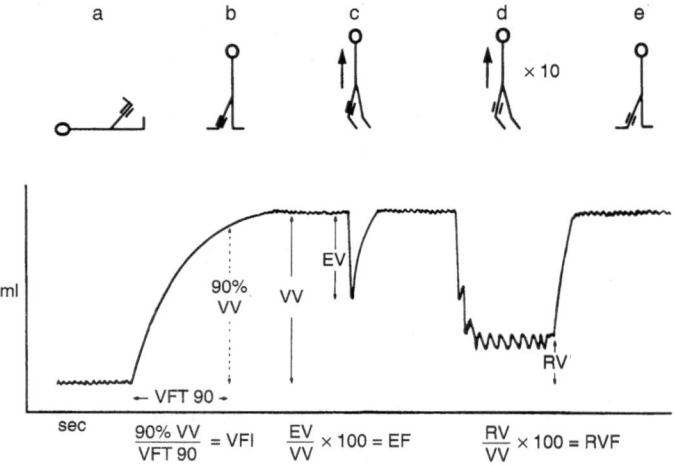

Figure 29.2. Typical recording of volume changes during a standard sequence of postural changes and exercise: patient in a supine position with the legs elevated 45° (a); patient standing with weight on the nonexamined leg (b); patient performing a single tiptoe movement (c); patient performing 10 tiptoe movements (d); patient again standing with weight on the nonexamined leg (e). VV, functional venous volume; VFT, venous filling time; VFI, venous filling index; EV, ejected volume; EF, ejected fraction; RVF, residual volume fraction. (Reprinted from Christopoulos DG, Nicolaides AN, Szendro G, et al. Airplethysmography and the effect of elastic compression on venous hemodynamics of the leg. J Vasc Surg 1987;5:148; and from Rutherford RB, ed. Vascular surgery. Philadelphia: Saunders, 1995:1838. Copyright © 1987 The Society for Vascular Surgery and The American Association for Vascular Surgery. With permission from The Society for Vascular Surgery and The American Association for Vascular Surgery.)

Treatment

Conservative, nonoperative, treatment for chronic venous insufficiency has been and remains the primary therapy. This form of therapy generally focuses on decreasing lower extremity venous hypertension. **Bed rest with elevation** is very effective in relieving symptoms of CVI, but it generally is not practical for more than a very short period.

Due to the limitation of bed rest and elevation, some form of **compression** is prescribed. The most common compression garment is a commercially made, graduated compression stocking that provides increased compression at the level of the ankle, but less compression as it ascends the leg. Patients with active venous ulceration can be treated with any of a number of layered compression dressings. The most common is the paste gauze dressing developed by the German dermatologist Paul Unna in 1896. The current **Unna's boot** consists of dome paste dressing, containing calamine, zinc oxide, glycerin, sorbitol, and magnesium aluminum silicate. The dressing is applied with graduated compression from the foot to the knee. An additional layer of an elastic wrap is then added. The dressing is kept in place for several days and frequently for up to a week. The therapy effectively facilitates healing of venous stasis ulcers about 70% of the time. Once healed, the patient should convert to lifelong compression stocking use.

Multiple pharmacologic agents have been tried for the treatment of CVI and venous ulcerations. Most have little or no significant benefit. Diuretics, ironically, provide little benefit for patients with CVI, although they may benefit patients with systemic causes of lower extremity swelling, such as cardiac failure and renal insufficiency.

Surgical intervention rarely is indicated as a first line of therapy for patients with CVI. Commonly performed procedures include ligation and stripping of varicose veins, subfascial ligation of perforating veins, and, uncommonly, venous reconstruction. While vein ligation and stripping address only the superficial venous system, they frequently do provide significant symptomatic relief. Linton and others described procedures involving ligation of perforating veins for the treatment of CVI.[13] Currently, a newer technique is available to accomplish this, **subfascial endoscopic perforator vein surgery (SEPS)**. Retrospective analysis of the procedure demonstrates ulcer healing in 88% of cases treated with SEPS.[14]

More aggressive venous reconstructions have been described for patients with advanced CVI. The operations have included venous valve repair, valve transplantation, and venous bypass procedures. The results of these procedures are encouraging, but the procedures should be reserved for extreme cases.

The patient presented at the beginning of this chapter may have chronic venous insufficiency. If she does not have chronic ulcerations,

---

[13] Linton RR. The postthrombotic ulceration of the lower extremity: its etiology and surgical treatment. Ann Surg 1953.

[14] Gloviczki P, Bergen JJ, Menewat SS, et al. Safety, feasibility, and early efficacy of subfascial endoscopic perforator surgery: a preliminary report from the North American registry. J Vasc Surg 1997;25:94–105.

she most likely could be treated successfully with a compression stocking.

Lymphedema

Lymphedema represents another possible cause of a swollen lower extremity. The swelling of lymphedema is caused by an abnormality in the lymphatic drainage of the leg. It may be secondary to a congenital abnormality of the lymphatic system, leading to **primary lymphedema**, or it may be due to some acquired abnormality, leading to **secondary lymphedema**. Primary lymphedema has no demonstrable precipitating cause. Secondary lymphedema results from well-described causative mechanisms, such as recurrent infection or surgical or radiation therapy for tumor or trauma, all of which can lead to obliteration of the lymphatic vessels. Secondary lymphedema is the more common of the two forms. Tropical elephantiasis caused by infection with *Wuchereria bancrofti* is the most common form of secondary lymphedema internationally. Its incidence in the United States fortunately is low.

The diagnosis of lymphedema generally is based on **history and physical exam**. Careful **history of trauma and chronic infections** to the lower extremity should be elicited. A **history of surgery or radiation to the pelvis or extremity** obviously would lead one to think that the swelling was secondary to injury or obliteration of the lymphatic vessels.

The swelling from lymphedema generally starts at the level of the foot and ankle and progresses in a cephalad direction. The distribution of the edema produces a characteristic shape. In the lower extremity, the edema usually involves the forefoot and spares the metatarsophalangeal joint, so that, on lateral view, the foot and ankle resemble a buffalo hump. With more extensive edema, the limb assumes a tree trunk–link appearance. The edema usually does involve the digits, which rarely are involved when the edema is secondary to other causes. The edema may be pitting particularly early in the process, but it may lose the pitting with the onset of significant subcutaneous fibrosis. Unlike in venous insufficiency, the skin changes in lymphedema lack the dark pigment changes. Lymphedema certainly is part of the differential of the patient in the case presented here, particularly if the patient provides a history of previous surgery or infection.

A limited number of diagnostic tests may be helpful. It certainly is reasonable to obtain a **lower extremity duplex scan** to rule out DVT or CVI as etiologies of the swelling. Other studies, such as **CT scans or magnetic resonance imaging (MRI)**, may be helpful in assessing possible secondary etiologies of the lymphedema and in helping rule out lymphangiosarcoma. **Lymphangiography** rarely is indicated. **Lymphoscintigraphy** using radiolabeled albumin, gold colloid, and technetium colloid can be performed to assess lymphatic function and largely has replaced lymphangiography.

Treatment

Lymphedema, whether it is primary or secondary, is a chronic condition and has no cure. Treatment, therefore, is palliative. The primary goal of therapy is to decrease limb volume in order to reduce discomfort, provide cosmesis, and avoid infection.

The noninterventional methods of treating lymphedema represent the first line of therapy, and, in fact, they are used to treat the vast majority of patients. The therapeutic interventions include **adequate skin care, elevation and compression of the extremity, the use of pneumatic compression garments, manual lymph drainage and bandaging, the use of benzopyrones, and aggressive treatment of infections**. Benzopyrones, theoretically, act by increasing protein lysis by macrophages in the interstitium. This action may decrease limb volume moderately and improve the softness of the skin. The other modalities mentioned above attempt to reduce limb volume via mechanical compression or manual massage.

The **surgical forms of therapy**, which generally are reserved for only the extreme cases, fall into one of two categories: **physiologic or excisional**. The physiologic procedures attempt to reestablish lymphatic drainage. Examples of physiologic procedures include lymphangioplasty, omental transposition, enteromesenteric bridge, lymphovenous anastomoses, and lympholymphatic anastomoses. It is important to note, however, that all of the above-mentioned procedures rarely are performed, and most vascular surgeons have seldom, if ever, performed any of them. Excisional procedures include total skin and subcutaneous excision, the Charles procedure, buried dermal flap, the Thompson procedure, and subcutaneous excision underneath flaps, the modified Homans procedure. These procedures are aggressive and have relatively high complication rates. Success rates are modest, in the range of 65%, and therefore these procedures should be reserved only for those patients who have not responded to measures that are more conservative.

Some of the important points to remember when dealing with lymphedema are that the condition is chronic, some form of compression garment is necessary, and any form of infection within the affected extremity should be treated aggressively. Patients need to be educated as to the signs and symptoms of infection and instructed to seek medical attention immediately if they develop signs of infection. Many physicians provide their patients suffering from lymphedema with a prescription for an appropriate antibiotic to avoid any delays in initiation of therapy.

If the patient in the case presented has lymphedema, she should be treated conservatively with compression of the affected extremity and education regarding the signs and symptoms of infection.

Summary

The presentation of a patient with a swollen leg is a rather common event. Most patients present with chronic symptoms and can be treated conservatively. The etiology generally is related to a systemic, venous, or lymphatic abnormality. Few patients present with potentially life-threatening problems (e.g., an acute DVT), and they warrant urgent and aggressive treatment. A thorough history and a thorough physical examination coupled with noninvasive testing lead to the appropriate diagnosis in the majority of cases. If a patient is found to have an acute DVT, aggressive therapy is indicated. Fortunately, with the advent of LMWHs, many of these patients can be treated safely as outpatients or with a relatively short hospital stay. Ironically, a vascular surgeon frequently is consulted when a patient presents with a swollen leg. The role of surgery is limited in the treatment of patients with swollen legs, but it may be useful in small subsets of patients. A reasonable understanding of the pathophysiology of the swollen leg as described in this chapter greatly assists a physician in making the correct therapeutic decisions regarding these sometimes difficult patients.

Selected Reading

Foley MI, Moneta GL. Venous disease and pulmonary embolism. In: Norton JA, Bollinger RR, Chang AE, et al, eds. *Surgery: Basic Science and Clinical Evidence*. New York: Springer-Verlag, 2001.

30

Skin and Soft Tissues

M. Nerissa Prieto and Philip D. Wey

Objectives

1. To understand indications for and methods of biopsy, and to establish diagnoses for patients with skin lesions.
2. To describe characteristics of nonmelanoma skin cancers (basal cell and squamous cell carcinoma).
3. To develop a management plan for a patient with basal cell carcinoma.
4. To develop a management plan for a patient with squamous cell carcinoma.
5. To describe characteristics of atypical and dysplastic nevi.
6. To describe characteristics of malignant melanoma.
7. To develop a management plan for a patient with malignant melanoma.
8. To understand indications for and methods of biopsy for soft tissue masses.
9. To develop a management plan for a patient with possible soft tissue sarcoma.

Cases

Case 1

A 52-year-old woman presents with a lesion that has persisted for 1 year and slowly has become larger and more raised over time. There is no family history of skin cancer. Physical exam reveals a flesh-colored raised nodule on the left cheek at the nasolabial fold measuring approximately 7mm in diameter. The lesion has a pearly appearance and is smooth with rolled borders and surface telangiectasia.

Case 2

A 60-year-old man with a long history of sun exposure presents for evaluation of a nonhealing wound of the forehead of approximately 18 months' duration. Physical examination reveals widespread actinic sun damage to the skin, with multiple scaly patches measuring 2 to 3 mm. Facial skin is deeply wrinkled, with a few small tan macules 3 to 4 mm in diameter. On the forehead is a 15-mm erythematous, indurated, slightly raised plaque with distinct borders and central ulceration.

Case 3

A 25-year-old woman presents with multiple pigmented lesions of the arms and trunk. She states that they have been present nearly all her life and have not changed in appearance. She is concerned because a distant family member recently was diagnosed with melanoma. Exam reveals multiple discrete 2- to 4-mm homogeneously colored brown to black lesions, some of which are slightly raised.

Case 4

Further examination of the patient described in **Case 3** reveals an 8-mm homogeneously pigmented, dark brown lesion on her abdomen. It is asymmetric in shape with scalloped borders and is slightly raised with a variegated surface texture.

Case 5

A 45-year-old man presents with a pigmented lesion on his shoulder. It first appeared in his thirties and slowly enlarged over many years before nearly doubling in size and becoming more raised and nodular over the past year. He is fair-skinned, and his natural hair color is sandy blond. He is an avid outdoorsman, but he does not wear sunscreen. His father has been diagnosed with melanoma. Examination reveals an 18-mm raised, nodular, darkly pigmented lesion with variegated color and surface texture with scalloped borders. There is no palpable lymphadenopathy.

Case 6

A 37-year-old man presents with painless swelling of the right thigh, with rapid progression over the past 4 to 6 months. Physical exam reveals a poorly circumscribed mass measuring 10 × 8 cm over the proximal anterior right thigh. It is deep and firm on palpation, nonfluctuant, and immobile.

Skin Lesions

Introduction

Most skin lesions are benign and can be diagnosed on examination based solely on physical characteristics. The identification and diagnosis of malignant skin lesions, however, is critical given their morbidity, mortality, and frequency. It is estimated that nearly half of all persons who live to the age of 65 will have one or more skin cancers in their lifetime. Well over one million new cases of skin cancer were identified in 2001, and that number was expected to rise slightly in 2002, accounting for approximately half of all new cancer diagnoses and making the skin the most common site of human malignancy.

When distinguishing malignant from benign lesions, the patient's history, ethnicity, and genetic predisposition, as well as the physical characteristics of the lesion on exam, may serve to raise or lower the clinician's index of suspicion. The distinction often is still difficult to make, and, ultimately, **biopsy of the lesion and pathologic assessment are necessary for diagnosis when there is concern of malignancy.**

General Evaluation

Elements of the patient's history that should raise suspicion of malignancy include changes in color, surface texture, shape or elevation of a lesion, appearance of a new lesion with suspicious characteristics, family or personal history of skin cancer, and history of sun or toxic exposure. Focused examination of the presenting lesion should follow. In addition, the physician should perform a **thorough examination of the entire skin surface**, including scalp, palms, soles, and nail beds, noting any atypical lesions and documenting their size and appearance for future comparison.

While close observation of a lesion may be appropriate in some instances, **biopsy of suspicious lesions is highly recommended.** One also should understand approaches to precancerous lesions, since biopsy is indicated in some but not in others. **Small lesions may be biopsied by full excision, while large lesions may be approached with full-thickness incisional biopsy or punch biopsy.** Techniques that compromise pathologic evaluation, such as shave biopsy, which often is used in the treatment of benign lesions, are contraindicated in the workup of potentially malignant lesions.

Basal Cell Carcinoma

The patient described in **Case 1** exhibits a facial lesion that fits the classic description of basal cell carcinoma (BCC) of the nodular type, the most commonly occurring of the four clinical subtypes of BCC described in **Table 30.1. Basal cell carcinoma is the most common**

Table 30.1. Four clinical subtypes of basal cell carcinoma.

Superficial	Erythematous scaly macules that may exhibit ulceration, crusting, or atrophic scarring
Sclerosing or morpheaform	Poorly defined, firm, yellow-white plaques
Nodular	Flesh-colored nodule with telangiectasia, with or without central ulceration and pearly borders
Pigmented	May be deeply pigmented, often confused with melanoma

malignancy in the general population, usually occurring on the head and neck. Sun exposure is considered to be a primary causative factor, similar to other skin cancers, and patients almost always are fair-skinned Caucasians. Tumors of the nasolabial fold (as in this patient), medial and lateral canthi, and postauricular regions often are associated with worse outcomes. **Skin biopsy of suspected BCC is mandatory to confirm diagnosis and would be an appropriate next step in the management of this patient.**

Since this is the patient's first presentation, the physician should elicit the **patient's history of sun exposure and history of predisposing medical conditions**, including such rare conditions as xeroderma pigmentosum and basal cell nevus syndrome. Since patients with BCC may develop multiple tumors over time and since recurrent disease is not uncommon, personal history of BCC and other skin cancers should be obtained. **Physical examination should be performed meticulously**, since different types of BCC may mimic scar tissue or dermatitis, and should include examination of local lymph node basins.

Basal cell carcinoma expands locally over long periods of time, and the tendency for metastasis is low: only 2% of cases involve regional lymph nodes. **As a result of its indolent and nonaggressive behavior, excisional biopsy of localized primary BCC with 2- to 3-mm margins is curative in 95% of cases.** Pathologic assessment of frozen sections intraoperatively can provide preliminary confirmation of complete excision of the tumor. Alternatively, **Mohs' micrographic excision**, usually performed by a dermatologist, is highly effective as well, with a similar cure rate. This technique involves progressive excision and mapping of the tumor bed by microscopic examination of tissue as it is excised until a clear margin is identified. It commonly is reserved for lesions in anatomically sensitive areas such as the lip, nasal rim, and eyelid. Using Mohs' technique, the amount of normal tissue removed in the course of excision is minimized. Other methods also have been used to treat BCC; these typically are reserved for patients with contraindications to surgery or for patients with multiple tumors in whom numerous excisions would be unfeasible. **Electrodesiccation and curettage** is one such method, used for ablation of a lesion <2 cm in diameter. **Radiation therapy** also is acceptable if tissue preservation is important. Both of these techniques are associated with a lower cure rate and accordingly are not appropriate as first-line treatment.

Squamous Cell Carcinoma

The patient described in **Case 2** exhibits several manifestations of significant sun damage to the skin, including solar lentigo (tan macules), deep wrinkling, and actinic keratosis (scaly patches and plaques). **Actinic keratoses** are the result of ultraviolet damage to epidermal cells, and, while they may persist in a benign state for long periods of time, they may progress to **squamous cell carcinoma** (SCC). Alternatively, they may regress with cessation of sun exposure. The physician should monitor this patient closely and consider treatment of extensive actinic keratoses with topical fluorouracil, cryosurgery, electrodesiccation and curettage, dermabrasion, or laser therapy. Biopsy should be performed if actinic lesions exhibit suspicious changes, including increasing erythema or induration, enlargement, ulceration, or bleeding. In this patient, whose nonhealing wound likely represents SCC, malignancy may have developed from a preexisting site of actinic keratosis.

A nonhealing wound or ulcer is a classic presentation of SCC. But SCC also may appear as an indurated, erythematous papule or plaque, which can be hyperkeratotic, as in this case, or smooth, with or without ulceration. Invasive SCC has a 5-year metastasis rate of 5%, although the likelihood of metastasis is two to three times greater with lesions >2 cm and location on the lip or ear. Similarly at high risk of recurrence and metastasis are lesions of mucous membranes, nose, scalp, forehead, and eyelid. Malignant transformation to SCC can occur within nonhealing wounds of various etiologies, as in scar tissue following burn or trauma (Marjolin's ulcer), tissue damaged by radiation therapy, or at sites of chronic infection or draining sinus tracts; these tumors also tend to be particularly aggressive. **Table 30.2** summarizes characteristics of SCC that confer high risk of metastasis and poor outcome.

As in other skin cancers, **sun exposure is a primary causative factor in SCC.** Other risk factors include toxic exposure to arsenic, nitrates, or hydrocarbons, as well as immunosuppression, particularly in organ transplant patients. Premalignant lesions that may degenerate into SCC include actinic keratosis, as described in the patient in **Case 2**, Bowen's

Table 30.2. Features of cutaneous squamous cell carcinoma (SCC) associated with increased risk of recurrence and metastasis.

Feature	Approximate relative risk[a] of:	
	Recurrence	Metastasis
Clinical		
Rapid growth	+	+
Size >2 cm	2	2
Location on lip	2	3
Location on ear	2	3
Immunosuppression	+	2
History of radiation therapy	+	+
History of treatment for SCC	3	4
Histologic		
Tumor depth >4 mm or to Clark level IV or V[b]	2	5
Poorly differentiated	2	3
Infiltrative margins	+	+
Spindle cell or acantholytic features	+	+
Perineural invasion	5	5

[a] Relative risk of 1 is defined as the likelihood of recurrence or metastasis of a small primary SCC.
[b] Tumor invasion to Clark level IV involves the reticular dermis, to Clark V involves the subcutaneous fat.
+ Indicates association with increased risk, but lacking sufficient data to calculate relative risk.
Source: Reprinted from Alam M, Ratner D. Primary care: cutaneous squamous cell carcinoma. N Engl J Med 2001;344(13):975–983, with permission. Copyright © 1994 Massachusetts Medical Society. All rights reserved.

disease (SCC in situ), and keratoacanthoma. There also is a significant association between cutaneous SCC and human papillovirus infection, particularly types 6 and 11 in SCC of the genital region and type 16 in periungual tumors.

Early detection of SCC is critical, since early disease is largely curable and late disease has a dismal prognosis. The physician should perform **a thorough history of potential predisposing conditions, including sun or other radiation exposure, exposure to carcinogens, immunosuppression, and family and personal history of skin cancer.** Patients with a positive skin cancer history or extensive actinic skin damage should undergo **regular screening examinations** for new or changing lesions.

Physical examination of the patient in **Case 2** should include examination of the entire skin surface and palpation of regional nodal basins surrounding questionable lesions. **Given this patient's history of sun exposure and evidence of extensive sun damage and because of the suspicious size and characteristics of the presenting lesion, a full-thickness biopsy is warranted.** Radiologic and laboratory tests are not indicated unless there are symptoms of or reason to suspect metastasis.

Treatment of this patient's low-risk lesion would involve surgical resection with 4-mm margins, with frozen section to confirm clear margins. This approach is associated with a 95% chance of a cure. As in BCC, **Mohs' excision** also would be an appropriate first-line treatment and is, in fact, the procedure with the highest rate of cure for high-risk primary or recurrent lesions. Acceptable alternative therapies for limited low-risk SCC include **electrodesiccation and curettage, cryosurgery, and radiation.** Indications may include inoperable tumors, large lesions in cosmetically sensitive areas, or patient contraindications to surgery.

Nevi (Moles)

Many patients present for evaluation of nevi (**melanocytic nevocellular nevi or moles**). Moles are extremely common in all races, and it is not uncommon to find several dozen on a single individual. While most such lesions are entirely benign, the incidence of and mortality from malignant melanoma has increased markedly over recent years, bringing to the forefront the importance of the physician's ability to recognize suspicious lesions.

Freckles (ephelides) should be distinguished from nevi. These tan to light brown, small macules with irregular borders are lesions of the basal and upper dermis that result from increased melanin production by nonneoplastic melanocytes. They are benign and require no treatment.

The common nevi seen in the patient presented in **Case 3** are made up of benign neoplastic melanocytes, called nevus cells, and are classified according to the site of nevocellular proliferation. They are typically small, well-circumscribed macules or papules that, with the exception of the dermal nevus described below, regress spontaneously by the sixth decade of life. History of childhood sunburn may increase the likelihood of developing a greater number of nevi, and those with numerous nevi (more than 40) have a greater likelihood of developing melanoma and should be monitored closely. **The vast majority of nevi do not undergo malignant transformation.**

All three of the **common benign nevus types** are represented among the many lesions of this patient. In **junctional nevi**, nevus cells are clustered at the dermal–epidermal junction above the basement membrane. These are dark brown to black, macular to slightly raised lesions that appear in young children after age 2. They are round to oval, with smooth regular borders. **Compound nevi** are composed of nevus cells both at the dermal–epidermal junction and within the dermis. They also are brown to black in color, are usually slightly raised, and are frequently hairy, with sharply defined but often irregular borders and smooth to slightly papillary surfaces. A compound nevus surrounded by an area of hypopigmentation is called a **halo nevus. Intradermal nevi** are made up of nevus cells primarily occupying the dermis, sometimes extending into subcutaneous fat. These are flesh-colored to brown, raised, fleshy papules that distort normal skin anatomy, with hairs and dark flecks sometimes present on the surface. The occasional presence of telangiectasia may make differentiation from BCC difficult. **Malignant transformation of any of these nevi is rare when they are small in size (<6 mm), stable in appearance over time, and lacking suspicious characteristics, including ulceration, bleeding, or pruritis.** No intervention is indicated for this patient's lesions at this time, although she should be instructed to monitor their appearance and to follow up with her physician for periodic screening exams.

Atypical and Dysplastic Nevi

Case 4 describes a specific lesion on the same young woman as in **Case 3**. Unlike the many pigmented lesions on her arms and trunk that easily are classified as benign, this particular lesion should come to the physician's attention because of its size and irregular shape and surface texture. This lesion is termed atypical on the basis of its gross clinical characteristics. **Any nevus is classified as clinically atypical if relatively large in size, i.e., >6 mm, asymmetric, or having an irregular, raised surface or color variegation. While often referred to as dysplastic nevi, atypical nevi may or may not demonstrate histologic dysplasia.**

A single atypical nevus can be found in 5% of whites in the United States, and, in the absence of family history of melanoma, this finding is associated with a 6% lifetime risk of developing melanoma. **In persons with one or more atypical nevi and a strong family history, the risk of developing melanoma may be as high as 80%.** In these persons, the atypical nevus itself may undergo malignant transformation, or disease may develop *de novo* elsewhere; hence, **annual skin screening exams by a physician strongly are recommended**. In all patients with a single atypical nevus or nevi, education regarding melanoma risk and self-examination is essential. **Because atypical nevi**

Table 30.3. Elements of history to consider in evaluation for melanoma.

Intermittent but intense exposure to sunlight
Blistering sunburns in childhood
Tendency to sunburn rather than tan
Living in sunny climates close to the equator
Positive family history of melanoma
Positive personal history of melanoma or other skin cancer
History of atypical nevi
Recent changes in mole(s)

are associated with increased risk of developing melanoma, full-thickness biopsy of this patient's lesion should be performed.

Melanoma

The lesion of the patient described in **Case 5** is worrisome for several reasons. He has a significant history of sun exposure and sunburn, which is a strong risk factor in fair-complexioned individuals. Intermittent but intense sunlight exposure in particular appears to increase risk. Additionally, melanoma in a first-degree relative, in this case his father, increases risk by at least eight times. The patient also reports a recent history of rapid change in the size and texture of the lesion, which should alert the physician to the likelihood of a malignant process. Other suspicious changes not seen in this patient include changes in color, ulceration, bleeding, or pruritis. Given the high likelihood of malignant melanoma in this patient, one also should question him about recent weight loss or other constitutional symptoms that may be indicative of metastatic disease. **Table 30.3** summarizes **elements of a patient history that should be considered significant in the evaluation of a possible melanoma.**

On exam, this patient's lesion possesses many characteristics typical of malignant melanoma, including heterogeneous color and nodularity and relatively large (1.8 cm) diameter. **The mnemonic ABCDE as described in Table 30.4 summarizes key characteristics of pigmented lesions that should raise suspicion of malignancy. Table 30.5** lists other physical findings that the physician also should take into con-

Table 30.4. The ABCDE of melanoma: characteristics of pigmented lesions suggestive of melanoma.

A: Asymmetry
B: Border irregularity
C: Color variation or variegation
D: Diameter greater than 6 mm
E: Elevated area or palpable nodule within a formerly flat lesion
Also: ulceration, inflammation, bleeding, satellite nodules, local lymphadenopathy

Table 30.5. Elements of physical examination to consider in evaluation for melanoma.

Caucasian, fair skin with freckles
Red or blond hair, blue eyes
Presence of atypical nevi
Evidence of sun-induced skin damage
The ABCDE (see Table 30.4)

sideration. The ABCDE mnemonic is a useful guideline, and the diagnosis of melanoma based on history and physical exam alone is highly sensitive when made by an experienced physician. Nonetheless, not all melanomas are clinically obvious, as different histologic types present very differently. Amelanotic melanoma, for instance, is a dangerous, albeit rare entity, because of its tendency to go unrecognized, and hence, it tends to be diagnosed at a later stage when therapy becomes more problematic.

Besides a complete history and examination of the suspect lesion, a thorough examination of the skin over the entire body is essential to the initial evaluation and follow-up of this high-risk patient. While 60% of melanomas arise **de novo** from epidermal melanocytes, 40% arise from malignant degeneration of a preexisting atypical or dysplastic nevus. Identification and monitoring of atypical nevi permits early detection and intervention, which are critical, since **the depth of melanoma invasion at the time of diagnosis is the most accurate predictor of survival. Regional lymph node basins also should be palpated for clinical evidence of nodal involvement.**

Given the highly suggestive appearance and suspect history of the presenting lesion, further evaluation is mandatory. The management of this patient would begin with **excisional biopsy**, to include a 1- to 2-mm margin of grossly normal skin and subcutaneous tissue. **Incisional or punch biopsy** also would be an acceptable approach and would be indicated for larger lesions or those in cosmetically sensitive areas. **Full-thickness biopsy techniques are absolutely necessary to provide adequate tissue for pathologic assessment and staging,** while allowing for reexcision at the site should the malignancy be confirmed. **Shave biopsy, cryosurgery, and electrodesiccation should not be used,** since they compromise histologic assessment and primary staging of disease, which are the cornerstones of establishing prognosis and defining treatment.

An excisional biopsy of the patient's shoulder lesion in **Case 5** was performed. The biopsy results showed superficial spreading melanoma of intermediate thickness at 2.8 mm.

Superficial spreading melanoma is the most common type of melanoma, accounting for approximately 70% of all cases. It begins as a brown, slightly elevated lesion, progressing to have irregular, raised borders, a variegated brown to black color pattern, and a diameter of 2 to 3 cm, sometimes with central pigment loss. It exhibits a prolonged radial growth phase, with lateral extension confined to the epidermis and papillary dermis. This noninvasive growth pattern can last as long as a decade, and, as a result, it generally is associated with a good prognosis. In this patient's case, however, increasing nodularity may be indicative of vertical growth into deeper layers of skin and increased likelihood of metastasis.

There are three other distinct histologic types of melanoma, each exhibiting its own characteristic features, growth patterns, and prognoses. **Nodular melanoma** represents 8% to 10% of all melanomas, with characteristically uniform gray-blue to brown or black color, although they also can be nonpigmented. These demonstrate almost immediate vertical growth, and hence, they are associated with early metastasis and poor prognosis. **Lentigo maligna melanoma** accounts for approximately 10% of cutaneous melanomas. They are typically flat, tan macules of up to 3 cm or more in diameter that grow slowly and radially within the upper dermis. Elevated nodules and irregular areas of dark brown or black pigmentation arising within these lesions may represent invasive melanoma. The precursor lesion is known as lentigo maligna (Hutchinson's freckle). **Acral-lentiginous melanoma** represents only 1% of melanoma cases and occurs exclusively on the palms, soles, and nail beds. Its prognosis ranges from good to poor. Unlike the other subtypes, it occurs with equal frequency among Caucasians and dark-skinned persons. Lesions generally are flat with irregular borders, variably pigmented brown-black to black, but they also may be amelanotic.

As in other forms of cancer, **disease staging of melanoma using a TNM (tumor-node-metastasis) classification scheme** is ideally predictive of prognosis and useful in guiding therapy. The most recent TNM classification and staging system for melanoma of the American Joint Committee on Cancer (AJCC) was published in 2002 and is shown in **Tables 30.6** and **30.7.**

Depth of tumor invasion as measured in millimeters (Breslow depth) is the defining variable in determining the next appropriate step in this patient's management. Lesion thickness has been found to be inversely related to survival, and it is a good predictor of prognosis in node-negative patients. Melanomas are referred to as thin (less than 1 mm thick), intermediate (1.0 to 4.0 mm thick), and thick (greater than 4 mm) with regard to prognosis and management. The **Clark level (Table 30.8)** describes the level of invasion relative to the histologic layers of the skin. While these levels correlate reasonably well with Breslow depth, the basis of the Clark system is flawed, in that no true barriers to tumor invasion exist in the subepidermal layers and, in that dermal thickness varies greatly in different parts of the body. It is, however, an independent prognostic feature of thin (T1, i.e., <1.0 mm) melanomas. **Chest x-ray, serum alkaline phosphatase, and lactate dehydrogenase are recommended as screening measures for pulmonary and liver metastasis in patients with melanoma greater than 1 mm thick.**

Treatment of Melanoma

Definitive treatment of melanoma is surgical control of both local and metastatic disease. The recommended surgical approach to the

Table 30.6. Melanoma TNM classification.

T classification	Thickness	Ulceration status
T1	≤1.0 mm	a: without ulceration and level II/III
		b: with ulceration or level IV/V
T2	1.01–2.0 mm	a: without ulceration
		b: with ulceration
T3	2.01–4.0 mm	a: without ulceration
		b: with ulceration
T4	>4.0 mm	a: without ulceration
		b: with ulceration
N classification	**No. of metastatic nodes**	**Nodal metastatic mass**
N1	1 node	a: micrometastasis*
		b: macrometastasis†
N2	2–3 nodes	a: micrometastasis*
		b: macrometastasis†
		c: in-transit met(s)/satellite(s) without metastatic nodes
N3	4 or more metastatic nodes, or matted nodes, or in-transit met(s)/satellite(s) with metastatic node(s)	
M classification	**Site**	**Serum lactate dehydrogenase**
M1a	Distant skin, subcutaneous, or nodal mets	Normal
M1b	Lung metastases	Normal
M1c	All other visceral metastases	Normal
	Any distant metastasis	Elevated

* Micrometastases are diagnosed after sentinel or elective lymphadenectomy.
† Macrometastases are defined as clinically detectable nodal metastases confirmed by therapeutic lymphadenectomy or when nodal metastasis exhibits gross extracapsular extension.
Source: Reprinted from Balch CM, Buzaid AC, Soong SJ, et al. Final version of the American Joint Committee on Cancer staging system for cutaneous melanoma. J Clin Oncol 2001;19(16):3635–3648. Review. With permission from the American Society of Clinical Oncology.

patient's primary lesion of intermediate thickness (2.8 mm) is **excision with a margin of 2 cm** (Intergroup Melanoma Surgical Trial, level I evidence),[1] which may be performed at the time of initial diagnostic biopsy, or the recommended margin may be taken as a reexcision at the biopsy site once malignant pathology is confirmed. As in **Case 5**, intermediate-thickness lesions demonstrate a 15% to 45% chance of regional nodal involvement with no distant metastasis. Recommended surgical margins for excision of melanomas of various thicknesses are summarized in **Table 30.9**.

Surgical excision of a primary melanoma lesion and any diseased lymph nodes may be curative in the absence of distant metastasis, and

[1] Balch CM, Urist MM, Karakousis CP, et al. Efficacy of 2-cm surgical margins for intermediate-thickness melanomas (1–4 mm): results of a multi-institutional randomized surgical trial. Ann Surg 1993;218:262–267.

Table 30.7. Proposed stage groupings for cutaneous melanoma.

	Clinical staging[a]			Pathologic staging[b]		
	T	N	M	T	N	M
0	Tis	N0	M0	Tis	N0	M0
IA	T1a	N0	M0	T1a	N0	M0
IB	T1b	N0	M0	T1b	N0	M0
	T2a	N0	M0	T2a	N0	M0
IIA	T2b	N0	M0	T2b	N0	M0
	T3a	N0	M0	T3a	N0	M0
IIB	T3b	N0	M0	T3b	N0	M0
	T4a	N0	M0	T4a	N0	M0
IIC	T4b	N0	M0	T4b	N0	M0
III[c]	Any T	N1	M0			
		N2				
		N3				
IIIA				T1–4a	N1a	M0
				T1–4a	N2a	M0
IIIB				T1–4b	N1a	M0
				T1–4b	N2a	M0
				T1–4a	N1b	M0
				T1–4a	N2b	M0
				T1–4a/b	N2c	M0
				T1–4b	N1b	M0
				T1–4b	N2b	M0
				Any T	N3	M0
IV	Any T	Any N	Any M1	Any T	Any N	Any M1

[a] Clinical staging includes microstaging of the primary melanoma and clinical/radiologic evaluation for metastases. By convention, it should be used after complete excision of the primary melanoma with clinical assessment for regional and distant metastases.
[b] Pathologic staging includes microstaging of the primary melanoma and pathologic information about the regional lymph nodes after partial or complete lymphadenectomy. Pathologic stage 0 or stage 1A patients are the exception; they do not require pathologic evaluation of their lymph nodes.
[c] There are no stage III subgroups for clinical staging.
Source: Reprinted from Balch CM, Buzaid AC, Soong SJ, et al. Final version of the American Joint Committee on Cancer staging system. J Clin Oncol 2001;19(16):3635–3648. Review. With permission from the American Society of Clinical Oncology.

the technique of **sentinel node biopsy** (SNB) described below can be used to identify patients with positive nodes who would benefit from full lymph node dissection. Prior to or at the same time as wide excision of the primary lesion, isosulfan blue and radioactive tracer are injected into the lesion or biopsy site. These are allowed time to drain to the node or nodes that provide primary lymphatic drainage to the

Table 30.8. Clark's classification of melanoma tumor depth

Level I: Confined to the epidermis (melanoma in situ)
Level II: Invades papillary dermis
Level III: Penetrates up to junction of papillary and reticular dermis
Level IV: Invades the reticular dermis
Level V: Extends into subcutaneous fat

Table 30.9. Current recommendations for excision margins for cutaneous melanomas.

Location	Tumor thickness	Recommended margin	Evidence	Reference
Trunk and proximal extremity	≤1 mm	1 cm	Randomized trial[a]	Veronesi et al.[e], Veronesi et al.[f]
	1–2 mm	2 cm if able to be closed primarily, otherwise 1 cm	Randomized trials[a]	Karakousis et al.[d], Veronesi et al.[e], Veronesi et al.[f], Balch et al.[g]
	2–4 mm	2 cm	Randomized trial[a]	Karakousis et al.[d], Balch et al.[g]
	>4 mm or with satellitosis	At least 2 cm	Nonrandomized clinical series[b], Accepted surgical practice[c]	Heaton et al.[h]
Head and neck and distal extremity	≤1 mm	1 cm	Randomized trial[a]	Veronesi et al.[e], Veronesi et al.[f]
	>1 mm	At least 1 cm	Accepted surgical practice[c]	

[a] Level I evidence.
[b] Level II evidence.
[c] Level III evidence.
[d] Karakousis CP, Balch CM, Urist MM, Ross MM, Smith TJ, Bartolucci AA. Local recurrence in malignant melanoma: long-term results of the multi-institutional randomized surgical trial. Ann Surg Oncol 1996;3:446–452.
[e] Veronesi U, Cascinelli N, Adamus J, et al. Thin stage I primary cutaneous malignant melanoma. Comparison of excision with margins of 1 or 3 cm. N Engl J Med 1988;318:1159–1162.
[f] Veronesi U, Cascinelli N. Narrow excision (1-cm margin): a safe procedure for thin cutaneous melanoma. Arch Surg 1991;126:438–441.
[g] Balch CM, Urist MM, Karakousis CP, et al. Efficacy of 2 cm surgical margins for intermediate-thickness melanomas (1–4 mm): results of a multi-institutional randomized surgical trial. Ann Surg 1993;218:262–269.
[h] Heaton KM, Sussman JJ, Gershenwald JE, et al. Surgical margins and prognostic factors in patients with thick (>4 mm) primary melanoma. Ann Surg Oncol 1998;5:322–328.

Source: Reprinted from Sondak VK, Margolin KA. Melanoma and other cutaneous malignancies. In: Norton JA, Bollinger RR, Chang AE, et al, eds. Surgery: Basic Science and Clinical Evidence. New York: Springer-Verlag, 2001, with permission.

Note: Level I evidence is defined as prospective, randomized clinical trials.
Level II evidence is defined as clinical trials without randomization or case-controlled retrospective studies.
Level III evidence is defined as retrospective analyses without case controls, accepted clinical practice, or anecdotal case reports.

disease-affected region, called the "sentinel" nodes, of which there is at least one but sometimes as many as four. These sentinel nodes then are identified easily by the presence of radioactivity and dye and are removed selectively. If the sentinel node is free of melanoma, the remainder of the regional lymph basin will be disease-free in more than 95% of cases, and full lymph node dissection usually is not indicated. Full lymph node dissection is reserved for patients with positive sentinel nodes and, in the absence of distant metastases, may be therapeutic, although therapeutic efficacy is unproven to date. Nonetheless, **SNB is widely used in clinical practice in the treatment of intermediate-thickness melanomas (1–4 mm) and in selection of patients for adjuvant therapy.** For the patient in **Case 5**, then, excision and simultaneous SNB with possible lymph node dissection would be the next step in management.

For the patient with clinically appreciable lymphadenopathy, **fine-needle aspiration (FNA)** of regional lymph glands also is an appropriate means of evaluating the nodal basin. As with SNB, identification of a positive node is indication for full nodal basin dissection in melanoma of intermediate thickness.

In a melanoma thicker than 4 mm, full lymph node dissection after positive SNB or FNA usually is not indicated, as metastasis to distant sites is highly likely, eliminating any advantage of lymph node dissection in preventing disease progression. **Thick melanomas should be excised with 2- to 3-cm margins** (M.D. Anderson and Moffitt Cancer Centers, level II evidence).[2]

Thin melanomas (<1 mm), on the other hand, have a very low likelihood (<5%) of nodal involvement, and SNB typically does not play a role, **since excision of thin melanoma lesions with 1-cm margins has been shown to be largely curative** (World Health Organization Melanoma Trial, level I evidence).[3]

Staging and Treatment of Metastatic Disease

Sentinel node biopsy or fine-needle aspiration of clinically involved nodes is necessary for disease staging in melanomas >1 mm thick and has implications for outcome and future management. Chest x-ray, serum alkaline phosphatase, and lactate dehydrogenase, which, as stated previously, are recommended for melanomas >1 mm thick, also contribute to the metastatic workup for melanoma. A number of chemotherapeutic and immunotherapeutic agents have been tested for use as adjuvant therapy in the treatment of metastatic melanoma. **Only interferon-alpha-2b has shown demonstrated efficacy and was approved for use by the Food and Drug Administration (FDA) in 1996 in therapy of resected high-risk melanoma.** A high-dose regimen was demonstrated in randomized controlled studies (Eastern Cooper-

---

[2] Heaton KM, Sussman JJ, Gershenwald JE, et al. Surgical margins and prognostic factors in patients with thick (>4 mm) primary melanoma. Ann Surg Oncol 1998;5: 322–328.

[3] Veronesi U, Cascinelli N. Narrow excision (1-cm margin). A safe procedure for thin cutaneous melanoma. Arch Surg 1991;126:438–441.

ative Oncology Group, level I evidence)[4] to have a positive effect on survival in patients with a single positive node or thick primary tumor. Although no direct evidence of efficacy has been demonstrated in patients with in-transit metastases, local recurrent satellite nodules, or stage IV disease, these patients may be offered adjuvant interferon therapy as well. No benefit of interferon therapy has been shown in node-negative patients.

Malignant Soft Tissue Lesion: Sarcoma

Sarcomas are a group of histologically diverse, albeit rare, tumors of mesodermal and occasionally ectodermal origin, affecting soft tissue or bone. They are grouped together because of their similar biologic features and responses to treatment. Sarcomas of the soft tissue account for approximately 1% of adult malignancies and 15% of pediatric malignancies; 50% or more of all cases are ultimately fatal. **Figure 30.1** demonstrates the diversity of soft tissue sarcomas with regard to anatomic site and histology.

Case 6 describes a patient with a rapidly expanding, poorly circumscribed, deep leg mass. A detailed history may elucidate risk factors in this patient. The most common nongenetic **predisposing conditions are previous irradiation and chronic lymphedema, either acquired, as after lymphadenectomy, or congenital. Exposure to alkylating chemotherapeutic agents, phenoxy acetic acids, vinyl chloride, arsenic, and other toxins is associated with development of sarcoma.** Certain **genetic conditions** also impart increased risk, including neurofibromatosis, familial retinoblastoma, and Li-Fraumeni and Gardner's syndromes. Despite the recognition of numerous factors that confer increased risk, most patients with soft tissue sarcoma present with no identifiable etiology.

Approximately half of all sarcomas affect the extremities, with two thirds presenting as a painless mass, as in the patient described in **Case 6**. The differential diagnosis of an extremity mass includes benign soft tissue tumor, most often lipoma, as well as hematoma or muscle injury, all of which are extremely common. With the exception of peripheral nerve tumor transformation in neurofibromatosis, benign tumors do not typically degenerate into malignancy.

Physical exam should include an assessment of the size and mobility of the presenting lesion and its relationship to the fascia, i.e., superficial versus deep. **In this patient, the clinical findings of immobility, large size (>5 cm), history of rapid growth, and persistence should raise suspicion of a malignant process and warrant biopsy of the lesion.** Indications for biopsy are summarized in **Table 30.10**.

Local radiologic studies [computed tomography (CT) or magnetic resonance imaging (MRI)] are sometimes performed before biopsy

---

[4] Kirkwood JM, Strawderman MH, Ernstoff MS, et al. Interferon alpha-2b adjuvant therapy of high-risk resected cutaneous melanoma: the ECOG Trial EST 1684. J Oncol 1996;14(1):7–17.

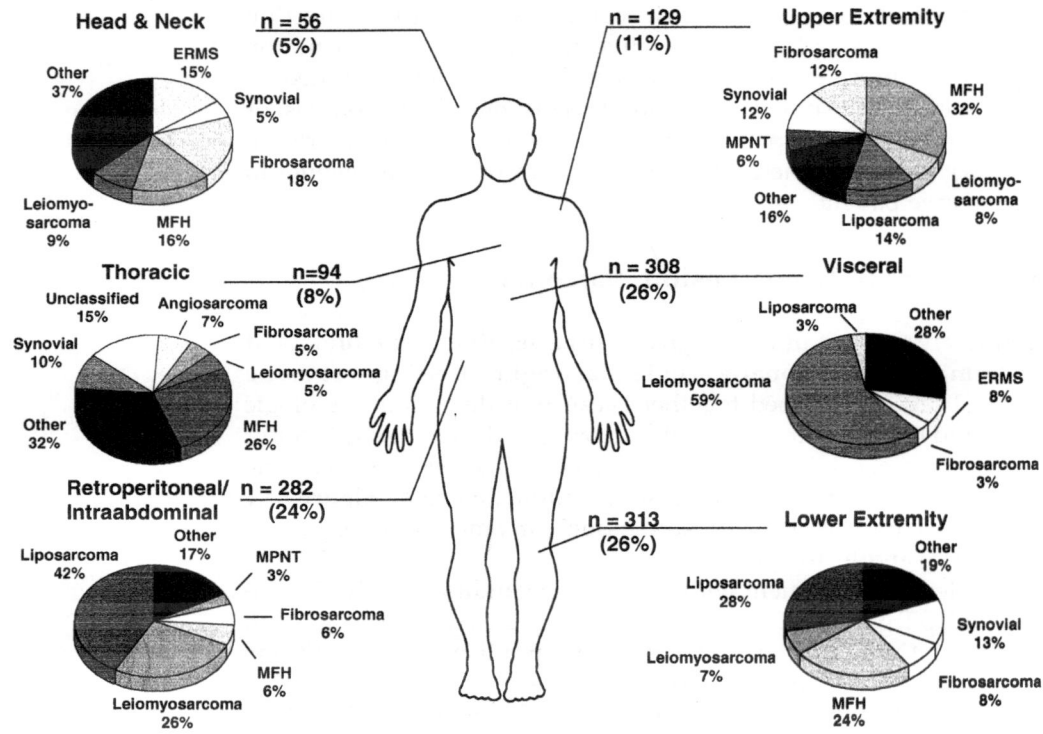

Figure 30.1. Anatomic distribution and site-specific histologic subtypes of 1182 consecutive patients with soft tissue sarcomas seen at the University of Texas M.D. Anderson Cancer Center (University of Texas M.D. Anderson Cancer Center Sarcoma Database, June 1996–December 1998). MFH, malignant fibrous histiocytoma; ERMS, embryonal rhabdomyosarcoma; MPNT, malignant peripheral nerve sheath tumor. (Reprinted from Pisters PWT. Soft tissue sarcoma. In: Norton JA, Bollinger RR, Chang AE, et al, eds. Surgery: Basic Science and Clinical Practice. New York: Springer-Verlag, 2001, with permission.

to elucidate the extent and compartmentalization of the tumor and to clarify the involvement of neurovascular and other surrounding structures. These studies often can rule out a benign process such as a lipoma and provide anatomic information that may help determine the best biopsy approach. Magnetic resonance imaging has been regarded as the study of choice because of its ability potentially to differentiate tumor and muscle, while providing clear definition of fascial planes and neurovascular structures. The advantage of MRI over CT, however, remains controversial. Computed tomography is indeed a cost-effective option and has been reported to provide as much clinically useful information as MRI in the diagnosis and staging of soft tissue tumors.

Because of its large size, suspicious history, and deep location, this patient's lesion should be biopsied by percutaneous core needle

Table 30.10. Indications for biopsy of a soft tissue lesion.

Noticeable enlargement
Size >5 cm
Persistence beyond 4–6 weeks
Deep location on exam

biopsy, a widely used method of biopsy that usually provides adequate tissue for diagnosis while being minimally invasive. **Fine-needle aspiration** is used by some, **but tissue obtained using this method can be difficult to assess,** and this technique typically is reserved for diagnosis of suspected recurrence. Many surgeons performing these biopsies tattoo the biopsy site for later excision, since tumor recurrence within the biopsy needle tract has been reported. The position of the biopsy site for these and other techniques is of significance, since sarcomas exhibit regional morphologic variation, and, as a result, multiple samples may be required for diagnosis.

Incisional or excisional biopsy of a suspicious soft tissue mass may be performed when definitive diagnosis cannot be achieved by less invasive means. Small, superficial lesions lend themselves to excisional biopsy, if not located nearby critical anatomic structures that would compromise appropriate surgical margins or in turn be compromised by such excision. For both excisional and incisional biopsy, incisions should be placed over the most superficial point of the tumor and should be oriented longitudinally along the axis of the extremity to facilitate wide local excision of the biopsy site and remaining tumor at a later time. Local hemostasis is critical to prevent seeding of tumor cells into adjacent tissues by hematoma.

With more than 30 histologic subtypes and with the anatomic heterogeneity and rarity of soft tissue sarcomas, a meaningful **staging system** that accurately describes all forms of the disease is in evolution. **The American Joint Committee on Cancer–International Union Against Cancer (AJCC-UICC) system is used widely and incorporates the standard tumor-node-metastasis (TNM) classification as well as histologic grading** ranging from well-differentiated to undifferentiated and substaging based on tumor location relative to fascia **(Table 30.11)**.[5] It is important to note that, although node status is included in this classification scheme, sarcomas metastasize hematogenously, and, as such, node involvement has no specific prognostic significance except as a site of distant metastasis.

Tissue biopsy of the patient's lesion in **Case 6** revealed a grade 2, moderately differentiated liposarcoma. **Staging of this patient's disease calls for detailed imaging studies if not performed prior to biopsy: CT or MRI of the affected extremity to look for skip metastases or local bone involvement and plain film or CT of the chest.** Spread hematogenously, sarcomas of the extremities metastasize most frequently to the lungs. **The grade of a sarcoma as determined by biopsy is related to the likelihood of metastasis.** Generally, low-grade lesions are an indication for chest x-ray, while chest CT usually is indicated in high-grade lesions. Bone metastases are the second most common type of distant disease associated with soft tissue sarcoma; accordingly, **technetium bone scanning** also might be used by some in staging disease.

Treatment of extremity sarcoma has centered on surgical resection, which, until 10 to 20 years ago, entailed amputation of the affected

---

[5] Greene FL, Page DL, Fleming ID, et al, eds. AJCC Cancer Staging Manual, 6th ed. New York: Springer-Verlag, 2002.

Table 30.11. American Joint Committee on Cancer staging system for soft tissue sarcomas.

T0	No evidence of primary tumor			
T1	Tumor 5 cm or less in greatest dimension			
T1a	Superficial tumor			
T1b	Deep tumor			
T2	Tumor more than 5 cm in greatest dimension			
T2a	Superficial tumor			
T2b	Deep tumor			
N0	No regional lymph node metastasis			
N1	Regional lymph node metastasis			
M0	No distant metastasis			
M1	Distant metastasis			
G1	Well differentiated			
G2	Moderately differentiated			
G3	Poorly differentiated			
G4	Undifferentiated			
Stage I	T1a,1b,2a,2b	N0	M0	G1–2
Stage II	T1a,1b,2a	N0	M0	G3–4
Stage III	T2b	N0	M0	G3–4
Stage IV	Any T	N1	M0	Any G
	Any T	N0	M1	Any G

Source: Reprinted from Greene FL, Balch CM, Fleming ID, et al, eds. American Joint Committee on Cancer AJCC Cancer Staging Manual, 6th ed. New York: Springer-Verlag, 2002, with permission.

limb. Prospective randomized studies have shown, however, that **limb-sparing surgery with postoperative radiation therapy yields overall survival rates comparable to those achieved with amputation** (National Cancer Institute, level I evidence),[6] **and that this approach results in superior local control of disease compared to surgical resection alone (Table 30.12).** Limb-sparing surgery requires full excision of the mass with wide margins rather than enucleation of the tumor pseudocapsule, which is associated with very high local recurrence rates. No studies to date have defined the ideal margin of resection, but 2 cm is an arbitrary and commonly used margin. It also should be noted that there is evidence that primary soft tissue sarcomas <5 cm may be treated with resection alone without radiotherapy.

Other therapies used in the treatment of localized soft tissue sarcoma of the extremities include **chemotherapy**, whose role remains controversial despite decades of randomized trials, **combined chemotherapy and radiotherapy protocols**, and **hyperthermic isolated limb perfusion**, which has shown usefulness in some settings and is currently in clinical trials.

The most effective treatment to date of soft tissue sarcoma metastasis, which occurs most frequently in the lungs, is surgical resection of pulmonary lesions. Unfortunately, metstatectomy benefits only a

---

[6] Rosenberg SA, Tepper J, Glatstein E, et al. The treatment of soft tissue sarcoma of the extremities: prospective randomized evaluations of (1) limb sparing surgery plus radiation therapy compared with amputation and (2) the role of adjuvant chemotherapy. Ann Surg 1982;196:305–315.

Table 30.12. Phase III trials of adjuvant radiotherapy for localized extremity and trunk sarcomas stratified by grade (level I evidence).

Histologic grade	First author/ institution	Treatment group	Radiation dose (Gy)	No. of patients	No. with local failure	LRFS	OS
High grade	Pisters/MSKCC[b]	Surgery + BRT	42–45	56	5 (9%)	89%	27%
		Surgery	—	63	19 (30%)	66%	67%
	Yang/NCI[a]	Surgery + XRT	45 + 18 (boost)	47	0 (0%)	100%	75%
		Surgery	—	44	9 (20%)	78%	74%
Low grade	Pisters/MSKCC[b]	Surgery + BRT	42–45	22	8 (36%)	73%	96%
		Surgery	—	23	6 (26%)	73%	95%
	Yang/NCI[a]	Surgery + XRT	45 + 18 (boost)	26	1 (4%)	96%	NR
		Surgery	—	24	8 (33%)	63%	NR

LRFS, local recurrence-free survival; OS, overall survival; MSKCC, Memorial Sloan-Kettering Cancer Center; BRT, brachytherapy; NCI, National Cancer Institute; XRT, external-beam radiation therapy.
[a] Yang JC, Chang AE, Baker AR, et al. A randomized prospective study of the benefit of adjuvant radiation therapy in the treatment of soft tissue sarcomas of the extremity. J Clin Oncol 1998;16:197–203.
[b] Pisters PWT, Harrison LB, Leung DHY, et al. Long-term results of a prospective randomized trial of adjuvant brachytherapy in soft tissue sarcoma. J Clin Oncol 1996;14:859–868.
Source: Reprinted from Pister PWT. Soft tissue sarcoma. In: Norton JA, Bollinger RR, Chang AE, et al, eds. Surgery: Basic Science and Clinical Practice. New York: Springer-Verlag, 2001, with permission.

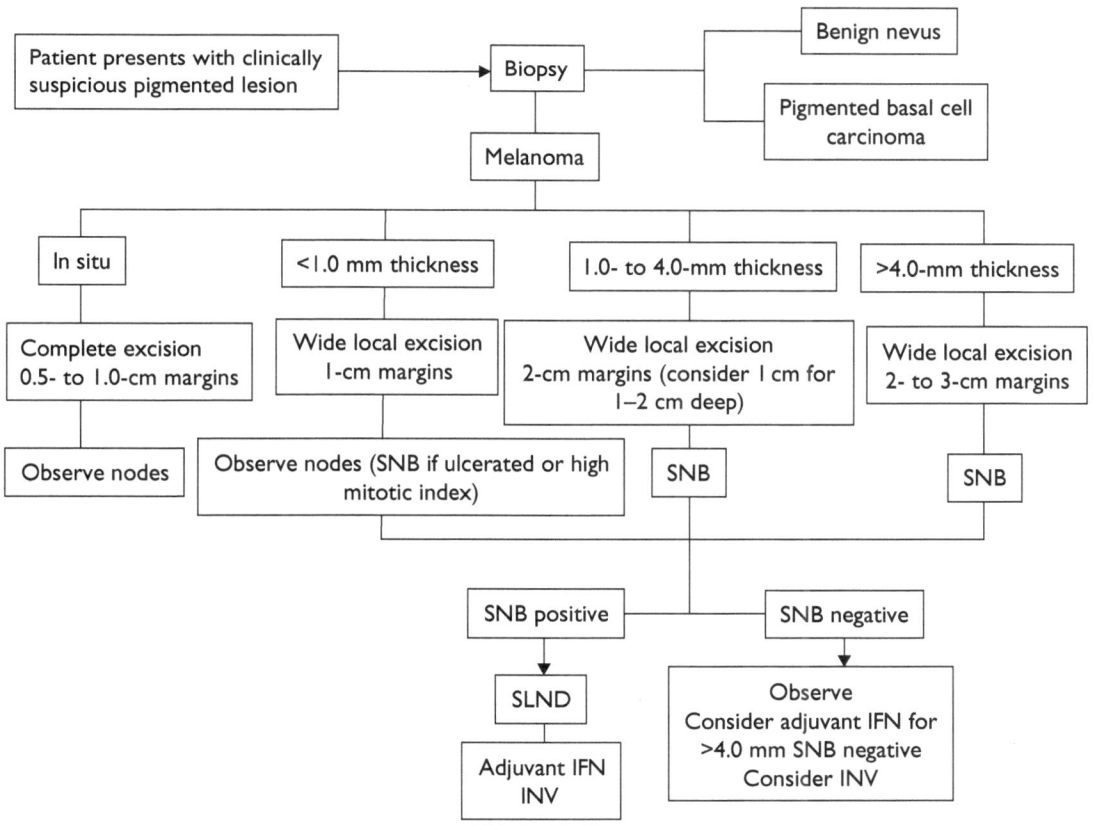

Algorithm 30.1. Management of localized cutaneous melanoma. *SNB,* sentinel node biopsy; *SLND,* selective complete lymphadenectomy; *IFN,* high-dose adjuvant interferon alpha-2b: *INV,* investigational therapies. (Wagner JD, Gordon MS, et al. Current therapy of cutaneous melanoma. Plast Reconstr Surg 2000;105(5):1774–1801. April 2000. With permission from Lippincott Williams and Wilkins.)

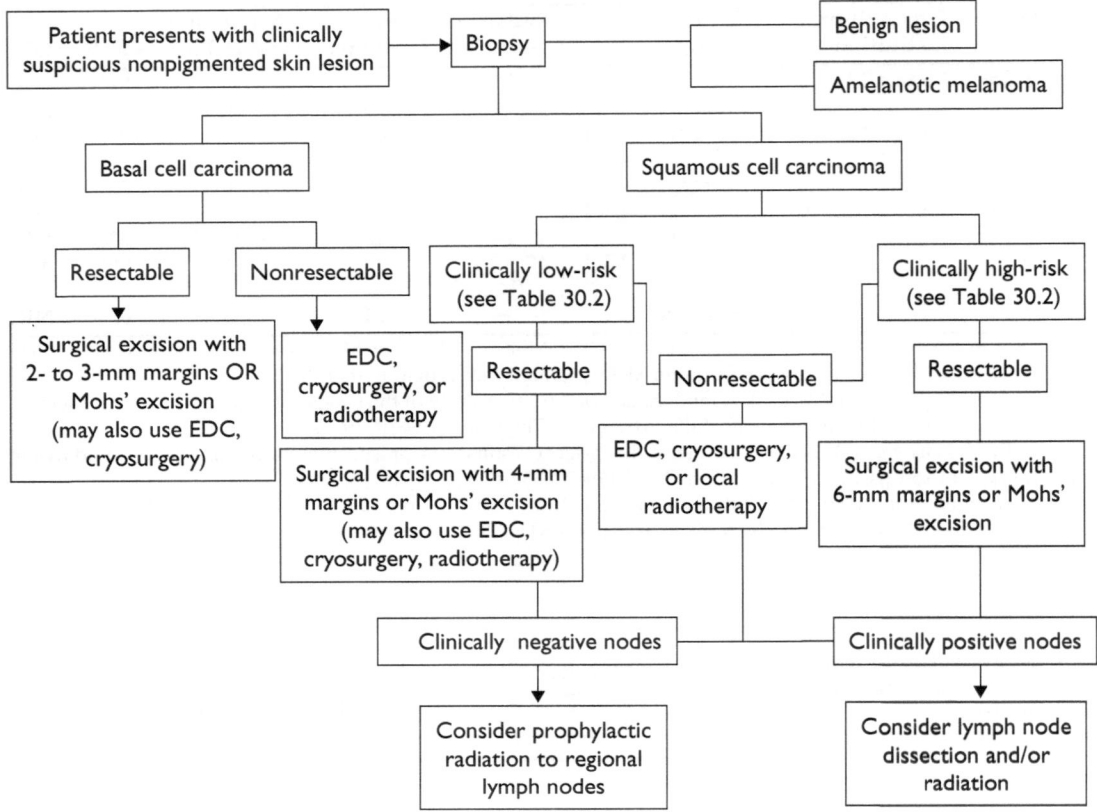

Algorithm 30.2. Management of nonmelanoma skin cancer. *EDC*, electrodesiccation and curettage.

small fraction of such patients (<15%), and hence it is critical that patient selection for pulmonary resection be conducted in an extremely cautious manner. The following commonly are accepted as criteria for patient selection: (1) the primary tumor is controlled or controllable, (2) there is no extrathoracic disease, (3) the patient is an appropriate medical candidate for thoracotomy and pulmonary resection, and (4) complete resection of all metastatic disease seems possible. In this way, the morbidity of thoracotomy can be limited to the few patients most likely to benefit from this aggressive procedure.

Retroperitoneal sarcomas are relatively rare, accounting for approximately 15% of all sarcomas. Their diagnosis, treatment, and management are beyond the scope of this chapter.

Summary

Given the extremely common presentation of skin lesions by patients to surgeons and general practitioners alike, it is vital that all physicians be comfortable differentiating those lesions that are thoroughly benign, those that are somewhat questionable, and those that are most likely malignant. Given the rise in incidence of all forms of skin cancer and given the dismal outcomes associated with late diagnosis of squamous cell carcinoma and melanoma, recognizing the "red flags" of malignant skin lesions and knowing when to refer to a specialist for biopsy are essential skills. The general approach to the management of skin lesions is summarized in **Algorithms 30.1** and **30.2**.

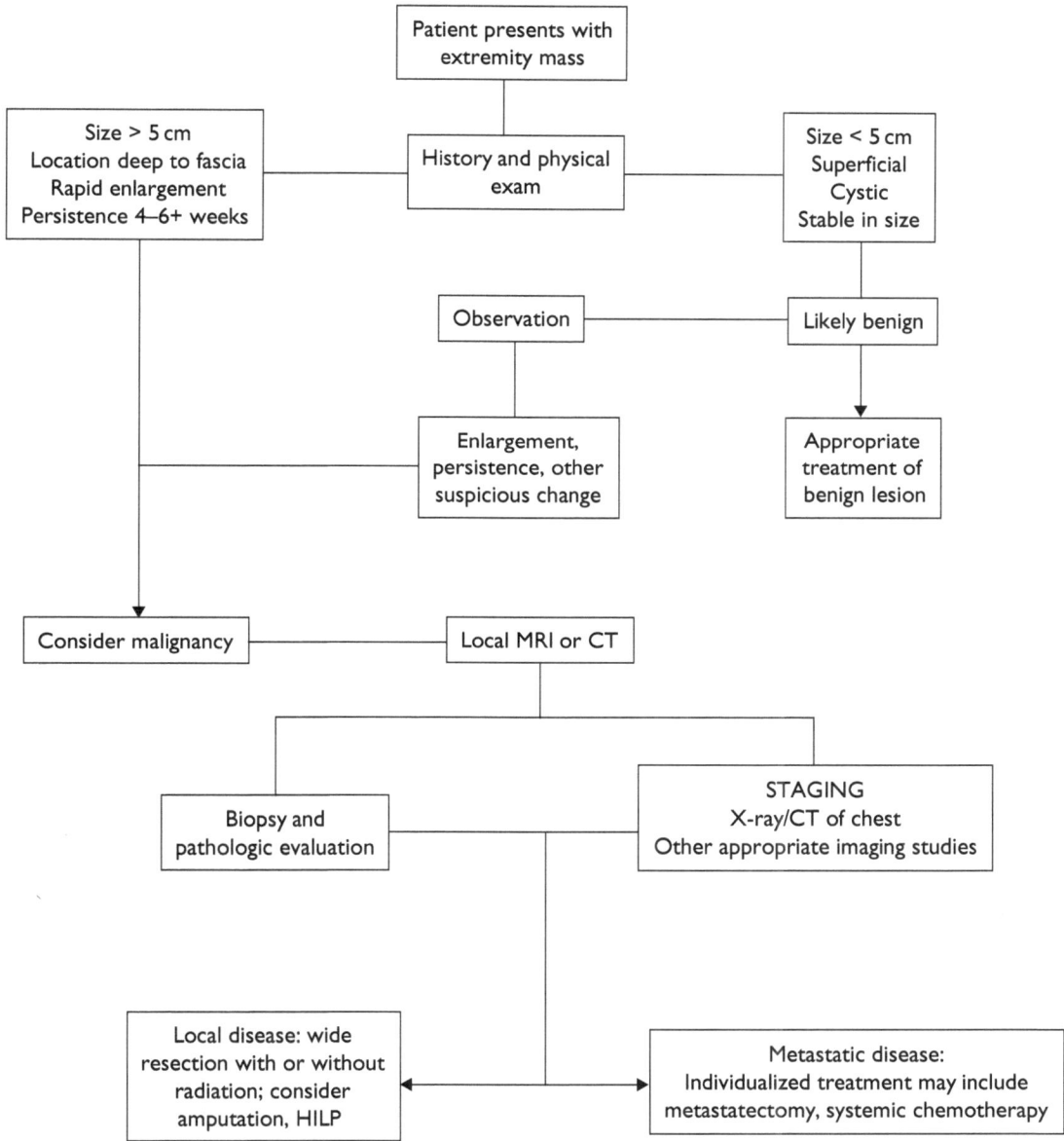

Algorithm 30.3. Initial management of extremity mass and soft tissue sarcoma. *HILP,* hyperthermic isolated limb perfusion. (Adapted from Pisters PWT. Ann Surg Oncol 1998;5:464–472. With permission of Lippincott Williams & Wilkins. Adapted from Peabody TD, Gibbs CP, Simon MA. Current Concepts Review-Evaluation and Staging of Musculoskeletal Neoplasms. J Bone Joint Surg Am 80A(8):1204–1218, August 1998. With permission of The Journal of Bone and Joint Surgery. Adapted with permission from Pisters PWT. Soft Tissue Sarcoma. In: Norton JA, Bollinger RR, Chang AE, et al, eds. Surgery. Basic Science and Clinical Evidence. New York: Springer-Verlag, 2001.)

A similar statement can be made regarding soft tissue masses. Certainly, benign soft tissue lesions of the extremities in the form of lipomas or hematomas are extremely common, but it is the essential role of the physician or surgeon to recognize the symptoms and presentation of sarcoma, a disease that, while it may be relatively uncommon, is associated with extremely high rates of morbidity and mortality despite early recognition. **Algorithm 30.3** outlines an approach to the initial evaluation of an extremity mass and to soft tissue sarcoma.

Selected Readings

Alam M, Ratner D. Primary care: cutaneous squamous cell carcinoma. N Engl J Med 2001;344(13):975–983.

Balch CM, Buzaid AC. Finally a successful adjuvant therapy for high-risk melanoma. J. Clin Oncol 1996;14:1.

Bickels J, Jelinek JS, et al. Biopsy of musculoskeletal tumors: current concepts. Clin Orthop Rela Res 1999;368:212–219.

Bruce AJ, Brodland DG. Overview of skin cancer detection and prevention for the primary care physician. Mayo Clin Proc 2000;75(5):491–500.

Lewis JJ, Brennan MF. Soft tissue sarcomas. Curr Probl Surg 1996;33:817–880.

Morton DL, Wen DR, et al. Technical details of intraoperative lymphatic mapping for early stage melanoma. Arch Surg 1992;127:392.

Peabody TD, Gibbs CP, Simon MA. Evaluation and staging of musculoskeletal neoplasms. J Bone Joint Surg 1998;80A(8):1204–1218.

Pisters PWT. Soft tissue sarcoma. In: Norton JA, Bollinger RR, Chang AE, et al, eds. Surgery: Basic Science and Clinical Evidence. New York: Springer-Verlag, 2001.

Reintgen DS, Cox EB, et al. Efficacy of elective lymph node dissection in patients with intermediate primary thickness melanoma. Ann Surg 1983;198:379.

Rosenberg SA, Tepper J, Glatstein E, Bruce AJ, Brodland DG. The treatment of soft tissue sarcomas of the extremities: prospective randomized trial of limb-sparing surgery plus radiation compared with amputation and the role of adjuvant chemotherapy. Ann Surg 1982;196:305–315.

Sondak VK, Margolin KA. Melanoma and other cutaneous malignancies. In: Norton JA, Bollinger RR, Chang AE, et al, eds. Surgery: Basic Science and Clinical Evidence. New York: Springer-Verlag, 2001.

Wagner JD, Gordon MS, et al. Current therapy of cutaneous melanoma. Plast Reconstr Surg 2000;105(5):1774–1802.

31

Trauma Fundamentals

Jeffrey Hammond

Objectives

1. To describe the priorities and sequences of trauma patient evaluation.
2. To describe the four classes of hemorrhagic shock and their clinical recognition.
3. To describe the initial management of the trauma resuscitation, including fluid management, assessment of central nervous system (CNS) status, spine protection, and triage.
4. To describe the diagnostic tools available in evaluation of abdominal trauma (ultrasound, computed tomography, peritoneal lavage).
5. To describe the differential diagnosis in thoracic trauma.
6. To discuss the pertinent issues related to alcohol as they pertain to trauma.
7. To discuss the economic and public health impact of trauma.

Case

You are working in an emergency department when a 46-year-old man arrives after a motor vehicle crash. The paramedics relate the history of a possibly intoxicated driver in a single car crash. The unrestrained driver was ejected partially from the vehicle after it struck a tree. An airbag was not present. The patient has been semiconscious en route, groaning frequently, and not responding to questions. His level of consciousness appeared to deteriorate in the ambulance. His last set of vital signs reveals a pulse rate of 120, systolic blood pressure of 100, and respiratory rate of 28 per minute. He arrives immobilized on a spine board and in a cervical collar. There appears to be an obvious deformity of the left thigh. An 18-gauge peripheral intravenous (IV) line has been established by the paramedics. No medical history is available.

What are your initial interventions and priorities? This chapter provides a framework for case workup.

Introduction

The history of surgery is, in many respects, the history of the development of trauma management. Today, trauma is a principal public health problem in every society, stretching across cultural and socioeconomic groups. **Trauma remains the leading cause of death in all age categories from infancy to middle age (1 to 44 years of age) in the United States.** In 1984, trauma exceeded cancer and heart disease combined as a measure of years of potential life lost (YPLL) as determined by the Centers for Disease Control and Prevention. By 1988, the estimated total annual cost of accidental trauma, including lost wages, expenses, and indirect losses, was estimated to be $180 billion in the United States alone. **At the end of the 1990s, with over 100,000 trauma deaths annually in the United States and three permanent disabilties for each death, trauma-related costs exceeded $400 billion annually.**

Trauma mortality has a trimodal pattern. The first cohort, approximately 50% of trauma deaths, occurs in the immediate postinjury period and represents death from overwhelming injury such as high spinal cord transection, aortic disruption, or massive intraabdominal injuries. Recognizing that there is little that sophisticated treatment systems can do to salvage these patients, efforts should be directed at prevention.

It is in the **second peak** in the trimodal distribution, however, that trauma systems and trauma centers perhaps can make their greatest contributions. Deaths in this group, usually caused by severe traumatic brain injury or uncontrolled hemorrhage, occur within hours of the injury and represent perhaps one-third of all trauma deaths. Institution of a trauma system or trauma center development can result in a reduction in preventable death rates of 20–30% to 2–9%. The **third peak** occurs 1 day to 1 month postinjury and comprises approximately 10% to 20% of deaths. It is most often due to refractory increased intracranial pressure subsequent to closed head injury or pulmonary complications. With aggressive critical care, nonpulmonary sources of sepsis, renal failure, and multiple organ failure as a cause of death are declining.

The management of the case presented at the beginning of this chapter is implicit in the discussion of trauma fundamentals that follows.

Trauma Triage

A cornerstone of trauma care is the timely identification and transport to a trauma center of those patients most likely to benefit from trauma care; this is the principle of triage. Triage, adapted from a

French military concept, is at its simplest the sorting of patients based on need for treatment and an inventory of available resources to meet those needs. This may take place in the field or within the institution. Trauma triage is founded upon the recognition that the nearest emergency room may not be the most appropriate destination. **On a more complex level, triage involves the development of an algorithm that seeks to avoid undertriage (and possible adverse outcome) while minimizing overtriage (and overloading the system).**

Multiple prehospital scoring mechanisms have been suggested to assist in the triage decision. It has been hoped that some scoring technique would facilitate identification of the 5% to 10% of trauma patients estimated to require the sophisticated trauma center. **Current triage schema tend to assess the potential for life- or limb-threatening injury utilizing physiologic, anatomic, or mechanism of injury criteria. In general, physiologic criteria offer the greatest yield, while anatomic criteria are intermediate yield predictors and mechanism criteria are the lowest yield predictors.** The best criteria of major trauma include prolonged prehospital time, pedestrians struck by vehicles moving at speeds greater than 20 mph, associated death of another vehicular occupant, systolic blood pressure less than 90 mm Hg, respiratory rate less than 10 or greater than 29 breaths per minute, and Glasgow Coma Scale score of less than 13.

The Trauma Survey

The basic tenets of trauma resuscitation focus on addressing the management decisions and treatment algorithms that are present for the patient who survives to reach the emergency department. To focus on this, **the revised Advanced Trauma Life Support (ATLS) course retains the mnemonic ABC**. Efforts during the initial or **primary survey** are directed at establishing a secure **airway**, using techniques of rapid sequence intubation if necessary, identifying that the patient has adequate **breathing** by ruling out or treating immediately life-threatening chest injuries (**Table 31.1**), and ensuring adequate **circulation** by control of obvious hemorrhage. **Expeditious hemorrhage control**, through operative and nonoperative means, has received increased emphasis over volume normalization through fluid administration and blood pressure maintenance in the new iteration. Simply put, **the best way to maintain or reestablish blood pressure is to stop the bleeding rather than to use pressors or large-volume administration.** These treatment principles hold true in both the prehospital environment (emergency medical services, EMS) and the trauma center setting. In fact, effective trauma care is predicated on a seamless transition of care from EMS to the hospital team. This requires coordination, communication, and treatment plans that are integrated and follow a logical sequence.

The medical history obtained during the primary survey also focuses on the essential information. A more detailed history can be taken as time permits after the primary survey. The **mnemonic AMPLE**

Table 31.1. Life-threatening chest/thoracic injuries.

Immediately life threatening
  Airway occlusion
  Tension pneumothorax
  Sucking chest wound (open pneumothorax)
  Massive hemothorax
  Flail chest
  Cardiac tamponade

Potentially or late life threatening
  Aortic injury
  Diaphragmatic tear
  Tracheobronchial injuries
  Pulmonary contusion
  Esophageal injury
  Blunt cardiac injury ("myocardial contusion")

Source: Used/Reproduced from American College of Surgeons' Committee on Trauma. Advanced Trauma Life Support R for Doctors, Student Course Manual, 6th ed. Chicago: American College of Surgeons, 1997, p. 125, with permission.

is useful (**Table 31.2**). Prehospital personnel should be questioned about vital signs en route and other details that could enhance understanding of the patient's physiologic state.

The Primary Survey

The **primary survey** (see **Algorithm 31.1**) is brief, requiring no more than a few minutes. **A cornerstone of the primary survey concept is the dictum to treat life-threatening injuries as they are identified.** This deviates from the traditional conceptual approach to the patient taught in medical school, wherein treatment is delayed until a thorough history is obtained, a physical examination performed, and all differential diagnoses are entertained. Management during the primary survey relies heavily on knowledge of the expected patterns of injury based on the mechanism of transfer of kinetic energy. Laboratory tests and diagnostic radiology are not emphasized at this point. X-rays should be ordered judiciously and should not delay resuscitative efforts or patient transfer to definitive care. Appropriate basic monitoring includes pulse oximetry and cardiac rhythm monitoring.

Extending the alphabetical mnemonic to D, evaluation of **disability**, directs the resuscitation team **to assess neurologic function and assign a Glasgow Coma Scale** (GCS) score. The GCS was designed to translate a subjective impression of altered mental status (e.g., terms

Table 31.2. The AMPLE mnemonic.

A: Allergies
M: Medications
P: Past medical history
L: Last meal (when?)
E: Environment (of event)

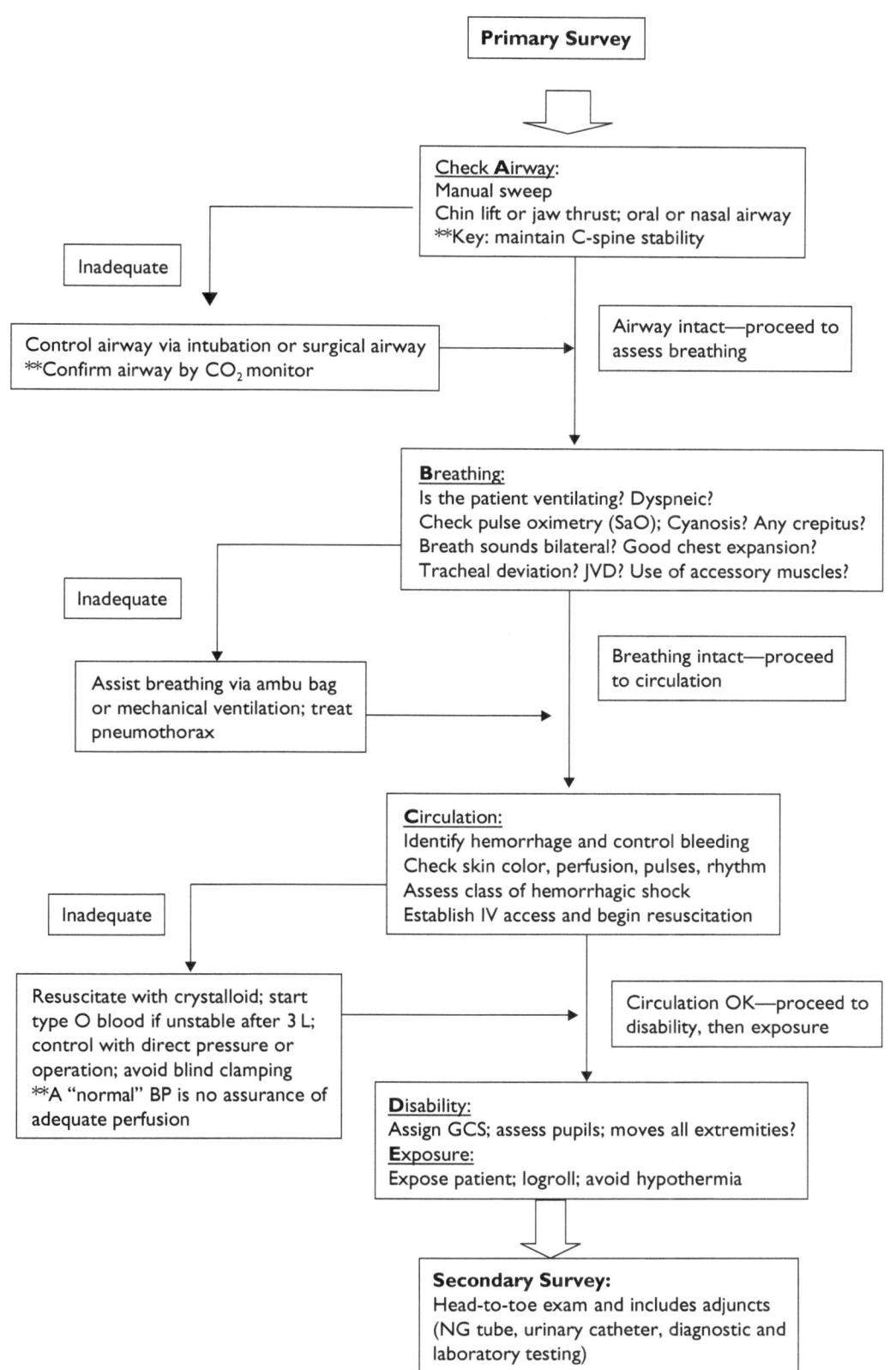

Algorithm 31.1. Algorithm for conduct of primary survey in trauma patient. BP, blood pressure; GCS, Glasgow Coma Scale; JVD, jugular venous distention; NG, nasogastric.

Table 31.3. Glasgow Coma Scale.

Component	Score
Best eye opening	
Spontaneously	4
To verbal command	3
To pain	2
No response	1
Best verbal response	
Oriented and converses	5
Disoriented	4
Inappropriate words	3
Incomprehensible sounds	2
No response or sounds	1
Best motor response	
Obeys commands	6
Localizes pain	5
Flexion-withdrawal	4
Decorticate flexion	3
Decerebrate extension	2
No motor response	1

such as lethargy, stupor, or somnolence) into an objective scoring mechanism. The score derives from assessment of the patient's best motor, verbal, and eye opening responses (**Table 31.3**). The patient always is assigned the most favorable score (e.g., if the patient is decorticate on one side and decerebrate on the other, the higher motor score is assigned), so that the score is reported as a finite number and not a range. This is extremely important, since it allows early detection of progression of neurologic deficit. If, on the other hand, the GCS were reported as a range, for example as 9 to 10, then one could not determine if a subsequent report of a GCS of 8 to 9 represented no change or a drop of two points. Often, the trauma patient arrives in the emergency department intubated or therapeutically paralyzed. In these cases, the preintubation GCS should be elicited from the field personnel for use as the treatment baseline. Alternatively, the verbal component of the score can be predicted from the motor and eye opening components using the following formula:

$$\text{Derived verbal score} = -0.3756 + (\text{Motor score} \times 0.5713) + (\text{Eye score} \times 0.4233)$$

Implicit in this neurologic assessment is the assumption that a spine injury is present until proven otherwise, dictating the need for vigilance in spine immobilization. This especially is true when concomitant head injury is present, and the head and neck axis should be considered as a single unit. Evidence of significant intracranial edema or space-occupying lesion, such as a GCS less than 8 or focal findings on cranial nerve exam, dictates early diagnostic imaging and neurosurgical consultation.

Extending the alphabetical mnemonic to E, exposure, directs the examiner to remove all clothing and log roll the patient to fully evaluate for injuries.

The Secondary Survey

The **secondary survey** naturally follows the primary survey, and it is here that a more **thorough head-to-toe examination** is performed. **The secondary survey does not begin until the primary survey is completed and resuscitation is well under way.** This stage can be thought of as "tubes and fingers in every orifice." Rectal and vaginal examination and both urinary catheterization and gastric tube placement occur during the secondary survey. In this survey, a complete neurologic examination is performed. Frequent reassessment of vital signs is emphasized.

Definitive hemorrhage control rather than normalization of volume status again is emphasized as the target of shock management. Blood loss may be estimated through assessment of blood pressure, heart rate, and skin color (**Table 31.4**). Invasive monitoring is not warranted. Hypovolemic hypotension requires 15% to 40% blood volume loss, but it may be a late sign in younger patients with good compensatory mechanisms. **Failure to correct hypotension or tachycardia after rapid infusion of 2 to 3 L of crystalloid solution suggests a volume deficit of greater than 15% or ongoing losses.** Blood transfusion, using type O if type specific is not available, should be considered when blood loss exceeds 1 L or when greater than 3 L of crystalloid are needed to maintain blood pressure. Type O-positive blood can be given safely to most patients, reserving often difficult-to-inventory O-negative blood for women of childbearing age who may benefit from the reduced risk of antigenicity. Attention must be directed toward avoiding the creation of a secondary injury or insult, primarily by **avoiding hypotension or hypoxia.** This especially is true in the management of closed head injury. The Traumatic Coma Data Bank indicates that even a single episode of hypotension results in poorer outcomes after head injury.

Prophylactic antibiotics should be started for penetrating trauma or open fractures. The **tetanus immunization** status of the patient must be ascertained. If the immunization status is uncertain or if the patient has a tetanus-prone wound, tetanus immunoglobulin should be administered with the tetanus toxoid booster. Tetanus-prone wounds include those greater than 6 hours old, crush injuries, burns, electrical injuries, frostbite, high-velocity missile injuries, devitalized tissue, denervated or ischemic tissue, or direct contamination with dirt or feces.

Great care should be exercised during resuscitation efforts to **protect against transmission of blood-borne diseases to the healthcare staff.**

Table 31.4. Estimated blood loss based on physical exam.

	Class I	Class II	Class III	Class IV
Blood loss (mL)	Up to 750	750–1500	1500–2000	>2000
Blood loss (% volume)	Up to 15%	15–30%	30–40%	>40%
Pulse rate	<100	>100	>120	>140
Blood pressure	Normal	Normal	Decreased	Decreased
Respiratory rate	14–20	20–30	30–40	>40
Urine output (mL/hr)	>30	20–30	5–15	Negligible
Mental status	Slightly anxious	Mild anxiety	Anxious, confused	Lethargic

Between 1% and 16% of trauma patients are infected with the human immunodeficiency virus (HIV) at time of presentation. The incidence increases with the percentage of penetrating trauma within the case mix. The prevalence and risk of hepatitis B is even greater. Nevertheless, adherence to the principle of **universal precautions**, i.e., the practice of strict barrier techniques applied in all cases based on the presumption that all patients are infected, is poor. Compliance with infection control standards cannot be achieved by passive informational techniques, but it requires active and continuous in-service and supervision.

During the secondary survey, injuries are cataloged and potentially life-threatening or disabling injuries are identified. A treatment plan and priorities are set. A basic principle of trauma resuscitation is the need for **continual reevaluation and reassessment**. A **tertiary survey** can identify up to a 5% to 10% missed injury rate. While the majority of these delayed diagnoses are not life- or limb-threatening, some in fact will be significant.

Finally, the leader of the resuscitation team also must be able to **accurately assess the facility's ability to render definitive care and arrange for transfer to a tertiary facility or trauma center if warranted**. Transfer to a higher level of care must be accomplished through physician-to-physician communication in a timely fashion and can be facilitated by preexisting transfer agreements.

Evaluation of the Abdomen

The approach to the diagnosis of blunt abdominal trauma is undergoing evolution (**Table 31.5**). **Diagnostic peritoneal lavage** (DPL) became the preferred method of evaluating the abdomen through the 1970s. It is highly sensitive, approaching 97% in blunt trauma and 93% in penetrating trauma, with a 99% specificity. Its high sensitivity was both an advantage as well as a disadvantage, however, as concern grew over the phenomenon of "nontherapeutic laparotomy." While most of the morbidity of nontherapeutic laparotomy for trauma is transient, such as atelectasis, ileus, hypertension, or urinary tract infection, a rate of between 2.5% and 4% has been identified for this complication. This concern has been accentuated by the trend to nonoperative management of solid organ injury, borrowed from the spleen-saving approach and experience of surgeons managing pediatric trauma.

Improvements in speed and resolution of **computed tomography** (CT) led to this modality becoming the favored diagnostic approach for the **stable trauma patient**. Advantages of CT investigation of abdominal trauma include visualization of solid organ anatomy, including retroperitoneal structures, and the ability to grade and quantify injury. This feature permits an expectant nonoperative approach to solid organ injury. Disadvantages include the need to transport patients from the relative safety of the emergency department (ED) resuscitation area to the radiology suite and the possible complications of administering a dye load, such as allergic reaction or renal impairment. Moreover, the

Table 31.5. Comparison of diagnostic methods to evaluate abdominal trauma.

	Diagnostic peritoneal lavage (DPL)	Ultrasound	Computed tomography (CT) scan
Sensitivity/ specificity	97–99% sensitive and specific for blunt trauma; poorer specificity (44–86%) for penetrating trauma	82–97% sensitivity; 95–100% specificity	85–100% sensitivity; 95–100% specificity
Accuracy	Poor; only indicates presence of blood; does not indicate if bleeding ongoing	Same as DPL	Very accurate; permits solid organ injury grading; demonstrates retroperitoneum
Speed	Fast, but >10 minutes and training required	Fast, taking 5–6 minutes	>20 minutes; requires time and patient transport
Risk	≤1% if done open/ semiopen and proper technique	None	Risk related to contrast (allergy, renal insufficiency)
Advantages	Very sensitive; objective; guidelines for both blunt and penetrating trauma	Noninvasive, sensitive; can be performed in resuscitation bay while other activities ongoing	Very specific with good sensitivity; good for evaluating posterior injuries
Disadvantages	Not recommended if prior laparotomy; not useful for retroperitoneal injuries	Operator dependent; requires equipment; not useful for penetrating trauma	May miss intestinal or diaphragmatic injuries; suitable only for stable patients

grading or staging of solid organ injury based on CT findings alone may correlate poorly with anatomic findings and should be considered in the context of vital signs indicative of hemodynamic status, such as pulse and blood pressure.

Building on the experience of European surgeons, Rozycki et al[1] have begun to popularize **ultrasound as a replacement for DPL in the unstable patient**. Advantages of the **focused abdominal sonogram for trauma (FAST)** technique include its speed and immediacy; however, its true utility has not been established yet. It remains an operator-dependent technique that, like DPL, is sensitive but not specific. It has the potential to make DPL obsolete, but the inability of FAST to demonstrate subtle injuries often seen on CT, such as occult pneumothorax, pulmonary contusion, and solid organ hematomas, may render it inferior to CT in the hemodynamically stable patient or in patients with pelvic ring fractures.

Laparoscopy has not proven efficacious, with the exception of investigating penetrating trauma to the flank or back to rule out diaphragmatic injury, a condition for which DPL, CT, and FAST are not accurate.

[1] Rozycki G, Ochsner MG, Feliciano D, et al. Early detection of hemoperitoneum by ultrasound examination of the right upper quadrant: a multicenter study. J Trauma 1998;45:878–883.

Traumatic Brain Injury

The **nonoperative management of traumatic brain injury (TBI)** is predicated on reducing brain edema in the absence of a space-occupying lesion that can be surgically attacked. **Evidence-based medicine (EBM) guidelines developed by the American Academy of Neurosurgery (AAN) and the Brain Injury Foundation** reflect current literature and have standardized the approach to the care of the head-injured patient.[2] However, available class I data were sparse and could support the recommendation of only one treatment standard, which was the contraindication of use of steroids in the therapy of traumatic brain injury.

The AAN guidelines advocate, based on strong class II data, the use of **intracerebral pressure monitoring for patients with GCS less than or equal to 8.** Ventriculostomies appear to be more efficacious than subarachnoid bolt monitors. This is coupled with **a recommendation against overaggressive hyperventilation**, to levels below a P_{CO_2} of 25 mm Hg. Remaining areas of controversy, however, include the value of more modest levels of hyperventilation, the efficacy of mild-to-moderate systemic hypothermia, and whether the appropriate end point for measurement of medical management of TBI should be intracerebral pressure (ICP) or cerebral perfusion pressure (CPP).

The **role of CT scanning in so-called mild or minor head trauma** (GCS 13–15) is unclear. Increasingly, patients with brief loss of consciousness as an isolated injury are being discharged from the emergency department rather than admitted for observation. Proponents of CT for mild closed head injury cite the significant minority of patients with a skull fracture or operative lesion, while detractors cite poor cost-effectiveness of CT as a screening tool. Grading of concussion is underutilized, contributing to the poor understanding of the pathophysiology and sequelae of concussion. **Use of the American Academy of Neurology classification system for concussion (Table 31.6) and neuropsychological follow-up are indicated.**

Spinal Cord Injury

The use of steroids for acute spinal cord injury (SCI) remains a source of controversy. While the **National Acute Spinal Cord Injury Study (NASCIS)** was established in 1975 to study the potential effects of drug therapy in SCI, the issue remains unresolved. The anticipated benefits of steroids in SCI include inhibition of lipid peroxidation and reduction of arachidonic acid metabolites. The **NACSIS II study**, released in 1990, often is cited as demonstrating a positive effect of methylprednisolone when administered as a bolus of 30 mg/kg followed by a 24-hour infusion of 5.4 mg/kg, if administered within 8 hours of injury. Patients in the treatment arm were found to have better sensory levels

---

[2] Brain Trauma Foundation. Guidelines for the management of severe head injury. J Neurotrauma 1996;13:638–734.

Table 31.6. Grades of concussion.

Grade 1
1. Transient confusion
2. No loss of consciousness
3. Concussive symptoms or mental status abnormalities resolve in *less* than 15 minutes

Grade 2
1. Transient confusion
2. No loss of consciousness
3. Concussive symptoms or mental status abnormalities (including amnesia) last *more* than 15 minutes

Grade 3
1. Any brief loss of consciousness
   a. Brief (seconds)
   b. Prolonged (minutes)

Source: Reprinted from Kelly JP, Rosenberg J. Practice parameter. The management of concussion in sport. Report of the Quantity Standards Committee. Neurology 1997;48:581–585. With permission from Lippincott Williams & Wilkins.

and higher motor scores than the control arms at 6-month follow-up. However, this study, now the basis for the wide adoption of steroid use in SCI, was flawed by its retrospective analysis, potential selection bias, questionable end points, and failure to address the potential negative side effects of steroids. Class II data (nonblinded, historical controls) suggest that pneumonia is more prevalent and hospitalization extended in steroid-treated patients.[3]

A follow-up study, **NASCIS III**, published in 1997, included a 48-hour trial as well as another lipid peroxidation inhibitor, tirilazad. There was a reported advantage of the prolonged dosing of steroids in the subset in which treatment was begun between 3 and 8 hours postinjury, but there was no difference if steroids were started within 3 hours of injury. There was no difference in overall Functional Independence Measure (FIM) scores among the three groups. Moreover, as in NASCIS II, randomization was not equivalent, raising the issue of selection bias affecting validity of the conclusions. Additionally, patients in the 48-hour methylprednisolone group had a higher incidence of severe sepsis and pneumonia than patients in the other two arms, again raising the question of whether the questionable marginal benefits outweigh the risks.[4]

Trauma and Alcohol

Alcohol consumption is a major etiologic factor in both intentional and unintentional trauma. Both acute alcohol use and chronic alcohol use have a significant impact on mortality, and, with regard to motor

---

[3] Nesathurai N. Steroids and spinal cord injury: revisiting the NASCIS 2 and NASCIS 3 trials. J Trauma 1998;45:1088–1093.
[4] Nesathurai N. Steroids and spinal cord injury: revisiting the NASCIS 2 and NASCIS 3 trials. J Trauma 1998;45:1088–1093.

vehicle trauma, the link between alcohol use and death follows a dose-response curve. It has been estimated that one alcohol-related fatality occurs every 22 minutes. One half of the cost of motor vehicle crashes in the U.S. is attributable to alcohol.

Failure to recognize the role alcohol plays in trauma represents an opportunity lost. Among the myths related to alcohol use are the following two: that alcohol protects against serious injury and that most people injured after consuming alcohol are social drinkers. While intoxication is a legal issue, set in most states at a blood alcohol level (BAL) of 100 mg/mL, impairment can be demonstrated at levels of 0.05%. Other than BAL, biochemical markers, such as gamma-glutamyltransferase (GGT), are not sensitive to acute changes in BAL and better reflect chronic use. **Screening tests, such as the World Health Organization (WHO) Audit filter, the CAGE (see below), the Short Michigan Alcohol Screening Test (SMAST), and the TWEAK,** are more effective assays to identify the problem drinker at risk for future alcohol-related trauma.

The Audit is a WHO-sponsored test focusing on the patient at serious risk for hazardous driving. Validated in six nations, it combines a 10-item questionnaire with a lab test (GGT) and a physical examination. The SMAST uses a 13-item questionnaire to detect behavioral correlates of alcoholism. It focuses on the consequences of problem drinking and the patient's perception of his/her problem. The TWEAK assay originally was developed to identify at-risk pregnant drinkers. Five questions specifically address tolerance, symptoms, and daily use. The CAGE survey derives its name from the four questions posed to the patient:

1. Have you ever felt the need to CUT DOWN on drinking?
2. Have you ever felt ANNOYED by criticism of drinking?
3. Have you ever felt GUILTY about drinking?
4. Have you ever taken a morning EYE-OPENER?

Two or more "yes" answers are considered positive. Studies indicate little difference in the sensitivity and selectivity among these screening tests. The CAGE generally is used more widely as a tool since it can be administered by nonmedical personnel (e.g., social workers), can be given quickly even in an ED setting, and is easy to use and interpret.

The value of **early identification** cannot be overemphasized, however, and must be coupled with **early intervention**. The best time to initiate therapy is after a crisis. Gentillello and colleagues[5] at Harborview Medical Center, reported on the creation of a trauma center–based intervention team. After even one inpatient contact, professional treatment can obtain long-term (defined as 1 year) abstinence rates as high as 64% to 74%, compared to abstinence rates of 10% when treatment is delayed until referral after hospital discharge.

[5] Gentillello LM, Duggan P, Drummond D, et al. Major injury as a unique opportunity to initiate treatment in the alcoholic. Am J Surg 1988;156:558–561.

Trauma in Pregnancy

Trauma complicates 6% to 7% of all pregnancies. Important and predictable anatomic and physiologic changes occur with pregnancy. Domestic violence often increases during pregnancy. Attention to these details are required to ensure optimal outcome for both patients—the mother and the fetus. The pregnant trauma patient is treated best by a multidisciplinary team. **A general maxim, however, is that to care best for the fetus, one must take care of the mother.**

The basic principles of trauma care essentially remain the same. However, there are some differences. The signs of shock may be masked by the physiologic maternal hypervolemia. Additionally, systolic blood pressure and diastolic blood pressure decrease 15 to 20 mm Hg in the first two trimesters; the pulse rate increases by 15 to 20 beats/minute by the third trimester. Fetal distress predates maternal distress since the maternal circulation is maintained preferentially. Beyond the 20th week of pregnancy, the gravid uterus may compress the vena cava, resulting in reduced venous return and hypotension. This can be relieved by manual distraction of the uterus or logrolling the patient into the left lateral decubitus position. Fetal heart monitoring should be initiated on all patients beyond the 20th week of gestation as soon as possible. Diagnostically, ultrasound can be considered a "noninvasive DPL." Radiographs should be individualized, shielding the uterus when possible. The effects of radiation exposure are greatest from 2 to 7 weeks; there is little risk of teratogenesis after 17 weeks, although there is an increased relative risk of childhood malignancies. The current recommendation is to limit exposure to less than 5 rad, with most radiographic studies delivering millirad doses (**Table 31.7**).

Current Controversies

Not all trauma management decisions fit neatly into the paradigm described in this chapter. Within the EMS community, **the debate over "scoop and run" versus "stay and play" attempts at stabilization in the field continues.** This debate extends to use of helicopters for civilian trauma. The success of Vietnam War era aeromedical evacuation has not been demonstrated fully in an urban setting, and its greatest utility has been demonstrated in rural areas.

Table 31.7. Radiation exposure from common radiographic studies.

Study	Dose to fetus in mRads
Chest x-ray	<1–8
C-spine	1–10
Pelvis	200–350
Extremity	<1–3
Head CT	50
Abdomen CT	1000–9000

While use of the military antishock garment (MAST) suit has waned since the 1980s, and its use is now discouraged, **the manner and means of the optimal fluid resuscitation regimen in the hypotensive patient is controversial**. Recent work by Bickell and colleagues[6] supports the radical approach of limiting crystalloid infusion, even in the face of hypotension, in favor of a more rapid evacuation to a location for definitive care. Their approach was advocated for penetrating as opposed to blunt trauma, and their favorable results may have been assisted by the selection bias as well as by an unusually well-organized urban EMS service. Conversely, Buchman and colleagues[7] demonstrated a significant decrease in resuscitation times and increase in unexpected survival for the 5% of patients presenting in class III/IV shock utilizing a rapid infuser. More to the point, Feero and colleagues[8] identified that unexpected survival correlated with reduced scene time, stressing the importance of triage and transport over interventions that may increase scene time.

Summary

Trauma is more of a disease of modern times than ever before. It is a public health problem of epidemic proportions that transcends geographic boundaries and affects all age groups. It is the most common cause of preventable death in the United States. An organized and methodologic approach to both trauma care and prevention has proven to be successful wherever practiced.

Selected Readings

Alyono D, Morrow CE, Perry JF. Reappraisal of diagnostic peritoneal lavage criteria for operation in penetrating and blunt trauma. Surgery 1982;92: 751–757.

American College of Surgeons Committee on Trauma. Advanced Trauma Life Support. Chicago: American College of Surgeons, 1997.

Ballard RB, Rozycki GS, Newman PG, et al. An algorithm to reduce the incidence of false negative FAST examination in patients at high risk for occult injury. J Am Coll Surg 1999;189:145–151.

Bickell WH, Wall MJ Jr, Pepe PE, et al. Immediate versus delayed fluid resuscitation for hypotensive patients with penetrating torso injuries. N Engl J Med 1994;331:1105–1109.

Brain Trauma Foundation. Guidelines for the management of severe head injury. J Neurotrauma 1996;13:638–734.

Buchman TG, Menker JB, Lipsett P. Strategies for trauma resuscitation. Surg Gynecol Obstet 1991;172:8–12.

---

[6] Bickell WH, Wall MJ Jr, Pepe PE, et al. Immediate versus delayed fluid resuscitation for hypotensive patients with penetrating torso injuries. N Engl J Med 1994;331: 1105–1109.

[7] Buchman TG, Menker JB, Lipsett P. Strategies for trauma resuscitation. Surg Gynecol Obstet 1991;172:8–12.

[8] Feero S, Hedges JR, Simmons E, Irwin L. Does out-of-hospital EMS time affect trauma survival? Am J Emerg Med 1995;13:133–135.

Eastern Association for the Surgery of Trauma. Practice Management Guidelines for prophylactic antibiotics in penetrating abdominal injury and in open fractures. Web site: www.east.org, 1998.

Eastman AB. Blood in our streets: status and evolution of trauma care systems. Arch Surg 1992;127:677–681.

Enderson BL, Reath DB, Meadors J, et al. The tertiary trauma survey: a prospective study of missed injury. J Trauma 1990;30:666–669.

Feero S, Hedges JR, Simmons E, Irwin L. Does out-of-hospital EMS time affect trauma survival? Am J Emerg Med 1995;13:133–135.

Flint L, Babikian G, Anders M, et al. Definitive control of mortality from severe pelvic fracture. Ann Surg 1990;211:703–711.

Gentillello LM, Duggan P, Drummond D, et al. Major injury as a unique opportunity to initiate treatment in the alcoholic. Am J Surg 1988;156:558–561.

Hammond JS. Trauma: priorities, controversies and special situations. In: Norton JA, Bollinger RR, Chang AE, et al, eds. Surgery: Basic Science and Clinical Evidence. New York: Springer-Verlag, 2001.

Hammond JS, Eckes JM, Gomez GA, et al. HIV, trauma and infection control: universal precautions are universally ignored. J Trauma 1990;30:555–561.

Kelly JP, Rosenberg J. Practice parameter: The management of concussion in sport. Report of the Quality Standards Committee. Neurology 1997;48: 581–585.

Mackersie R. Abdominal trauma. In: Norton JA, Bollinger RR, Chang AE, et al, eds. Surgery: Basic Science and Clinical Evidence. New York: Springer-Verlag, 2001.

Malangoni M, Cue J, Fallat M, et al. Evaluation of splenic injury by computed tomography and its impact on treatment. Ann Surg 1990;211:592–599.

Nesathurai N. Steroids and spinal cord injury: revisiting the NASCIS 2 and NASCIS 3 trials. J Trauma 1998;45:1088–1093.

Pevec WC, Peitzman AB, Udekwu AO, et al. Computed tomography in the evaluation of blunt abdominal trauma. Surg Gynecol Obstet 1991;173: 262–267.

Rozycki G, Ochsner MG, Feliciano D, et al. Early detection of hemoperitoneum by ultrasound examination of the right upper quadrant: a multicenter study. J Trauma 1998;45:878–883.

Sutyak JP, Chiu WC, D'Amelio LF, et al. Computed tomography is inaccurate in estimating the severity of adult splenic injury. J Trauma 1995;39:514–518.

Wisner DH. History and current status of trauma scoring systems. Arch Surg 1992;127:111–117.

32

Evaluation and Management of Traumatic Brain Injury

Scott R. Shepard

Objectives

1. To describe the physiology of intracranial pressure (ICP) and cerebral perfusion pressure (CPP).
2. To understand the effects of blood pressure, ventilatory status, and fluid balance on ICP and CPP.
3. To describe the evaluation and management of different types of head injury.

Case

A 22-year-old man is brought to the emergency room following a high-speed motorcycle accident. The paramedics report that the patient struck a tree and that there was a 5-minute loss of consciousness. On arrival, the patient has the following vital signs: respiratory rate, 12; blood pressure, 150/75; heart rate, 92. He opens his eyes to painful stimuli, follows simple commands, and answers questions with inappropriate words.

Introduction

Traumatic brain injury (TBI) continues to be a major public health problem despite the technologic revolution in medicine. The annual incidence of TBI has been estimated to be approximately 200 cases per 100,000 persons in the United States (550,000 annually in the U.S.). The majority of head injuries (80%) are mild head injuries, with the remainder divided equally between moderate and severe head injuries. The majority of those with severe TBI and many of those with moderate TBI are disabled permanently, resulting in an annual expenditure in the U.S. of $25 billion to cover the care of these individuals.

Table 32.1. Glasgow Coma Scale (GCS).

Eye opening (E)	Motor response (M)	Verbal response (V)
Spontaneous (4)	Follows commands (6)	Oriented (5)
To voice (3)	Localizes (5)	Confused (4)
To painful stimuli (2)	Withdraws (4)	Inappropriate words (3)
None (1)	Abnormal flexion (3)	Moaning (2)
	Extension (2)	None (1)
	None (1)	
GCS = E + M + V		

Source: Reprinted from Gustilo RB, Anderson JT. Prevention of infection in the treatment of 1025 open fractures of long bones. J Bone Joint Surg 1976; 58(A), 453, with permission.

Initial Evaluation

Initial Systemic Trauma Evaluation, Focused Head Injury Evaluation, and Neurologic Assessment

The primary evaluation of the TBI patient involves a thorough **systemic trauma evaluation** according to the Advanced Trauma Life Support (ATLS) guidelines. After completion of the initial trauma evaluation and if the patient is hemodynamically stable, a **focused head injury evaluation** should be initiated. It is important to attempt to obtain a **thorough history** of the mechanism of the trauma as well as of the events immediately preceding the trauma, because specific information, such as the occurrence of syncope prior to the accident, necessitates an evaluation for the etiology of such an event.

After a sufficient history has been obtained, the **neurologic assessment** begins. The first part of the neurologic evaluation is the **Glasgow Coma Scale (GCS) (Table 32.1). Although the GCS is part of the initial trauma evaluation, it should be repeated periodically to assess for neurologic deterioration.** The GCS was developed by Teasdale and Jennett[1] and is used to describe the general level of consciousness of TBI patients as well as to define the severity of head injuries. It is important to remember that the GCS is a screening exam and does not substitute for a thorough neurologic exam. The GCS is divided into three categories: **eye opening (E)**, **motor response (M)**, and **verbal response (V)**. The score is determined by the sum of the score in each of the three categories, with a maximum score of 15 and a minimum score of 3. Since patients who are intubated cannot be assessed for a verbal response, they are evaluated only with eye opening and motor scores, and the suffix "T" is added to their GCS to indicate that they are intubated. Mild head injuries are defined as TBI patients with a GCS of 13 to 15, and moderate head injuries are defined as those with a GCS of 9 to 12. A GCS of 8 or less defines a severe head injury. These definitions are not rigid and should be considered as a general guide to the level of injury. In the case presented above, the patient's eye opens to stimuli (E = 2), and the patient follows simple commands (M = 6) and uses inappropriate words (V = 3), resulting in a GCS of 11 (2 + 6 + 3).

---

[1] Teasdale G, Jennett B. Assessment of coma and impaired consciousnes. A practical scale. Lancet 1974;2:81–84.

The neurologic assessment of the TBI patient should include a complete brainstem exam (pupillary exam, ocular movement exam, corneal reflex, gag reflex), a motor exam, and a sensory exam. Many TBI patients have significant alterations of consciousness and/or pharmaceuticals present that will limit the neurologic exam.

Brainstem Exam

Pupillary Exam: A careful **pupillary exam** is an essential part of the evaluation of the TBI patient, especially in patients with severe injuries. When muscle relaxants have been administered to a patient, only the pupillary exam is available for evaluation. Several factors can alter the pupillary exam. Narcotics cause pupillary constriction, and medications or drugs that have sympathomimetic properties cause pupillary dilation. These effects often are strong enough to blunt or nearly eliminate pupillary responses. Prior eye surgery, such as cataract surgery, also can alter or eliminate pupillary reactivity.

A normal pupillary exam consists of bilaterally reactive pupils that react to both direct and consensual stimuli. Bilateral, small pupils may be caused by narcotics or pontine injury (disruption of sympathetic centers in the pons). Bilateral fixed and dilated pupils are secondary to diffuse cerebral hypoxia, which may result from either severe elevations of ICP, preventing adequate blood flow to the brain, or diffuse systemic hypoxia. A unilateral fixed (unresponsive) and dilated pupil has two potential causes. If the pupil does not constrict when light is directed at the pupil but constricts when light is directed into the contralateral pupil (intact consensual response), this usually is the result of a traumatic optic nerve injury. If a unilateral dilated pupil does not respond to either direct or consensual stimulation, this usually is a sign of transtentorial herniation. Unilateral pupillary constriction usually is secondary to Horner's syndrome, in which the sympathetic input to the eye is disrupted. Horner's syndrome may be caused by a disruption of the sympathetic system, either at the apex of the lung or adjacent to the carotid artery.

Ocular Movement Exam: When there is a significant alteration in the level of consciousness, there often is a loss of voluntary eye movement, and abnormalities in ocular movements may occur. Ocular movements involve the coordination of multiple centers within the brain, including the frontal eye fields, the parapontine reticular formation (PPRF), the medial longitudinal fasciculus (MLF), and the III and VI cranial nerve nuclei. When voluntary eye movements cannot be assessed, **oculocephalic and oculovestibular testing** may be performed.

Oculocephalic testing (doll's eyes) assesses the integrity of the horizontal gaze centers and involves observation of eye movements when the head is rotated rapidly from side to side. This maneuver is contraindicated in any patient with a known or suspected cervical spine injury. Oculocephalic testing is performed by elevating the head 30 degrees and briskly rotating it from side to side. A normal response is for the eyes to rotate away from the direction of the movement as if they are fixating on a target that is straight ahead, similar to the way a doll's eyes move when its head is turned. If the eyes remain fixed in position and do not rotate, this is indicative of dysfunction in the lateral gaze centers and is referred to as negative doll's eyes.

Oculovestibular testing (cold water calorics) is another method for the assessment of the integrity of the gaze centers. Oculovestibular testing is performed with the head elevated to 30 degrees and requires the presence of an intact tympanic membrane. In oculovestibular testing, ice-cold water slowly is instilled into the external auditory canal. This causes an imbalance in the vestibular signals and initiates a compensatory response. Cold water irrigation in the ear of an alert patient results in a fast nystagmus away from the irrigated ear and a slow, compensatory nystagmus toward the irrigated side. If warm water is used, the opposite will occur. This is the basis for the acronym **COWS** (cold—opposite, warm—same) and refers to the direction of the fast component of nystagmus. As the level of consciousness declines, the fast component of nystagmus gradually fades, and, in the unconscious patient, only the slow phase of nystagmus is present. If there is a normal oculocephalic response to cold water calorics (eye deviation toward the side of irrigation), this indicates that the injury is rostral to the upper brainstem and that the PPRF, the MLF, and third and sixth cranial nerve nuclei are intact.

Corneal Reflex and Gag Reflex: The **corneal reflex** is assessed by gently stroking the cornea with a soft wisp of cotton. The normal response is a single blink on the side of stimulation. The corneal reflex is mediated by the fifth and seventh cranial nerves, and intact corneal reflexes indicate integrity of the pons. The **gag reflex**, in which gentle stimulation of the posterior oropharynx results in elevation of the soft palate, assesses the integrity of the lower brainstem (medulla).

Motor Exam and Sensory Exam

After the brainstem exam has been completed, a **motor exam and a sensory exam** should be performed. A thorough motor or sensory exam is difficult to perform in any patient with an altered level of consciousness. When a patient is not alert enough to cooperate with strength testing, the motor exam is limited to an assessment for asymmetry. This may be demonstrated by an asymmetric response to central pain stimulation or a difference in muscle tone between the left and right side. If there is asymmetry in the motor exam, this may be indicative of a hemispheric injury and may raise the suspicion for a mass lesion. It often is difficult to perform a useful sensory exam in the TBI patient. Patients with altered levels of consciousness are unable to cooperate with sensory testing, and a sensory exam may not be reliable in intoxicated or comatose patients.

Diagnostic Evaluation

After the patient has been stabilized and an appropriate neurologic exam has been performed, the diagnostic evaluation may begin.

Radiographic Evaluation

X-Rays

Skull x-rays rarely are used today in the evaluation of closed head injury. They occasionally are used in the evaluation of penetrating head trauma and can provide a rapid assessment of the degree of foreign-body penetration in nonmissile penetrating head injuries (e.g., stab wounds).

Computed Tomography

Computed tomography (CT) scan is the diagnostic study of choice in the evaluation of TBI because it has a rapid acquisition time, it is universally available, and it accurately demonstrates acute hemorrhage.

The subject in the case presentation would undergo a head CT scanning during his evaluation. The standard CT scan for the evaluation of acute head injury is a noncontrast scan with three data sets: bone windows, tissue windows, and subdural windows. The bone windows provide a survey of bony anatomy, and the tissue windows allow for a detailed survey of the brain and its contents. The subdural windows provide better visualization of intracranial hemorrhage. **Table 32.2**

Table 32.2. Checklist for interpreting a trauma head computed tomography (CT) scan: features to examine.

Soft tissue windows: start inferiorly and work up to the vertex
  1. **Fourth ventricle: is it shifted? compressed? blood in it?**
  2. **Cerebellum: bleed or infarct?**
  3. **Brainstem cisterns obliterated? check the quadrigeminal and ambient cisterns**
  4. **Check lateral ventricles for blood (especially in occipital horns), size (especially temporal horns), and mass effect**
  5. **Extraaxial blood: EDH is lens-shaped, does not cross sutures; SDH crosses sutures; SAH channels into sulci and fissures; measure maximum thickness of clot in millimeters; check circle of Willis, sylvian fissure for SAH**
  6. **Look for intraparenchymal hematomas and contusions, especially frontal and temporal tips, inferior frontal lobes, and under any fractures (measure clot thickness in mm)**
  7. **Measure midline shift in millimeters at level of septum pellucidum**
  8. **Check top cuts for effacement of sulci, often a subtle sign of mass effect**

Bone windows
  1. **Check five sets of sinuses (ethmoid, sphenoid, frontal, mastoid, maxillary) for fracture or opacification; the maxillary sinuses may only be partially seen on standard head cuts**
  2. **Look for fracture of orbital apex (? CN II compression), petrous temporal bone (? basilar skull fracture), or convexities (if depressed, is it more than a table's width? measure the depression in mm)**
  3. **Check for intracranial or intraorbital air; this is much easier to see on bone windows than soft tissue windows**

CN, cranial nerve; EDH, extradural hematoma; SAH, subarachnoid hemorrhage; SDH, subdural hematoma.
Source: Reprinted from Starr P. Neurosurgery. In: Norton JA, Bollinger RR, Chang AE, et al, eds. Surgery: Basic Science and Clinical Evidence. New York: Springer-Verlag, 2001, with permission.

Table 32.3. CT classification of head injury.

Injury level	Midline shift	Basal CSF cisterns	Hematoma or contusions
I	None	Cisterns widely patent	Minimal, if any
II	Not present or shift	Cisterns widely patent	No lesion with volume >25 mL
III	Shift < 5 mm	Partial compression or absent	No lesion with volume >25 mL
IV	Shift > 5 mm	Partial compression or absent	No lesion with volume >25 mL

CSF, cerebrospinal fluid.

provides a suggested checklist for the evaluation of the head CT in a TBI patient.

It is important to use a systemic approach when reviewing a CT scan and to follow the same protocol each time. Consistency is much more important than the specific order used. First, the bone windows should be examined for fractures, beginning with the cranial vault itself, and then the skull base and the facial bones should be examined. Next, the tissue windows should be examined for the presence of any of the following: extraaxial hematomas (e.g., epidural or subdural hematomas), intraparenchymal hematomas, or contusions. Next, the brain should be surveyed for any evidence of pneumocephalus, hydrocephalus, cerebral edema, midline shift, or compression of the subarachnoid cisterns at the base of the brain. Finally, the subdural windows should be examined for any hemorrhage that may not be visualized easily on the tissue windows.

Computed tomography scans may be used for classification as well as for diagnostic purposes. There is a classification scheme published by Marshall et al[2] that classifies head injuries according to the changes demonstrated by CT scan. This system defines four categories of injury, from diffuse injury I to diffuse injury IV (**Table 32.3**). These levels of injury are based on the presence of three different abnormalities— midline shift, patency of cerebrospinal fluid (CSF) cisterns at the base of the brain, and presence of a contusion or a hematoma—seen on the CT scan.

Skull Fractures: Skull fractures are classified as either nondisplaced (linear) fractures or comminuted fractures. Linear skull fractures sometimes are difficult to visualize on the individual axial images of a CT scan. The scout film of the CT scan, which is the equivalent of a lateral skull x-ray, often demonstates linear fractures, which may be difficult to appreciate on the axial views of a CT scan. Comminuted fractures are complex fractures with multiple components. A comminuted fracture may be displaced inward, which is defined as a depressed skull fracture.

Intracranial Hemorrhages: Intracranial hemorrhages are divided into two broad categories: **extraaxial hematomas** and **intraaxial hematomas (Table 32.4)**. On CT, acute hemorrhage is hyperintense when compared with the brain and usually appears as a bright white signal.

[2] Marshall LF, Marshall SB, Klauber MR. A new classification of head injury based on computerized tomography. J Neurosurg 1991;75:S14–S20.

Table 32.4. Intracranial hemorrhages.

Intraaxial hematomas	Extraaxial hematomas
Intracerebral hematoma	Epidural hematoma
Subarachnoid hemorrhage	Subdural hematoma
Cerebral contusion	

Extraaxial hematomas include **epidural and subdural hematomas**. **Epidural hematomas** are located between the inner table of the skull and the dura. They typically are biconvex in shape because their outer border follows the inner table of the skull, and their inner border is limited by locations where the dura is firmly adherent to the skull (**Fig. 32.1**). Epidural hematomas usually are caused by injury to a dural-based artery, although 10% of epidurals may be venous in origin. Epidural hematomas, especially those of arterial origin, may enlarge rapidly. **Subdural hematomas** are located between the dura and the brain. Their outer edge is convex, while their inner border usually is irregularly concave (**Fig. 32.2**). Subdural hematomas are not limited by the intracranial suture lines, and this is an important feature that aids in their differentiation from epidural hematomas. Subdural hematomas usually are venous in origin, although some are due to arterial bleeding.

Intraaxial hematomas are defined as hemorrhages within the brain parenchyma. These hematomas include **intraparenchymal**

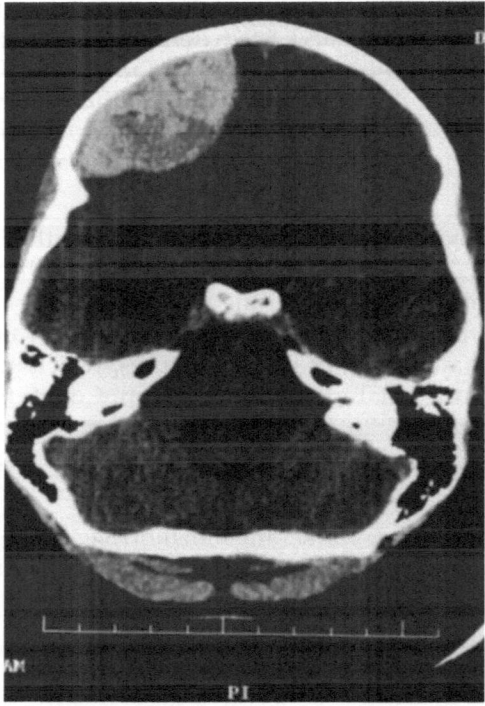

Figure 32.1. Computed tomography (CT) of epidural hematoma.

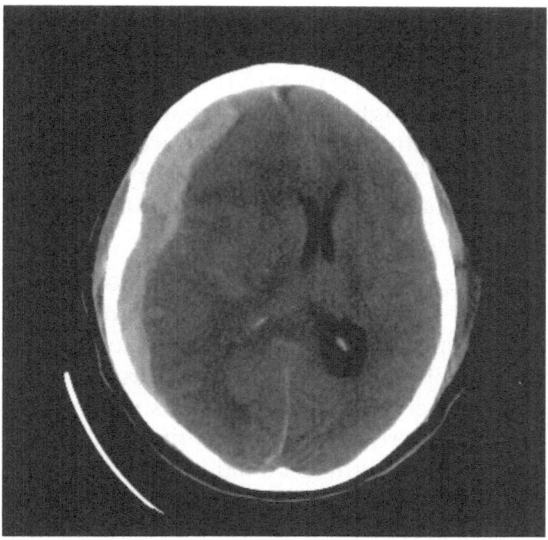

Figure 32.2. CT of subdural hematoma.

hematomas, cerebral contusions intraventricular hemorrhages, and subarachnoid hemorrhages. Intraparenchymal hemorrhages are homogeneous regions of hyperintense signal on CT (Fig. 32.3). Cerebral contusions are posttraumatic lesions in the brain that appear as irregular, heterogeneous regions in which hyperintense changes (blood) and low-density changes (edema) are intermixed (Fig. 32.4).

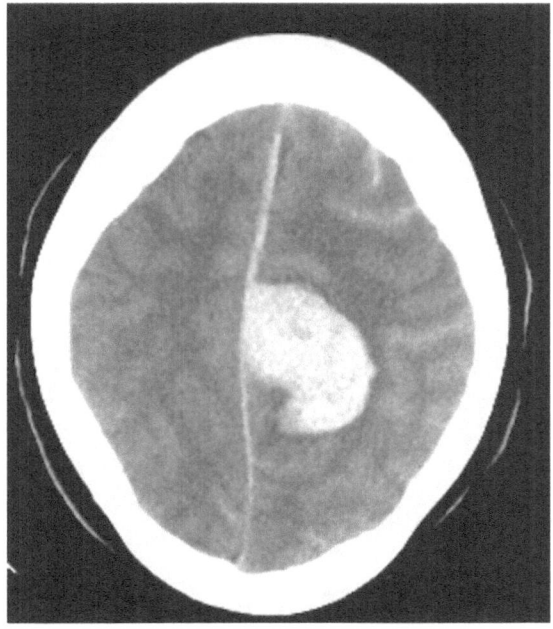

Figure 32.3. CT of intraparenchymal hematoma.

Intraventricular hemorrhages are regions of high intensity within the ventricular system. **Subarachnoid hemorrhages** that occur as a result of trauma typically are located over gyri on the convexity of the brain. These are thin layers of high-intensity signal located on the surface of the cortex. They are distinct from the subarachnoid hemorrhages that occur as the result of a ruptured cerebral aneurysm, which usually are located in the arachnoid cisterns at the base of the brain.

Magnetic Resonance Imaging
Magnetic resonance imaging (MRI) has a limited role in the evaluation of acute head injury. Although MRI provides extraordinary anatomic detail, it commonly is not used to evaluate acute TBI. This is due to its long acquisition time and the difficulty of using it in the critically ill. **It may be used to evaluate patients with unexplained neurologic deficits.** It is superior to CT for identifying diffuse axonal injury (DAI) and small strokes. Diffuse axonal injury is defined as neuronal injury in the subcortical gray matter or the brainstem as a result of severe rotation or deceleration. It often is the explanation for a depressed level of consciousness in a patient with normal intracranial pressure and without evidence of significant injury on CT scan. Magnetic resonance angiography may be used in some TBI patients to assess for vascular injury.

Angiography
Prior to the development of CT, **cerebral angiography** was used to demonstrate the presence of an intracranial mass lesion. **Currently, angiography is used in acute head injury only when there is the suspicion of a vascular injury.** This includes patients with evidence of a

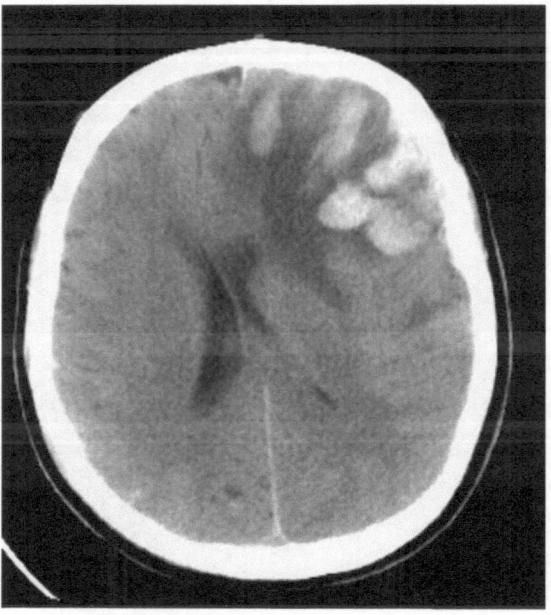

Figure 32.4. CT of cerebral contusion.

Table 32.5. Relative volume of intracranial components.

Brain	85% to 90%
Intravascular blood	8% to 10%
CSF	2% to 3%

potential carotid injury (hemiparesis without a significant hematoma or the presence of Horner's syndrome) and patients with temporal bone fractures that traverse the carotid canal.

Pathophysiology

Intracranial Compliance

Appropriate management of TBI requires an appreciation of some of the anatomic features of the brain. The brain floats in CSF within the skull, a rigid and inelastic container. The skull cannot expand to accommodate any increases in volume of the brain, thus, only small increases in cerebral volume can be tolerated before ICP begins to rise dramatically. This concept is defined by the **Monro-Kellie doctrine**, which states that the total intracranial volume is fixed.[3] The intracranial volume (V i/c) is equal to the sum of its components: **V i/c = V (brain) + V (CSF) + V (blood)**. The brain comprises 85% to 90% of the intracranial volume, while intravascular cerebral blood volume accounts for 8% to 10% and CSF accounts for the remainder, 2% to 3% (**Table 32.5**). When cerebral edema is present, it increases the relative volume of the brain. Since the intracranial volume is fixed, unless there is some compensatory action, such as a decrease in the volume of one of the other intracranial components, the intracranial pressure will rise. This is related intimately to intracranial compliance, which is defined as the change in pressure due to changes in volume. The brain has very limited compliance and cannot tolerate significant increases in volume that can result from diffuse cerebral edema or significant mass lesions, such as a hematoma. Individual treatments for elevated ICP are designed to decrease the volume of one of the intracranial components, thereby improving compliance and decreasing ICP.

Cerebral Perfusion Pressure

A second crucial concept in TBI pathophysiology is the concept of **cerebral perfusion pressure (CPP)**, which is defined as the difference between the mean arterial pressure (MAP) and the ICP: **CPP = MAP − ICP**. In the noninjured brain, cerebral blood flow (CBF) is constant in the range of CPP between 50 and 150 mm Hg due to autoregulation by the arterioles. When the CPP is less than 50 mm Hg or greater than 150 mm Hg, the autoregulation is overcome, and blood flow becomes

[3] Chestnut RM, Marshall LF. Treatment of abnormal intracranial pressure. Neurosurg Clin North Am 1991;2(2):267–284.

entirely dependent on the CPP, a situation defined as pressure passive perfusion. In pressure passive perfusion, the CBF is no longer constant but proportional to the CPP. Thus, when the CPP falls below 50 mm HG, the brain is at risk of ischemia due to insufficient blood flow. Autoregulation also is impaired in the injured brain, and, as a result, there is pressure passive perfusion within and around injured regions of the brain.

Herniation

Elevated ICP is deleterious because it can decrease CPP and CBF, which may result in cerebral ischemia. Also, uncontrolled ICP may result in **herniation**, a process that involves the movement of a region of the brain across fixed dural structures, resulting in irreversible and often fatal cerebral injury. The intracranial compartment is divided into three compartments by two major dural structures, the falx cerebri and the tentorium cerebelli. When there is a significant increase in ICP or a large mass lesion is present, the brain may be displaced across the edge of the falx or the tentorium, a phenomenon known as herniation. As the brain slides over these dural edges, it compresses other regions of the brain (e.g., the brainstem) and cause neurologic injury. There are five types of herniation: **transtentorial herniation, subfalcine herniation, central herniation, cerebellar herniation**, and **tonsillar herniation**. **Transtentorial herniation** occurs when the medial aspect of the temporal lobe (uncus) migrates across the free edge of the tentorium. This compresses the third cranial nerve, interrupting parasympathetic input to the eye and resulting in a dilated pupil. This unilateral dilated pupil is the classic sign of transtentorial herniation and usually (80%) occurs ipsilateral to the side of the transtentorial herniation. The changes that occur in the other types of herniation are listed in **Table 32.6.**

Treatment

The treatment of TBI may be divided into **the treatment of closed head injury and the treatment of penetrating head injury.** While there is significant overlap in the treatment of these two types of injury, there are some important differences that are discussed later in this chapter. Closed head injury treatment is divided further into the treatment of mild and moderate/severe head injuries. See **Algorithm 32.1** for initial management of the traumatic brain injury patient.

Table 32.6. Herniation syndromes.

Herniation syndrome	Mechanism
Transtentorial herniation	Medial temporal lobe is displaced across the tentorial edge
Subfalcine herniation	Medial frontal lobe is displaced under the falx
Central (downward) herniation	Cerebral hemisphere(s) is displaced down through the tentorial incisura
Cerebellar (upward) herniation	Cerebellum is displaced up through the tentorial incisura
Tonsillar herniation	Cerebellar tonsils are displaced through the foramen magnum

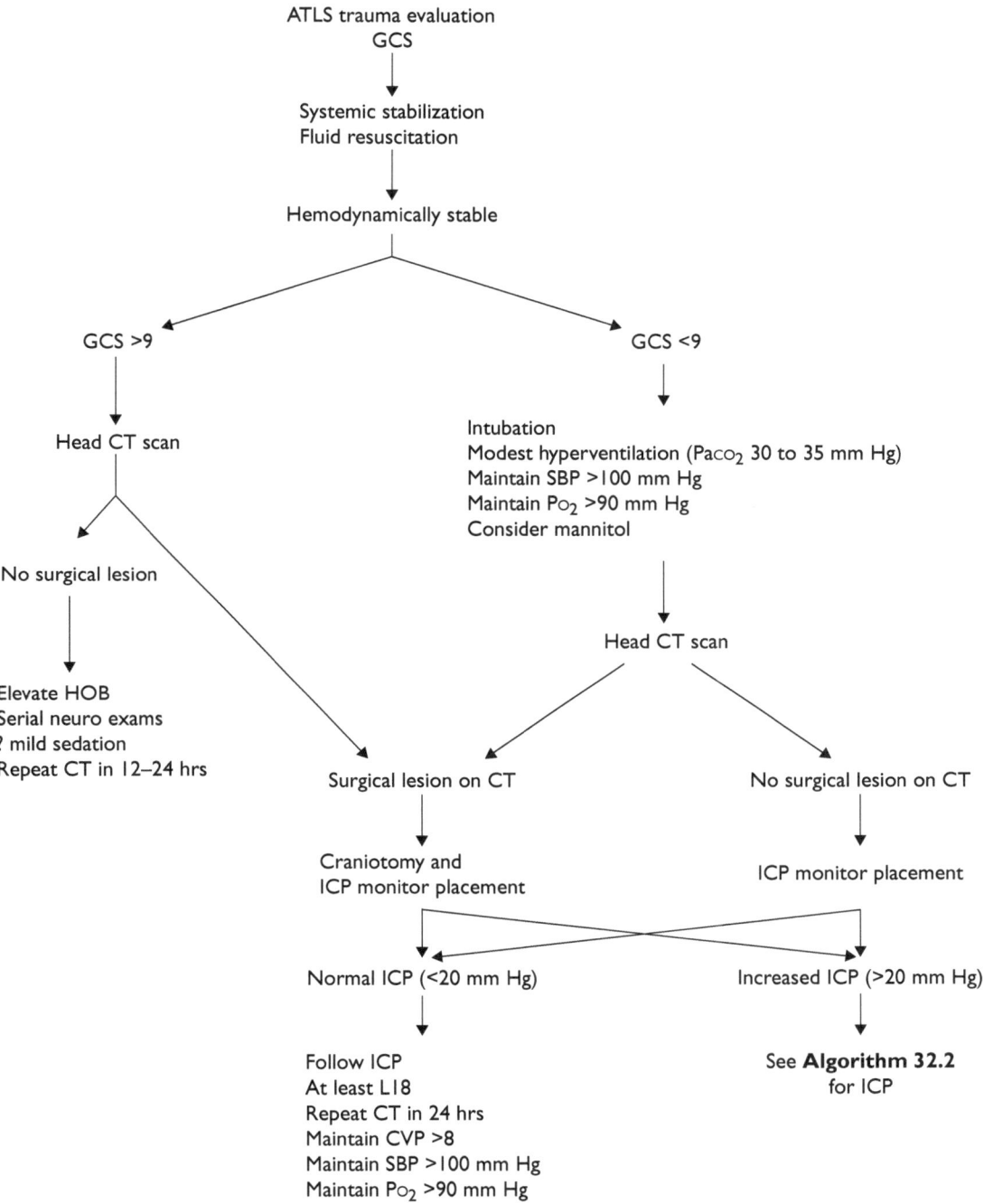

Algorithm 32.1. Initial management of the traumatic brain injury patient. ATLS, Advanced Trauma Life Support; CT, computed tomography; GCS, Glasgow Coma Scale; HOB, head of bed; ICP, intracranial pressure; SBP, systolic blood pressure. Reprinted from Bullock R, Chestnut R, Clifton G, et al. Guidelines for the management of severe head injury. Brain Trauma Foundation, American Association of Neurological Surgeons, Joint Section on Neurotrauma and Critical Care. J Neurotrauma 1996 Nov; 13(11):641–734. Copyright © 1995, Brain Trauma Foundation. With permission of Mary Ann Leibert, Inc., Publishers.

Closed Head Injury

Mild Head Injury Treatment

The majority of head injuries are **mild head injuries**. Most people presenting with mild head injuries do not have any progression of their head injury; however, up to 3% of mild head injuries progress to more serious injuries.

Patients with mild to moderate headaches, dizziness, and nausea are considered to have a low-risk injury. Most of these patients require only observation after they have been assessed carefully, and many do not require radiographic evaluation. These patients may be discharged if there is a reliable individual to monitor them at home. After a mild head injury, those displaying persistent emesis, severe headache, anterograde amnesia, loss of consciousness, or signs of intoxication by drugs or alcohol should be evaluated with a head CT scan.

Patients with mild head injuries typically have concussions. A **concussion** is defined as physiologic injury to the brain without any evidence of structural alteration, as in the case presented. Loss of consciousness frequently occurs in concussions, but it is not part of the definition of concussion. Concussions may be graded on a scale of I to V based on criteria such as length of confusion, type of amnesia following the event, and length of loss of consciousness (**Table 32.7**).

As many as 30% of patients who experience a concussion develop a **postconcussive syndrome (PCS)**, which occurs when there is a persistence of any combination of the following after a head injury: headache, nausea, emesis, memory loss, dizziness, diplopia, blurred vision, emotional lability, and sleep disturbances. The PCS may last between 2 weeks and 6 months. Typically, the symptoms peak from 4 to 6 weeks following the injury. On occasion, the symptoms of PCS last for a year or longer, and some patients are disabled permanently by PCS.

Moderate and Severe Head Injury Treatment

The treatment of **moderate and severe head injuries** begins with initial cardiopulmonary stabilization by ATLS guidelines. **The initial resuscitation of a head-injured patient is of critical importance to prevent hypoxia and hypotension.** Analysis of the Traumatic Coma Data Bank, a database of 753 severe head injury patients, revealed that TBI patients who presented to the hospital with hypotension had twice the

Table 32.7. Classification of concussion.

Concussion Grade	Confusion or disorientation	Type of amnesia	Loss of consciousness
I	Transient	None	None
II	Brief	Anterograde	None
III	Prolonged	Retrograde	<5 minutes
IV	Prolonged	Retrograde	5 to 10 minutes
V	Prolonged	Retrograde	>10 minutes

Table 32.8. Surgical indications in nonpenetrating head trauma.

Subdural/epidural hematoma resulting in midline shift >5 mm
Intracerebral hematoma >30 cc
Temporal or cerebellar hematoma with diameter >3 cm
Open skull fracture
Skull fracture with displacement >1 cm

mortality rate of those patients who were normotensive on presentation[4]. The combination of hypoxia and hypotension resulted in a mortality rate two-and-one-half times greater than if both of these factors were absent. After **initial stabilization** and assessment of the GCS, a **neurologic exam** as described earlier should be performed.

After a thorough neurologic assessment has been performed, a **CT scan of the head** is obtained. If there is a surgical lesion present, then arrangements are made for immediate transport to the operating room. Although there are no strict guidelines for defining surgical lesions in head injury, most neurosurgeons consider any of the following to represent **indications for surgery** in the head-injured patient: extraaxial hematoma with midline shift greater than 5 mm, intraaxial hematoma with volume >30 cc, an open skull fracture, or a depressed skull fracture with more than 1 cm of inward displacement (**Table 32.8**). Also, any temporal or cerebellar hematoma that is greater than 3 cm in diameter usually is evacuated prophylactically because these regions of the brain do not tolerate additional mass as well as other regions of the brain.

If there is no surgical lesion present on the CT scan, or following surgery if one is present, **medical treatment** of the head injury begins. The first phase of treatment is to institute general supportive measures. After appropriate fluid resuscitation has been completed, intravenous fluids are administered to maintain the patient in a state of euvolemia or mild hypervolemia. A previous tenet of head injury treatment was fluid restriction, which was thought to limit the development of cerebral edema and increased ICP. Fluid restriction decreases intravascular volume and decreases cardiac output. A decrease in cardiac output often results in decreased cerebral flow, which results in decreased brain perfusion and may cause an increase in cerebral edema and ICP. Thus, **fluid restriction is contraindicated in the TBI patient**.

Another supportive measure used to treat TBI patients is **elevation of the head**. When the head of the bed is elevated to 30 degrees, the venous outflow from the brain is improved, and this helps to reduce ICP. If a patient is hypovolemic, elevation of the head may cause a drop in cardiac output and cerebral blood flow. Therefore, the head of the bed is not elevated in hypovolemic patients. Also, the head should not be elevated in patients in whom a spine injury is suspected or until an unstable spine has been stabilized.

---

[4] Marshall LF, Gautille T, Klauber M, et al. The outcome of severe closed head injury. Neurosurgery 75:S28–S36, 1991.

Table 32.9. Indications for ICP Monitoring in TBI Patients.

GCS < 9
Patient requiring prolonged deep sedation or muscle relaxants
TBI patient undergoing prolonged general anesthesia

GCS, Glasgow Coma Scale; ICP, intracranial pressure; TBI, traumatic brain injury.

Sedation often is necessary in TBI patients. Some patients with head injuries are significantly agitated and require sedation. Also, patients with multisystem trauma often have painful systemic injuries that require analgesics, and most intubated patients require sedation. Short-acting sedatives and analgesics should be used to accomplish proper sedation without eliminating the ability to perform periodic neurologic assessments. This requires careful titration of medication doses and periodic weaning or withholding of sedation to allow for neurologic assessment.

The use of **anticonvulsants** in TBI is a controversial issue. There is no evidence that the use of anticonvulsants decreases the incidence of late-onset seizures in patients with either closed head injury or traumatic brain injury. Temkin et al[5] demonstrated that the routine use of Dilantin in the first week following TBI decreases the incidence of early-onset (within 7 days of injury) seizures, but it does not change the incidence of late-onset seizures. Also, the prevention of early post-traumatic seizures does not improve the outcome following TBI. Therefore, the prophylactic use of anticonvulsants is not recommended for more than 7 days following TBI and is considered optional in the first week following TBI.

Intracranial Pressure Monitoring: After general supportive measures have been instituted, the issue of ICP is addressed. Intracranial pressure monitoring consistently has been shown to improve outcome in head-injured patients. It is indicated for any patient with a GCS <9 or for any patient in whom serial neurologic examinations cannot be performed (e.g., any patient with a head injury who requires prolonged deep sedation/pharmacologic relaxants or any head injury patient undergoing extended general anesthesia) (**Table 32.9**).

Intracranial pressure monitoring involves the placement of an invasive probe. Intracranial pressure may be monitored by means of an **intraparenchymal monitor or an intraventricular monitor (ventriculostomy)**. **Intraparenchymal ICP monitors** are devices that are placed into the brain parenchyma and measure ICP by means of fiberoptics, strain gauge, or other technologies. These monitors are very accurate; however, they do not allow for drainage of CSF. A **ventriculosotomy** is a catheter placed into the lateral ventricle through a small twist drill hole in the skull. The ICP is then measured by transducing the pressure in a fluid column. Ventriculostomies allow for the drainage of CSF, which can be effective in decreasing the ICP.

[5] Temkin NR, Dikmen SS, Wilensky AJ, et al. A randomized, double-blind study of phenytoin for the prevention of post-traumatic seizures. N Engl J Med 1990;323(8): 497–502.

Once an ICP monitor has been placed, ICP is monitored continuously. The normal range of ICP in the adult is 0 to 20 mm Hg. The normal ICP waveform is a triphasic wave in which the first peak is the largest peak and the second and third peaks progressively are smaller. When intracranial compliance is abnormal, the second peak becomes larger than the first peak. Also, when intracranial compliance is abnormal, pathologic waves may appear. Lundberg et al[6] described three types of abnormal ICP waves: A, B, and C. Lundberg A waves (plateau waves) have a duration of between 5 and 20 minutes and an amplitude up to 50 mm Hg over the baseline ICP. After an A wave dissipates, the ICP is reset to a baseline level that is higher than when the wave began. Lundberg A waves are a sign of severely compromised intracranial compliance. The rapid increase in ICP caused by these waves can result in a significant decrease in CPP and may lead to herniation. Lundberg B and C waves have a shorter duration and a lower amplitude than A waves, and, as a result, these waves are not as deleterious as A waves.

Treatment of Increased ICP: The goal of treatment of increased ICP is to optimize conditions within the brain to prevent secondary injury. Maintaining ICP within the normal range is part of an approach designed to optimize both CBF and the metabolic state of the brain. There are many potential interventions used to lower ICP, and each of these is designed to improve **intracranial compliance**, which results in improved CBF, increased CPP, and decreased ICP. The **Monro-Kellie doctrine** provides the framework for understanding and organizing the various treatments for elevated ICP.[7] In the TBI patient with increased ICP, the volume of one of the three components of intracranial volume must be reduced in order to improve intracranial compliance and decrease ICP. If there is an intracranial mass lesion greater than 30 cc in volume, it should be evacuated prior to initiating treatment of increased ICP. The discussion of the different treatments for elevated ICP will be organized according to which component of intracranial volume they affect. **Algorithm 32.2** provides an overview of the treatment of increased intracranial pressure.

Management of elevated ICP involves using a combination of some of the treatments. Although there are no rigid protocols for the treatment of head injury, there are many algorithms published that provide treatment schema. The American Association of Neurologic Surgeons published a comprehensive evidence-based review of the treatment of traumatic brain injury called the **Guidelines for the Management of Severe Head Injury**.[8] In these guidelines, there are three different categories of treatments: standards, guidelines, and options (**Table 32.10**).

---

[6] Lundberg N, Troup H, Lorin H. Continuous recording of ventricular pressure in patients with severe acute traumatic brain injury. J Neurosurg 1965;22:581–590.
[7] Chestnut RM, Marshall LF. Treatment of abnormal intracranial pressure. Neurosurg Clin North Am 1991;2(2):267–284.
[8] Bullock R, Chestnut R, Clifton G, et al. Guidelines for the management of severe head injury. Brain Trauma Foundation, American Association of Neurological Surgeons, Joint Section on Neurotrauma and Critical Care. J Neurotrauma 1996;13(11):641–734.

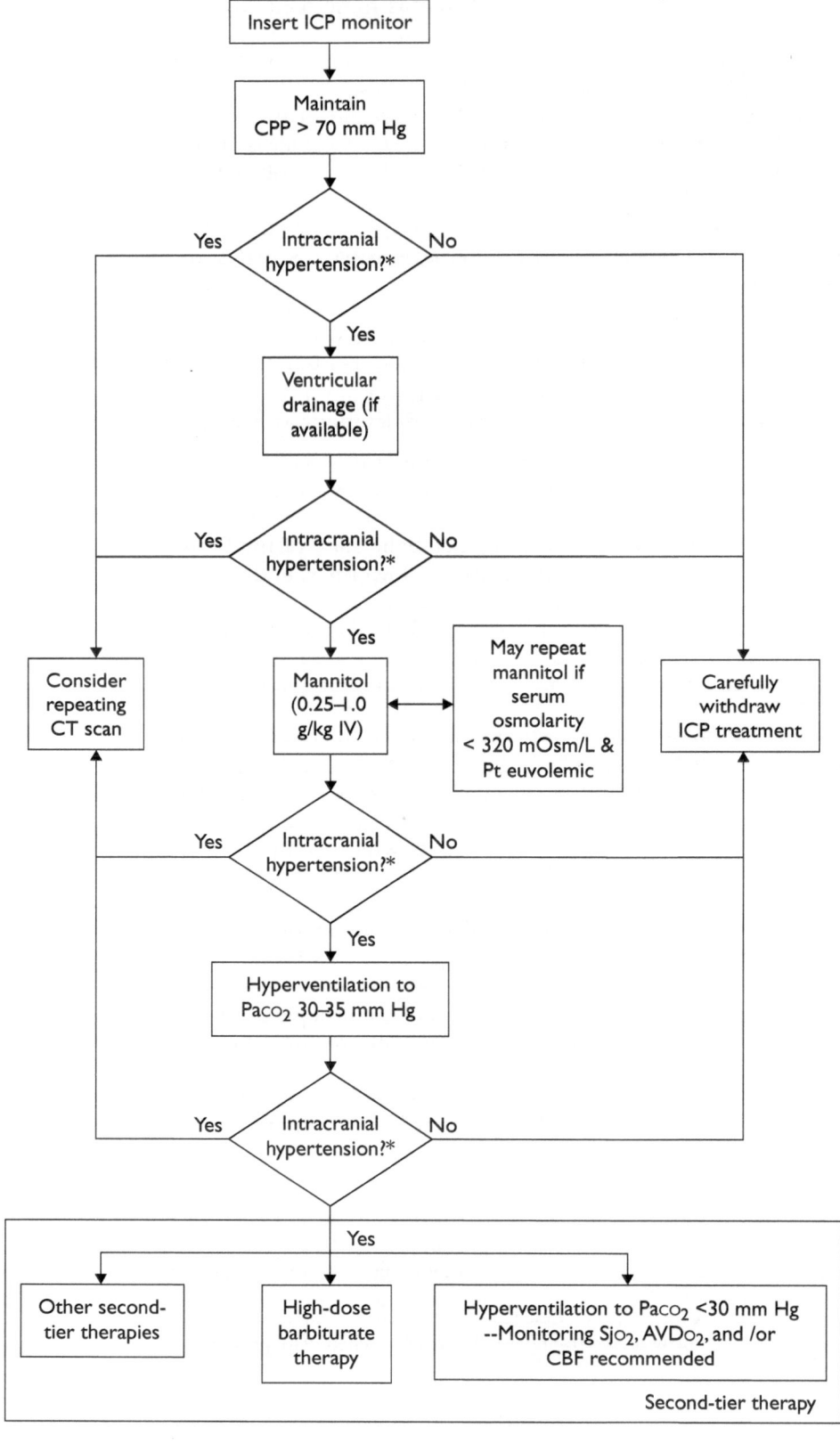

Table 32.10. Techniques for controlling elevated intracranial pressure (ICP) (level II and level III evidence).

Technique	Description	Level of evidence
Surgical evacuation of mass lesions	When a mass lesion is >30 mL and is surgically accessible, craniotomy for removal will contribute to ICP control	III
Head elevation	The head should be elevated to 30 degrees or greater, slightly extended, and not rotated	III
Optimize venous drainage	Loosen devices that constrict venous return in the neck, such as a cervical collar or an excessively tight tie, for the endotracheal tube	III
Intravenous mannitol	Osmotic diuretics such as mannitol may be given to keep serum osmolarity at 290–310 mOsm/dL; diuresis beyond 320 mOsm/dL is counterproductive as it diminishes cerebral perfusion and may cause renal failure	II[a]
CSF drainage	Drainage performed by ventriculostomy, *not* by spinal tap or spinal drain; may be impractical when ventricles are very small; increasingly performed, but not yet convincingly supported by class I evidence	II[b]
Sedation	Indicated for patients with elevated ICP who are agitated and straining against mechanical ventilation; may use 2% propofol infusion; shown to lower ICP (day 3) in comparison with controls; increasingly performed, but not yet convincingly supported by class I evidence	II[a]
Mild temporary hyperventilation	For temporary control of elevated ICP, mild reduction of PCO_2 to 30–35 may be useful; however, randomized studies have shown that long-term or aggressive hyperventilation is harmful because it lowers cerebral perfusion, and efficacy of mild temporary hyperventilation for improved outcomes has not been demonstrated	III[b]
Pentobarbital coma	Load 10 mg/kg over 30 min, then 5 mg/kg q 1 h for 3 doses, then 1 mg/kg/h; titrate to keep serum pentobarbital level 3–4 mg/dL, or to maintain a "burst suppression pattern" on a portable EEG (only some randomized studies have supported the effectiveness of pentobarbital coma for lowering ICP)	II[a,c]
Mild hypothermia	Now under study for severely elevated ICP in head trauma; preliminary class II evidence suggests efficacy	II[a]

[a] Allen CH, Ward JD. An evidence-based approach to management of increased intracranial pressure. Crit Care Clin 1998;14:485–495.
[b] Poungvarin N, Boopat W, Viriyavejakul A, et al. Effects of dexamethasone in primary supratentorial intracerebral hemorrhage. N Engl J Med 1987;316:1229–1233.
[c] Ward JD, Becker DP, Miller JD, et al. Failure of prophylactic barbiturate coma in the treatment of severe head injury. J Neurosurg 1985;62:383–388.
Source: Reprinted from Starr P. Neurosurgery. In: Norton JA, Bollinger RR, Chang AE, et al, eds. Surgery: Basic Science and Clinical Evidence. New York: Springer-Verlag, 2001, with permission.

Algorithm 32.2. Critical pathway for treatment of intracranial hypertension in the severe head injury patient. CPP, cerebral perfusion pressure. (Reprinted from Bullock R, Chestnut R, Clifton G, et al. Guidelines for the management of severe head injury. Brain Trauma Foundation, American Association of Neurological Surgeons, Joint Section on Neurotrauma and Critical Care. J Neurotrauma 1996;13(11):641–734. Copyright © 1995, Brain Trauma Foundation.)

Blood, CSF, and Brain Components: The first component of total intracranial volume to be considered is the **vascular component**. This includes both the venous and arterial compartments. Elevation of the head, as discussed earlier, increases venous outflow and decreases the volume of venous blood within the brain. This results in a small improvement in intracranial compliance, and therefore, it has only a modest effect on ICP. Another component of intracranial vascular volume is the arterial blood volume. This may be reduced by mild to moderate **hyperventilation**, in which the Pco_2 is reduced to between 30 and 36 mm Hg. This decrease in Pco_2 causes vasoconstriction at the level of the arteriole, which decreases cerebral blood volume enough to reduce ICP. The effect of hyperventilation has a duration of action of approximately 2 to 3 days, after which the cerebral vasculature resets to the reduced level of Pco_2. This is an important point because, **once hyperventilation is implemented, the Pco_2 should not be returned rapidly to normal,** as this may cause rebound vasodilatation, which can result in increased ICP. Severe hyperventilation was, at one time, an important component of the treatment of TBI and increased ICP. It has been shown that reducing Pco_2 to 25 mm Hg or lower, causes enough vasoconstriction that CBF is reduced to the point where there is a high probability of developing cerebral ischemia. Thus, **prolonged severe hyperventilation is not used routinely to treat elevated ICP.** Brief periods of severe hyperventilation may be used to treat patients with transient ICP elevations due to pressure waves or in the initial treatment of the patient in neurologic distress until other measures can be instituted. There are rare instances in which ICP elevations are due to excessive CBF, a condition known as hyperemia. When hyperemia is the cause of increased ICP, severe hyperventilation may be utilized. This requires the use of jugular venous saturation monitoring to evaluate for excessive cerebral oxygen extraction, which indicates that the degree of hyperventilation is too severe and may cause cerebral ischemia.

Cerebrospinal fluid represents the second component of total intracranial volume and accounts for 2% to 3% of total intracranial volume. Total CSF production in the adult is approximately 20 cc per hour. In many TBI patients with elevated ICP, a ventriculostomy may be placed, and CSF may be drained. Cerebrospinal fluid drainage frequently results in significant improvement in ICP.

The third and largest component of total intracranial volume is the **brain or tissue component**, which comprises 85% to 90% of the total intracranial volume. When there is significant brain edema, it causes an increase in the tissue component of the total intracranial volume and results in decreased compliance and an increase in ICP. Treatments for elevated ICP that reduce total brain volume are diuretics, cerebral perfusion pressure augmentation (CPP strategies), metabolic suppression, and decompressive procedures.

Diuretics: Diuretics are very powerful in their ability to decrease brain volume and therefore decrease ICP. **Mannitol**, an osmotic diuretic, is the most common diuretic used. Mannitol draws water out of the brain into the intravascular compartment. It has a rapid onset of action and an average duration of 4 hours. Mannitol is more effective when given in intermittent boluses than if it is used as a continuous infusion. The standard dose is between 0.25 g/kg and 1.00 g/kg given every 4 to 6 hours. Electrolytes and serum osmolality must be monitored carefully during its use. Also, sufficient hydration must be administered to maintain euvolemia. Mannitol should not be given if the serum Na is >147 or if the serum osmolarity is >315. There is a maximum dose of 4 g/kg of mannitol/day. At doses higher than this, mannitol can cause renal toxicity.

Cerebral Perfusion Pressure (CPP) Management: Cerebral perfusion pressure (CPP) management involves artificially elevating the blood pressure to increase the MAP and the CPP. Because there is impaired autoregulation in the injured brain, there is pressure passive cerebral blood flow within these injured areas. As a result, these injured areas of the brain often have insufficient blood flow, and there will be tissue acidosis and lactate accumulation. This causes vasodilation, which increases cerebral edema and ICP. When the CPP is raised to 65 or 70 mm Hg, the ICP often is lowered because increased blood flow to injured areas of the brain results in better perfusion and decreases the tissue acidosis. This often results in a significant decrease in ICP.

Metabolic Therapies: Metabolic therapies are designed to decrease the cerebral metabolic rate, which, in turn, decreases the ICP. Metabolic therapies are a powerful means of reducing ICP, but they are reserved for situations in which other therapies have failed to control ICP because of their many potential adverse effects. Some of these adverse effects are hypotension, immunosuppression, coagulopathies, arrhythmias, and myocardial suppression. Metabolic suppression may be achieved through drug-induced metabolic inhibition or induced hypothermia.

Barbiturates are the most common class of drugs used to suppress cerebral metabolism. Barbiturate coma typically is induced with pentobarbital. A loading dose of 10 mg/kg is given over 30 minutes, and then 5 mg/kg/hr is given for 3 hours. A maintenance infusion of between 1 and 2 mg/kg/hr is begun after loading is completed. The infusion is titrated to provide burst suppression on continuous electroencephalogram (EEG) monitoring and serum level of 3 to 4 mg/dL. Typically, the barbiturate infusion is continued for 48 hours, and the patient is weaned off the barbiturates. If the ICP again escapes control, the patient may be reloaded with pentobarbital and weaned again in several days.

Hypothermia also may be used to suppress cerebral metabolism. The use of mild hypothermia involves decreasing the core temperature to 34° to 35°C for 24 to 48 hours and then slowly rewarming the patient over 2 to 3 days. Hypothermia patients also are at risk for hypotension and systemic infections.

Decompressive Procedures: Another treatment that may be used in the TBI patient with refractory ICP elevation is **decompressive craniectomy**. This is a surgical procedure in which a large section of the skull is removed and the dura is expanded.

Penetrating Trauma

There are two main aspects of the **treatment of penetrating brain injuries**. The first is the **treatment of the traumatic brain injury caused by the penetrating object**. Penetrating brain injuries, especially from high-velocity missiles, frequently result in severe ICP elevations. This aspect of penetrating brain injury treatment is identical to the treatment of closed head injuries. The second aspect of penetrating head injury treatment involves **debridement and removal of the penetrating objects**. Bullet wounds are treated by debridement of as much of the bullet tract as possible, dural closure, and reconstruction of the skull as needed. If the bullet can be removed without significant risk of neurologic injury, it should be removed to decrease the risk of subsequent infection. Penetrating objects, such as knives, require removal to prevent further injury and infection. If the penetrating object is either near or traverses a major vascular structure, an angiogram is necessary to assess for potential vascular injury. When there is the possibility of vascular injury, penetrating objects should be removed only after appropriate vascular control is obtained.

Penetrating brain injuries are associated with a high rate of infection, both early infections as well as delayed abcesses. Appropriate debridement and irrigation of wounds help to decrease the infection rate. Late-onset epilepsy is a common consequence of penetrating brain injuries and can occur in up to 50% of patients with penetrating brain injuries. There is no evidence that prophylactic anticonvulsants decrease the development of late-onset epilepsy.

Head Injury in Children

There are several ways in which **head injury in children** differs from head injuries in adults. Children tend to have more diffuse injuries than adults, and traumatic intracerebral hematomas are less common in children than in adults. Also, early posttraumatic seizures are more common in children than in adults.

When a child with a head injury is being evaluated, **nonaccidental trauma must be ruled out**. Traumatic brain injury is the most common cause of morbidity and mortality in nonaccidental trauma in children. Radiographic signs of nonaccidental trauma include unexplained multiple or bilateral skull fractures, subdural hematomas of different ages, cortical contusions and shearing injures, cerebral ischemia, and retinal hemorrhages. If any of these are present, the case should be referred to the proper child welfare agency.

Complications

Neurologic complications resulting from TBI are quite common and include neurologic deficits, hydrocephalus, seizures, cerebrospinal fluid fistulas, vascular injuries, infections, and brain death.

The **neurologic deficits** that result from TBI include focal motor deficits, cranial nerve injuries, and cognitive dysfunction. Common cranial nerve deficits following TBI include olfactory nerve dysfunction, hearing loss, and facial nerve injury. Facial nerve injuries are common when there is a temporal bone fracture and occur in 10% to 30% of longitudinal temporal bone fractures and 30% to 50% of transverse fractures.

Hydrocephalus is a common, late complication of TBI. Posttraumatic hydrocephalus may present as either ventriculomegaly with increased ICP or as normal pressure hydrocephalus. Those patients with increased ICP secondary to posttraumatic hydrocephalus demonstrate the typical signs of hydrocephalus including headaches, visual disturbances, nausea/vomiting, and alterations in level of consciousness. Normal pressure hydrocephalus usually presents with memory problems, gait ataxia, and urinary incontinence. Any patient who develops neurologic deterioration following TBI should be investigated for the possibility of hydrocephalus.

Posttraumatic seizures are a complication of TBI and are divided into three categories: early, intermediate, and late. Early seizures occur within 24 hours of the initial injury; intermediate seizures occur between 1 and 7 days following injury; and late seizures occur more than 7 days after the initial injury. Posttraumatic seizures are very common in those with a penetrating cerebral injury, and late seizures occur in as many as one half of these patients.

Cerebrospinal fluid fistulas, either rhinorrhea or otorrhea, may occur in as many as 5% to 10% of patients with basilar skull fractures. Approximately 80% of acute cases of CSF rhinorrhea and 95% of CSF otorrhea resolve spontaneously within 1 week. There is a 17% incidence of meningitis with CSF rhinorrhea and a 4% incidence of meningitis with CSF otorrhea. Prophylactic antibiotics have not been demonstrated to decrease this meningitis risk. When acute CSF fistulas do not resolve spontaneously, potential treatments include CSF drainage by means of a lumbar subarachnoid drain or craniotomy for dural repair.

Vascular injuries are uncommon sequelae of traumatic brain injury. Arterial injuries that may occur following head trauma include arterial transections, posttraumatic aneurysms, dissections, and carotid-cavernous fistulas (CCFs).

Intracranial infections in uncomplicated closed head injury also are uncommon. When basilar skull fractures or CSF fistulas are present, there is an increased risk of infection as discussed above. As expected, there is a higher incidence of infection in penetrating cerebral injuries and open depressed skull fractures.

Brain death can result from either massive initial injury or prolonged severe elevations of ICP. Brain death is defined as the absence of any voluntary or reflex cerebral function. **A strict protocol is necessary to prove that brain death has occurred.** It must be established that there are no sedating medication or neuromuscular blocking agents present. The patient's electrolytes, blood count, body temperature, and arterial blood gas all must be within the normal range. The neurologic exam should demonstrate the absence of all brainstem reflexes and no response to central painful stimuli. The lack of any neu-

Table 32.11. Glasgow Outcome Scale.

Assessment	Definition
Good recovery (G)	Patient returns to preinjury level of function
Moderately disabled (MD)	Neurologic deficits but able to look after self
Severely disabled (SD)	Unable to look after self
Vegetative (V)	No evidence of higher mental function
Dead (D)	

rologic response is not sufficient to establish brain death, and confirmatory testing must be performed. Confirmatory tests include the apnea test, cerebral nuclear blood flow study, angiogram, and EEG. Two neurologic exams and two confirmatory tests are required to establish brain death.

Outcome

The outcome of traumatic brain injury, as one would expect, is related to the initial level of injury. While the initial GCS provides a description of the initial neurologic condition, it does not correlate tightly with outcome. The **Glasgow Outcome Scale (GOS)** is the most widely used tool to follow TBI patient outcomes.[9] This scale divides outcome into five categories: good, moderately disabled, severely disabled, vegetative, and dead (**Table 32.11**). Many methods have been devised in an attempt to predict the outcome of TBI. These algorithms often are complex, and few are able to accurately predict the outcome of TBI. There is one simplified model that uses three factors: age, motor score of the GCS, and pupillary response (normal, unilateral unresponsive pupil, or bilateral unresponsive pupil); it provides a reasonable assessment of outcome. While it is extremely difficult to predict the outcome of TBI, several factors have been identified that correlate with poor outcomes. The Traumatic Coma Data Bank analyzed 753 patients with TBI and identified five factors that correlated with a poor outcome[10]: age >60; initial GCS <5; presence of a fixed, dilated pupil; prolonged hypotension or hypoxia early after injury; and the presence of a surgical intracranial mass lesion.

Summary

Traumatic brain injury is a common problem in the United States, affecting approximately 550,000 people annually. Patients with TBI should be evaluated by the ATLS protocol and serial GCS assessments, followed by a thorough neurologic exam when they are systemically stable. Head CT is the diagnostic imaging modality of choice in the

---

[9] Jennet B, Bond M. Assessment of outcome after severe brain damage: a practical scale. Lancet 1975;1:480–484.

[10] Marshall LF, Gautille T, Klauber M, et al. The outcome of severe closed head injury. Neurosurgery 75:S28–S36, 1991.

evaluation of TBI, and MRI scanning is used only in special situations. Some patients with mild head injuries may not require CT scanning; however, patients with moderate or severe injuries must be evaluated with a CT scan. If no surgical lesion is present or following surgery if one is present, specific treatment of the head injury begins. Patients with a GCS of 8 or less require placement of an ICP monitor. If the ICP is elevated, these patients are treated with some or all of the following: CSF drainage, modest hyperventilation, and diuretics. These strategies are designed to decrease the volume of one of the three intracranial components (brain, blood, and CSF) in order to improve intracranial compliance and decrease ICP. If these strategies are not effective in controlling ICP, then other treatment modalities, such as barbiturate coma, hypothermia, or decompressive craniectomy, may be utilized. There are many potential neurologic complications of head injury including cranial nerve deficits, seizures, infections, hydrocephalus, and brain death. While patients with mild head injury usually do well, some of those who develop a postconcussive disorder are disabled permanently. It is very difficult to predict the outcome of moderate and severe head injuries, and most algorithms devised for this purpose do not reliably predict outcome. As expected, many of these patients have poor outcomes.

Selected Readings

American Association of Neurological Surgeons. Joint Section on Neurotrauma and Critical Care. Management guidelines for traumatic head injury. J Neurotrauma 17(6–7):469–537.

Bullock R, Chestnut R, Clifton G, et al. Guidelines for the management of severe head injury. Brain Trauma Foundation, American Association of Neurological Surgeons, Joint Section on Neurotrauma and Critical Care. J Neurotrauma 1996;13(11):641–734.

Chestnut RM, Marshall LF. Treatment of abnormal intracranial pressure. Neurosurg Clin North Am 1991;2(2):267–284.

Choi SC, Narayan RK, Anderson RL, Ward JD. Enhanced specificity of prognosis in severe head injury. J Neurosurg 1988;69(3):381–385.

Ingebrigsten T, Rommer B, Kock Jensen C. Scandinavian guidelines for the initial management of minimal, mild & moderate head injury. Scandinavian Neurotrauma Committee. J Trauma 2000;48(4):760–766.

Marshall LF, Marshall SB, Klauber MR. A new classification of head injury based on computerized tomography. J Neurosurg 1991;75:S14–S20.

Rosner MJ, Rosner SD, Johnson AH. Cerebral perfusion pressure: management protocol and clinical results. J Neurosrug 1995;83(6):949–962.

Starr P. Neurosurgery. In: Norton JA, Bollinger RR, Chang AE, et al., eds. Surgery: Basic Science and Clinical Evidence. New York: Springer-Verlag, 2001.

Sumas ME, Narayan RK. Head injury. In: Principles of Neurosurgery. 1999; 117–171.

33

Musculoskeletal Injuries

Charles J. Gatt, Jr.

Objectives

1. To describe the principles of muscle contusions, lacerations, and strains.
2. To describe the principles of tendon injuries and tendonopathies.
3. To describe the anatomy of long bones.
4. To describe common fracture patterns.
5. To describe evaluation of an isolated fracture.
   a. Obtain a pertinent musculoskeletal history.
   b. Perform a physical examination as it pertains to the musculoskeletal system.
   c. Present a case of an isolated musculoskeletal injury using appropriate terminology.
6. Describe the commonly encountered muscle, tendon, and skeletal injuries that occur in the upper and lower extremities as well as the pelvis and spine.

It is assumed that the reader understands the basic anatomy of the musculoskeletal, circulatory, and peripheral nervous systems.

Case

A 35-year-old man sustained an isolated injury to his right lower leg as a result of direct trauma from an exploding truck tire. The patient did not lose consciousness, and, other than right lower leg pain, he had no complaints of pain in other body regions.

Introduction

The musculoskeletal system consists of the bony skeleton, ligaments, joint capsules, and muscle tendon units. Each individual segment of the skeleton is connected to adjacent segments by ligaments and joint capsules. The ligaments and capsules are considered static restraints, and they have no contractile ability. Consequently, they cannot generate motion between adjacent segments. However, as static restraints, the ligaments and capsules control motions between adjacent skeletal segments. The muscle tendon units derive their structural support from the underlying skeleton. The muscle tendon units, having the ability to contract, generate motion between skeletal segments. Thus, the musculoskeletal system consists of three general components that rely on each other in order to function properly. **Injury to one component may lead to dysfunction of and ultimately to deterioration of the other two components.** In addition, the musculoskeletal system relies on and supports the circulatory system and the nervous system. Musculoskeletal injuries can result in damage to either of these two systems, and **damage to the circulatory and or nervous system can result in dysfunction or deterioration of the musculoskeletal system**.

This chapter focuses on musculoskeletal injuries. First, basic principles of musculoskeletal injuries and disorders are reviewed. Then, common musculoskeletal injuries are highlighted by body region. Upon completion of the chapter, the reader should have a familiarity with basic principles of musculoskeletal injuries as well as a general knowledge base of specific musculoskeletal injuries.

Muscles: Contusions, Lacerations, and Strains

A **muscle contusion** occurs when muscular tissue sustains a direct blow. This can be a high- or low-energy injury. As a result of the trauma, intramuscular capillaries are injured. Bleeding and a hematoma can form deep within the muscle tissue, and this usually results in surrounding edema. Since muscle tissue is surrounded by a layer of fibrous tissue, or compartment, that has limited expansile ability, pressure can build up within the muscle compartment, leading to pain and sometimes to neurovascular compromise, resulting in a compartment syndrome. Compartment syndrome is discussed in detail later in the chapter.

Muscle lacerations result in damage to myofibers, nerves, and blood vessels. Lacerations heal with formation of scar tissue, and, consequently, the continuity of muscle fibers is disrupted permanently. In addition, neurologic damage at the site of the laceration results in denervation of the muscle fibers distal to the site of the laceration.

Muscle strain injuries occur at the musculotendinous junction. They usually occur during an eccentric contraction of a muscle (i.e., the muscle is contracting while elongating). This injury results in localized inflammation at the musculotendinous junction, with the result being pain. In the vast majority of these cases, the injuries **heal spontaneously and result in minimal, if any, permanent dysfunction.**

Tendon Injuries and Tendonopathies

Tendon avulsions occur as a result of trauma as well as a result of attritional failure. Avulsions almost always occur at the tendon–bone interface. Traumatic tendon avulsions usually are associated with an eccentric muscular contraction. The muscle tendon unit is being elongated usually by an external force, while the muscle tendon unit is contracting to oppose the external force. Since the anchor of the tendon to the bone is lost, the muscle continues to contract and pulls the tendon end further away from its normal site of attachment. Consequently, the opportunity for spontaneous healing is minimal, and these injuries often require surgical repair. Attritional or atraumatic tendon avulsions also occur, but usually they are the consequence of age-related degeneration or a consequence of systemic disorders. Even in the atraumatic tendon avulsions, the muscular component continues to contract, thus pulling the tendon further away from its site of attachment to the bone. If the tendon avulsion results in dysfunction, this also requires surgical repair to restore normal function.

Tendon laceration can occur as a result of penetrating trauma, such as a knife wound. If a tendon is lacerated only partially, the appropriate positioning of adjacent joints can minimize tension on the partially lacerated tendon and allow for spontaneous healing. However, if a tendon is lacerated completely, the proximal aspect of the tendon usually retracts as a result of muscular contraction, producing a significant gap between the two tendon ends and making spontaneous healing unlikely. These injuries usually require surgical repair to restore normal function.

Tendinopathies are very common. They can occur spontaneously, as a result of repetitive use or as a result of repetitive trauma. The patients usually present complaining of pain and sometimes swelling around the tendon. Although tendonopathies often are described as tendonitis, **histologic evaluation in many cases demonstrates no evidence of an inflammatory response.** These cases usually demonstrate mucoid degeneration of tendinous tissue, and it is more appropriate to **refer to tendonopathy as tendonosis.** In cases in which inflammation is present, tendonitis is an inappropriate description. These injuries are **treated with rest and temporary immobilization, and they usually resolve spontaneously.**

Joint Injuries and Arthropathies

Adjacent segments of the skeleton are connected by ligament and joint capsules. In some cases, the ligaments are distinct, identifiable structures, and, in other cases, the ligaments may be only a thickening of the joint capsule. **A sprain is a traumatic injury to the joint capsule**

and/or ligament. Sprains often are graded as a function of the severity of the injury. A grade I sprain results in microtrauma to the capsular and ligamentous tissue. There is a minimal to no permanent elongation of the structures. A grade II sprain usually is considered a partial disruption of the capsule or ligamentous tissue. There is a minimal but detectable elongation of the tissue, yet the overall integrity of the ligament and capsule remain intact. A grade III sprain results in complete disruption of the joint capsule and ligament tissue (**Fig. 33.1**). Grade I and II sprains usually result in minimal joint dysfunction. However, grade III sprains may have significant impact on joint function. Since the capsule and ligaments serve as static restraints to the joint motion, disruption may result in irregular motion between the adjacent skeletal segments. An extreme example of this is a joint dislocation when the articulation between two adjacent skeletal segments is disrupted completely. If not corrected, irregular motion is allowed to continue at the joint and results in deterioration of the articular cartilage and ultimate posttraumatic arthropathy of the joint.

Joints also can be affected by **primary arthropathy. Osteoarthritis** is the most common and can affect one or multiple joints. It involves loss of articular cartilage and capsular thickening, as well as chronic

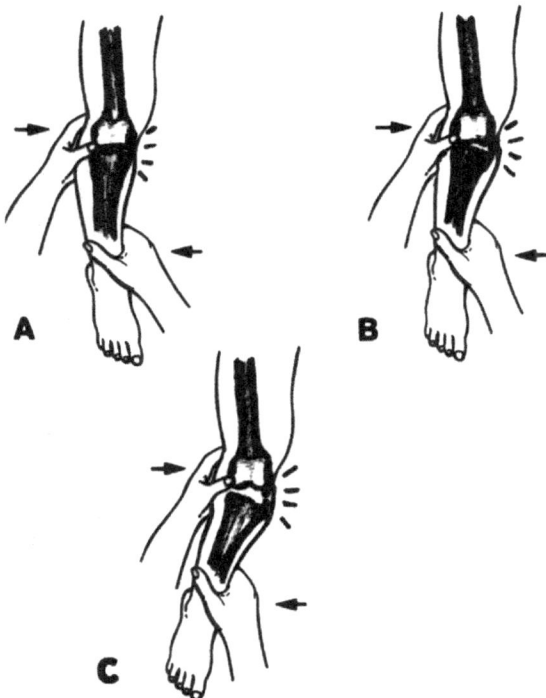

Figure 33.1. Clinical examination of joint sprain: (A) Grade I sprain with microtearing of ligament fibers. (B) Grade II sprain with partial tearing of ligament fibers. (C) Grade III sprain with complete tear of ligament. (Reprinted from Almekinders LC. Soft Tissue Injuries in Sports Medicine. Cambridge, MA: Blackwell Science, 1996, with permission.)

inflammation within the joint. This is a consequence of extrinsic and intrinsic factors. Some patients have a genetic predisposition to the development of osteoarthritis, and, in these cases, multiple joints usually are involved. **Inflammatory arthropathy**, such as **rheumatoid arthritis and psoriatic arthritis**, is due to autoimmune disorders. **Crystalline arthropathy**, such as **gout or pseudogout**, which involve deposition of uric acid crystals and calcium pyrophosphate crystals, respectively, also can lead to joint deterioration over time. **Septic arthritis** can be due to penetrating trauma that introduces foreign material into the joint or can be due to seeding of the joint from hematogenous spread from a nonsterile site, such as the mouth. **Septic arthritis, once diagnosed, requires urgent treatment, which includes aspiration, cultures, and formal irrigation of the joint.**

Fractures

Bone is strongest in compression and weakest in tension and torsion. As a consequence, the majority of **fractures** are due to bending and torsion. In the case of bending, the bone fails on the tension side, and then it finally fails on the compression side. However, in many cases, bending is combined with torsion, resulting in a combination of these forces, leading to failure of the osseous structure. Thus, the external forces that lead to the fracture can be determined by the proper evaluation of the fracture pattern (**Fig. 33.2**). A simple **transverse fracture** is evidence of a fracture caused by axial tension, such as in an **avulsion fracture** at a tendon or ligament attachment site. Transverse fractures also can result from repetitive axial loading, such as in a **stress fracture**. A **spiral fracture** is a result of a torsional stress to the bone. This occurs as a result of high- or low-energy trauma. **In some pediatric cases, spiral fractures of long bones should be a warning sign of abuse. Oblique fractures** are a consequence of bending, as the bone initially fails on its tension side and then fails on its compression side. In some cases, failure on the compression side of the bone results in multiple fracture lines, referred to as a **comminution fracture. Spiral oblique fractures** are the consequence of bending and torsional forces and, in some cases, have comminution on the compression side of the bone. Finally, in cases due to high-energy trauma, the fracture pattern is one of extensive **comminution with multiple fragments**. This fracture pattern is demonstrated in the case presentation. **Compression fractures** usually occur in vertebral bodies and can be the consequence of high-energy trauma, or they can occur in pathologic bone in cases of tumors, metabolic disorders, or osteoporosis.

Anatomy of the Bone

Understanding of the **gross anatomy** of the bone is helpful in fracture evaluation (**Fig. 33.3**). First, a distinction must be made between the **skeletally mature bone and the skeletally immature bone**. The description of the bone regions is the same for the two subsets, with the exception that the skeletally immature bone usually has two active

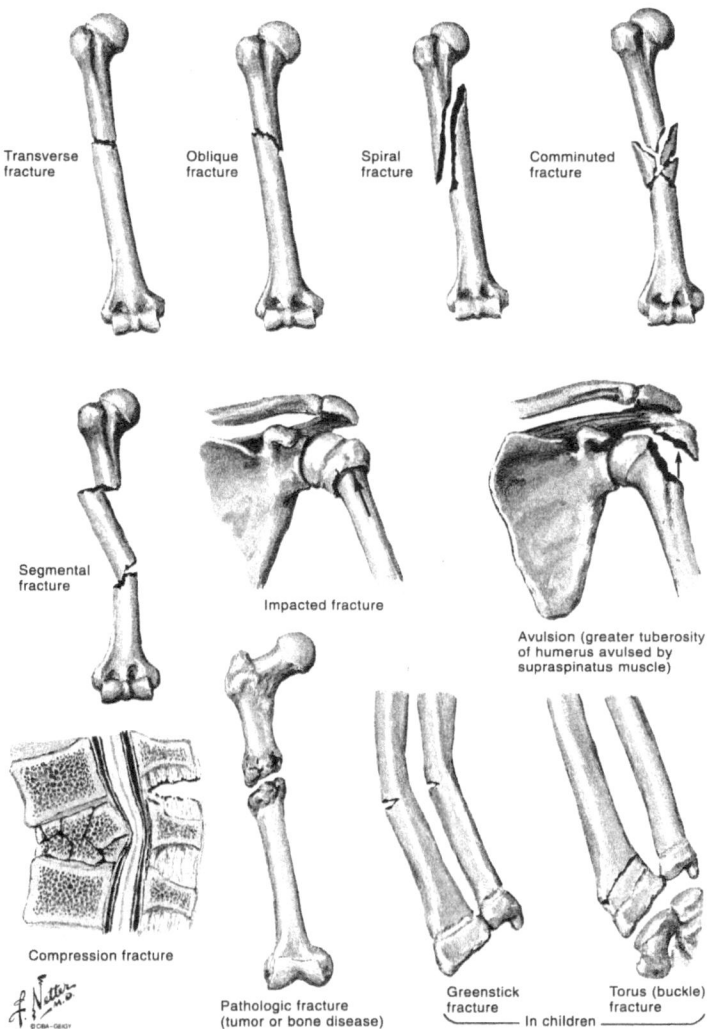

Figure 33.2. Common fracture patterns. (Reprinted from Netter PH. The Ciba Collection of Medical Illustrations, Volume 8: Musculoskeletal System. Part III: Trauma, Evaluation, and Management. West Caldwell, NJ: Ciba-Geigy Corporation, 1993. Netter illustrations used with permission from Icon Learning Systems, a division of MediMedia USA, Inc. All rights reserved.)

growth centers. The two ends of the long bone are referred to as the epiphysis. The end of the epiphyseal region usually is covered with articular cartilage. In the skeletally immature bone, the boundary of the epiphysis is the growth plate or physeal plate, commonly referred to as the physis. The physis is where longitude bone growth occurs. In skeletally mature bone, a remnant of the physis exists, referred to as a physeal scar, and usually is visible radiographically and represents a delineating line between bone regions. On the other side of the physis is the metaphysis. This region of the bone has a relatively thin cortex with a relatively large circumference that tapers down to a smaller

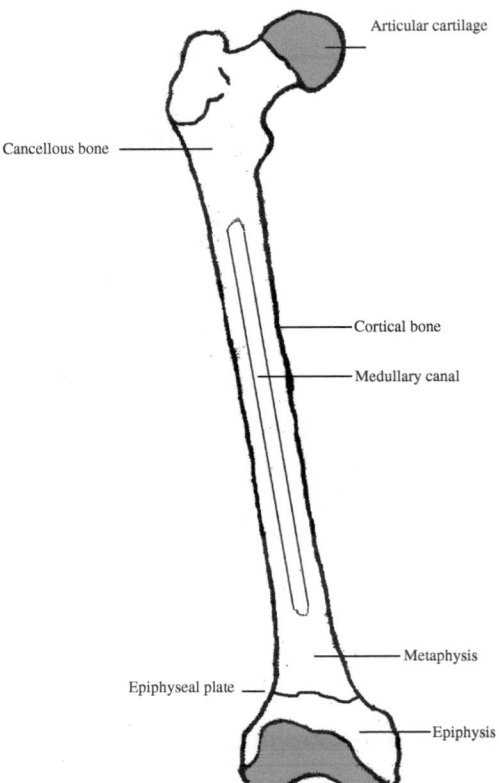

Figure 33.3. Gross anatomy of a long bone.

circumference with a thicker cortex. The central portion of the bone is long and tubular with a thick cortex and is referred to as a diaphysis. The cancellous bone in this region is relatively sparse compared to the density of the cancellous bone in the metaphyseal region.

Patient Evaluation

Care for the patient with a suspected fracture begins with the **usual history and physical examination**.

When the patient is awake and alert, a history should be obtained. The mechanism of injury should be determined. If the injuries were sustained as a result of high-energy trauma, such as motor vehicle accident or a fall from a height, loss of consciousness, mental status change, cardiopulmonary symptoms, and abdominal symptoms should be addressed. In the case of isolated musculoskeletal trauma, patients usually are distressed and unwilling to give a detailed history. However, from a brief history, mechanism of injury can be determined, as can locations of maximum pain and discomfort.

The physical examination in the patient who sustained musculoskeletal trauma can be performed based on the history obtained. If the patient has sustained high-energy trauma, a complete musculoskeletal physical examination should be performed after breathing and circulation have been evaluated. The much more common patient is the one who sustained isolated musculoskeletal trauma to one extremity. In this case, the examination focuses on the involved extremity. Initial inspection of the extremity reveals obvious deformities and breaks in the skin. Peripheral pulses should be evaluated, as well as capillary refill. Motor and sensory examinations, especially distal to the site of injury, should be performed. **When complete evaluation of the extremity has been performed, the injured extremity should be splinted.** Splinting of the injured extremity makes the patient more comfortable and also minimizes further trauma to surrounding soft tissues as a result of a fracture or dislocation. However, if there is an obvious deformity that is grossly malaligned, **longitudinal traction on the affected extremity often provides improvement of the position of the extremity, alleviates pressure on neurovascular structures, and makes the patient more comfortable**. Once improved position has been obtained, a splint can be applied. In the upper extremities and the lower extremities below the knee, it is easy to apply a padded plaster splint. **In general, the splint should incorporate the joint above and below the site of injury.** For femur fractures, skeletal traction or temporary traction applied to the soft tissues may be necessary.

See **Algorithm 33.1** for general fracture care.

Open Fractures

If evaluation of the injured extremity demonstrates a break in the skin, an **open fracture** should be suspected. Open fractures, commonly referred to as **compound fractures**, occur when the injured bone communicates with the outside world through a skin wound. This can be the case even when the skin has only a very small, pinhole-sized wound. At the time the injury occurs, the displacement of the fracture ends may be much greater than the displacement at the time of evaluation. Therefore, bone fragments that penetrate the skin and retract back into the wound can pull outside debris deep beneath the skin. If the soft tissue injury is significant enough, examination of the soft tissues can reveal a path directly down to the fracture site. In the occurrence of soft tissue injury around a joint, it may be difficult to evaluate whether the soft tissue injury path is in continuity with the joint. In these cases, injecting the joint with an appropriate volume of sterile fluid and observing for evidence of fluid extravasation from the nearby soft tissue wound will confirm continuity between the soft tissue trauma and the articular environment.

Open fractures can be classified into **three grades** (**Table 33.1**). Grade 1 open fractures have a relatively small associated soft tissue injury, usually less than 1 cm in length. Grade 2 open fractures have larger wounds, with the length of the skin damage 1 cm or longer and no significant soft tissue loss. In the case presented at the beginning of the chapter, the patient sustained a grade 2 open fracture of the tibia. Grade

3 open fractures usually are the result of high-energy trauma and involve significant soft tissue damage. Grade 3 fractures are subdivided into three subtypes: grade 3A is a significant soft tissue injury with no significant soft tissue loss; grade 3B is a significant soft tissue injury, including periosteal stripping, with loss of soft tissue, thus usually

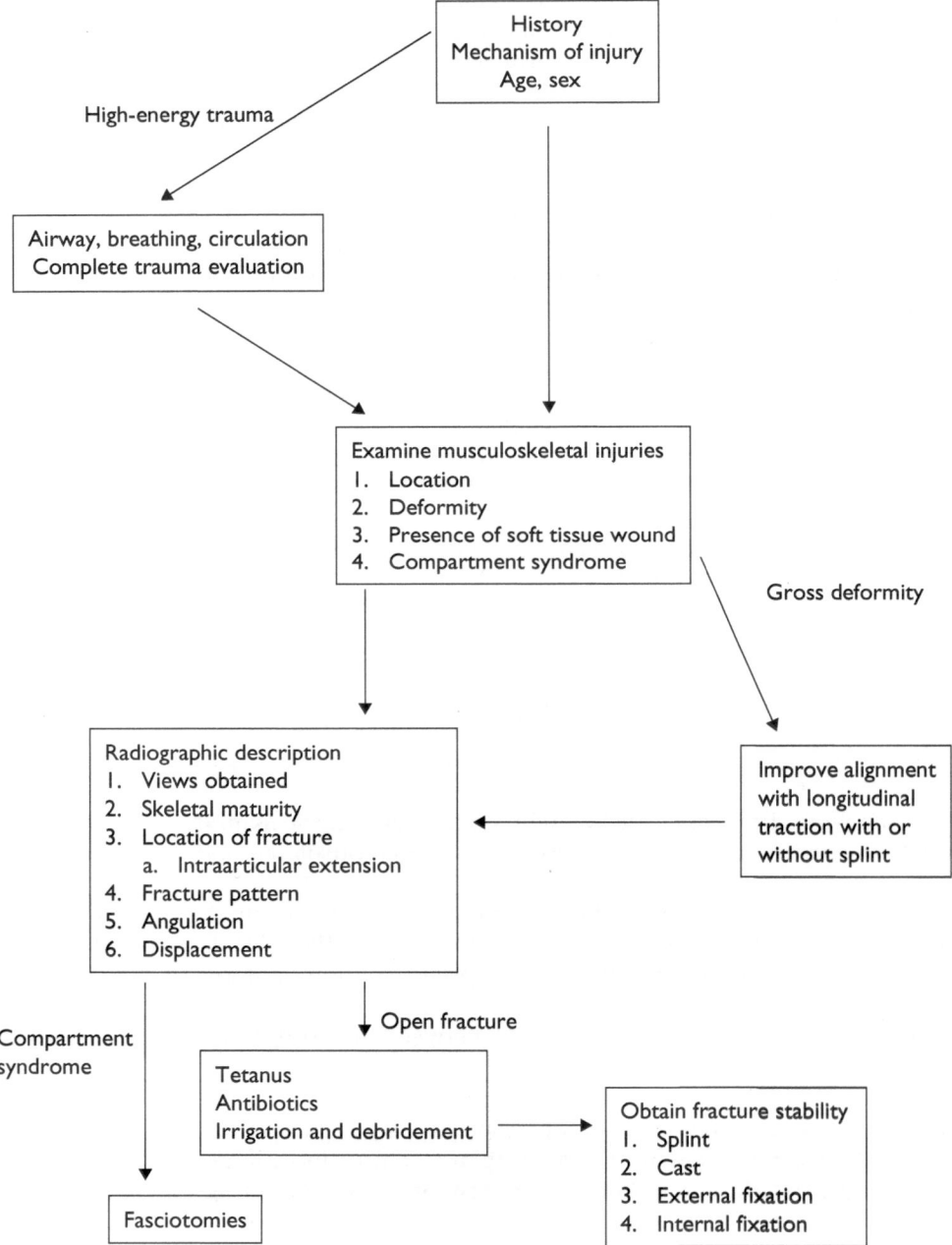

Algorithm 33.1. Algorithm for general fracture care.

Table 33.1. Gustilo and Anderson classification of open fractures.

Open fracture grade	Description
1	Low-energy injury Wound <1 cm in length
2	Moderate-energy injury Wound 1–10 cm in length
3A	High-energy injury Wound <10 cm in length; requires no major soft tissue procedure for wound closure
3B	As above, but more extensive soft tissue injury with wound requiring major soft tissue procedure for closure
3C	Like grade 3B injury, but in addition with major arterial injury requiring revascularization for limb salvage

Source: Reprinted from Gustilo RB, Anderson JT. Prevention of infection in the treatment of 1025 open fractures of long bones. J Bone Joint Surg 1976;58(A);453. Lowenberg DW, Fang A. Orthopaedic surgery. In: Norton JA, Bollinger RR, Chang AE, et al, eds. Surgery: Basic Science and Clinical Evidence. New York: Springer-Verlag, 2001.

requiring a separate procedure for coverage; grade 3C has an associated arterial injury that requires repair.

Open fractures are given extra consideration due to the **risk of infection** of the fracture site. Once evaluated thoroughly, an **open fracture should be treated urgently in the operating room with formal irrigation and debridement**. The routine treatment is direct exposure of the fracture site, debridement and removal of any debris that may have entered the fracture site, irrigation with 10 L of pulsatile lavage, stabilization of the fracture, and appropriate treatment of soft tissues. In most cases, **primary closure is not performed at the time of initial fracture management**. Multiple irrigations and debridements may be required to remove all debris and minimize the risk of infection, and, ultimately, if soft tissue injury is significant enough, coverage procedures, such as rotational or free flaps, may be necessary. **Tetanus prophylaxis** should be administered if appropriate, and **intravenous antibiotics** also should be administered for at least 24 and as long as 48 hours.

Compartment Syndrome

Even in low-energy, isolated musculoskeletal trauma, **compartment syndrome** can occur. This can be one of the more serious complications of extremity trauma. In general, compartment syndrome is an increase in muscular compartment pressure that ultimately prevents or inhibits perfusion of muscular and neural tissue. **Classic signs of pain, pallor, pulselessness, and paresthesias are not always present.** In general, an extremity that appears **massively swollen with tense skin, diminished distal sensation, and potentially diminished peripheral pulses** should be inspected for compartment syndrome. Compartment syndrome is an evolving process and should be monitored very carefully. **Repeat clinical examinations should be the hallmark of management. Measuring intracompartmental pressures with**

a monitor provides documentation and quantitative data regarding compartment syndrome. Pressure measurement techniques that demonstrate true intracompartmental pressure within 20 mm Hg of the diastolic pressure indicate the presence of compartment syndrome. However, it can be difficult to perform compartment pressure measurement accurately, and equipment often is unavailable. Therefore, it is emphasized that **repeat clinical examinations remain the hallmark of management**. If it is determined that a patient does have a compartment syndrome based on clinical examination or compartment pressure measurements, **the patient should be treated urgently with fasciotomies**. At that time, stabilization (provisional or definitive) of the fracture should be performed to minimize further damage to soft tissues.

Radiographic Evaluation

Once an appropriate history has been obtained, a physical examination has been performed, and initial fracture management has been instituted, **radiographic evaluation** provides definitive information regarding the fracture. **All fractures should be evaluated with orthogonal radiographs.** This means at least two radiographic views should be obtained from two different angles. This allows for an estimation of the three-dimensional deformity resulting from the injury. In some cases, such as fractures of the vertebral column or the acetabulum, a computed tomography (CT) scan may prove beneficial in evaluating the fracture completely.

Injury Descriptions

After the history, physical examination, and radiographic evaluation are completed, a **description of the injury** can be formulated. For some reason, fracture description often proves difficult and leads to confusion in the relaying of information from one practitioner to another. However, following simple guidelines should allow for a **clear and concise description of the injury** and fracture with no confusion. This description should address:

1. Age
2. Sex
3. Whether the injury is isolated or one of multiple injuries in a traumatized patient
4. Location of injury(ies), presence of deformity
5. Presence and description of soft tissue wound
6. Radiographic description
   a. Radiographic views obtained of the affected bone
   b. Whether the patient is skeletally mature or skeletally immature
   c. Location of the fracture with mention of intraarticular extension
   d. Fracture pattern

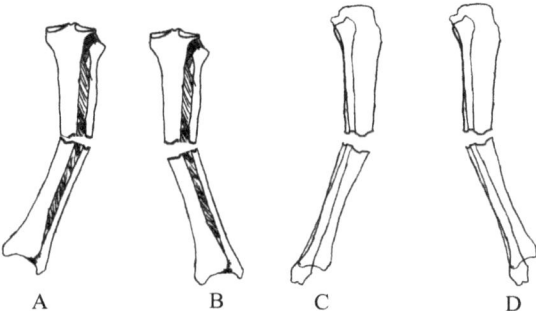

Figure 33.4. Fracture deformities. (A) Tibia fracture with varus angulation (apex lateral). (B) Tibia fracture with valgus angulation (apex medial). (C) Tibia fracture with procurvatum angulation (apex anterior). (D) Tibia fracture with recurvatum angulation (apex posterior).

    e. Angulation (**Fig. 33.4**)
    f. Displacement (**Fig. 33.5**)

Joint Dislocations

High- and low-energy trauma can result in **dislocation of the joint**. On physical examination, this usually is clinically evident. Although not truly necessary, most joint dislocations are evaluated radiographically prior to institution of treatment. Diagnosed joint dislocations should be addressed promptly. In general, neurovascular structures pass in close proximity to articular locations and often are stretched as a result of the dislocation. A prompt reduction or restoration of the joint congruity alleviates stress on the nearby structures and also minimizes trauma to the articular cartilage of the involved joint. Neurovascular status should be reassessed after reduction.

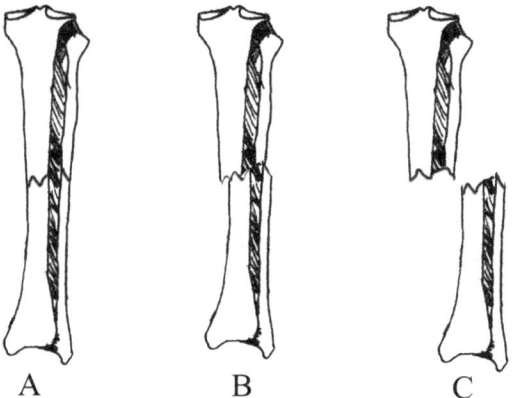

Figure 33.5. Fracture displacement. (A) Tibia fracture nondisplaced. (B) Tibia fracture 50% displaced. (C) Tibia fracture 100% displaced.

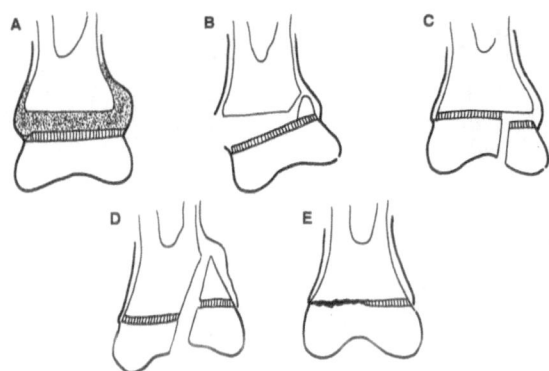

Figure 33.6. Salter-Harris fracture classification. (A) Salter-Harris type I—usually a nondisplaced fracture. (B) Salter-Harris type II. (C) Salter-Harris type III. (D) Salter-Harris type IV. (E) Salter-Harris type V—a crush injury to the physeal plate. (Reprinted from Evarts CM. Surgery of the Musculoskeletal System. New York: Churchill Livingstone, 1983. Copyright © 1983 Elsevier Inc. With permission from Elsevier.)

Pediatric Fractures

Fractures are common in children. Their bones are not as strong as those of adults. Their bones are more plastic and have the ability to bend without breaking. This can result in a **torus fracture**, which commonly is referred to as a **buckle fracture**. This usually occurs in a metaphyseal region of the bone and has the appearance of a minimally angulated fracture with a buckling of one cortex. In high-energy injuries, the bone may compress at one side and fail in tension on the other cortex, leading to a **greenstick fracture**, in which the bone appears bent, as would occur when trying to break a live branch from a tree.

Another important aspect of pediatric fractures is the **involvement of the growth plate**. The **Salter-Harris classification describes the injury through the growth plate of long bones (Fig. 33.6).** In a Salter-Harris type I fracture, the injury occurs through the growth plate without radiographic evidence of damage to the metaphyseal or epiphyseal bone. In the type II injury, the fracture line extends through the growth plate with a metaphyseal fragment of bone remaining with the epiphyseal fragment. In the type III injury, the fracture line goes through the growth plate and then through the epiphysis of the bone. Consequently, this is an intraarticular injury. In a type IV injury, the fracture line extends through the metaphysis, the growth plate, and the epiphysis, and, again, this is an intraarticular injury. The type V injuries are difficult to recognize. They involve compression of the growth plate with no obvious fractures in the metaphyseal or epiphyseal region. **Type III and IV injuries pose an increased risk for growth disturbance and usually require anatomic reduction to minimize the risk of disturbance of longitudinal growth of the bone.** Type V injuries also carry an increased risk of growth disturbance, although it is difficult to change the clinical outcome.

Common Musculoskeletal Injuries by Body Region

Shoulder

The skeletal anatomy of the shoulder consists of the humerus, the scapula, and the clavicle. The lone skeletal connection of the upper extremity to the axial skeleton consists of the articulation between the proximal clavicle and the sternum. The scapula articulates with the distal end of the clavicle at the acromioclavicular joint, but the body of the scapula has no true skeletal articulation with the rib cage. The humerus articulates with the scapula at the glenoid, forming the glenohumeral joint. Although the body of the scapula does not form a true joint with the axial skeleton, it is fastened securely to the chest wall by surrounding musculature. The glenohumeral joint does not have tremendous osseous stability, since the articular surface area of the humeral head is much greater than that of the glenoid, yet, the radius of curvatures of both articular surfaces is identical.

The external musculature of the shoulder certainly is prone to muscle strain injury. Since the external muscles, such as the deltoid, pectoralis major, trapezius, and latissimus dorsi, are used to position the arm in space, injuries from lifting heavy objects and protecting oneself from a fall are quite common. A tendon injury that commonly occurs around the shoulder is a **rupture of the proximal biceps tendon**. The biceps muscle actually has two origins, one from the superior aspect of the glenoid and one from the coracoid process. **Rupture of the long head**, the tendon that attaches to the superior glenoid tubercle, is common in the older population. This usually occurs with routine daily activities and generally is the result of attritional tearing of the biceps tendon. The result is a biceps muscle belly that retracts distally. This injury does not require surgical treatment. There is essentially no effect on elbow supination strength, and elbow flexion strength also is maintained by the brachialis muscle. Rupture of the biceps proximally usually is indicative of preexisting rotator cuff pathology.

The **rotator cuff** is formed by four muscles: the supraspinatus, the infraspinatus, the subscapularis, and the teres minor. These four muscles form a conjoined tendinous cuff that attaches to the proximal humerus. Rotator cuff muscles take their origin from the scapula and essentially pull the humeral head into the glenoid. **Rotator cuff strains** can occur as a result of lifting relatively light as well as heavy objects. Repetitive use of the upper extremity also can lead to **inflammation of the rotator cuff**. In these cases, patients will note pain with forward elevation or abduction of the upper arm. Most strains and tendinopathy resolve with antiinflammatories and rehabilitative exercises. In some cases, the rotator cuff can tear away from the attachment on the proximal humerus. **Rotator cuff tears most commonly involve the supraspinatus tendon.** In these cases, patients notice pain and weakness with forward elevation and abduction of the shoulder. Small tears of the rotator cuff can be managed conservatively, using nonsteroidal antiinflammatory drugs and rehabilitative exercises. In a patient who does not respond to conservative measures or has evidence of a large tear of the rotator cuff, surgical intervention usually is indicated. The usual treatment involves removal of the anterior portion of the acromion, release of the coracoacromial ligament, and repair of the torn rotator cuff to its humeral attachment.

As stated earlier, the **glenohumeral joint** does not have tremendous osseous stability. Consequently, the glenohumeral capsule and ligaments provide an important role as static stabilizers to the glenohumeral joint. **Dislocation of the glenohumeral joint usually results in detachment of the capsule and ligaments from the rim of the glenoid.** In the most common dislocation, the humeral head dislocates in an anterior and inferior direction in relation to the glenoid face. However, isolated inferior dislocations and posterior dislocations of the glenohumeral joint also occur. **Inferior glenohumeral dislocations** are referred to as luxatio erecta, and the patient presents with the arm fully abducted. **Posterior glenohumeral dislocations** usually result from a seizure, an electrical shock, or a fall onto the anterior aspect of the shoulder. **Anterior dislocations of the glenohumeral joint** are significantly more common than the other two types (**Fig. 33.7**). These usually occur as a result of trauma to the shoulder while the arm is held in an abducted and externally rotated position or as a result of a direct blow to the posterior aspect of the shoulder.

When evaluating a patient with a **shoulder dislocation, the axillary nerve function should be evaluated prior to reduction**, since this can be injured at the time of the dislocation. Injury to the axillary nerve would result in decreased sensation near the distal insertion of the deltoid muscle as well as diminished deltoid function. In the elderly population, recurrence of glenohumeral dislocation is quite rare, although attention should be paid to the function of the rotator cuff during early recovery after the dislocation. If there is evidence of rotator cuff tear early after a glenohumeral dislocation, consideration should be given to surgical repair. In the younger, more athletic population, glenohumeral dislocation frequently can lead to **glenohumeral**

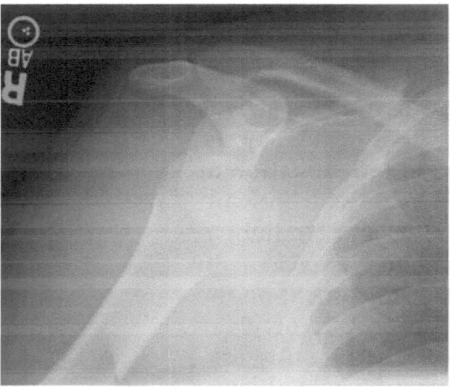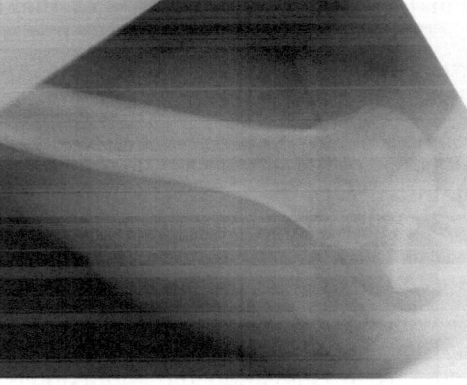

Figure 33.7. Radiographs of an anterior glenohumeral dislocation: anteroposterior (AP) and axillary views.

instability. **The risk of redislocation of the glenohumeral joint after a primary traumatic dislocation ranges from 70% to 90%.** The subsequent dislocations usually require less trauma than the index dislocation. In many cases, recurrent instability of glenohumeral joint requires surgical intervention. The treatment usually consists of repairing the anterior inferior capsule and the inferior glenohumeral ligament complex to the rim of the glenoid.

The **acromioclavicular (AC) joint** commonly is injured by a direct blow to the lateral aspect of the shoulder. This occurs when patients fall on the lateral side of their upper arm or run into a hard object, such as an outfield wall in baseball. It commonly is referred to as a **shoulder separation**. In the clinical evaluation of the AC joint separation injury, it appears as if the clavicle has migrated superiorly. However, the clavicle is fixed rigidly by the sternoclavicular joint and really does not rotate significantly. In the AC joint separation, the ligaments between the distal clavicle and the acromion are disrupted, and the scapula rotates. In grade I and grade II AC joint separations, the AC ligaments are disrupted. In grade III separations, the AC ligaments are disrupted, as are the coracoclavicular ligaments. In the vast majority of cases, surgical intervention rarely is indicated. Patients do quite well with AC joint separations. However, in more significant injuries, disruption of the ligaments is accompanied by penetration of the deltotrapezial fascia by the distal clavicle. In this case, the distal clavicle is in a subcutaneous position and will lead to chronic pain. In these cases, surgical intervention is indicated. The usual treatment is for repair or reconstruction of the coracoclavicular ligaments and repair of the deltotrapezial fascia.

Fractures to the scapula are of little consequence. The scapula body is encased completely by muscle and heals very rapidly. Although there is initial dysfunction of the shoulder, the scapula body heals, and good return of function is expected. The only fracture of the scapula that may require surgical intervention is an intraarticular fracture of the glenoid that involves greater than 30% to 40% of the articular surface with a significant step-off on the joint surface, or a fracture of the glenoid neck in conjunction with a fracture of the clavicular shaft that allows for medial migration of the shoulder.

Clavicular fractures are quite common. They are the result of a fall onto the lateral aspect of the upper arm. The majority of clavicle fractures occur in the midshaft region. Since this portion of the bone is in a relatively subcutaneous position, deformities are visually obvious. Healing usually occurs without surgical intervention. Improvement in the position of fracture fragments usually is not required. This injury can be treated with a sling or a figure-of-eight strap, which attempts to retract the shoulders and to help align the fracture fragments. However, the figure-of-eight strap is difficult to wear and often not well tolerated by patients. Restoration of essentially normal shoulder function is expected as clavicle fractures heal.

Fractures of the proximal humerus are very common in the elderly population. Due to the osteopenic condition of their bone, the proximal humerus is susceptible to fracture as the result of a fall onto the lateral side of the arm or onto an outstretched hand. In the majority of these injuries, the fractures are displaced minimally and often heal uneventfully, although shoulder stiffness or adhesive capsulitis can be a complicating factor during the recovery. Usually, in high-energy injuries to the proximal humerus, **displacement** occurs as a result of the fracture. In these cases, the fracture fragments usually are determined by muscular attachment. The greater tuberosity becomes one fracture fragment. The lesser tuberosity, which serves as a subscapularis attachment, becomes another. The articular surface of the humeral head is an individual fracture fragment and can be dislocated in an anterior or posterior direction.

The **junction between the humeral shaft and the humeral neck is another commonly involved fracture site.** In cases in which there is significant displacement of the tuberosity fragments, surgical intervention is indicated to restore glenohumeral function. In cases in which the articular surface of the humeral head is displaced in conjunction with the tuberosity and shaft fractures or in the case where the articular surface is dislocated, it is difficult to obtain adequate healing even with surgical intervention. Usually, a shoulder hemiarthroplasty is the treatment of choice.

Fracture of the humeral shaft usually occurs as a result of a twisting injury to the upper arm. **Spiral fractures of the humeral shaft in the pediatric population can be a sign of physical abuse.** In an isolated injury, this fracture rarely requires surgical treatment. It often heals in acceptable alignment with splint immobilization. It is important to **assess the integrity of the radial nerve in conjunction with humeral shaft fractures,** especially if the fracture has occurred between the junction of the middle and distal thirds of the humeral shaft. In the majority of cases of humeral shaft fracture with radial nerve injury, the radial nerve function returns spontaneously, and surgical exploration of the nerve rarely is indicated unless the fracture is an open fracture and surgical treatment is instituted for the prevention of infection. At that time, the radial nerve can be explored.

Elbow and Forearm

The skeletal anatomy of the elbow consists of the humerus, ulna, and radius. There are three articulations at the elbow joint. The proximal ulna forms the hinge joint with the distal humerus. The head of the radius articulates with the distal humerus at the capitellum. There also is a joint between the radial head and the proximal ulna. The joint between the radial head and the capitellum allows for rotation about the long axis of the radius, thus allowing the pronation and supination of the **forearm.**

Muscle strain injuries around the elbow are common, since the muscles around the elbow tend to set the wrist and forearm into a position of power for daily activities. **Avulsion of the biceps tendon** from its attachment on the radial tuberosity has a dramatic presentation. The injury usually occurs during eccentric contraction of the biceps. The patient presents with the biceps musculature migrated proximally in the arm. Although some patients believe that this injury leads to a loss of elbow flexion strength, this is not the case. The strongest flexor of the elbow is the brachialis muscle. Patients who avulse their biceps from its distal insertion actually note a loss in forearm supination strength. In the younger patient, especially in those involved in strenuous manual labor or those concerned with body symmetry, surgical reattachment usually is indicated. In the older patient, nonoperative treatment consisting of range of motion and strengthening usually provides an excellent functional outcome, and surgery can be avoided. **Triceps avulsions from the olecranon** are much rarer and almost always require surgical treatment to restore elbow extension strength.

Dislocations of the elbow joint almost always occur as a result of a fall onto an extended arm. As the elbow is forced into hyperextension, the joint dislocates such that the proximal ulna and the radial head lie posterior to the distal humerus. When evaluating a patient with an elbow dislocation, a complete neurovascular examination should be performed prior to reduction, since the brachial artery and the median, ulnar, and radial nerves all pass in close proximity to the elbow joint and can be injured at the time of the dislocation. Associated fractures of the radial head are detected on radiographic evaluation of the dislocation. Once the elbow joint has been reduced, a repeat neurovascular examination should be performed, particularly to ensure no nerve entrapment has occurred during the reduction maneuver. As opposed to the shoulder, the elbow joint tends to be stable after dislocation, and the risk of recurrent dislocation is very low. The primary concern after an elbow dislocation is regaining motion of the elbow. Posttraumatic contractures are not uncommon and can be prevented with early motion and rehabilitation.

Fractures about the elbow usually are the result of a fall with a direct blow to the elbow or a fall onto the outstretched hand. **Fractures of the distal humerus** involving the articular surface or the supracondylar region tend to be high-energy injuries with extensive comminution (**Fig. 33.8**). These usually require open reduction and internal fixation. **Fractures of the proximal ulna**, referred to as olecranon fractures, result in disruption of the elbow extensor mechanism, and these require surgical internal fixation if displaced. **Fractures of the radial head** tend to occur as a result of a fall onto on outstretched arm. In general, these tend to be lower energy injuries and often have minimal displacement. The primary treatment of these is early motion to prevent posttraumatic contracture. However, if the radial head fragment is displaced severely and results in mechanical block to full motion, the fragment may need to be reduced and fixed or excised surgically. **A Monteggia fracture is a fracture of the proximal ulna with a dislocation of the radial head.** This injury requires surgical intervention. Anatomic reduction of the ulnar shaft fracture almost always results in reduction of the radial head with good stability. **Fractures of the shaft of the radius and ulna** occur as a result of a direct blow to the forearm or a fall onto an outstretched hand. These injuries usually are displaced and angulated. In general, these injuries require open reduction and internal fixation, since healing in a nonanatomic

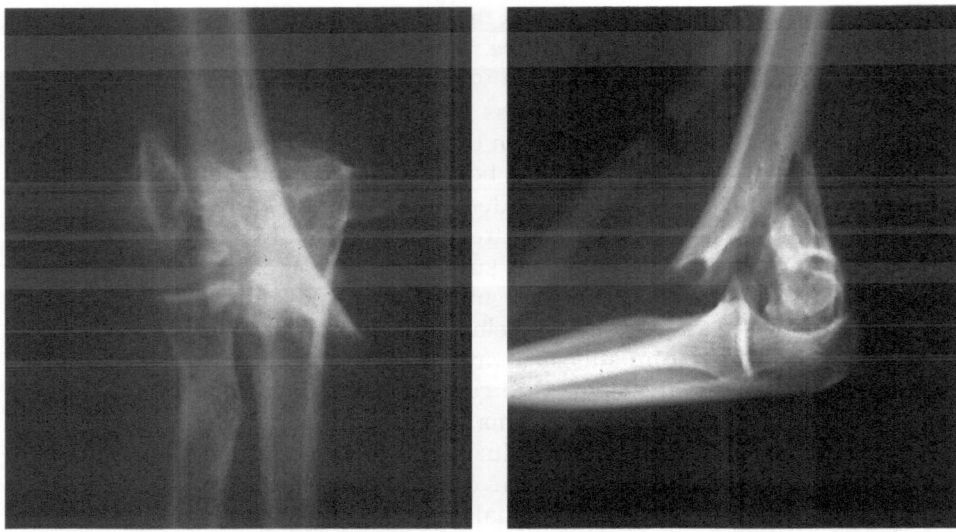

Figure 33.8. Radiographs of a supracondylar humerus fracture: AP and lateral views.

position results in loss of pronation and supination of the forearm (**Fig. 33.9**).

Hand and Wrist

The wrist joint consists of the distal radius, the distal ulna, and the carpal bones: scaphoid, lunate, triquetrum, trapezoid, trapezium,

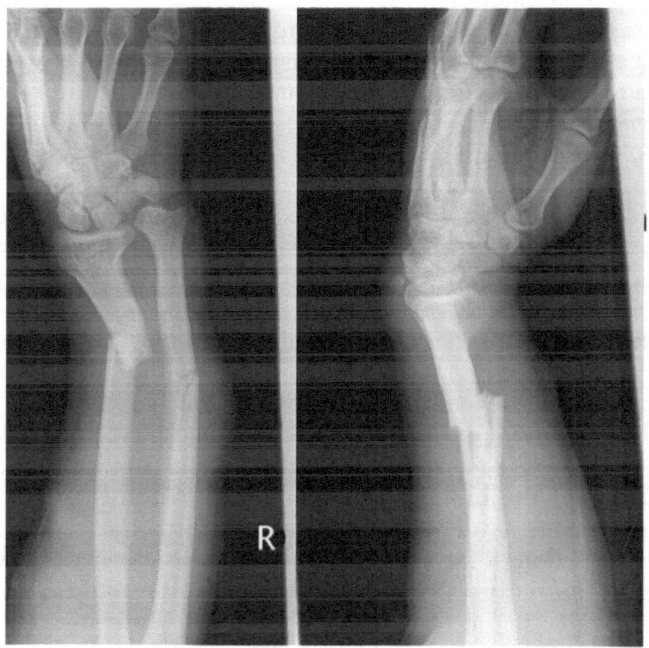

Figure 33.9. Radiographs of a forearm fracture: AP and lateral views.

capitate, hamate, and pisiform. Distal to the carpus, the hand consists of the metacarpals and phalanges. As opposed to the muscle injuries that occur in the rest of the upper extremity, **soft tissue injuries around the wrist and hand tend to involve injuries to the tendons**. **Extensor tendon injuries** usually are the result of lacerations. Cut tendon ends often can be identified in an emergency setting and primarily repaired with good results. In contrast, **flexor tendon injuries** tend to be avulsions of the flexor tendons from their distal insertions and usually are the result of forced extension of the finger while the finger flexor is contracting. **These injuries usually require surgical intervention with meticulous surgical technique**. Poor handling of the flexor tendons during surgical repair can result in excessive scar formation and significant loss of finger motion.

Dislocations of the wrist usually are the result of a fall onto an outstretched hand. Despite the significant trauma to the wrist, this injury is missed in the emergency setting. There is certainly diffuse soft tissue swelling and pain as a result of the injury, but radiographic evaluation of the injury can be confusing. However, careful evaluation of a lateral radiograph of the wrist documents the injury (**Fig. 33.10**). In a wrist

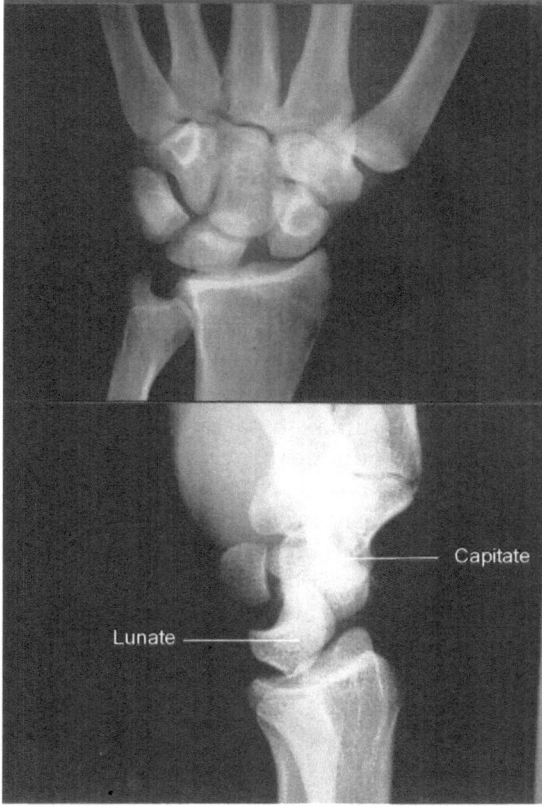

Figure 33.10. Radiographs of a perilunate dislocation: AP and lateral views. Note on the lateral view that the lunate is dislocated. This radiograph is commonly misinterpreted.

dislocation often referred to as a perilunate dislocation, the base of the capitate is dislocated from its articulation with the lunate. Either the lunate is dislocated in a volar direction and the capitate appears to articulate with the distal radius, or the lunate maintains its articulation with the distal radius and the capitate and the rest of the carpus have dislocated in a dorsal direction. This **injury results in significant pressure on the median nerve** as it passes through the carpal tunnel; it requires prompt treatment **and almost always requires open reduction** and internal fixation due to the multiple ligament injuries that occur between the various carpal bones. More common dislocations involve the metacarpocarpal joints, the metacarpophalangeal joints, and the interphalangeal joints. Many of these dislocations can be treated with closed reduction with longitudinal traction, and maintained with appropriate positioning of the hand. The carpometacarpal dislocations usually require cast treatment to maintain the reduction. Dislocations of the metacarpophalangeal joints and the interphalangeal joints usually require only minimal immobilization, followed by restoration of motion.

Fractures of the distal radius are one of the most commonly encountered injuries. Although a **Colles' fracture describes a comminuted fracture of the distal radius that extends to the articular surface and includes a fracture of the ulnar styloid, the term commonly is used to describe all distal radius fractures**. The typical patient with a distal radius fracture is an elderly woman with osteoporosis who has fallen onto her outstretched hand. In these injuries, the distal fragment usually is displaced dorsal relative to the proximal fragment, and the clinical deformity associated with this injury sometimes is referred to as a silver-fork deformity. The majority of these injuries can be treated with a closed reduction and cast immobilization. In the younger patient who sustains a high-energy injury with significant disruption of the articular surface, surgical intervention is required.

Fracture of the scaphoid is another injury that occurs as a result of a fall onto an outstretched hand. Clinically, this injury often does not present without much swelling. However, the patient tends to have tenderness in the anatomic snuffbox to palpation. If a scaphoid fracture is suspected, **radiographs should be inspected carefully, since up to 20% of these injuries are not diagnosed at the initial evaluation.** If the clinical examination is consistent with a scaphoid fracture and the **initial radiographs do not demonstrate a fracture, the patient should be immobilized in a thumb spica splint and follow-up should be arranged, since radiographic evidence of the injury may not be present until 2 to 3 weeks after the injury.** This injury does have a high incidence of nonunion, especially if the injury is not immobilized in the early stages or if there is displacement of the fracture. **A fracture of the fifth metacarpal neck** is referred to as a boxer's fracture and usually occurs as a result of the patient's striking a hard object with a clenched fist. This particular injury should be inspected carefully for a **laceration over the head of the metacarpal**. The laceration can be the result of the clenched fist hitting the tooth of another person. Consequently, this particular injury is at **significant risk for infection** and requires thorough irrigation in addition to treatment of the fracture. **Antibiotics should provide coverage for *E. corrodens* in addition to routine skin flora.** This injury presents with apex dorsal angulation at the level of the metacarpal neck distally, and this almost always can be successfully reduced and held in good position with cast immobilization.

Pelvis and Hip

The osseous anatomy of the pelvis forms a closed circle. In the posterior aspect, the sacrum, which contains the distal spinal nerve roots, articulates with the ilium on either side. The circle is closed anteriorly at the pubic symphysis. The **hip joint** is formed by the articulation between the head of the proximal femur and the acetabulum. In contrast to the "ball and socket" joint of the shoulder, the round head of the femur is well contained in the deep socket of the acetabulum. The large muscles around the hip certainly are susceptible to **contusion injury**. Falls can lead to **contusion of the gluteus maximus**. In sports events, high-energy direct blows to the anterior thigh can lead to **quadriceps contusions and hematomas**. This particular injury can be very painful and lead to a very tense-appearing thigh. However, compartment syndrome with this injury is extremely rare. The size of the hematoma formation can be controlled by early splinting of the leg with the knee held in hyperflexion, putting the quadriceps muscle on stretch. Since myositis ossificans at the site of the quadriceps injury is a troublesome sequela, minimizing the size of the hematoma formation is beneficial.

Another sports-related injury that often has a dramatic presentation is **avulsion of the sartorius muscle from the anterosuperior iliac spine or avulsion of the rectus femoris from the anteroinferior iliac spine**. In either of these injuries, patients report feeling a pop in their hip and present with significant pain with ambulation. Physical examination usually does not demonstrate an obvious muscle deformity. However, palpation over the appropriate iliac spine helps diagnose the site of the injury.

Dislocations of the hip joint usually are caused by high-energy trauma, such as a motor vehicle accident or a fall from a height, although they can occur in sporting injuries. **The most common dislocation is a posterior dislocation of the femoral head from the acetabulum. In this case, the patient presents with the hip flexed, adducted, and internally rotated.** When the dislocation is anterior, the patient presents with the hip held in abduction, flexion, and external rotation. Prior to reduction, a neurovascular examination should be performed with attention paid to sciatic nerve function, since this nerve can be injured, especially with posterior dislocations. Radiographs should be evaluated for other associated injuries, such as **acetabular wall fractures, femoral head fractures, or fractures of the femur**. Reduction of hip dislocation usually requires some form of sedation, followed by application of longitudinal traction in line with the deformity. Once reduced, a repeat neurologic examination should be performed, again paying attention to the function of the sciatic nerve. After the reduction has been performed, a radiographic evaluation should include a CT scan to detect any loose fragments that may be in the hip joint. Recurrent dislocation after hip dislocation is rare. **Avascular necrosis of the femoral head can occur in up to 40% of patients who sustain dislocations of the hip** and may present as late as 18 months after the injury. Protection from early weight bearing has not been shown to change the incidence of avascular necrosis.

Low-energy fractures of the pelvis occur commonly as a result of a fall in elderly patients. Fractures usually occur through the superior or inferior pubic ramus, and patients present complaining with groin pain and painful ambulation. Routine radiographs commonly demonstrate the fracture. However, in cases of significant osteoporosis with minimal displacement, the fracture can be difficult to detect, and a bone scan may be necessary to confirm the diagnosis. These injuries are stable and respond to protected weight bearing. **High-energy fracture of the pelvis** can be a life-threatening injury. Most notable is the **"open-book" fracture** of the pelvis as a result of anterior-posterior compression of the pelvis (**Fig. 33.11**). In this case, the pubic symphysis is disrupted, allowing the opening of the pelvic ring anteriorly, and, in the posterior aspect of the pelvic ring, the sacroiliac joint usually is disrupted. As a consequence, the venous plexus that lies anterior to the sacroiliac joint is damaged, and excessive bleeding can occur. Since the pelvis volume is increased as a result of the pubic symphysis diastasis, **significant blood loss can occur.** Physical examination demonstrates the instability of the pelvis as obvious motion is detected with compression of the iliac wings together. **This injury requires urgent treatment to stabilize the pelvis.** The situation can be temporized in the emergency room setting either with straps or percutaneous tongs. Once cleared, the **patient should be brought to the operating room for application of an external fixator** that closes down the pelvis and prevents excessive

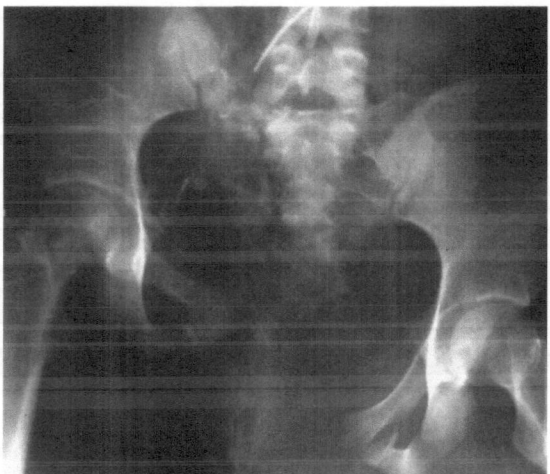

Figure 33.11. Radiograph of an open-book pelvis injury. Note the extreme diastasis of the pubic symphysis.

blood loss. This can be a lifesaving procedure and should not be delayed unless absolutely necessary. **High-energy lateral compression injuries** to the pelvis also result either in disruption of the pubic symphysis of the pubic rami on the anterior aspect of the pelvis and disruption of the sacroiliac joint or a crush injury of the sacral body on the posterior aspect of the pelvis. Although blood loss is expected with this injury, the pelvic volume is not expanding, and, consequently, urgent stabilization of the pelvis rarely is required.

Fractures of the hip are divided into two categories: intracapsular and extracapsular. Intracapsular fractures are fractures of the femoral neck. In elderly patients, a fracture of the femoral neck can result in an impacted valgus position of the fracture fragments, and this is treated routinely with screw fixation. When a fracture of the femoral neck is displaced, the blood supply to the femoral head usually is disrupted, and there is a significant risk of avascular necrosis of the femoral head. Consequently, many of these injuries are treated with primary hemi-arthroplasty in the elderly patient. However, in the younger patient, a displaced femoral neck fracture should be treated with more aggressive attempts to achieve a reduction of the fracture to a near-anatomic position and fixation with screws. **Extracapsular or peritrochanteric fractures of the femur** can result in significant blood loss into the thigh. This needs to be recognized, especially in the elderly patient with a low cardiac reserve. These injuries generally require surgical treatment with screw and side plate fixation or intermedullary fixation. **Fractures in the intertrochanteric region** heal readily while **fractures to the subtrochanteric region of the femur** have a much higher significance of nonunion and hardware failure. In cases of peritrochanteric fractures of the hip, avascular necrosis is not a concern.

Fractures of the femoral shaft are the result of high-energy injuries, such as motor vehicle accidents or falls from a significant height. Physical examination of the thigh should be thorough to be sure that there is not an open wound associated with the femoral shaft fracture. These injuries require surgical fixation, and this usually is done in an intermedullary fashion. **Fixation of these fractures within 24 to 48 hours from the time of injury has been shown to decrease the incidence of adult respiration distress syndrome (ARDS), especially in the multi-trauma patient population.**

Knee and Lower Leg

The osseous anatomy of the knee consists of the distal femur, the proximal tibia, and the proximal fibula. The distal femur articulates only with the proximal tibia. This often is considered a hinged joint, although rotations do occur about the longitudinal axis and in the coronal plane. The proximal fibula articulates with the proximal tibia, but this occurs distal to the femorotibial articulation. The fibula does not articulate with the femur. The patella is a sesamoid bone within the extensor mechanism of the knee. Its deep surface is covered with articular cartilage, and the patella articulates with the femur. The primary role of the patella is to increase the length of the extensor moment arm.

Since very little muscle tissue overlies the knee joint, **muscle contusions are not common**. In general, **significant contusions tend to occur in the posterior aspect of the lower leg** as a result of direct blows to the gastrosoleus complex. These injuries can lead to significant swelling, and neurovascular status should be assessed in association with these injuries.

The most dramatic muscle injuries around the knee are **disruptions of the extensor mechanism**. In the younger population, **patellar tendon ruptures** can occur while jumping or while landing from a jump. These injuries present with a high-riding patella, referred to as patella alta, and a palpable defect at the inferior pole of the patella. The majority of these injuries are **avulsions of the patellar tendon** from the distal pole of the patella. **Ruptures of the quadriceps tendon** tend to occur in the middle-aged and elderly population. These often are low-energy injuries and can occur with an activity as simple as ascending or descending the stairs. In these cases, the patient presents with a swollen knee, a low-riding patella referred to as patella baja, and a palpable defect at the superior pole of the patella. Similar to patellar tendon ruptures, quadriceps ruptures usually occur as **avulsions of the quadriceps tendon** from the superior pole of the patella. Both of these injuries usually require primary surgical repair of the tendon avulsion injury in order to restore normal knee function.

Dislocations of the knee joint can occur as a result of high-energy trauma, such as motor vehicle accidents, or as a result of lower energy trauma, such as sporting injuries. In these dislocations, the anterior and posterior cruciate ligaments usually are disrupted, as is the medial and/or lateral collateral ligament. Because the popliteal artery and tibial and peroneal nerves lie close to the posterior knee capsule, this injury does have a high incidence of neurovascular injury. Since the soft tissue envelope around the knee joint is relatively thin, the deformity is obvious to inspection. This injury should be reduced rapidly to minimize the risk of neurovascular damage. However, even after a prompt reduction, **a lower extremity angiogram is indicated to evaluate the integrity of the popliteal artery and its intimal layer**. Knee dislocations usually are treated with primary repair of injured ligamentous structures. Instability after dislocation usually is less of a problem than posttraumatic stiffness of the knee joint.

Dislocations of the proximal tibiofibular joint are rare. In general, the fibula dislocates in an anterior direction. The most common mechanism is landing from a jump, and this injury is seen in parachute landings. This injury can be difficult to detect both clinically and radiographically, but, once diagnosed, closed reduction usually is achieved easily with direct pressure on the proximal fibula in the appropriate direction.

Fractures of the distal femur usually occur through the supracondylar region of the distal femur with both high- and low-energy injuries in this region. It is not uncommon to see a vertical extension of the fracture that splits the medial and lateral femoral condyles. These injuries usually require internal fixation with intermedullary implants or open reduction and internal fixation with plate and screws.

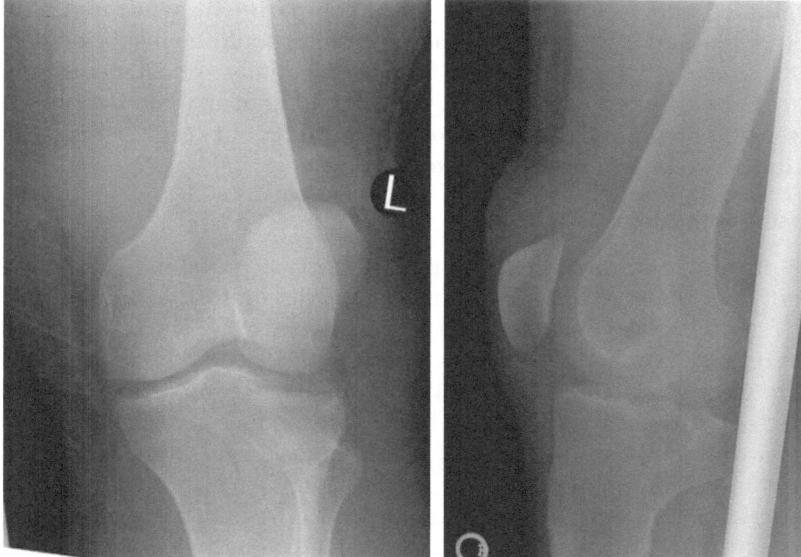

Figure 33.12. Radiographs of a tibial plateau fracture: AP and lateral views.

Fractures of the proximal tibia, referred to as tibial plateau fractures, usually involve damage to the lateral compartment of the tibial plateau (**Fig. 33.12**). At times, these injuries can be difficult to visualize on routine radiographs, and further imaging studies, such as **a CT scan, may be necessary to evaluate depressions of the tibial articular surface**. When the joint surface has been depressed greater than 1 cm, surgical intervention usually is indicated and involves elevation of the tibial articular surface back to its anatomic position with plate and screw stabilization.

Fractures of the patella result from a fall onto a flexed knee. Many patellar fractures are simple transverse fractures. When the fracture fragments are displaced, there is disruption of the extensor mechanism, and open reduction and internal fixation is indicated to restore normal knee function.

Fractures of the shaft of the tibia and fibula are relatively common. Low-energy injuries can occur from simple falls and sport activities. Even with low-energy injuries, significant swelling in the lower leg can occur. Since there is no significant fascial disruption, the patient should be evaluated and followed for a potential compartment syndrome. The lower energy injuries usually can be reduced into a near-anatomic position with closed manipulation and can be controlled in a long leg cast. If the fracture line has a high degree of obliquity, the fracture should be followed for excessive shortening even in a long leg cast. If this is the case, intermedullary nail fixation is appropriate to maintain length. Higher energy fractures of the tibial and fibular shaft usually result in comminuted fractures that are unstable, and it is difficult to maintain acceptable length even in a long leg cast. These injuries usually are managed with intermedullary nail fixation. However, in these injuries, significant soft tissue swelling can occur, and **the patient should be**

evaluated and followed for potential compartment syndrome. With both high- and low-energy injuries, the skin should be inspected carefully. The medial border of the tibia is essentially subcutaneous, and fractures easily can penetrate the skin, resulting in an open fracture. As discussed previously, **open fractures require urgent surgical irrigation and debridement to prevent osteomyelitis.**

Case Discussion

On physical examination, the patient in the case presented was awake, alert, and oriented, but he was in obvious discomfort. Examination of his right lower leg demonstrated minimal deformity. There was a 7-cm soft tissue wound on the anterior aspect of the leg, and bone fragments were palpable in the depths of the wound. The compartments of the affected extremity were soft. There were no neurovascular deficits distal to the injury site. The rest of musculoskeletal examination was unremarkable.

Figure 33.13 demonstrates anteroposterior (AP) and lateral views of the right tibia and fibula in a skeletally mature individual. The radiographs demonstrate a comminuted segmental fracture of the diaphysis of the tibia and fibula without intraarticular extension. There is mild varus and apex posterior deformity and moderate displacement of the fracture fragments. (This is an example of **a clear, short, and concise description of an orthopedic injury and should allow for clear communication between physicians.**)

Tetanus toxoid and intravenous antibiotics were administered in the emergency department. The patient was brought urgently to the

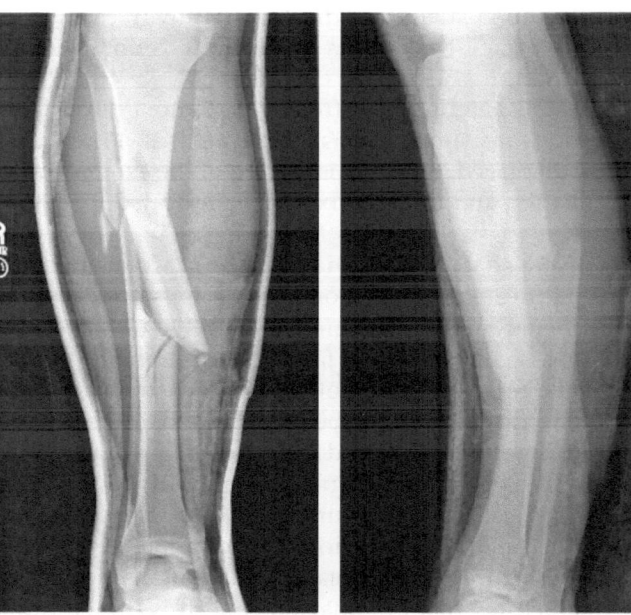

Figure 33.13. AP and lateral radiographs of an open tibia fracture. There is a segmental fracture of the tibia. There is mild varus angulation on the AP view and apex posterior (recurvatum) angulation on the lateral view.

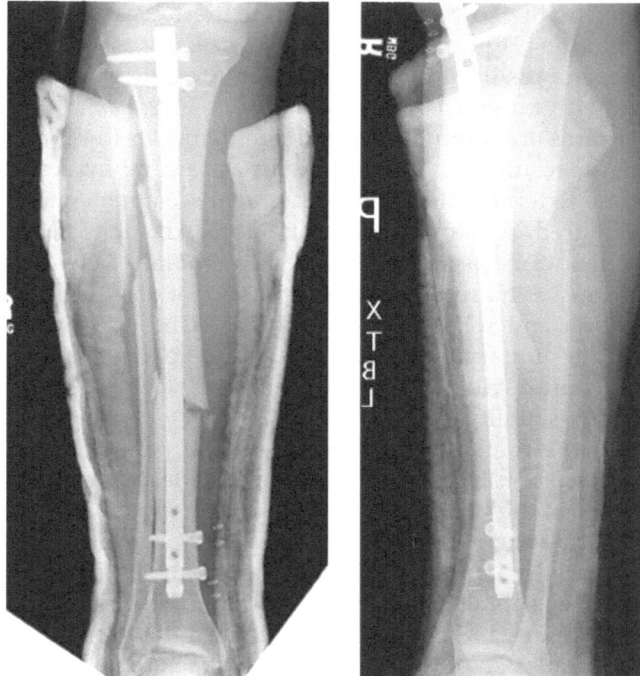

Figure 33.14. AP and lateral radiographs of an open tibia fracture after intramedullary nailing.

operating room for a debridement of his wounds followed by an intramedullary nailing of the tibia (**Fig. 33.14**).

Foot and Ankle

The ankle joint is formed by the articulation of the distal tibia, fibula, and talus. The body of the talus fits between the medial malleolus, a medial extension of the distal tibia, and the lateral malleolus. This joint acts primarily as a hinge, although rotation in the coronal and transverse planes does occur. In addition, vertical translation occurs between the tibia and fibula. The foot can be divided into three segments: the hindfoot, the midfoot, and the forefoot. The hindfoot consists of the talus and calcaneus. The midfoot is created by the tarsal bones. The forefoot consists of the metatarsals and phalanges.

Muscle strain injuries about the ankle most commonly are associated with sprains of the ankle joint. In general, these sprains of either the peroneal muscles or tibialis posterior muscle are mild sprains and resolve with minimal treatment. The most notable muscle injury is **rupture of the Achilles tendon**. This injury usually occurs in middle-aged individuals during recreational sporting events. The history reveals a sudden pain and sometimes a "pop" in the back of the ankle. There rarely is a history of preexisting Achilles tendonitis. Physical examination demonstrates minimal soft tissue swelling and a palpable defect in the region of the Achilles tendon. The Thompson squeeze test is performed with the patient prone and the knees flexed. **With an Achilles tendon rupture, manually squeezing the gastrosoleus muscle does not result in plantarflexion of the ankle (a positive test), but it does with an intact Achilles tendon.**

Ankle sprains are commonly encountered injuries to the ankle. They usually are the result of an inversion injury or a combination of abduction force and external rotation. The lateral ankle ligaments most commonly are injured. With more substantial force, the deltoid ligament as well as the syndesmosis and interosseous membrane between the tibia and fibula can be injured. Treatment consists of short-term or partial immobilization and rehabilitative exercises. True dislocations of the talus from the ankle mortise are rare. Once reduced, these injuries usually are quite stable, and posttraumatic stiffness is more of a concern than instability.

Sprains of the foot can affect one or several joints of the hindfoot, midfoot, or forefoot. In general, these injuries lead to significant soft tissue swelling at the site of the injury. They usually can be treated with a stiff-soled shoe and progression to full weight bearing as symptoms allow. **Dislocations** also can affect one or several joints of the foot. Dislocations such as subtalar dislocations and midtarsal dislocations have obvious deformities and can be closed reduced with longitudinal traction and manipulation of the distal segment back to an anatomic position. Since the soft tissue coverage over the dorsum of the foot is thin, these dislocations should be treated promptly to prevent soft tissue loss due to prolonged tension. In rare cases, nearby tendons can block a closed reduction, and these require surgical treatment.

Fractures of the ankle occur as a result of inversion or eversion stress on the ankle combined with axial rotation. They also can result from high-energy axial loads on the lower extremity. Low-energy stable injuries to the ankle result in a fracture of one malleolus and no significant ligamentous injury. On the other hand, unstable fractures of the ankle result in bimalleolar fractures or lateral malleolar fracture with a significant ligamentous injury resulting in translation of the talus from its anatomic position beneath the distal tibia. Radiographs should be carefully scrutinized for evidence of medial clear space widening (**Fig. 33.15**). Although the unstable injuries can be treated by closed manipulation and casting, open reduction and internal fixation usually are recommended. **Fractures of the distal tibia with extension into the ankle joint** commonly are referred to as pilon fractures. These usually are high-energy injuries that result in significant soft tissue swelling at the site of the fracture. As a consequence, many of these injuries are treated with a combination of external fixation and limited internal fixation. This technique avoids the soft tissue dissection necessary for open reduction and internal fixation.

Calcaneal fractures usually are the result of a fall from a height, such as a ladder. As with most high-energy injuries, they usually are associated with significant soft tissue swelling. **It is important to examine the patient for signs of lumbar spine injury, since 10% of patients with calcaneal fractures have an associated lumbar spine fracture.**

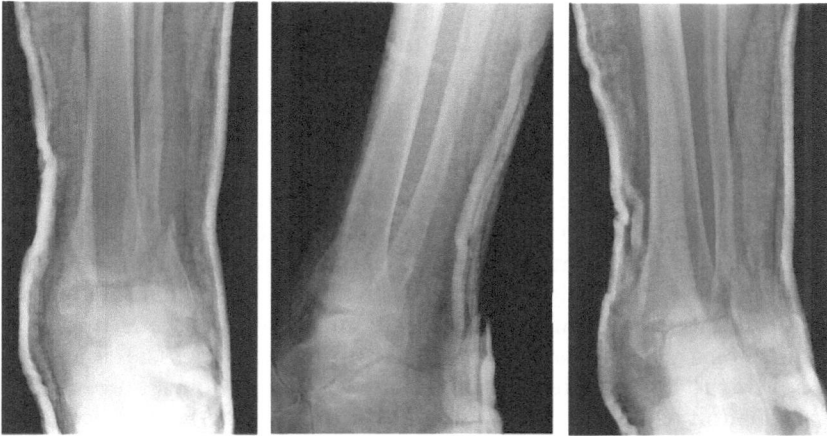

Figure 33.15. Radiographs of a bimalleolar ankle fracture: AP, lateral, and oblique views.

In the past, surgical treatment for displaced calcaneal fractures was rare. However, surgical intervention is becoming increasingly more common in the hope of improving the long-term outcome of this sometimes devastating injury.

Displaced fractures of the talar neck usually are high-energy injuries. In some cases, the fracture is associated with a dislocation of the talar body from the ankle joint. These injuries have a relatively high incidence of avascular necrosis of the talar body. Open reduction and internal fixation usually are indicated for displaced fractures.

Of the metatarsals, **fracture of the fifth metatarsal** seems to cause the most confusion. **Fractures of the proximal tuberosity of the fifth metatarsal** result from inversion injuries to the foot. These are extremely common, and minimal treatment is indicated. On the other hand, a **fracture of the proximal metaphyseal-diaphyseal junction**, referred to as a Jones' fracture, can be a troublesome fracture. This injury is treated best by prolonged non–weight bearing and sometimes internal fixation with an intramedullary screw.

Lawn-mower injuries to the foot are worth mentioning. These can be devastating injuries. There usually are multiple fractures and associated soft tissue loss. Prevention of infection is paramount in the treatment. Despite early and aggressive treatment, amputation is not uncommon.

Spine

The spine is a long column of vertebral bodies that serve to protect the spinal cord. There are seven cervical vertebrae, 12 thoracic vertebrae, and five lumbar vertebrae. Below the lumbar spine is the sacrum, consisting of fused vertebrae, and then the coccygeal segments. Rotational motion of the head occurs through rotation in the upper cervical segments. Flexion and extension of the neck occur through motion in the middle and lower cervical segments. Due to articulation with the ribs, little motion occurs through the thoracic segments. Trunk rotation occurs through the upper lumbar segments, and flexion and extension occur through the lower lumbar segments. Each vertebra articulates with the vertebra above and below via two facet joints and the intervertebral disk.

Muscle strain injuries in the cervical and lumbar spine are common. Symptoms generally are localized to the paraspinal region, and radicular symptoms are rare. The history may reveal minimal to no trauma that results in significant pain. Physical examination demonstrates obvious discomfort and muscle guarding. Signs of neurologic compromise, such as sensory deficits or muscle weakness, are rare and should alert the examiner to potential disk herniation. Radiographic examination usually is normal except for routine age-related degenerative findings at the facet joints or disk spaces. Findings on magnetic resonance imaging (MRI) do not demonstrate soft tissue edema, and the disk bulges commonly detected are not necessarily evidence of disk disease. These muscle strain injuries are self-limiting and resolve with rest and rehabilitative exercises.

Facet joint dislocations occur in the cervical spine as a result of motor vehicle accidents, but they also can occur in sports-related injuries. The patient complains of significant cervical pain. However, radicular complaints are not always present. Physical examination demonstrates muscle guarding, point tenderness to palpation, and limited painful motion of the cervical spine. Neurologic deficits are not always present. Radiographic evaluation should include AP, lateral, and odontoid views that show the cervical spine from C1 to C7. Facet joint dislocations may demonstrate anterior translation of the superior vertebral body in relation to the inferior and acute angulatory change in the longitudinal axis of the cervical spine. However, some facet dislocations can be overlooked on initial review of the radiographs. Enlargement of the soft tissue shadow anterior to the vertebral body may be an indication of ligamentous spine injury. Also, if the patient is awake and alert, flexion-extension lateral radiographs of the cervical spine may be helpful. Otherwise, CT scan usually diagnoses the dislocation of the facet joint. An MRI of the cervical spine prior to treatment helps diagnose associated disk injury. Treatment is by a prompt reduction of the dislocation. A reduction can be performed with the patient awake by applying longitudinal traction with skeletal tongs in the skull. This technique should be done with radiographic and neurologic monitoring and may be safer than open treatment with the patient under anesthesia. Once reduced, these injuries require some form of surgical stabilization.

Fractures of the spinal column without displacement usually are stable and often present with no neurologic compromise. These injuries are amenable to brace treatment. Higher energy injuries can result in fracture fragments encroaching on the neural elements, such as the spinal cord in the cervical and thoracic spine and nerve roots in the lumbar spine (**Fig. 33.16**). A careful physical examination demonstrates the level and extent of neurologic involvement. In cases of incomplete

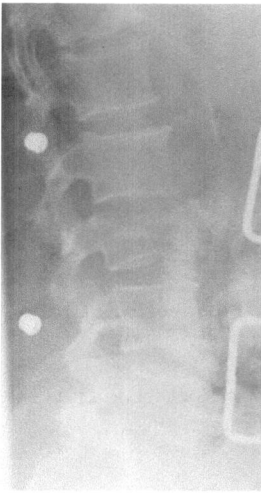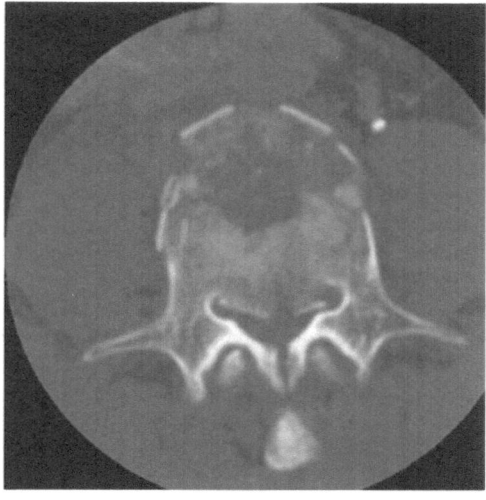

Figure 33.16. Lateral radiograph and computed tomography (CT) scan of a lumbar burst fracture. Note encroachment of spinal canal by vertebral body fragment.

spinal cord injury and nerve root injury, decompression and stabilization should be performed promptly. When complete loss of function below a spinal cord injury occurs, the prognosis for return is poor, but stabilization usually is required to prevent further deformity and to facilitate care for the patient.

Summary

Proper function of the musculoskeletal system is dependent on the proper form and function of skeletal, musculotendinous, ligamentous, vascular, and neural structures. Injury to even one of these elements usually leads to malfunction and deterioration of one or more of the remaining components. Thus, a thorough understanding of all of these components is necessary to diagnose and treat musculoskeletal injuries.

Assessment of the patient who has sustained musculoskeletal trauma should be systematic. Airway, breathing, and circulation (ABC) are assessed, followed by a comprehensive history. Then a comprehensive or focused physical examination should be performed. The examination should include evaluation of musculoskeletal, vascular, and neural components. Then diagnostics, such as radiographs, should be performed. Urgent treatment should be employed in cases of compartment syndrome. Appropriate traction and immobilization techniques should be employed. With this systematic approach to patient evaluation, communication of injuries and patient status should not be a source of confusion. After an appropriate evaluation and stabilization of the patient, a definitive treatment plan that leads to an optimal outcome can be implemented.

Selected Readings

Bucholz RW. Orthopaedic Decision Making. St. Louis: Mosby, 1996.

Greene WB. Essentials of Musculoskeletal Care, 2nd ed. Rosemont, IL: American Academy of Orthopaedic Surgeons, 2001.

Ivevson LD. Manual of Acute Orthopaedic Therapeutics, 4th ed. Boston: Little, Brown, 1994.

Lowenberg DW, Fang A. Orthopaedic surgery. In: Norton JA, Bollinger RR, Chang AE, et al, eds. Surgery: Basic Science and Clinical Evidence. New York: Springer-Verlag, 2001.

Rizzo M, Levin LS. Hand surgery. In: Norton JA, Bollinger RR, Chang AE, et al, eds. Surgery: Basic Science and Clinical Evidence. New York: Springer-Verlag, 2001.

Rockwood CA Jr, Green DP, Bucholz RW, Heckman JD. Rockwood and Green's Fractures in Adults, 4th ed. Philadelphia, JB Lippincott, 1996.

34

Burns

Jeffrey Hammond

Objectives

1. To describe the assessment of the burn wound, including total body surface area and depth, and to explain how this assessment relates to the early management of a major burn.
2. To discuss fluid resuscitation, including choice of fluid and rate of administration.
3. To discuss the recognition and management of inhalation injury.
4. To describe the options for wound coverage.
5. To discuss the role of rehabilitation therapists in the patient's recovery.

Case

A 65-year-old man sustained a burn injury in a housefire. He was semi-conscious when pulled from the house by firefighters. He has blistering burns to the face, to half of both the chest and back, and to both upper extremities, including the hands. The wounds to the arms cover at least 75% of the circumference of the arms. The firefighters removed his smoldering clothing and wrapped him in clean sheets. They placed a peripheral intravenous line in the antecubital fossa through the burn wound and started supplemental oxygen via a face mask. The patient now is responding to questions, is groaning in pain, is hoarse, and is appearing somewhat anxious. He is coughing carbonaceous sputum, but he denies shortness of breath. He has a history of "high sugar" controlled by weight loss and diet. He is a social drinker and has a 40 pack per year smoking history, but he stopped 10 years ago. His last set of vital signs, performed 10 minutes prior to emergency department arrival, revealed a systolic blood pressure of 110, a heart rate of 105, and a respiratory rate of 26.

Introduction

Thermal injuries entail destruction of the skin envelope as a result of the transfer of energy in the form of heat, cold, chemicals, radiation, or electricity. Burn injury represents a formidable public health problem. Each year in the United States, 300,000 people are burned seriously enough to warrant medical care. Of these, approximately 6000 will die. One third of these deaths are in children less than 15 years of age. For each death, three serious disabilities result, and each burn victim carries significant physical and psychological scars.

Treatment of the injuries requires knowledge not only of the management of the local burn wound, but also of fluid resuscitation and hemodynamic, fluid, and electrolyte management, of rational use of antibiotics and infection control, of nutritional support, of pain management, of physical medicine and rehabilitation, and of psychosocial intervention. Regionalization of burn care into burn centers has led to improved results. However, all surgeons and emergency medicine specialists may be challenged with the initial care and resuscitation of burn patients and, occasionally, with long-term care of smaller or more moderate injuries. Discussion in this chapter is limited to the more common heat-related thermal injury. See **Algorithm 34.1** for an initial approach to burn care.

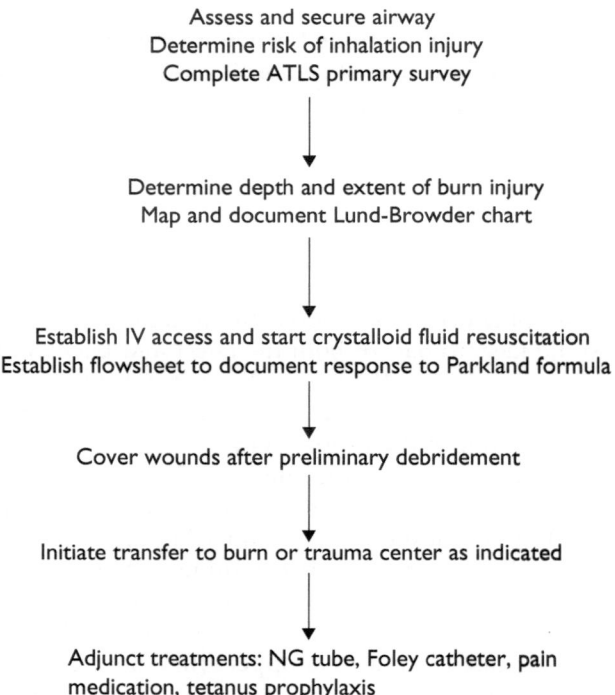

Algorithm 34.1. Algorithm of an initial approach to burn care. ATLS, Advanced Trauma Life Support; NG, nasogastric.

First Principles

The initial response and approach to the burn patient set the stage for further care and outcome. **First, remember that the burn victim is a *trauma* victim.** One must consider the possibility of associated injuries and not focus solely on the external manifestation of the burn. **The ABC of trauma care (airway, breathing, and circulation), as outlined in the Advanced Trauma Life Support (ATLS) course, should be followed, beginning with when the patient is first seen.** Burn injuries do not bleed in the acute phase, and therefore evidence of **blood indicates an associated injury**.

The integrity of the airway must be ensured. The burn patient rapidly can become edematous, even at areas distant to the burn wound. Upper airway edema may or may not be associated with an inhalation injury. Obvious perioral or intraoral burns, stridor, hoarseness, or use of accessory muscles of respiration are good indicators to protect the airway with endotracheal intubation. Because of the increased mortality associated with emergency tracheostomy in the burn patient, it is important to err on the side of safety. This is true especially for patients requiring interfacility transport. An endotracheal tube always can be removed later. **Once an adequate airway has been assured and the primary trauma survey has been completed, the burn wound must be assessed.** In the case presented above, the patient, who was burned in an enclosed space, has facial burns and hoarseness suggestive of early onset of upper airway edema.

The Language of Burn Care

What sets burns apart from other forms of trauma is the damage to and loss of the protective shell that keeps the outside out. Skin is more than a passive envelope, however; it is a dynamic organ that has active biologic and immunologic functions. **The response to injury and resultant treatment decisions depend in great measure on the *size*—expressed as the percent of the total body surface area (TBSA)—and *depth* of the burn.** These are the key components of the language of burn care. An accurate assessment of burn size is critical to the selection of an appropriate fluid resuscitation regimen, nutritional support calculations, decisions on transfer to tertiary facilities, and prognosis for survival.

Dermatopathologists divide the skin into more than a dozen layers, but, for practical purposes, skin is composed of three zones: **epidermis, superficial dermis, and deep dermis**. These are of importance in burn care since the depth of burn determines the potential for primary skin regeneration versus scarification (the need for surgical coverage by skin grafting or flap rotation).

First-degree burns involve the epidermis only. These injuries present as painful, reddened wounds similar to a severe sunburn. While painful and requiring analgesia, they have no physiologic significance and **should *not* be counted in the TBSA calculation.**

Second-degree burns involve the superficial dermis and produce a painful and moist or blistered wound. These wounds generally close, that is, reepithelialize, in 7 to 10 days. Note that a *closed* wound is not the same as a *healed* burn wound, since a burn wound may require 3 to 18 months to mature.

Third-degree burns involve the deep dermal layer and may penetrate into the subcutaneous fat. These wounds have the appearance of parchment or tanned hide. Coagulated vessels may be seen through the burn wound, called an eschar. These wounds usually are painless, because of the destruction of dermal pain corpuscles, but sensation to touch may be preserved. Because the skin appendages, such as hair follicles and sweat glands from which skin regeneration occurs, are destroyed, these wounds close only with scar tissue produced by epithelial migration from wound edges. For the best cosmetic and functional results, third-degree burns require skin grafting or flap closure.

So-called fourth-degree burns, involving bone or periosteum, are the result of charring or high-voltage electrical injury.

Assessment of burn depth is a clinical decision. A burn wound is not homogeneous. Factors that are significant predictors of depth include location of the burn, patient age, preexisiting medical conditions, and etiology of the burn injury. Hot water scalds usually are second-degree wounds, while immersion burns, due to the longer contact time, are third degree. Flame burns generally are third degree, and grease or tar burns can be deceptively deep. The burn is a dynamic rather than a static wound, and serial inspection over several days may reveal that the burn wound has "progressed" in depth as marginally viable skin tissues in the zone of injury die.

The *"rule of nines"* often is taught as a rapid evaluation of burn size. This method divides the body into multiples of 9% TBSA. The head, for example, is 9%, while both the anterior and posterior torso are 18% each. The problem with this methodology is that it is highly inaccurate and frequently leads to overestimation of burn size by factors of 100%. This especially is true in children, for whom the head has a larger percentage of TBSA and the limbs a smaller percentage. It is best used as a "quick and dirty" field assessment.

A more formal and accurate method of burn size calculation is to use standard body nomograms, such as the Lund-Browder chart. This nomogram is accurate for 95% of the population. Using such a chart (Fig. 34.1) facilitates documentation. Since adult proportions are reached at about age 12, separate nomograms exist for adults and children. For burns that are highly irregular in shape, such as tar injuries or grease splatters, a "hand count" method may be helpful. Each individual's hand is approximately 1.25% of his/her TBSA.

Inhalation Injury

The presence or absence of inhalation injury is a major determinant of survival in burns. Inhalation injury is associated with mortality rates of as high as 78%. True respiratory burns of the lower pulmonary

ROBERT WOOD JOHNSON
UNIVERSITY HOSPITAL
New Brunswick, New Jersey

EMERGENCY DEPARTMENT
BURN TRAUMA SHEET

DATE / TIME	DATE / TIME OF INJURY	PATIENT AGE	SEX ☐ MALE ☐ FEMALE	WEIGHT ☐ LB ☐ KG

ETIOLOGY (CHECK)
☐ Flame ☐ Scald ☐ Grease ☐ Dry Heat ☐ Explosion ☐ Chemical ☐ Tar ☐ Electrical (>500v.) ☐ Electrical (<500v.)

BURN INJURY CHECK LIST

R/O Inhalation:
closed space ☐ yes ☐ no
explosion ☐ yes ☐ no
burning plastics ☐ yes ☐ no
carbonaceous sputum ☐ yes ☐ no
singed nares ☐ yes ☐ no
dyspnea ☐ yes ☐ no
dysphonia (voice) ☐ yes ☐ no
oral mucosa involved ☐ yes ☐ no
Possible escharotomy
circumferential burn ☐ yes ☐ no
pulses intact ☐ yes ☐ no
(note: remember to remove rings)
Electrical injury (high voltage)
electrical contact ☐ yes ☐ no
loss of consciousness ☐ yes ☐ no
arrhythmia ☐ yes ☐ no
rhythm_____
myoglobinuria ☐ yes ☐ no
Medical History
alcohol use ☐ yes ☐ no
Drug / ETOH screen sent
time_____
drug abuser ☐ yes ☐ no
COPD ☐ yes ☐ no
heart disease ☐ yes ☐ no
hypertension ☐ yes ☐ no
diabetes ☐ yes ☐ no
sickle cell anemia ☐ yes ☐ no
Recent exposure to
communicable dx ☐ yes ☐ no
If yes explain _____
_____
other_____
ALLERGIES ☐ yes ☐ no
list _____
_____
Status of TET. TOX ☐ <5yr ☐ >5yr
MEDICATIONS
_____
_____
_____
_____
_____
Associated injuries:
_____
_____
_____
_____
Pregnant ☐ yes ☐ no
LMP_____
Eye injury ☐ yes ☐ no
singed eyebrows ☐ yes ☐ no
singed eye lashes ☐ yes ☐ no
irrigate ☐ yes ☐ no
soln _____

RELATIVE % OF AREAS AFFECTED BY GROWTH (circle age used)

AREA	AGE	0	1	5	10	15	ADULT
A = 1/2 HEAD		9 1/2	8 1/2	6 1/2	5 1/4	4 1/2	3 1/2
B = 1/2 THIGH		2 3/4	3 1/4	4	4 1/4	4 1/2	4 2/4
C = 1/2 LEG		2 1/2	2 1/4	2 3/4	3	3 1/4	3 1/2

CODE:
2° ▨▨▨▨▨▨▨▨   3° ■■■■■■■■

FLUID RESUSCITATION (Parkland Formula)
4cc RL × % burn × wt. (kg) =

_____ cc/RL/d.

÷24= _____ cc/RL/hr.
(note children under 2 have limited
glycogen stores, use D5RL)

EST % BURN BY AREA

AREA	3°	TOTAL
HEAD		
NECK		
ANT. TRUNK		
POST. TRUNK		
GENITALS		
BUTTOCKS		
UPPER ARM		
FOREARM		
HANDS		
THIGHS		
LEGS		
FEET		
SUM		

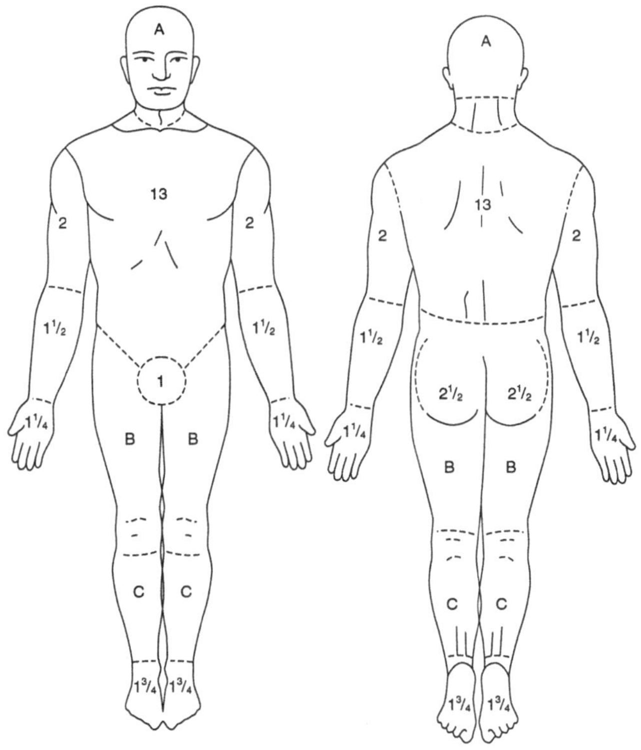

SIGNATURE _____ ,MD

DESIGNED BY MADISON BUSINESS FORMS 11/17/93 REJBURN rev 6/21/95

Figure 34.1. Example of emergency department "burn sheet."

tract are rare, generally occurring only with the inhalation of super-heated steam. What commonly is thought of as a respiratory "burn" is a response to inhalation of the products of combustion, or carbon monoxide toxicity. Incomplete products of combustion, such as aldehydes, nitrogen dioxide, and hydrochloric acid, can cause direct parenchymal lung damage. Carbon monoxide, with an affinity for oxygen more than 200 times that of hemoglobin, seriously can impair oxygen delivery to tissues.

Early diagnosis of inhalation injury can be difficult, and it usually is a clinical diagnosis supported by an index of suspicion. Classic signs such as singed nasal hairs and carbonaceous sputum are unreliable. The history of being burned in an enclosed space is a crucial element to elicit. **The strongest correlation for a pulmonary injury is a history of being burned in an enclosed space coupled with the presence of facial burns or the history of patient incapacitation from drugs or alcohol.**

The initial chest x-ray (CXR) or arterial blood gas (ABG) often are normal after inhalation injury. They should be viewed as screening tests and indicators of underlying pathology. The serum carbon monoxide level may be used to tailor therapy, but it may be unreliable if supplemental oxygen already has been administered. The concentration of carboxyhemoglobin is reduced by 50% for each 40-minute period of treatment with high-flow oxygen. Hyperbaric oxygen treatment is not routinely necessary and should be reserved for patients with CO levels greater than 40% or for those with neurologic symptoms. Bronchoscopy has been advocated as a diagnostic tool, but it adds little to the accuracy of the history and the physical examination. Direct laryngoscopy allows direct investigation for upper airway edema. Regardless of the CXR or ABG, the patient in the case presented very likely has an inhalation component based on the history of a burn in an enclosed space and the signs of facial burns, hoarseness, and carbonaceous sputum.

Since signs and symptoms of inhalation injury may appear over an 18- to 36-hour period, patients at risk or patients suspected of being at risk should be admitted for a 24-hour period of observation. Steroid therapy is not beneficial and carries a risk of superimposed infection; bronchodilator therapy and aggressive chest physiotherapy are advantageous. Prophylactic antibiotics are not recommended due to the risk of selection pressure for the emergence of resistant organisms. Ventilatory support may be necessary in severe cases. The preferred route is via endotracheal or nasotracheal intubation. The airway should be secured before edema necessitates a surgical airway; tracheostomy or cricothyroidotomy carries a higher morbidity and mortality rate.

Treatment: The First 24 Hours

The purpose of **fluid resuscitation** in the early postburn period is reexpansion of plasma volume within the extracellular space. Delivery of sodium ion into the extracellular space results in reestablishment of cellular membrane potentials and restores microvascular integrity. Controversy over the type and regimen of fluid resuscitation remains. All agree, however, that **restoration of plasma volume is essential in preventing renal failure and shock**.

The standard approach is to use the Parkland formula to establish daily needs (4 mL × weight in kg × % TBSA burned). The formula for estimating insensible water loss, expressed in milliliters per hour, is (25 + % TBSA burned) BSA. Access is via large-bore peripheral intravenous lines. As in the case presented at the beginning of the chapter, these lines may be placed through the burn wound if access sites are limited. Lactated Ringer's solution is the preferred crystalloid. Dextrose should not be used initially due to the risk of osmotic diuresis. This formula is a rough guide, however, and one fifth of patients need more and one fifth need less. The patient's response, as judged by urine output, guides therapy. For this reason, diuretics are to be avoided. Central venous or pulmonary artery pressures usually are unreliable. **The patient is the formula.**

Colloid generally is avoided in the first 24 hours. In some formulas, colloids in the form of albumin or fresh frozen plasma are added in the second 24 hours or when the capillary leak has stopped. A diuretic phase begins on the third to fifth postburn day with mobilization of the resuscitation fluid. During this phase, there is a risk of hypokalemia.

Emergency care of burns, either major or minor, requires **adequate tetanus prophylaxis**. The burn wound is anaerobic, and cases of clinical tetanus have been described even from superficial second-degree injuries. A booster of tetanus toxoid is recommended for patients already immunized. For those never immunized, both passive and active immunization using tetanus immune human globulin (Hyper-Tet) is suggested.

Efforts are directed at maintaining body temperature and preventing hypothermia. Iced saline is not used for initial debridement or wound coverage in the emergency department for that reason. Although application of cold decreases pain and edema, it may injure marginally viable cells and can induce hypothermia and increase metabolic demands if applied to greater than 10% TBSA.

Early in the management scheme, practitioners must determine if the patient **requires hospital admission** and whether resources for good burn care exist in their institution. Guidelines for admission have been developed by the American College of Surgeons and the American Burn Association (**Table 34.1**). **Transfer to a specialized burn center** is warranted if all components of the burn team are not available at the receiving institution.

Treatment: After the Emergency Department

The mainstay of burn treatment is good wound care, with attention to principles of infection control coupled with early wound closure and adequate nutritional support.

All blisters should be debrided except for those on the palms and soles if they are intact. In those areas, the skin is relatively thick, and

Table 34.1. Admission criteria.

Injury size:	Adult > 20% TBSA
	Child > 15% TBSA
	Third degree > 2% TBSA

Inhalation injury
High-voltage electrical injury
Chemical burns
Burns in the elderly
Circumferential limb injury
Suspicion of child abuse
Infected burns
Burns in special locations
   Face, neck, eyes, ears
   Hands, feet
   Flexor creases, joints
   Perineum, genitalia
Significant medical history
   Cardiac, renal, hepatic disease
   Hypertension
   Diabetes, sickle cell
Unable to care for self

TBSA, total body surface area.
Source: Adapted from American College of Surgeons Committee on Trauma. Advanced Trauma Life Support. Chicago: American College of Surgeons, 1997, with permission.

preservation of bullae reduces pain and speeds reepithelialization. Mechanical debridement is necessary; merely submerging the burn patient in a whirlpool is not sufficient.

Once the wound has been debrided, **topical drug therapy** controls bacterial colonization until spontaneous eschar separation and reepithelialization occur or until sharp debridement followed by surgical closure with skin grafts or flaps is completed. The advent of effective topical therapy significantly has reduced mortality from burn wound sepsis. The two major types of topical drug therapy currently in use are silver sulfadiazine (Silvadene, Flamazine) and mafenide acetate (Sulfamylon). *Silver sulfadiazine* is an all-purpose agent. It should be applied at least twice daily, removing old cream and cellular debris before each new application. If left for long periods, it may cake and produce a neo-eschar. It has only fair to poor eschar penetration, and it may not be effective in deeply burned or avascular areas. This property makes it more effective for prophylaxis rather than for therapy of burn wound infection. There are no significant metabolic side effects, but an infrequent hypersensitivity-type reaction may result in a transient leukopenia. Silver sulfadiazine should be discontinued if the white blood cell count falls below 2000. It generally is painless on application. *Mafenide acetate* is an alternative topical agent with excellent penetration into eschar. Its penetration properties make it a good choice for infected burns and burns in avascular areas, such as the ear. It has broad-spectrum antibacterial properties, but it predisposes to candidal overgrowth. Other disadvantages include pain on application and carbonic anhydrase inhibition. In large burns, systemic absorption may result in metabolic acidosis, with a compensatory hyperventilation. Pain on application can be lessened by making the thick cream into a slurry using saline, thus reducing the pH.

Early excision of the burn wound, popularized in the 1970s, has led to a decrease in complications and a decrease in patient length of stay. Early excision is defined as within the first 7 days postburn. **Tangential excision** is the sequential sharp removal of necrotic tissue until viable tissue is identified by the presence of punctate bleeding. This yields a better cosmetic and functional result than **full excision**, which is the removal of all tissue down to the underlying fascia. Tangential excision is associated with significant blood loss, and it is best performed with a planned, team approach. Excisions should be limited in time and should be TBSA debrided; several operative sessions may be required. **Circumferential injuries may create a vascular emergency.** The burn need not be totally circumferential or even full thickness. The inelastic burn wound (eschar) acts as a tourniquet; edema from the burn trauma and subsequent fluid resuscitation lead to increased compartment pressure. The **classic signs of pain, paresthesia, and pallor** may be difficult to assess. Loss of pulses or Doppler signals are seen late, and irreparable neurovascular damage already may have occurred. **Direct measurement of compartment pressure is the best way to determine the need for escharotomy.** This can be done with a 21-gauge needle connected to a transducer and pressure monitor by high pressure tubing. Pressures greater than 30 mm Hg are sufficient to occlude venous outflow. Individual compartments in the hand or leg can be measured selectively. Escharotomy involves incising the eschar down to underlying subcutaneous tissue. It is a bedside procedure, not to be confused with a fasciotomy. Escharotomy may need to be performed on both medial and lateral surfaces. Occasionally, eschar on the torso can create a restrictive respiratory insufficiency that can be relieved by chest escharotomy.

A number of **methods of wound closure** after debridement or excision are available. There is no substitute for the patient's own skin. Most burn wounds can be managed with **split-thickness skin grafts** 0.010 to 0.012 inch thick. Local or free flaps are the exception rather than the rule. Thicker skin grafts may provide better cosmetic and functional results, but they delay donor-site healing, which may be a factor in larger burns in which donor sites need to be reharvested. **Except for the face or other critical cosmetic areas, most skin grafts are meshed.** This allows for expansion and larger surface area coverage, and it permits fluid drainage, preventing subgraft seroma or hematoma collection. Skin meshing at a 1.5 : 1 ratio generally provide a good cosmetic result; if donor sites are sparse, meshing ratios of 3 : 1 and 6 : 1 can be employed. The most common cause of graft failure is poor adherence from movement. Closely conforming dressings and immobilizing splints maximize graft take. **In the absence of donor autograft, cadaver allograft, synthetic materials, or culture-derived skin have been used as substitutes. Wound closure also significantly decreases the dramatic metabolic demands imposed by a large burn.** Burns greater than 20% TBSA are associated with a hypercatabolic state characterized by increased oxygen consumption, increased nitrogen excretion, and loss of lean body mass. Metabolic rate, as calculated by the Harris-Benedict equation, may exceed baseline levels by 2 to $2^1/_2$ times. This hypermetabolism is both externally driven (evaporative losses) and internally driven (sympathetic discharge).

Another response to a burn injury greater than 20% TBSA is **ileus**, usually lasting 2 to 3 days. Once this has resolved, **enteral support** can begin. Establishing the minimum daily caloric needs has been controversial. The most commonly used estimate is the **Curreri formula**: $(25 \times kg) + (45 \times \% TBSA burn)$. This estimate, however, may **predict *maximal* caloric needs best, and strict adherence to the formula can result in overfeeding. A more realistic approach is to aim for levels approximately 60% to 70% of the Curreri formula** and to monitor nutritional outcomes by indirect calorimetry or urine nitrogen levels. Nitrogen requirements can be estimated at ratio of 1 g nitrogen to 150 calories.

How are Children Different from Adults?

Children are not merely "little adults." **The care of the pediatric burn patient is significantly different in fundamental ways from the care of the adult burn patient.** Estimation of burn size in the child requires a different nomogram, since the head comprises a greater surface area and the limbs comprise a lesser surface area in relation to the torso than in adults. Weight to surface area ratios are different as well, and this affects fluid requirements. A 7-kg child has one-tenth the weight of a 70-kg adult but one-fourth the surface area. Resuscitation formulas also must account for a higher ratio of total body water to body weight. Thus, in small children, the Parkland formula may not deliver enough fluid, and thus it should be supplemented by the daily maintenance dose. Unlike adults, children have limited glycogen stores, and thus, resuscitation fluid should contain glucose. The urine should be monitored for glycosuria in order to prevent osmotic diuresis.

Children have a higher rate of heat exchange than adults and poor heat conservation, making them susceptible to hypothermia. Limited renal and respiratory functions in the very young complicate electrolyte and nutrition management. Transient systolic hypertension has been described in up to one quarter of pediatric burn patients. Related to plasma renin, this phenomenon resolves with wound closure. Indications for treatment include hypertension persisting for greater than 24 hours, diastolic hypertension, or symptomatic hypertension.

As many as one third of burns in children are suspicious for **child abuse**, and 2% to 6% of pediatric burns requiring admission to the hospital can be proven to be nonaccidental. A suspicion of intentional burning warrants a social service investigation. Both historical and physical findings may alert the physician, nurse, or therapist to the possibility of child abuse (**Table 34.2**). Suspicion of a nonaccidental burn warrants admission to the hospital and a social service investigation, even if the burn itself could be managed on an outpatient basis.

Table 34.2. Historical and physical findings of child abuse by burning.

Historical clues
  Burn attributed to sibling
  Child brought to emergency room by nonrelated adult
  Inappropriate parental affect
  Treatment delay
  Differing historical accounts
  History of earlier accidents
  Inappropriate affect of the child or abnormal response to pain

Physical examination clues
  Injury inconsistent with history
  Injury inconsistent with child's developmental or chronologic age
  "Mirror image" injuries
  Burns localized to perineum, genitalia, or buttocks
  Injury appears older than stated age
  Unrelated injuries, old or new

Rehabilitation Issues

The importance of aggressive, early, and coordinated **rehabilitation therapy** to the ultimate outcome of the burn patient cannot be overemphasized. Passive range of motion and splinting begin immediately. **The burn wound will shorten by *contraction*, resulting in a *contracture* across flexor creases unless it is opposed.** The position of comfort is the position of contracture. **All joints should be positioned or splinted in an antideformity position.** Efforts to reduce edema facilitates range of motion. While survival is the primary goal, **physical and occupational therapy objectives** always are kept in mind. Since the goal is independent function, activities of daily living are stressed.

The risk of **hypertrophic scar formation** is reduced with early skin coverage. Burn scar in general and hypertrophic scar in particular are more tender and pruritic than superficial injuries or grafted areas. Patients often complain more about itching and heat intolerance than pain. Little can be done other than supportive care with skin moisturizers and analgesics or antihistamines. **Long-term treatment of hypertrophic scar involves pressure garments, steroid injection, and scar revision.** In the absence of functional disability, scar revision usually is delayed until the scar matures, a process that can take from 6 to 18 months.

Mental rehabilitation is as important as physical rehabilitation. The patient's cooperation and the cooperation of the family are essential to a successful outcome. Patient education should begin as early as possible. Depression, grief, and anger are common stages of the rehabilitation process. Social workers or other counselors are an integral part of the burn team.

Summary

Burn injury results in both physical and psychological trauma. Perhaps among all the trauma care disciplines, effective burn management demands an extended and interdisciplinary team. Optimal outcomes can be obtained only by a comprehensive and systematic approach. Attention to detail in burn assessment and early resuscitation set the stage. An accurate as possible assessment of burn size and depth is necessary for a rational resuscitation plan. It also facilitates decisions relating to possible transfer to a tertiary center and estimation of prognosis. Planning for early wound closure, adequate nutritional support to counter hypermetabolism, and coordinated rehabilitation and pain management efforts yield the best results.

Selected Readings

American Burn Association. Inhalation injury: diagnosis. JACS 2003;196:308–312.

American College of Surgeons Committee on Trauma. Advanced Trauma Life Support. Chicago: American College of Surgeons, 1997.

Hammond J, Perez-Stable A, Ward CG. Predictive value of historical and physical characteristics for the diagnosis of child abuse. South Med J 1991;84:166.

Hammond J, Ward CG. Transfers from emergency room to burn center: errors in burn size estimate. J Trauma 1997;27:1161.

Martin RR, Becker W, Cioffi WG, Pruitt BA Jr. Thermal injuries. In: Wilson R, Walt A, eds. Management of Trauma: Pitfalls and Practice, 2nd ed. Baltimore: Williams & Wilkins 1996.

Saffle J, Zeliff G, Warden GD. Intramuscular pressure in the burned arm: measurement and response to escharotomy. Am J Surg 1980;140:825.

Saffle JR. What's new in general surgery: burns and metabolism. JACS 2003; 196:267–289.

Sheridan RL. Burns. Crit Care Med 2002;30(11 suppl):S500–514.

Sheridan RL. Burn care: results of technical and organizational progress. JAMA 2003;290:719–722.

Ward CG, Hammond J. Burns. In: Kreis DJ Jr, Gomez GA, eds. Trauma Management. Boston: Little, Brown, 1989.

Yurt RW. Burns. In Norton J, Bollinger R, Chang A, et al, eds. Surgery: Basic Science and Clinical Evidence. New York: Springer-Verlag, 2001.

Principles of Perioperative Care of the Pediatric Surgical Patient

Randall S. Burd

Objectives

1. **To implement a unified approach to the pediatric surgical patient and his/her family.**
2. **To outline a basic nutritional program for infants and children in the perioperative period.**
3. **To understand the principles of adjusting fluids in, of evaluating fluid loss in, and of administering blood products and medications to the pediatric surgical patient.**

Case

You are asked to evaluate a 4-year-old boy for progressive abdominal distention and vomiting. He was well until 5 days ago, when he developed anorexia and a low-grade fever. Because his parents felt that he had a "stomach flu," they encouraged him to take liquids and gave him acetaminophen. Over the past day, he has had higher fevers at home and has developed increasing abdominal distention and vomiting. His parents estimate that he has lost several pounds during this recent illness. On examination, he has a temperature of 39°C, has a pulse rate of 110, is irritable, has sunken eyes, and has a distended tender abdomen. His white blood cell count is 19,000 with a left shift. A computed tomography (CT) scan of the abdomen is obtained that shows dilated loops of small bowel with inflammatory changes in the right lower quadrant, findings consistent with perforated appendicitis. An appendectomy is planned.

Introduction

Many medical students and surgical residents find their pediatric surgical rotation to be more difficult than their adult surgical rotations. **Because pediatric surgeons care for a wide range of children from**

Table 35.1. Principles for approaching the pediatric surgical patient.

Go slow
Children grow
The child's weight you should know

premature infants weighing less than a kilogram to nearly adult teenagers, a single approach or formula that comfortably can be learned when caring for adult patients often cannot be used when caring for the pediatric surgical patient. In addition, infants and younger children cannot present their symptoms themselves and may not be able to cooperate with medical evaluation and treatment, making history taking and physical examination a frustrating experiences. While a single approach to perioperative management of pediatric surgical patients of all ages and with all diagnoses is impossible, we have found that a few general strategies can be used to simplify the care of the pediatric surgical patients (Table 35.1). This chapter presents these strategies, and gives guidelines on how these strategies can be applied in everyday practice.

Principle 1: Go Slow

A "slow-down" approach is most productive and time efficient when examining the pediatric surgical patient. A hurried approach to history taking and examination is upsetting to the child, preventing accurate assessment and actually requiring additional time. The approach to pediatric surgical patients should be tailored to their ages and developmental stages. The first step in gaining the trust and the cooperation of the child during medical evaluation is to spend time in gaining the trust and cooperation of the parent. Parents understandably are anxious when their child is being evaluated for a possible surgical procedure, and even the smallest child easily can perceive this anxiety.

Infants and particularly toddlers are most difficult to examine for practitioners with no experience with children. A hurried approach particularly can be disruptive for this age group. Infants and toddlers often do not cooperate and do not understand the evaluation and the procedures that they are undergoing. Performing the physical examination slowly and out of order usually is helpful. It is more useful to proceed first with the abdominal examination while one has the trust of the child, and to perform evaluations that more typically are upsetting and may make the child cry, such as ear, nose, and throat examinations, at the end. It is useful to spend time having the child focus on a simple distraction, such as listening to the examiner's whispered voice, holding a toy, or watching bubbles being blown. When examining the child described in the case presented at the beginning of the chapter, using a calm voice, an unhurried approach, and a toy as a distraction may be useful.

Although attempts at detailed explanations of anatomy and procedures usually are not productive, time should be spent giving older children and teenagers a simple age-specific explanation of planned evaluations and treatments in order to gain their trust and cooperation. It also is useful to have children in these age groups participate with their parents in giving the medical history. Younger children are invited to provide additional information after their parents or caregivers have given the child's medical history, while teenagers should be the initial source of medical information in order to respect their growing autonomy. When possible, time should be spent with teenage patients in a second evaluation without a parent present, since important additional information may be obtained.

An additional aspect of a "slow-down" approach is to perform repeated examinations. If, during the initial encounter, the child is irritable or crying, making evaluation difficult, the examination may be repeated when the child gains comfort with the environment or examiner. In the case presented, a more accurate abdominal examination may be obtained on repeat examination than on an initial examination. Repeated evaluation particularly is useful in the emergency room evaluation of trauma, since the need for multiple simultaneous evaluations and interventions may make it difficult to get an accurate assessment of key aspects of the physical examination. Repeating the evaluation more than once usually proves to be an efficient use of time.

Principle 2: Children Grow

Nutritional Assessment

Nutritional assessment is an essential feature of the care of the pediatric surgical patient in the perioperative period. In addition to the usual goal in adults of replenishing and maintaining nutritional status, children have an additional goal of requiring sufficient nutritional support to continue their normal growth and development. This aspect of care is important particularly in premature infants who may be hospitalized for several weeks or months after surgery during this important growth phase. **The nutritional status of the hospitalized infant or child is evaluated on a daily basis to ensure that a plan is in place to meet the goals of replenishment, maintenance, or growth.**

Although most children seen by the pediatric surgeon are healthy and have adequate nutritional status, this observation should not prevent initial nutritional assessment in any child. The first step is to obtain an adequate **nutritional history**. The child's **medical history** is reviewed for acute illness (such as a viral illness associated with vomiting) or chronic illness (such as malignancy or metabolic disorders) that may affect adversely the child's baseline nutritional status. The child's **surgical history** also may be relevant if previous operations, such as intestinal resection, have been performed that adversely may affect gastrointestinal absorption and nutrition. The parent or caregiver should be asked to provide information about the child's **dietary history, food preferences, appetite, and recent weight changes**.

Nutritional assessment continues with measurement of the child's current **weight and height**. **Head circumference** also is included in the evaluation of infants and toddlers. Values are graphed on age-specific growth charts and compared to previous values whenever possible. Useful guidelines in evaluating the weight of infants is that newborn infants usually lose 10% of their birth weight in the first week due to normal postnatal diuresis, and infants will double their birth weight by 5 months and triple their birth weight by 1 year. Weight is most useful for acute nutritional deficiency, while height and head circumference are more useful for evaluating chronic nutritional changes. Although not required in most children, **biochemical tests** that can estimate nutritional status, such as albumin and transferrin levels, are useful when the initial history or examination suggests acute or chronic nutritional deficiency.

The Choice and Timing of Supplemental Nutrition

The decision whether or not to begin supplemental nutrition is made upon the child's hospital admission and is reassessed daily. Supplemental nutrition is not needed in most pediatric surgical patients, since initially most have adequate nutritional status and are hospitalized for only a few days. **Even if a decision initially is made to defer using supplemental nutrition, it is essential to reevaluate this decision on a daily basis and to document the reasons for this decision, since acute malnutrition after surgery can affect the outcome adversely in even healthy children. When it is anticipated that the child will not be able to resume a normal diet within 5 days, additional supplementation should be initiated (see Algorithm 35.1).** In the case presented at the beginning of the chapter, the clinical examination suggests recent weight loss due to anorexia and vomiting. While the child can be expected to resume normal oral intake several days after surgery, the child's weight on admission should be obtained and compared to his premorbid weight.

The route of administration of supplemental nutrition can be chosen using a simple algorithm (see **Algorithm 35.1**). An **enteral route** of nutrition generally is safest and least expensive. Evidence from adult and animal studies suggests that this route better preserves gut mucosal integrity and reduces the incidence of infectious and metabolic complications compared to using total parenteral nutrition. This route cannot be used when the gastrointestinal tract is not available because of recent abdominal surgery or in the presence of acute medical illnesses such as pancreatitis. When **parenteral nutrition** is begun, the reasons that require that choice should be reevaluated on a daily basis and a conversion to enteral nutrition should be started as soon as possible. In the case presented, the child's weight and oral intake should be followed carefully during hospitalization, and supplementation via an enteral or parenteral route should be initiated if a prolonged period of recovery is expected.

Estimating the nutritional requirements of infants and children often is an intimidating task for those not experienced with children.

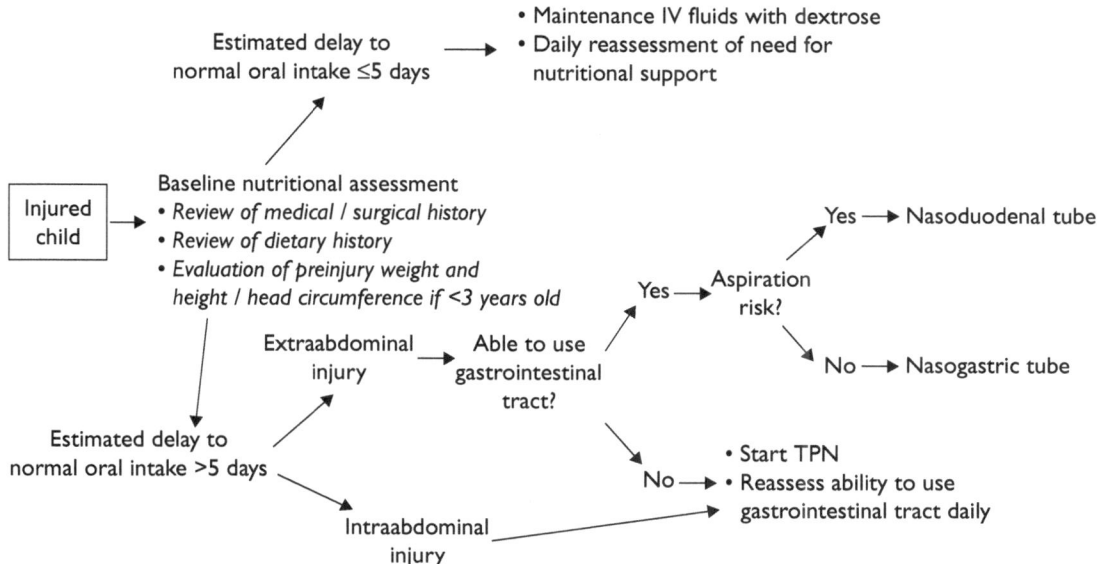

Algorithm 35.1. Algorithm for evaluating the timing and route of administration of nutritional support in pediatric trauma patients. TPN, total parenteral nutrition. (Reprinted from Burd RS, Coats RD, Mitchell BS. Nutritional support of the pediatric trauma patient: a practical approach. Respir Care Clin North Am 2001;7(1):79–96. Copyright © 2001 Elsevier Inc. With permission from Elsevier.)

Although requirements differ markedly depending on age, a step-wise approach can be used in most cases to simplify this task. A good starting point for estimating the caloric needs of a child are the recommended daily allowances (RDA) that have been established for different age groups by the Food and Nutritional Board of the National Academy of Sciences (**Table 35.2**). When this table is not readily available, **the RDA can be approximated quickly by using this equation: Estimated daily caloric requirements = [95 − (Age in years × 3)] kcal/kg/day.** The major limitation of this method is that it tends to over-

Table 35.2. Estimated caloric and protein requirements in infants and children.

Age (years)	Energy requirements (kcal/kg/day)	Protein (g/kg/day)
0–0.5	108	2.0–2.5
0.5–1	98	2.0–2.5
1–3	102	1.5–2.0
4–6	90	1.5–2.0
7–10	70	1.5–2.0
Male 11–14	55	1.0–1.5
Female 11–14	47	1.0–1.5

Source: Adapted from Siberry GK, Iannone R. Nutrition. In: The Harriet Lane Handbook, 15th ed. St. Louis, Mosby-Year Book, 1999. Reprinted from Burd RS, Coats RD, Mitchell BS. Nutritional support of the pediatric trauma patient: a practical approach. Respir Care Clin North Am 2001;7(1):79–96. Copyright © 2001 Elsevier Inc. With permission from Elsevier.

estimate the requirements in overweight or edematous patients and to underestimate requirements in malnourished patients. Although it is most useful to use the ideal body weight of the child, these methods provide a convenient starting point that can be reassessed as nutritional supplementation is given.

Monitoring Nutritional Supplementation

Weight should be evaluated on a daily basis in all children, and length and head circumference should be evaluated on a periodic basis in infants. Because of the inaccuracy of individual weight measurements in small premature infants, it is useful to consider the average weight change over longer periods in these patients. In general, sufficient nutritional supplementation should be given to achieve a gain of 15 to 30 g/day in infants and about 0.5% of current weight per day in older children. When weight assessment is difficult for children receiving long-term nutritional support because of factors such as fluid shifts or the addition of bandages or casts, weekly measurement of prealbumin values is useful to evaluate the adequacy of nutritional support.

Designing a Nutritional Program

The individual components of total **parenteral nutrition** are estimated and modified according to the infant or child's nutritional needs (see **Algorithm 35.2**). Adequate nitrogen usage usually can be achieved by providing 25 to 35 kcal of carbohydrate and lipid calories per gram of amino acids. Carbohydrates generally are given to provide 70% and lipids to provide 30% of nonprotein calories. The starting electrolyte composition of the formula is adjusted according to the child's age (**Table 35.3**). As with all aspects of nutritional supplementation, these parameters are reassessed regularly, and appropriate modifications are made for the child's current needs.

When an **enteral route** of nutrition is selected, direct modification of individual nutritional components usually is not needed, since most commonly used formulas have fixed and not modular components. Nevertheless, it is important to evaluate the key components of any given formula to ensure that individual components, particularly protein content, are met adequately in children receiving long-term support. Similar to breast milk, most commercially available infant formulas (e.g., Similar or Enfamil) contain 20 kcal per ounce of formula. Modified infant formulas suitable for premature infants that contain 24 kcal per ounce also are available. Breast milk almost always is preferred to formula and has been shown to afford a distinct outcome advantage for critically ill pediatric surgical patients. When additional calories are required, breast milk can be supplemented with commercially available fortifiers or by the addition of separate components, such as polycose or medium-chain fatty acid oils. Because the requirement for excess free water is unique to infants, formulas that provide one calorie per milliliter such as Pediasure or Pediatric Vivonex, usually are given to children older than 1 year. Because the solute

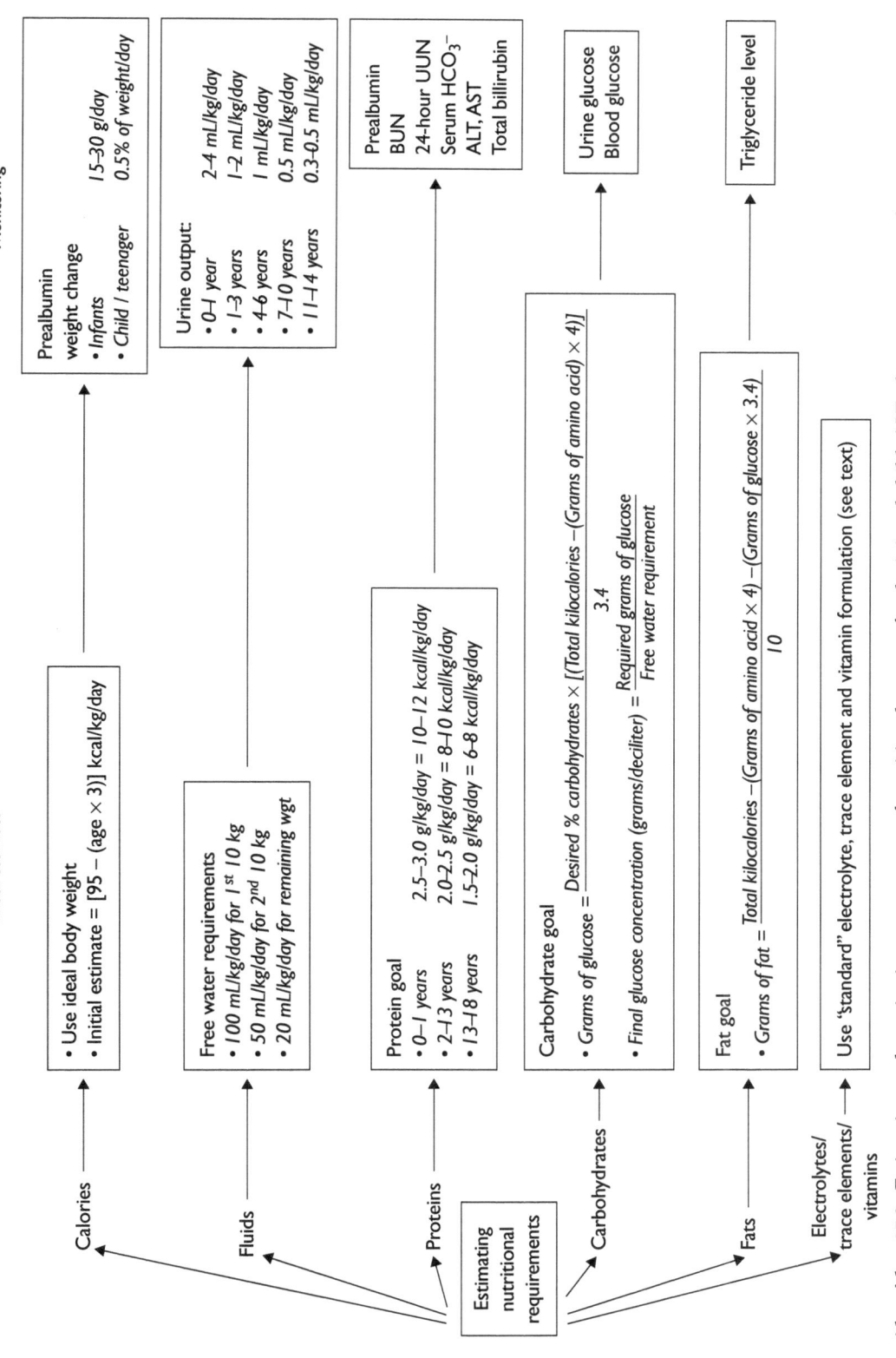

Algorithm 35.2. Estimating and monitoring components of nutritional support for the injured child. ALT, alanine aminotransferase; AST, aspartate aminotransferase; BUN, blood urea nitrogen; UUN, urinary urea nitrogen. (Reprinted from Burd RS, Coats RD, Mitchell BS. Nutritional support of the pediatric trauma patient: a practical approach. Respir Care Clin North Am 2001;7(1):79–96. Copyright © 2001 Elsevier Inc. With permission from Elsevier.)

Table 35.3. Recommended daily electrolyte and trace element requirements in infants and children.

Component		Daily requirement
Sodium		2–4 mEq/kg
Potassium		2–3 mEq/kg
Chloride		2–3 mEq/kg
Acetate		1–4 mEq/kg
Magnesium		0.25–0.5 mEq/kg
Calcium	Neonate:	300–500 mg/kg
	Infant:	100–200 mg/kg
	Child/adolescent:	50–100 mg/kg
Phosphorus	Neonate:	1–1.5 mM/kg
	Infant:	1.0 mM/kg
	Child/adolescent:	0.5–1.0 mM/kg
Zinc		50 µg/kg
Copper		20 µg/kg
Chromium		0.2 µg/kg
Manganese		1 µg/kg

Source: Reprinted from Burd RS, Coats RD, Mitchell BS. Nutritional support of the pediatric trauma patient: a practical approach. Respir Care Clin North Am 2001;7(1):79–96. Copyright © Elsevier Inc. With permission from Elsevier.

composition of these formulas may comprise up to about 30% of total volume, free water supplementation often is needed to achieve adequate fluid requirements and should be considered.

Principle 3: The Child's Weight You Should Know

The Importance of Initial Weight Assessment

Virtually all medical interventions in children, including nutritional support, fluids, medications, and tubes, are adjusted according to patient size. For this reason, it is important to weigh every child as soon as possible at the start of any evaluation. When immediate medical intervention, such as an emergency trauma setting, precludes obtaining the patient's weight, the child's weight can be approximated quickly using the following formula: (Age in years × 4) + 4 = Estimated weight in kilograms. Because the relative increase in weight observed in infants is greater than that observed in older children, adjustments based on weight changes may be needed on a daily basis in these patients.

Estimating Maintenance Fluid Rates

Maintenance fluids can be estimated rapidly using the 4-2-1 rule shown in Table 35.4. This method usually is easier to use than the 100-50-20 rule, since intravenous fluids generally are ordered on an hourly and not on a daily basis. With the premature infant, the fluid rate is modified on a nearly hourly basis, since fluid shifts due to insensible losses and seemingly minor additions and deletions, such as catheter flushes and blood draws, may create important fluid shifts. Fluid

Table 35.4. Calculation of maintenance fluid requirements.

Body weight (kg)	Fluid volume/hr
1–10	4 mL/kg
11–20	4 mL/kg + 2 mL/each kg over 10 kg
>20	60 mL + 1 mL/each kg over 20 kg

Source: Reprinted from Albanese CT. Pediatric surgery. In: Norton JA, Bollinger RR, Chang AE, et al, eds. Surgery: Basic Science and Clinical Evidence. New York: Springer-Verlag, 2001, with permission.

boluses also are tailored to a child's weight. Crystalloid boluses are given at a volume of 20 cc per kilogram, and boluses of colloids, such as albumin solutions, and fresh frozen plasma generally are given at a volume of 10 cc per kilogram.

Administration of Blood Product

Administration of blood products warrants special consideration. Several methods can be used to estimate the required volume of **packed red blood cells** needed to achieve a normal hematocrit. It is useful to calculate transfusion needs using more than one method in order to become familiar with each. **In an emergency setting when rapid transfusion is needed, an easy estimate of required transfusion volume is 10 cc per kilogram. A more accurate estimate can be obtained using the following equation:**

$$\text{Volume of cells (cc)} =$$
$$\frac{\text{Estimated blood volume (cc)} \times (\text{Desired} - \text{Actual hematocrit change})}{\text{Hematocrit of packed red blood cells}}$$

where the blood volume is estimated using Table 35.5 and the hematocrit of packed red blood cells is estimated as 65%. Regardless of the estimated volume, packed red blood cells are administered at a rate of about 2 to 3 cc/kg/hour. In small infants, the response to transfusion is evaluated after every 10 cc per kilogram volume in order to evaluate the need for additional transfusion and to avoid excessive transfusion.

The **volume of platelet transfusion** depends on the type of platelets that are used. "Random donor units" are the platelets obtained from a unit of blood. The blood is collected in the anticoagulant and spun

Table 35.5. Age-based estimation of blood volume.

Premature infants	85–100 mL/kg
Term newborns	85 mL/kg
Age >1 month to 3 months	75 mL/kg
Age 3 months to adult	70 mL/kg

Source: Adapted from Rowe PC, ed. In: The Harriet Lane Handbook, 11th ed. Chicago: Year Book Medical, 1987:25.

to give the platelet-rich plasma and the packed red blood cells. The platelet-rich plasma then is separated into a unit of fresh frozen plasma and a unit of platelets (about 50 cc). When using this type of platelet solution, 0.1 unit per kilogram or 1 unit for every 10 kg is given. In neonates, 5 to 10 cc per kilogram can be given. The other type of platelets that can be used are pheresed platelets. These come from a single donor and are obtained from donors by having their blood circulated through a machine that separates the platelets and returns the rest. This method results in a platelet preparation with a volume of about 200 to 250 cc per donor and is the equivalent of 6 to 8 random donor units. The advantage of using pheresed platelets is that the recipient is exposed to only one donor. For pheresed platelets, one-fourth unit can be given to a 5- to 25-kg patient, one-half unit to a 25- to 50-kg patient, and 1 unit to a nearly adult-sized teenage patient.

Estimate Fluid Status after Surgery

Monitoring of volume status in children in the perioperative period also is highly dependent on the patient's weight. Urine output is noted in cc per kilogram per hour and compared to the general guidelines shown in **Table 35.6.** Diapers can be weighed to estimate urine volume, which is useful in avoiding the potential trauma of bladder catheterization in small infants and children. **Other sources of fluid output** also are best evaluated, correcting for the child's weight (**Table 35.6**). Although each of these represent only estimates of expected output, it is useful to use these values when evaluating initial losses and when following ongoing losses.

Correct Dosing of Medications

Medication dosing also is critically dependent on the child's weight. Because seemingly small differences may lead to overdosing in a child, it is important that attention be paid to accurate dosing in children. Many children's hospitals have developed fail-safe mechanisms, such as administration forms, pharmacy verification, and double-checking protocols, to avoid inaccurate dosing of medications. Only pediatric medication manuals should be used to dose medications given to the child in the postoperative period. As is now being required at many

Table 35.6. Fluid management.

Other fluid ranges	
NGT output	0.5–2 cc/kg/h
Chest tube	2 cc/kg/d
Ileostomy output	<2 cc/kg/h
Intraoperative fluids	5–10 cc/kg/h
Urine output	
Newborn	2–4 cc/kg/h
Infant	1–2 cc/kg/h
Child	1 cc/kg/h
Teenager/adult	0.3–0.5 cc/kg/h

NGT, nasogastric tube.

hospitals, it is useful to note the patient's weight and the dose on a per kilogram basis on the patient order sheet whenever a new medication or new dosage of a medication is given.

Summary: Are Children Little Adults?

During fetal development, infancy, and childhood, rapid changes occur in physiology that usually are not observed in adult life. The unique physiology at each stage of development accounts for the occurrence of many diseases predominant in specific groups, such as necrotizing enterocolitis in premature infants, intussusception in toddlers, and appendicitis in older children and teenagers. The wide variations in physiology and the diversity of diagnoses that result from these changes account for the appeal of practicing pediatric surgery, but they can be an initial source of frustration for the student with initial experience only with adult patients. The use of principles for managing adults in the perioperative period frequently is not helpful for the pediatric surgical patient. Using principles that recognize the uniqueness of each stage of development can simplify the approach to the pediatric surgical patient.

Selected Readings

Albanese CT. Pediatric surgery. In: Norton JA, Bollinger RR, Chang AE, et al, eds. Surgery: Basic Science and Clinical Evidence. New York: Springer-Verlag, 2001.

Hansen A, Puder M. Manual of Neonatal Surgical Intensive Care. Hamilton, Ontario: BC Decker, 2003.

Moss L, Smith BM, Kosloske AM. Case Studies in Pediatric Surgery. New York: McGraw-Hill Professional, 2000.

36

Neonatal Intestinal Obstruction

Randall S. Burd

Objectives

1. To recognize the symptoms and signs of neonatal intestinal obstruction.
2. To understand a generalized approach to evaluating newborns with intestinal obstruction.
3. To be able to give a differential diagnosis for the causes of neonatal intestinal obstruction and to understand the general principles for treatment.

Case

You are asked to evaluate a 12-hour-old newborn male infant because of bilious vomiting. Polydramnios and a dilated stomach were noted on serial prenatal ultrasounds, but amniocentesis was not performed. The infant was born at 36 weeks by vaginal delivery to a 35-year-old mother without complication. The infant has been irritable and has vomited dark-green bilious material with each of two attempts at feeding. The infant is noted on examination to have findings consistent with trisomy 21 (Down syndrome) including poor muscle tone, oblique palpebral fissures, epicanthal folds, and abnormally shaped ears. The abdominal examination shows epigastric prominence, but it is otherwise normal, and the anus is in a normal position and appears patent. Duodenal atresia is suspected.

Introduction

A diverse range of diseases can lead to intestinal obstruction in the newborn infant (**Table 36.1**). While the etiology, pathophysiology, and treatment of surgical causes of intestinal obstruction in the neonate are varied, it is helpful to use a diagnostic approach that considers each disease, particularly since more than one may be present. Because **several of these diseases can be life-threatening or lead to lifelong disability if not treated promptly, the diagnostic evaluation should be rapid and follows a series of logical steps (see Algorithm 36.1).**

Presentation

The **initial presenting signs and symptoms** of neonatal intestinal obstruction are varied and include frothy oral secretions, poor feeding, bilious or nonbilious vomiting, abdominal distention, and absent or delayed passage of meconium. The **timing and nature** of each presenting finding can provide very useful information about the etiology of the intestinal obstruction. **Proximal intestinal obstructions, such as esophageal atresia or congenital causes of gastroduodenal obstruction, usually present within the first 24 to 48 hours of life. Distal obstructions, such as ileal or colorectal atresias, may present a few days after birth, while functional obstructions, such as Hirschsprung's disease, may present as late as a few weeks to years after birth.** Esophageal atresia presents with prominent oral and upper airway findings, including excessive frothy oropharyngeal secretions and repeated episodes of coughing, choking, or cyanosis that become apparent with attempts at feeding. Although poor feeding eventually is a feature of all causes of newborn intestinal obstruction, this finding may be delayed in patients with distal gastrointestinal tract or functional obstructions. **The absence of bile in the emesis suggests that the level of obstruction is proximal to the ampulla of Vater.** Bilious vomiting suggests a more distal obstruction and is an important finding, since about 25% of neonates with this finding eventually require abdominal surgery. In the case presented above, bilious emesis suggests an obstruction that is distal to the ampulla of Vater.

The presence and timing of onset of abdominal distention also can provide useful diagnostic information. **Abdominal distention that is present at birth can result from antenatal intestinal obstruction and perforation usually due to volvulus, intestinal atresia, meconium ileus (meconium peritonitis), an intraperitoneal mass (choledochal cyst, mesenteric cyst, duplication cyst, hydrometrocolpos, or ovarian cyst), a retroperitoneal mass (hydronephrosis or renal mass), or ascites.** Although epigastric fullness may be observed, generalized abdominal distention usually does not occur in neonates with gastroduodenal obstruction. Abdominal distention, however, can develop in the first hours after birth in neonates with esophageal atresia due to air passing through a concomitant tracheoesophageal fistula, particularly if the infant is ventilated mechanically. Neonates with malrotation and midgut volvulus also may develop abdominal distention due to dilatation of a closed segment of bowel distal to the usual site of duodenal obstruction. Abdominal distention usually is delayed in those infants with more distal or functional obstructions and may appear 24 hours or later after birth.

A mechanical or functional intestinal obstruction should be considered when passage of the first meconium stool is delayed or absent or

Table 36.1. Presentation of potential cause of neonatal intestinal obstruction.

Diagnosis	Usual presenting symptoms	Possible maternal ultrasound findings	Family history reported?	Abdominal examination
Esophageal atresia	Frothy oropharyngeal secretions, coughing, choking	Polyhydramnios, dilated esophageal pouch, absent gastric fluid	Yes	Usually normal
Pyloric atresia	Nonbilious emesis	Polyhydramnios, dilated stomach	Yes	Epigastric fullness, scaphoid lower abdomen
Duodenal atresia/ annular pancreas	Bilious emesis	Polyhydramnios, dilated stomach and duodenum	Yes	Epigastric fullness, scaphoid lower abdomen
Malrotation with midgut volvulus	Bilious emesis	None	Yes	Initially normal progressing to generalized distention and peritonitis
Jejunoileal atresia	Bilious emesis, abdominal distention	Polyhydramnios, variable amounts of dilated bowel	Yes	Generalized distention
Meconium ileus	Bilious emesis, abdominal distention, delayed or no passage of meconium	Echogenic meconium with proximal dilated bowel	Yes	Generalized distention
Meconium plug syndrome	Abdominal distention, delayed or no passage of meconium	Dilated bowel	No	Generalized distention
Small left colon syndrome	Bilious emesis, abdominal distention, delayed or no passage of meconium	Not reported	No	Generalized distention
Colorectal atresia	Bilious emesis, abdominal distention, delayed or no passage of meconium	Dilated bowel	No	Generalized distention

Table 36.1. *Continued*

Important associated anomalies and disorders	Findings on abdominal radiograph	Finding on barium enema	Additional studies needed to establish diagnosis	General treatment
VACTERL association, CHD, chromosomal anomalies	Gasless abdomen if no TEF, vertebral anomalies	Normal*	Chest x-ray with oroesophageal tube (see text)	Primary or delayed repair
Epidermolysis bullosa	Single bubble	Normal*	None	Primary repair
Trisomy 21, malrotation, CHD	Double bubble	Normal or malrotation*	None	Primary repair
Intestinal atresia	Double bubble	Malrotation	UGI series if diagnosis in doubt	Ladd procedure (see text)
Malrotation	Distended air-filled loops of intestine with absent distal air	Microcolon (in distal small-bowel atresias)	None	Primary repair
Cystic fibrosis	Dilated loops of intestine of variable caliber without air-fluid levels, ground-glass appearance	Empty microcolon with plugs within a narrow-caliber terminal ileum	None	Therapeutic contrast enemas, enterotomy with irrigation if unsuccessful
Prematurity	Multiple dilated loops of intestine	Obstructing intraluminal mass with proximal intestinal dilatation	Suction rectal biopsy to rule out Hirschsprung's disease	Therapeutic enemas
Infant of diabetic mother	Multiple dilated loops of intestine	Small caliber left colon with proximal intestinal dilatation	Suction rectal biopsy to rule out Hirschsprung's disease	Therapeutic contrast contrast enemas
None	Multiple dilated loops of intestine	Obstructing colorectal lesion	None	Primary repair

Continued

Table 36.1. *Continued*

Diagnosis	Usual presenting symptoms	Possible maternal ultrasound findings	Family history reported?	Abdominal examination
Hirschsprung's disease	Bilious emesis, abdominal distention, delayed passage of meconium	None	Yes	Generalized distention
Imperforate anus	Abdominal distention, no passage of meconium	Septated anechoic bowel in pelvis or lower abdomen	Yes	Generalized distention

CHD, congenital heart disease; TEF, tracheoesophageal fistula; UGI, upper gastrointestinal tract; VACTERL, vertebral, anal, cardiac, tracheoesophageal fistula, renal and limb anomalies.
* Contrast enema not usually needed for diagnosis or treatment.

only scant amounts of meconium are passed. **The initial passage of meconium usually occurs within the first 24 hours of life, but it may be delayed in normal premature infants without intestinal obstruction.** Delayed passage of meconium is a frequent finding in patients with distal intestinal obstruction and is observed in 90% of infants with Hirschsprung's disease. The passage of meconium does not indicate that a complete intestinal obstruction is not present, since meconium formed in utero distal to an obstruction may be evacuated.

The **maternal ultrasound** can provide important clues about the possible etiology of intestinal obstruction and should be reviewed when a neonate presents with signs or symptoms suggesting an intestinal obstruction. Amniotic fluid is normally swallowed by the fetus and absorbed from the gastrointestinal tract. Obstruction will impair intestinal absorption, leading to accumulation of amniotic fluid or polyhydramnios. As the length of intestine available for absorption decreases, the degree of polyhydramnios increases. **Polyhydramnios more likely is observed in the fetus with a proximal obstruction, such as esophageal atresia without tracheoesophageal fistula or duodenal atresia, and not those with a distal obstruction, such as distal ileal or colonic atresia (Fig. 36.1).**

Maternal ultrasound examination can provide other useful information. The sonographic findings of a dilated proximal esophageal pouch and lack of fluid in the stomach suggests esophageal atresia. Prominent upper abdomen fluid collections representing the fluid-filled stomach and duodenum suggest obstruction at the level of the duodenum, as in the case presented. Dilated loops of bowel with increased peristalsis may be observed in a fetus with distal intestinal obstructions, while

Table 36.1. *Continued*

Important associated anomalies and disorders	Findings on abdominal radiograph	Finding on barium enema	Additional studies needed to establish diagnosis	General treatment
Trisomy 21	Multiple dilated loops of intestine	Undilated rectum or distal colon with dilated proximal colon	Suction rectal biopsy	Resection of aganglionic intestine, anastomosis of ganglionic intestine to anorectum
Genitourinary anomalies, spinal/vertebral anomalies, CHD	Multiple dilated loops of intestine, possible vertebral anomalies	Not applicable	None	Primary or delayed repair

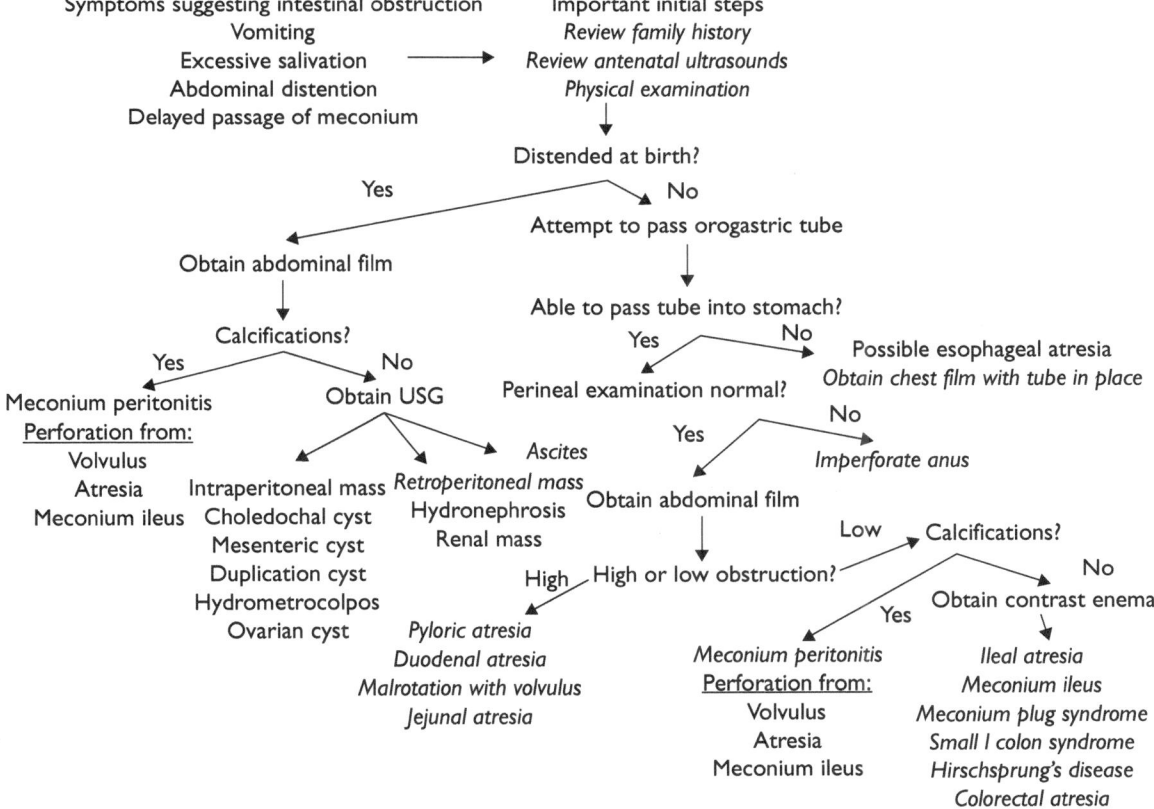

Algorithm 36.1. Algorithm to determine the etiology of neonatal intestinal obstruction. USG, ultrasonogram.

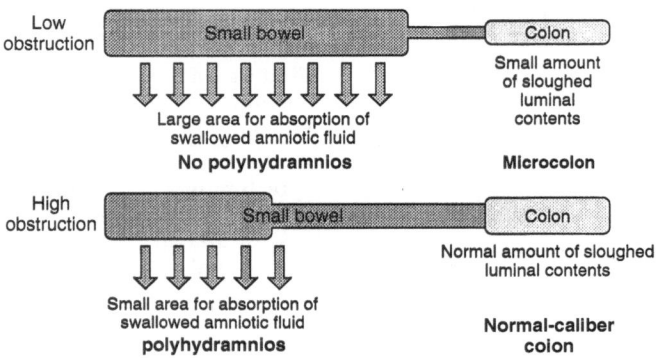

Figure 36.1. Polyhydramnios/microcolon.

dilated bowel associated with echogenic meconium has been observed in fetuses who later present with meconium ileus. Calcifications can form when the peritoneal cavity is exposed to meconium, and their presence suggests an antenatal intestinal perforation. Morphologic abnormalities suggesting a chromosomal defect also may have been observed, prompting amniocentesis and chromosomal testing. Chromosomal defects are found in about 5% of infants with esophageal atresia (most frequently trisomy 18 and 21) and about 30% of infants with duodenal atresia (most commonly trisomy 21).

Family and maternal history may provide additional insight into the cause of neonatal intestinal obstruction. Because a familial association has been reported for most causes, a family history of newborn or childhood surgery for intestinal obstruction should be sought, and the cause should be determined, if possible. Family members with disorders and anomalies outside of the gastrointestinal tract also may suggest an etiology of neonatal intestinal obstruction. For example, siblings of children with esophageal atresia may exhibit features of the VACTERL association (*v*ertebral, *a*nal, *c*ardiac, *t*racheo*e*sophageal fistula, *r*enal and *l*imb anomalies), or a family history of epidermolysis bullosa may be observed in neonates with pyloric atresia. Almost half of neonates with small left colon syndrome are infants of diabetic mothers.

Physical Examination

A **complete examination** is mandatory for all neonates with suspected intestinal obstruction. Particular attention should be focused on the abdominal examination, on the perineal inspection, and on identifying other anomalies, including features suggesting a chromosomal disorder. In the case presented at the beginning of the chapter, the presence of trisomy 21 provides indirect evidence supporting the diagnosis of duodenal atresia. The abdomen should be inspected for distention. Although difficult to observe in most cases, gastroduodenal or high jejunal obstruction may result in epigastric distention with a scaphoid lower abdomen, as described in the case presented. As discussed previously, mechanically ventilated neonates with esophageal atresia and a tracheoesophageal fistula also may exhibit abdominal distention. More distal obstructions produce progressive generalized abdominal distention. The abdomen should be examined for tenderness and masses, and the inguinal region should be inspected for hernia.

Examination of the perineum is important to rule out an imperforate anus. The main features to evaluate are the general perineal appearance and anal position and patency. The anal canal normally is positioned about halfway between the coccyx and base of the scrotum in males or the vestibule in females, and it is within a perineal depression surrounded by slightly pigmented skin. Variations from this standard suggest that a variant of imperforate anus may be present. Neonates with a short distance from the distal colon to the perineum (low imperforate anus) may have a perineal depression with pigmentation without a patent anal canal. With observation during the first 24 hours of life, meconium eventually may pass through a rectoperineal fistula and be seen exiting on the perineum anterior to the normal anal position or at midline raphe of the scrotum or penis in males or vestibule in females. Because meconium may be seen exiting on the perineum in patients with low imperforate anus, the examination should be performed carefully, since a normal anal canal may be confused by inexperienced observers with a low imperforate anus with a rectoperineal fistula. Neonates with a long distance from the distal colon to the perineum (high imperforate anus) have more remarkable perineal findings, including the absence of an anal opening, absence of a perineal depression ("flat bottom"), and lack of pigmented skin.

Additional screening maneuvers may be used to supplement the physical examination. To screen for esophageal atresia, a tube gently is passed through the mouth into the esophagus. In term infants with esophageal atresia, passage of the tube usually stops at about 10 cm (**Fig. 36.2**). If the tube successfully passes into the stomach, the gastric

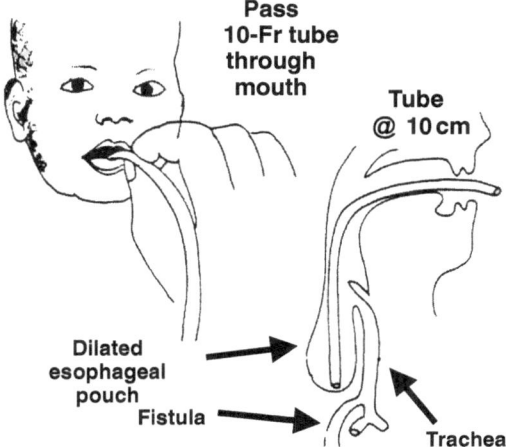

Figure 36.2. Passage of an oral tube to determine esophageal patency. (Adapted from Hutson JM, Beasley SW. The Surgical Examination of Children: An Illustrated Guide. Oxford: Heinemann Medical Books, 1988. Copyright © 1998 Elsevier Ltd. With permission from Elsevier.)

contents are aspirated and measured. Aspiration of more than 10 to 15 cc of bilious material suggests an intestinal obstruction and provides further support for pursuing additional workup for the cause.

Diagnostic Studies

At this point in the workup, the range of possible diagnoses may have been narrowed substantially, and minimal additional diagnostic studies may be required. When the clinical history, presentation, and examination suggest esophageal atresia, **posteroanterior and lateral chest radiographs** should be obtained while gently pushing an orogastric tube against the blind ending esophagus. The presence of a prominent esophageal air pouch containing a curled tube is observed in most cases of esophageal atresia. The **chest radiograph** also should be examined for an abnormal cardiac silhouette that may suggest concomitant congenital cardiac disease and for infiltrates attributable to aspiration of oropharyngeal secretions.

Posteroanterior and lateral decubitus abdominal radiographs should be obtained in all neonates with suspected intestinal obstruction. In the case presented at the beginning of the chapter, the next step is to obtain plain abdominal radiographs. In patients with esophageal atresia, the presence of air in the stomach confirms the presence of a tracheoesophageal fistula. Thoracic, lumbar, or sacral vertebral anomalies, including hemivertebrae and absent vertebrae, can be observed in patients with the VACTERL association and may provide further corroboration of the diagnosis of esophageal atresia. Neonates with pyloric atresia have a prominent dilated stomach. A "double bubble" corresponding to a dilated stomach and duodenum is characteristic of a duodenal obstruction and likely would be observed in the case presented. When duodenal obstruction is suspected but insufficient air has been swallowed to reveal this finding, it is useful to place 50 cc of air via a nasogastric tube and immediately obtain a prone abdominal radiograph. When few dilated loops of bowel are observed beyond the duodenum, jejunal atresia is most likely. When multiple loops of dilated bowel are observed, particularly at more than 24 hours of life, a more distal obstruction is likely (**Fig. 36.3**). Abdominal films demonstrating dilated loops of intestine without air-fluid levels and a ground-glass appearance, particularly in the right lower quadrant, produced by a mixture of air with thick meconium, is characteristic of meconium ileus. Scattered intraabdominal calcifications suggest antenatal perforation and possible obstruction related to meconium peritonitis. Among infants with imperforate anus, the frequency of vertebral anomalies, including lumbar hemivertebrae or absent vertebra and a deficient sacrum, increases as the distance from the perineum to the distal end of the rectum increases.

Plain radiographs together with the history and examination are sufficient to establish the likely diagnosis in most cases of proximal intestinal obstruction. **Upper gastrointestinal contrast** studies usually are not required before laparotomy. The main role of this type of study is to

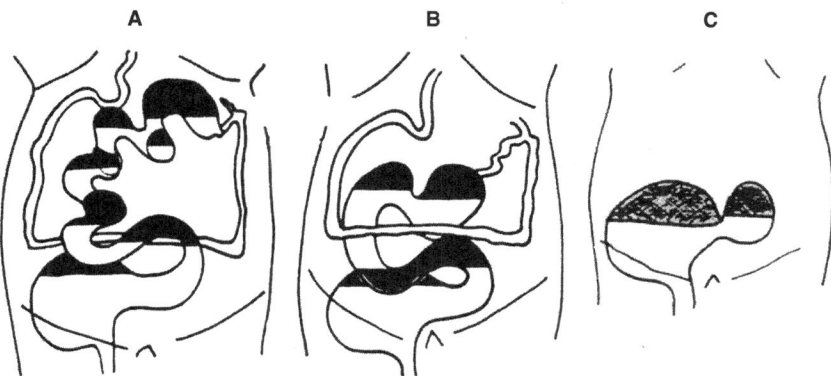

Figure 36.3. Characteristic abdominal film findings with high intestinal obstruction at the level of the duodenum (A), high obstruction at the level of the jejunum (B), and low obstruction at and distal to the ileum (C). (Adapted from Hutson JM, Beasley SW. The Surgical Examination of Children: An Illustrated Guide. Oxford: Heinemann Medical Books, 1988. Copyright © 1998 Elsevier Ltd. With permission from Elsevier.)

establish the diagnosis when it remains in doubt. An important use of this study is to distinguish duodenal atresia from malrotation and midgut volvulus when surgery is delayed because of the need to evaluate and manage suspected cardiac or other anomalies. In all cases of midgut volvulus, exploratory laparotomy should proceed expeditiously. Repair of duodenal atresia, however, may be delayed when it is likely that additional medical management will improve the postoperative course. An upper gastrointestinal contrast study performed to rule out malrotation is mandatory before discharge in all neonates with unexplained bilious vomiting and abdominal distention, since the failure to recognize malrotation before volvulus ensues can lead to midgut necrosis. Neonates with abdominal distention at birth usually should undergo abdominal sonography in addition to plain abdominal radiographs to evaluate for the previously mentioned intraperitoneal and retroperitoneal lesions.

A contrast enema is the most useful test to distinguish the varied causes of intestinal obstruction distal to the jejunum. The passage of intraluminal contents produced by antenatal mucosal shedding determines the degree of intestinal dilatation at birth. For this reason, a normal-caliber colon is observed in patients with proximal intestinal obstructions, and a microcolon is observed with complete obstruction at a point more distal to the jejunum. When meconium ileus is suspected, the contrast study should be performed with Gastrografin, which serves to draw fluid into the intestinal lumen and dislodge thick meconium because of its hyperosmolarity. The contrast study typically demonstrates an empty microcolon with meconium plugs within a narrow-caliber terminal ileum. Meconium plug syndrome is suggested by an obstructing intraluminal mass (usually inspissated meconium) with proximal intestinal dilatation. In small left colon syndrome, a narrow-caliber left colon and dilated proximal colon are observed.

Colorectal atresia may be demonstrated by failure to reflux contrast proximally past a point of obstruction.

The diagnosis of Hirschsprung's disease warrants special consideration. The barium enema in a typical case of Hirschsprung's disease shows an undilated rectum or distal colon with flow into a dilated proximal colon. The transition from ganglionic to aganglionic intestine is observed in the rectosigmoid colon in 85% of patients. When performed in the infant's first month of life, a barium enema may fail to demonstrate a clear transition zone. An abdominal film obtained 24 hours after the initial studies may show retention of barium in infants with Hirschsprung's disease even in the absence of an apparent transition zone. Although radiographic studies may suggest Hirschsprung's disease, a biopsy confirming aganglionic distal colon is needed before surgery. Sampling of the distal rectal mucosa and submucosa usually can be accomplished using a suction rectal device. Biopsy of the rectum probably is indicated in cases of meconium plug syndrome or small left colon syndrome before discharge, since these disorders can be confused with Hirschsprung's disease by clinical presentation and radiographic studies.

Differential Diagnosis

A range of medical conditions may present with symptoms and signs similar to the principal causes of neonatal intestinal obstruction. **Adynamic ileus due to sepsis is the most common mimicker of the surgical causes of intestinal obstruction and can be associated with poor feeding, bilious vomiting, and abdominal distention. Intracranial lesions, including hydrocephalus, subdural hemorrhage, and tumors, and renal diseases, such as genitourinary tract obstruction or renal agenesis, also may result in poor feeding and vomiting.** Evaluation for these nonsurgical disorders should be pursued promptly, and treatment should be begun when a surgical cause of obstruction is not identified.

Principles of Treatment

The surgical treatment of neonatal intestinal obstruction varies depending on the site of obstruction. In general, atresias are resected and gastrointestinal continuity is restored by anastomosis. In some cases, definitive treatment may need to be delayed for weeks or months to allow for further growth, such as in cases with infants with long-gap esophageal atresia or high imperforate anus. Malrotation with midgut volvulus is treated by immediate laparotomy and performing the Ladd procedure: derotation of the volvulus, division of aberrant peritoneal bands crossing the duodenum (Ladd's bands), straightening of the duodenum by mobilizing its retroperitoneal attachments, appendectomy, and placement of the cecum in the left lower quadrant. For meconium ileus and meconium plug syndrome, the contrast enema may be both diagnostic and therapeutic. When the obstruction fails to resolve with therapeutic enemas, surgical evacuation of the intraluminal obstruction may be needed with these two diagnoses. Small left colon syndrome most often improves with nonoperative management and requires surgical intervention only when obstructive symptoms persist or complications such as perforation are observed. The main indication for operation in meconium peritonitis is obstruction or perforation. Surgical repair varies depending on the etiology of the antenatal perforation and on the findings at laparotomy. The principal treatment for Hirschsprung's disease is resection of the aganglionic distal intestine and anorectal anastomosis using ganglionic intestine. Although a neonate with imperforate anus always undergoes repair, the method and timing of repair depend on the type of defect and presence of associated defects. The reader is referred to the selected readings for additional details of treatment of these disorders.

Summary

While the causes of newborn intestinal obstruction are diverse, a systematic approach can be used to differentiate the most common causes. The antenatal history, initial presentation, physical examination, and plain radiographs frequently can establish the diagnosis. The choice of additional diagnostic imaging, such as an upper or lower gastrointestinal series or ultrasound, should be based on the results of the initial workup. The basic principle of treating neonatal intestinal obstruction is to relieve the mechanical obstruction, whether the cause is due to luminal or extraluminal obstruction.

Selected Reading

Albanese CT. Pediatric surgery. In: Norton JA, Bollinger RR, Chang AE, et al., eds. Surgery: Basic Science and Clinical Evidence. New York: Springer-Verlag, 2001.

Oldham KT. Introduction to neonatal intestinal obstruction. In: Oldham KT, Colombani PM, Foglia RP, eds. Surgery of Infants and Children: Scientific Principles and Practice. Philadelphia: Lippincott-Raven, 1997.

Pena A. Atlas of Surgical Management of Anorectal Malformations. New York: Springer-Verlag, 1992.

37

Lower Urinary Tract Disorders

Michael Perrotti

Objectives

1. To discuss the evaluation and treatment options for men with benign prostatic hyperplasia and lower urinary tract symptoms (urinary frequency, nocturia, urgency, urinary retention).
   - Consider pertinent history and physical, diagnostic tests
2. To outline the evaluation and treatment options for patients with urinary incontinence.
3. To describe the potential etiologies of hematuria.
   - Consider age, presence of pain, character of bleeding, trauma
   - Consider occult versus gross hematuria
4. To discuss the diagnostic modalities available for evaluation of hematuria including risks, indications, and limitations.
   - Consider computed tomography (CT), cystoscopy, intravenous pyelogram, ultrasound, cystourethrogram, and retrograde pyelography
5. To discuss the etiologies and diagnostic evaluation of a patient with dysuria.
6. To discuss the etiologies and workup of a patient with pneumaturia.

Cases

Case 1

A 67-year-old woman may have a history of stress incontinence following the birth of her third child and reports a worsening at the time of menopause, but she seeks medical care at the present time because of inability to "hold my urine" 2 years after suffering a cerebral vascular accident. She has no other neurologic residua.

Case 2

A 17-year-old boy is brought to the emergency department after sustaining a bicycle accident. He is noted to have gross blood at the penile meatus. He has not voided since the time of his accident.

Case 3

A 22-year-old college student complains of burning with urination. He has a clear urethral discharge and recently has engaged in unprotected intercourse.

Introduction

Lower urinary tract disorders are intended to include those complaints related to the function of voiding that prompt a patient to seek the care of a physician. Such complaints may be a result of a **primary urinary tract etiology** (i.e., urinary tract infection) or of a **secondary urinary tract etiology** (i.e., bladder hyperreflexia following cerebral vascular accident). Hence, **a complete and accurate history and a complete and accurate physical examination remain of the utmost importance** in the evaluation of such patients.

This chapter discusses the presentation, workup, and treatment of common lower urinary tract disorders, including benign prostatic hyperplasia (BPH) and lower urinary tract symptoms (LUTS), urinary incontinence, hematuria, cystitis, dysuria, and pneumaturia.

Benign Prostatic Hyperplasia (BPH) and Lower Urinary Tract Symptoms (LUTS)

It is estimated that there are approximately 6 million patient visits annually among U.S. males for the evaluation of symptoms attributable to enlargement of the prostate gland. It is incumbent upon the evaluating physician to have a consistent approach to this disorder, to identify patients at increased risk of adverse event (i.e., acute urinary retention), and to initiate appropriate therapy in those patients in whom it is required. **It also is important to detect disease states that can mimic the symptoms of BPH.** The Agency for Health Care Policy and Research recommends that **all males with lower urinary complaints be administered a Prostate Symptom Questionnaire (Table 37.1).** This scoring system addresses six areas of voiding dysfunction that are scored from 0 (no symptoms) to 5 (severe symptoms), for a composite score ranging from 0 to 30.

Differential Diagnosis

It is important to rule out other etiologies of urinary symptoms in making the diagnosis of benign prostatic hyperplasia. The **presence of prostate cancer must be ruled out** since treatment of benign disease would be ineffective and would result in further disease

Table 37.1. American Urologic Association Prostate Symptom Index.

Symptom (each scored as 0–5)	Scale
Sense of incomplete emptying	0, not at all
Frequency	1, less than 1 in 5
Intermittency	2, less than 50% of time
Urgency	3, about half the time
Straining	4, greater than 50% of time
Nocturia	5, almost always

progression. **This can be accomplished with a well-performed digital rectal examination (DRE), a serum prostate-specific antigen (PSA) test, and reference to normal value ranges. It generally is recognized that a prostate biopsy is indicated in those men with either elevated serum PSA level (>4ng/mL) or a suspicious DRE finding before embarking upon a BPH treatment regimen (see Algorithm 37.1, Table 37.2).**

Irritative symptoms such as urinary frequency may be due to underlying urinary tract infection, bladder malignancy, primary bladder disorder (i.e., radiation cystitis), or neurologic disease such as history of cerebral vascular accident, multiple sclerosis, or Parkinson's disease (**Table 37.3**). Similarly, poor bladder emptying may be seen in primary neurologic disease and in the neuropathy associated with diabetes. In cases that are not diagnostically clear, urodynamic testing is performed to assess bladder function quantitatively. During this office procedure, the bladder is drained after voiding to measure postvoid residual, and then the bladder is filled at a determined rate and bladder pressure is

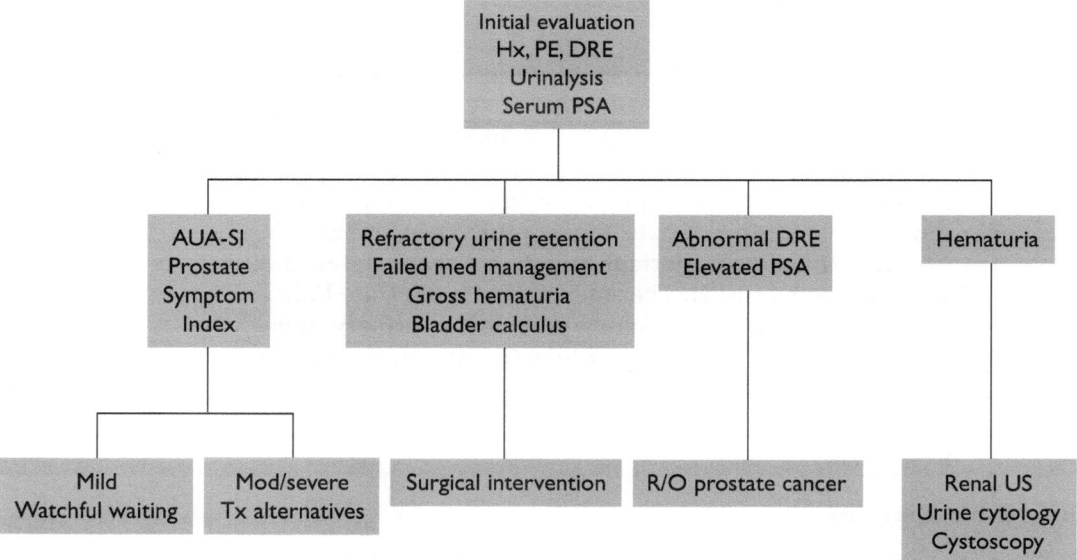

Algorithm 37.1. Algorithm for the evaluation and treatment of benign prostate hyperplasia. AUA-SI, American Urologic Association Prostate Symptom Index; DRE, digital rectal exam; Hx, history; PE, physical examination; PSA, prostate-specific antigen; R/O, rule out; US, ultrasound.

Table 37.2. Results of watchful waiting series for prostate cancer.

Author	n	Follow-up (years)	Overall mortality (%)	Dz-specific mortality (%)	CaP progression (%)	Level of evidence
Johansson[a]	223	10.2	56	8	34	III
Whitmore[b]	75	9.5	39	15	69	III
Hanash[c]	179	15	55	45	NA	III
George[d]	120	7	44	4	83	III
Madsen[e]	50	10	52	6	18	III

[a] Johansson J-E, Adami H-O, Andersson S-O, et al. High 10-year survival rate in patients with early, untreated prostatic cancer. JAMA 1992;267:2191–2196.
[b] Whitmore WF, Warner JA, Thompson IM. Expectant management of localized prostatic cancer. Cancer (Phila) 1991;67:1091–1096.
[c] Hanash KA, Utz DC, Cook EN, et al. Carcinoma of the prostate: a 15-year follow-up. J Urol 1972;107:450–453.
[d] George NJR. Natural history of localized prostatic cancer managed by conservative therapy alone. Lancet 1988;494–497.
[e] Madsen PO, Graverson PH, Gasser TC, et al. Treatment of localized prostatic cancer: radical prostatectomy versus placebo: a 15-year follow-up. Scand J Urol Nephrol Suppl 1988;110:95–100.
Source: Reprinted from Presti JC Jr. Urology. In: Norton JA, Bollinger RR, Chang AE, et al, eds. Surgery: Basic Science and Clinical Evidence. New York: Springer-Verlag, 2001, with permission.

measured. While performing this study, record is made of the bladder's response to filling (i.e., sensation, compliance, stability, capacity) and the peak strength of bladder pressure generation during voiding. The peak bladder voiding pressure is correlated with the electronically measured voiding urine flow measurement.

Cases of mixed disease states pose a management challenge. A patient may have poor bladder contractility secondary to diabetic nephropathy aggravated by bladder obstruction secondary to BPH. In such patients, results of BPH management often are suboptimal. In men with Parkinson's disease and bladder outlet obstruction secondary to BPH, transurethral resection of the prostate (TURP) is associated with a high rate of incontinence and is avoided, and maximal medical management is utilized.

Treatment

It generally is recommended that a discussion of treatment options be initiated in those men with moderate (8 to 19) or severe (≥20) symptom scores (**Table 37.4**). Treatment may include **surveillance alone, medical management, or surgical intervention, the gold standard being electrosurgical TURP.** After hearing a discussion of the potential risks and benefits of available therapies, most patients want medical management in an attempt to avoid a surgical procedure if possible.

Medical Management

Medical management consists primarily of **α-receptor blockade or 5α-reductase inhibition (Table 37.5).** Alpha-blocker agents (i.e., Cardura, Hytrin, Flomax) have been shown to decrease the tone of the α-innervated muscle of the prostatic stroma and bladder neck regions. These agents decrease the symptom score and improve urinary flow rates. As a result, the alpha-blockers are Food and Drug Administration

Table 37.3. Urodynamic findings in selected neurologic disorders.

Disorder	Common urodynamic finding
Suprapontine lesions	
Cerebral aneurysm	DH
Brain abscess	DH
Olivopontocerebellar degeneration	DH
Multiple system atrophy	DH, DA, ISD
Parkinson's disease	DH, DSD, ISD
Senile dementia	DH
Cerebral palsy	DH
Cerebral vascular disease	DH, DA (acute)
Cerebellar ataxia	DH
Bilateral lesions of the putamen	DH, DA
Normal pressure hydrocephalus	DH, DA
Huntington's chorea	DH
Hereditary ataxias	DH
Shy-Drager	DA, ISD
Spinal lesions	
Multiple sclerosis	DH, DA, DSD
Syringomyelia	DH, DSD
Herniated disk (cervical, thoracic)	DH, DSD
Herniated disk (lumbosacral)	DA, DH
Hereditary spastic paraparesis	DH
Tropical spastic paraparesis	DH
Myelomeningocele	DA, DH, DSD, ISD
Anterior spinal artery syndrome	DH, DA (nl sensation)
Sacral agenesis	DA, ISD
Tethered cord syndrome	DH, DA
Transverse myelitis	DH, DA, DSD
Mucopolysaccharidoses (including Hunter's syndrome)	DH
Lyme disease	DH
Congenital sensory neuropathy	DA (abnl sensation)
Neurosyphilis	DA (abnl sensation)
Guillain-Barré	DA, DH (+/– sensation)
Poliomyelitis	DA, DHIC
Tumor	DH, DA
AIDS	DH
Cauda equina/peripheral neuropathies	
Sacrococcygeal teratoma	DA
Caudal regression syndromes	DH, DA
Imperforate anus	DA, ISD
Diabetic neuropathy	DH (early), DA (late)
Alcoholic neuropathy	DH, DA (+/– sensation)
Uremic neuropathy	DH
Polyarteritis nodosa	DH
Porphyria	DH
Viral (Herpes zoster, Epstein-Barr, adenovirus, Coxsackie)	DA (+/– sensation)
Vitamin B_{12} deficiency	DA (abnl sensation)
Systemic lupus erythematosis	DH

abnl, abnormal; DH, detrusor hyperreflexia; DA, detrusor areflexia; DSD, detrusor sphincter dyssynergia; ISD, intrinsic sphincter deficiency; nl, normal.

Table 37.4. American Urologic Association Prostate Symptom Index (AUA-SI).

Classification	AUA-SI
Mild	0–7
Moderate	8–19
Severe	20–35

(FDA) approved for reduction of symptoms attributable to BPH. The other arm of medical therapy is the use of a 5α-reductase inhibitor. **Currently, there is only one 5α-reductase inhibitor—Proscar—available for use in the U.S. This agent reduces intraprostatic 5-hydroxy-testosterone, results in regression of the glandular component of BPH, and has been shown to reduce prostate volume by up to 20%.** Similar to alpha-blockers, 5α-reductase blockade reduces the symptom score, improves urinary flow rates, and is approved for this indication in men with BPH. Additionally, however, 5α-reductase inhibition has been shown to reduce the risk of acute urinary retention in men with moderate to severe symptoms of BPH in a well-conducted randomized prospective study and is approved for long-term use in men with BPH to prevent urinary retention. **There are data to indicate that risk reduction improves with increasing prostate size and advancing patient age at baseline, the very patients who are at the highest risk of urinary retention if not treated.** It is tempting to use both an alpha-blocker and 5α-reductase inhibitor simultaneously, given their differing mode of action. This is sometimes done in men with symptoms of BPH who are deemed not to be good surgical candidates secondary to significant comorbidities (i.e., recent myocardial infarction).

Surgical Management
Men who experience progression of symptoms despite medical management often are advised to undergo transurethral electrosurgical resection of the obstructing prostate tissue. This procedure is most effective in relieving the obstructive symptoms of BPH, allowing for markedly improved urinary flow and bladder emptying. Some men prefer surgical intervention to medical management due to severity of bladder outlet obstruction, medication adverse reaction, or cost-related issues. Newer thermal therapies are available that may provide symptom reduction with less attendant procedural risk compared to traditional electrosurgical resection.

Table 37.5. Agents used in the medical management of benign prostatic hyperplasia (BPH).

α-Receptor blockers	
Cardura	1–4 mg po qhs
Hytrin	Up to 10 mg po qhs
Flomax	0.4–0.8 mg po daily
5α-Reductase inhibitors	
Finasteride	5 mg po daily

Urinary Incontinence

Urinary incontinence is the involuntary loss of urine. This condition is seen in men and women and can have a variety of etiologies. It is important to obtain **a full medical history and to conduct a full physical examination, with special attention to urologic history, obstetrical and gynecologic history, and neurologic history (Table 37.3).** It often is helpful to approach the incontinent patient with the aim of classification based on a simplified approach that describes the bladder disorder (i.e., failure to store, as in a patient with stress incontinence) **(Table 37.6).**

Female Patient

In evaluating the female patient, as in Case 1, it is helpful first to determine whether the incontinence follows a pattern consis-

Table 37.6. Functional classification of urinary incontinence.

Failure to store
  Because of the bladder
    Detrusor hyperactivity
      Involuntary contractions
        Suprasacral neurologic disease
        Idiopathic
    Decreased compliance
      Fibrosis
      Idiopathic
    Sensory urgency
      Inflammation
      Infectious
      Neurologic
      Psychological
      Idiopathic
  Because of the outlet
    Stress incontinence
    Nonfunctional bladder neck/proximal urethra

Failure to empty
  Because of the bladder
    Neurologic
    Myogenic
    Psychogenic
    Idiopathic
  Because of the outlet
    Anatomic
      Prostatic obstruction
      Bladder neck contracture
      Urethral stricture
    Functional
      Smooth sphincter dyssynergia
      Striated sphincter dyssynergia

Table 37.7. Agents used in the medical management of detrusor hyperreflexia/overactive bladder.

Medication	Usual dose	Extended release available
Levsinex	0.375 mg po B.I.D.	Yes
Detrol	2 mg po B.I.D.	Yes
Ditropan	10 mg po T.I.D.	Yes

tent with stress urinary incontinence (i.e., leakage at bladder outlet with increases in intraabdominal pressure) or urgency urinary incontinence (i.e., leakage associated with the urge to void). Classically, a patient with stress urinary incontinence reports leakage of urine with sneeze, cough, or activities such as lifting, jogging, or brisk walking. The patient with urgency incontinence commonly reports accompanying urinary frequency and often is classified as having an "overactive" bladder. It is important to be aware that there may be overlap of these two broad categories, an example of which is illustrated by **Case 1**. Though this patient leaks urine with cough and sneeze, it is the urgency and urge incontinence following stroke that is interfering most with her activities of daily life. Detrusor hyperreflexia commonly is seen in cases of suprapontine cerebral disorders such as cerebrovascular accident (**Table 37.3**). Though bladder neck suspension would address the stress component of this patient's incontinence, what she really needs is **anticholinergic therapy** to control her detrusor hyperreflexia. In patients with stress urinary incontinence, options for management include **Kegel exercises, biofeedback, and operative suspension of the bladder neck**. There are a variety of techniques for bladder neck suspension, and, in most cases, a pubovaginal sling procedure is performed.

Male Patient

In the male patient with incontinence, it is important to rule out retention with urinary overflow incontinence. Retention may be due to BPH, primary bladder dysfunction as in diabetes, other neurologic etiology (i.e., multiple sclerosis), or a combination of factors. Retention of urine can be ruled out by measuring the postvoid bladder urine residual volume either with ultrasound or, more commonly, with bladder catheterization. Incontinent male patients may suffer from detrusor hyperreflexia with resultant urgency incontinence. Men with injury to the urinary sphincter show failure to store urine and a stress incontinence pattern.

Treatment of hyperreflexia consists of **anticholinergic therapy (Table 37.7)**. One must be cautious in the male patient not to induce urinary retention iatrogenically by weakening the detrusor too much. Risk of retention is due to the higher detrusor voiding pressure required in men to overcome the resistance of the prostatic urethra. In men with stress incontinence, treatment may be **conservative (i.e., Kegel, biofeedback) or may be operative**. Operative interventions include bladder neck injection with bulking agents such as collagen or implantation of artificial urinary sphincter.

Hematuria

Hematuria may be gross (visible to the naked eye), as in **Case 2**, or microscopic and can present alone or in combination with other symptoms. Etiologies include infection, urinary calculi, malignancy, and trauma. In **Case 2**, the patient experienced a traumatic event, resulting in gross hematuria. In this situation, urethral injury is likely. When pain is present, its location may point to the source of bleeding, indicating the importance of the patient history. Malignancy of the urinary tract is most common in smokers and in those over 40 years of age. It generally is recommended that, after the physical examination is performed, the patient provide urine for analysis and bacterial culture as well as for cytology testing for cancer cells. Results will direct further evaluation and treatment. (See Chapter 38, Evaluation of Flank Pain.)

Upper urinary tract imaging is required to rule out a renal etiology for hematuria, and renal ultrasound assesses for mass lesion, calculus, or other abnormality, such as hydronephrosis. Renal ultrasound is desirable given its safety and lack of need for contrast injection. It is limited, however, by its lack of ability to visualize the ureter wall. **Intravenous pyelogram (IVP)** provides anatomic imaging of the ureter's entire length, but it has been supplanted in most institutions by **computed tomography (CT) scanning.** Though CT lacks the fine ureteral lumen detail of IVP, it is far superior to IVP in imaging the kidneys, bladder, prostate, and surrounding structures.

In the nonacute setting, office fiberoptic cystoscopy is performed to inspect, under direct vision, the urethra, including the posterior prostatic urethra, and the bladder. Urine effluent from the left and right ureteral orifices is assessed for evidence of bleeding. Cystoscopy in the operating room under anesthesia is reserved for those with an abnormal finding on office fiberoptic cystoscopy and for those with gross bleeding requiring clot evacuation and fulguration. At the time of cystoscopy in the operating room, bladder biopsy, endoscopic tumor removal, retrograde pyelogram of the upper tracts, and ureteroscopy to evaluate the ureter and renal pelvis may be performed. Patients with gross hematuria may require hospitalization, prompt evaluation, and treatment for hemodynamic instability, significant drop in blood count, or inability to evacuate urinary tract (i.e., clot retention).

The evaluation of the trauma patient is coordinated with the trauma team. **The finding of gross blood at the penile meatus, as in our case study, requires evaluation of the urethra with retrograde urethrogram to rule out the presence of a urethral disruption.** In the event that a urethral disruption is documented, urethral catheterization of

Table 37.8. Urinalysis and intravenous urography in the diagnosis of ureteral injuries.

Reference	n^a	Urinalysis[b]	IVU[c]	Data class
Peterson[d]	18	10/13	7/11	III
Liroff[e]	20	9/13	N/A	III
Lankford[f]	10	9/9	8/8	III
Carlton[g]	39	N/A	17/21	III
Eickenberg[h]	17	N/A	7/9	III
Presti[i]	18	11/16	3/11	III
Steers[j]	18	14/16	7/8	III
Rober[k]	16	8/11	8/8	III
Campbell[l]	15	10/13	4/12	III
Total	171	71/91 (78%)	61/88 (69%)	

N/A, not available.
[a] Number of patients in study.
[b] Microscopic (>5 red cells/high-power field) or gross hematuria on initial urinalysis.
[c] Intravenous urography demonstrating ureteral injury.
[d] Peterson NE, Pitts JC. Penetrating injuries of the ureter. J Urol 1981;126:587–590.
[e] Liroff SA, Pontes JES, Pierce JM Jr. Gunshot wounds of the ureter: 5 years of experience. J Urol 1977;118:551–553.
[f] Lankford R, Block NL, Politano VA. Gunshot wounds of the ureter: a review of ten cases. J Trauma 1974;14:848–852.
[g] Carlton CE Jr, Scott R Jr, Guthrie AG. The initial management of ureteral injuries: a report of 78 cases. J Urol 1971;105:335–341.
[h] Eickenberg H, Amin M. Gunshot wounds to the ureter. J Trauma 1976;16:562–565.
[i] Presti JC Jr, Carroll PR, McAninch JW. Ureteral and renal pelvic injuries from external trauma: diagnosis and management. J Trauma 1989;29:370–374.
[j] Steers WD, Corriere JN Jr, Benson GS, et al. The use of indwelling ureteral stents in managing ureteral injuries due to external violence. J Trauma 1985;25:1001–1003.
[k] Rober PE, Smith JB, Pierce JM. Gunshot injuries of the ureter. J Trauma 1990;30:83–86.
[l] Campbell EW, Filderman PS, Jacobs SC. Ureteral injury due to blunt and penetrating trauma. Urology 1992;40:216–220.
Source: Reprinted from Presti JC Jr. Urology. In: Norton JA, Bollinger RR, Chang AE, et al, eds. Surgery: Basic Science and Clinical Evidence. New York: Springer-Verlag, 2001, with permission.

the bladder is avoided to prevent further urethral damage, and a suprapubic cystostomy tube is placed. In performing retrograde urethrogram, contrast is injected into the penile urethra under fluoroscopic guidance via a catheter placed in the fossa navicularis; 3 cc of saline placed in the retention balloon of the catheter provides an adequate seal. In the absence of contrast extravasation indicating that the urethra is intact, a Foley catheter may be passed into the bladder.

To rule out bladder perforation as a source of hematuria, a cystogram is performed. Contrast is instilled into the bladder under gravity via a Foley catheter, and a maximum of 400 cc is instilled. Imaging is achieved with either fluoroscopy or CT (i.e., CT cystogram). Extravasation of instilled contrast from the bladder indicates bladder perforation. The kidneys and ureters are evaluated most commonly with CT following intravenous contrast injection (**Table 37.8**). The kidneys are assessed to confirm blood flow and rule out renal parenchymal fracture. The integrity of each ureter is assessed from renal pelvis to bladder.

Cystitis

Cystitis denotes an inflammation of the urinary tract. By far the most common is bacterial cystitis, representing an inflammation in the bladder secondary to a bacterial infection. Bacterial cystitis may be accompanied by urinary frequency, dysuria, urgency, and foul-smelling or cloudy urine. There may be associated suprapubic discomfort, lower back pain, and low grade (i.e., <101°F) temperature elevation. Some patients present with hematuria due to marked bladder mucosal inflammation. It is preferable to obtain urine analysis and culture at the time of antibiotic initiation, though many patients are treated empirically. Commonly used first-line agents are Macrodantin and Bactrim, and success rates are approximately 60% and 75%, respectively. **Though required length of therapy remains poorly defined, it generally is agreed that 3 days is too short and 10 days probably unnecessary and associated with complications such as yeast vaginal overgrowth. Most patients are treated with 5 to 7 days of therapy.** In patients with persistent symptoms following antibiotic therapy, careful reevaluation of the urinary tract is required, starting with urinalysis and culture. Subsequent treatment and further evaluation are based on these results.

In the evaluation of patients with recurrent urinary tract infection (see **Algorithm 37.2**), it is important to differentiate between persistent and recurrent infection, to confirm that prior documented infection has been treated appropriately (i.e., appropriate antibiotic for sufficient duration), and to rule out predisposing factors such as structural abnormalities (i.e., bladder diverticulum, bladder outlet obstruction), potential nidus of infection (i.e., renal calculus), or host factors (i.e., postmenopausal state, immunosuppression). In patients with no discernible etiology, some success has been seen when bowel dysfunction (i.e., constipation) and voiding dysfunction (i.e., incomplete emptying; incontinence) are addressed. Complicated infections are those associated with temperature elevation above 101°F, structural abnormalities of the urinary tract, resistant organisms, or renal insufficiency. They pose a treatment challenge and often require advanced therapies.

Some patients have lingering bladder discomfort after infection has been treated appropriately. In these patients, the urinalysis is acellular, and culture results are negative. Often, such patients are treated with repetitive courses of antibiotics. However, in such patients, antispasmotic agents alone are effective (**Table 37.7**) for symptom relief.

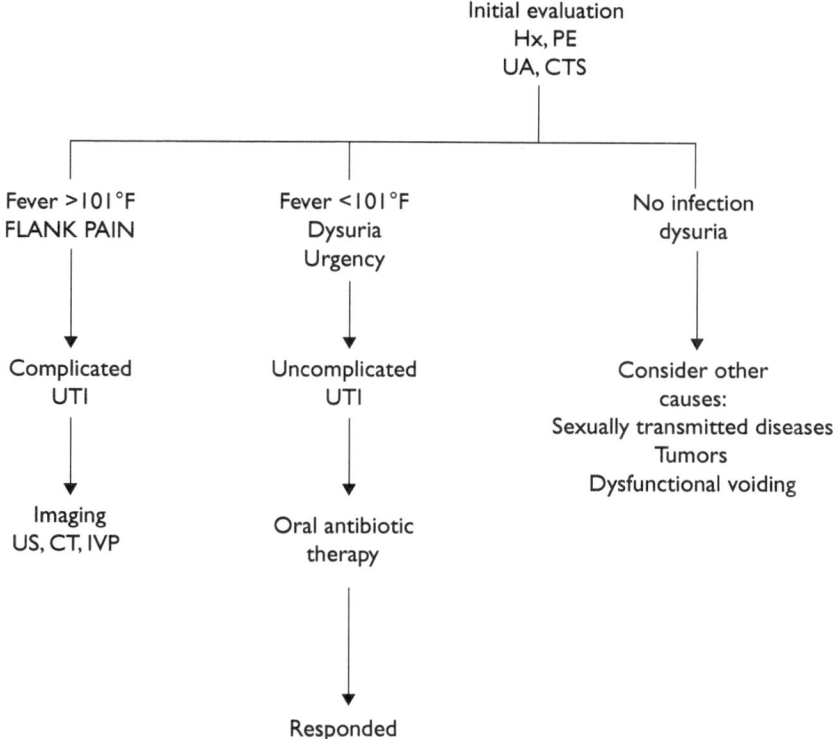

Algorithm 37.2. Algorithm for the evaluation of patient presenting with lower urinary tract in fection. C&S, culture and sensitivity; CT, computed tomography; IVP, intravenous pyelogram; UA, urinalysis; UTI, urinary tract infection.

Dysuria

Dysuria denotes painful urination and is common in bacterial cystitis. In some patients with dysuria, pyuria (i.e., white blood cells on urinalysis) are documented, but bacterial culture shows no growth. These patients, as in **Case 3**, may have a sexually transmitted urethritis (i.e., chlamydia), resulting in dysuria, and should be treated appropriately. As seen in **Case 3**, urethral discharge with dysuria is common with urethritis due to sexually transmitted disease. In patients with dysuria and hematuria only, an underlying bladder malignancy must be ruled out. These patients require evaluation with voided urinary cytology testing for cancer cells and office fiberoptic cystoscopy.

Pneumaturia

Pneumaturia rarely is seen in practice and denotes the sensation of passage of air with urination. The most serious underlying disorder is seen in cases of fistula formation between the gastrointestinal tract

and urinary tract. Most commonly, in cases of diverticular disease, a communication is seen between the colon and bladder. Less commonly, the etiology is colon cancer. The study of choice is a **CT scan of the abdomen and pelvis** to inspect the bladder for air. If the bladder has not been instrumented (i.e., cystoscopy, catheterization), no air should be within the bladder, and this finding on CT scan denotes presence of fistula until proven otherwise. Patients with enteric-vesical fistula have positive urine cultures refractory to antibiotic therapy, often with multiple organisms. In the absence of enteric-vesical fistula, pneumaturia may be due to urinary tract infection with a gas-producing organism. Other patients simply have "frothy" urine and need only to be reassured.

Treatment depends on etiology. In the case of urinary tract infection alone, appropriate **antibiotic therapy** is administered. In patients with enteric-vesical fistula, **formal evaluation of the gastrointestinal tract is required, often with barium enema and colonoscopy. Malignancy must be ruled out,** and colonic biopsy of any suspicious regions performed. Cystoscopy reveals a region of reddened, raised mucosa that may be biopsied. Repair is surgical, with primary treatment of the primary gastrointestinal process and simultaneous formal bladder repair.

Summary

Lower urinary tract symptoms result from abnormalities of the bladder and urethra. In males, benign hyperplasia is most common and may present with urinary frequency, urgency, or retention. In females, obstruction is uncommon; however, incontinence due to relaxation of the pelvic floor musculature is seen more often. The bladder and urethra are vulnerable to trauma and should be evaluated when blood is seen at the urethral meatus during trauma. Infection and tumor also can produce lower urinary tract symptoms, and cystoscopy is often needed to exclude the latter.

Selected Readings

Benign prostatic hyperplasia: diagnosis and treatment clinical practice guideline No. 8. AHCPR Publication No. 94-0582. February 1994.

Cohn DE, Rader JS. Gynecology. In: Norton JA, Bollinger RR, Chang AE, et al., eds. Surgery: Basic Science and Clinical Evidence. New York: Springer-Verlag, 2001.

Perrotti M, Fair WR. Prostate cancer: patient evaluation. In: Resnick MI, Thompson IM, eds. Surgery of the Prostate. New York: Churchill Livingstone, 1998:1–20.

Presti JC Jr. Urology. In: Norton JA, Bollinger RR, Chang AE, et al., eds. Surgery: Basic Science and Clinical Evidence. New York: Springer-Verlag, 2001.

Steers WD, Barrett DM, Wein AJ. Voiding function and dysfunction. B. Voiding dysfunction: diagnosis, classification and management. In: Gillenwater JY,

Grayhack JT, Howards SS, Duckett JW, eds. Adult and Pediatric Urology. St. Louis: Mosby-Year Book, Inc., 1996:1220–1325.

Zderic SA, Levin R, Wein AJ. Voiding function and dysfunction. A. Voiding function: relevant anatomy, physiology, pharmacology and molecular aspects. In: Gillenwater JY, Grayhack JT, Howards SS, Duckett JW, eds. Adult and Pediatric Urology. St. Louis: Mosby-Year Book, 1996:1159–1219.

38

Evaluation of Flank Pain

Joseph G. Barone

Objectives

1. **To discuss the potential etiologies of flank pain.**
2. **To discuss the imaging modalities available for the evaluation of flank pain.**
3. **To discuss the evaluation of a patient with flank pain.**
4. **To discuss the clinical presentation of a patient with urinary calculi.**

Case

You are asked to examine a 65-year-old woman with left flank pain. The pain is acute, severe, and radiates to the left lower quadrant. The patient complains of nausea, but there is no vomiting or diarrhea. Past medical history is significant only for hypertension. The patient does not smoke and denies alcohol and drug use.

On physical examination, the patient is afebrile, and the remaining vital signs also are normal. The only abnormality detected on physical examination is severe left costovertebral angle tenderness on percussion. Laboratory evaluations, including a complete blood count and serum chemistries, are normal. Urine Gram stain demonstrates no bacteria on an unspun specimen. Urinalysis demonstrates the presence of red blood cells and irregular crystals. An abdominal plain film demonstrates a 2-mm calcification at the level of the left pelvic brim.

Introduction

Flank pain often is due to a urologic etiology, such as renal calculus disease or acute pyelonephritis; however, cardiac, intraabdominal, musculoskeletal, and psychological causes also need to be considered. The quality and severity of the pain may provide a clue to its etiology. Flank pain that is due to infection, such as acute pyelone-phritis, usually is steady and dull, whereas pain that is due to an acutely obstructing calculus can be intense and sharp.

The kidney and its capsule are innervated by sensory fibers travel-ing to the T10-L1 spinal cord. Pain that originates from the kidney often is felt just lateral to the sacrospinalis muscle beneath the 12th rib pos-teriorly. The pain often radiates anteriorly, but it also may be referred to the inguinal, labial, penile, or testicular areas. It is not uncommon for a man with a ureteral calculus to complain of pain at the tip of the penis or for a women with the same problem to experience labial pain.

Flank pain that originates from urinary tract pathology may be caused by obstruction, inflammation, or mass. Hydronephrosis occurs when there is obstruction of the urinary tract that results in dilation of the renal collecting system. Dilation of the renal collecting system leads to distention of the renal capsule, and this distention results in flank pain. In the case presented above, flank pain accompanied by crystals in the urine is suggestive of hydronephrosis due to an obstructing renal calculus.

When evaluating a patient with flank pain, **the severity of the pain generally correlates inversely with the duration of the problem.** That is, chronic, gradual distention of the renal capsule over a long period of time due to a slowly enlarging ureteral tumor often is associated with mild to moderate flank pain. The pain is mild or dull because it results in gradual but possibly severe distention of the renal collecting system and capsule. In contrast, the acute flank pain that is associated with an obstructing renal calculus often is severe, since it results in sudden distention of the renal collecting system and capsule. In the case presented, it is likely that an obstructing calculi is causing the patient's symptoms. **Severe flank pain caused by an acute urinary tract obstruction is termed renal colic.**

It is important for the clinician to determine if the pain represents an emergency or if the problem can be managed in the outpatient setting. In this regard, it is important to determine if there is associated fever, dehydration, nausea, or vomiting. Comorbid medical conditions, such as diabetes, immunocompromise, or pregnancy, also need to be considered. When flank pain presents in association with any one of these factors, hospital admission may be necessary to prevent possible complications, such as pyelonephritis or urosepsis, from developing. In the case presented, none of these factors are present, so this patient can be managed in the outpatient setting.

Since a prime objective for the clinician is to determine if the flank pain represents an emergent medical problem, it is helpful to consider the differential diagnosis of flank pain (see **Algorithm 38.1**).

Differential Diagnosis of Flank Pain

Urinary Calculi

One of the most common causes of acute, severe flank pain is **sudden distention of the renal collecting system and capsule secondary to an**

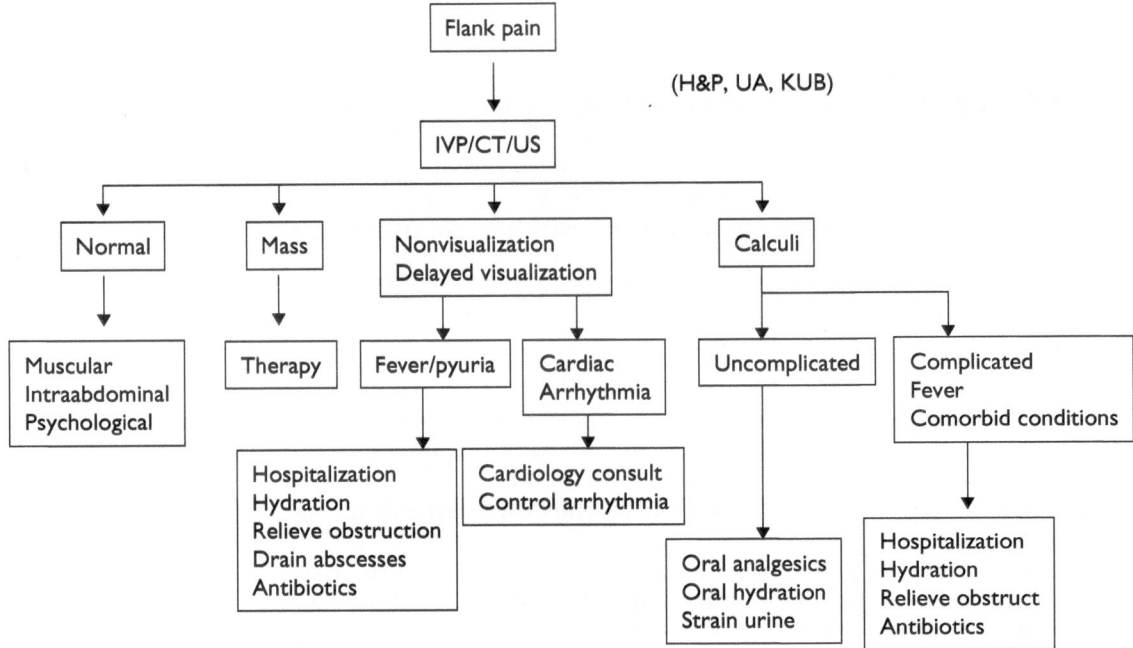

Algorithm 38.1. Algorithm for the clinical evaluation of the patient presenting with acute flank pain. CT, computed tomography; H&P, history and physical examination; IVP, intravenous pyelogram; KUB, kidney and urinary bladder; UA, urinalysis; US, ultrasound.

obstructing urinary calculi. Most urinary calculi cause pain only when they obstruct the flow of urine from the kidney into the bladder. A nonobstructing stone usually does not cause significant flank pain. Since the patient in the case presented has pain, it is probable that obstruction is present. Typically, the stone becomes caught in the renal pelvis or ureter and causes obstruction of urine flow. The back pressure results in pain and hydronephrosis.

Types of Urinary Calculi
The most common type of urinary tract calculus is composed of calcium oxalate. Oxalate is found in many green leafy vegetables and teas, and it is considered to be an inducer of stone formation. When urine becomes supersaturated with calcium or oxalate, precipitation of crystals can result in stone formation. Causes for supersaturation with calcium or oxalate include excess bone resorption of calcium from immobility, intestinal hyperabsorbtion of calcium from sarcoidosis, and renal leak of calcium seen with renal tubular acidosis. However, **most individuals who form calcium oxalate stones do not drink enough fluids**, which results in concentrated urine. This facilitates crystal precipitation and stone formation. Even though the patient in the case presented has a family history of calcium oxalate calculi, dehydration is the most likely cause of her stone formation. For this reason, calcium oxalate stones are more common in the summer months and in the

southern United States "stone belt," where it is hot and where dehydration is more likely to occur.

Other common types of stones include magnesium ammonium phosphate and carbonate apatite stones. These stones sometimes are called infection stones, since they form secondary to urinary tract infections with urea splitting bacteria. Urea splitting bacteria raise the pH of the urine, and this facilitates the formation of infection stones by lowering the solubility of magnesium-ammonium and phosphate. Common urea splitting bacteria include *Escherichia coli* and *Proteus mirabilis*. **Infectious stones can enlarge quickly and sometimes can fill the entire renal collecting system to form a staghorn calculus.** The term **staghorn calculus** indicates that the stone is a large stone, but it does not imply stone composition. All urinary calculi have the potential to form staghorn calculi; however, infection stones result in staghorn formation most often.

Some stones, including uric acid and cystine stones, form secondary to metabolic abnormalities. These stones are seen less commonly in clinical practice, but they should be suspected in patients with a history of gout or homozygous cystinuria. **It is estimated that 25% of patients with uric acid stones have gout.** Uric acid is an end product of purine metabolism. Hyperuricosuria may be seen in gout, myeloproliferative disorders, idiopathic hyperuricosuria, and patients with increased dietary purine. **Uric acid stones are clinically unique, since they cannot be seen on a standard abdominal x-ray. They can, however, be visualized on ultrasound or computed tomography (CT) scan.** Since the formation of uric acid stones is very dependent on the pH of the urine, they generally form only if the urine pH is consistently below 5.5. Uric acid stones have been dissolved successfully by raising urinary pH to 6.5 or slightly above. Typically, an oral urinary alkalinizing agent, such as potassium citrate, is used to raise urine pH and dissolve uric acid stones. Cystine stones are uncommon and form only in patients who are homozygous for cystinuria. **Cystinuria is an inherited defect of the renal tubule causing loss of cystine, ornithine, arginine, and lysine.** The loss of cystine is the only clinical problem patients suffer, since they excrete over 250 mg of cystine per liter of urine. This high urinary cystine level is problematic, since stone formation results in urinary cystine levels of 170 mg per liter of urine at pH 5. Patients who are heterozygous for cystinuria excrete less urinary cystine and generally do not suffer from cystine stone formation.

Risk Factors
Some of the common risk factors for developing urinary calculi include inadequate fluid intake, excess sodium intake, metabolic abnormalities, inflammatory bowel disease, dehydration, and family history.
Patients with inflammatory bowel disease form stones composed of calcium oxalate by a unique mechanism. Fat malabsorption caused by the inflammatory bowel disease results in excess fats in the gut, which bind to calcium. This creates a situation in the gut in which oxalate, which normally binds to calcium, enters the bloodstream in its ionic

form. The oxalate then is excreted by the kidneys, and hyperoxaluria results. Since oxalte is a stone inducer, it binds with urinary calcium and facilitates calcium oxalate stone formation.

Other medical conditions increase the risk for stone formation by causing hypercalciuria, which is excess calcium in the urine. These medical problems include renal tubular acidosis, sarcoidosis, hyperparathyroidism, chronic immobility, and paralysis. In these conditions, hypercalciuria results when excess calcium is absorbed from bone or the gut and ultimately is excreted by the kidneys. In renal tubular acidosis, the renal tubule leaks calcium directly into the urine.

Chronic urinary tract infection also can lead to stone formation due to urea splitting bacteria, which lead to an elevated urine pH. Urease catalyzes the hydrolysis of urea into ammonia and carbon dioxide. These end products cause a rise in urinary pH, which facilitates infectious stone formation. *P. mirabilis* and *E. coli* are the most common urea splitting bacteria that are associated with urinary tract infection and urinary calculi formation. These bacteria raise the pH of the urine, and this allows the precipitation of magnesium-ammonium-phosphate or apatite stones. **Patients with infected urine and flank pain due to an obstructing calculi may require hospitalization to prevent urosepsis.**

Management

As illustrated in the case presented, most patients who present with flank pain secondary to acutely obstructing urinary calculi can be managed on an **outpatient basis. Cornerstones of therapy include adequate hydration, pain relief, and control of any associated nausea or vomiting.**

If the pain is severe enough to require intravenous morphine sulfate or if there is associated fever or dehydration due to nausea or vomiting, **hospital admission** may be necessary. Again, one of the most important decisions the clinician has to make is to determine if the patient can be treated as an outpatient or if the patient needs hospital admission. There are several indications for hospital admission, and **fever is a common indicator for admission (Table 38.1).** As Table 38.1 indicates, appropriate **blood and urine cultures** need to be performed, and other causes of infection need to be considered. **Fever in the presence of obstructing urinary calculi can be an ominous clinical finding that suggests an accumulation of purulent urine proximal to an obstructing stone.** This is an especially serious situation if the patient has **comorbid medical conditions,** such as diabetes. **Emergent intravenous antibiotics, aggressive intravenous fluid hydration, and percutaneous or transureteral drainage of the infected urine** usually are necessary in these situations. **Patients with fever and obstructing urinary calculi should not be discharged from the emergency room, as urosepsis and septic shock can develop quickly.**

Following the acute event, it is suggested that all patients who form urinary stones undergo **a metabolic evaluation consisting of a complete blood count, urinalysis, serum chemistry profile, and a 24-hour urine collection for calcium, phosphorus, uric acid, creatinine, citrate, and oxalate levels.** This evaluation can be done on an outpatient basis.

Table 38.1. Evidence-based practice management guideline for the evaluation of fever in critically ill adult patients.[a]

Temperature measurement	
Level I:	Record the temperature and the site of measurement in the patient's medical record. The nosocomial spread of pathogens must be avoided when using temperature measurement devices.
Level II:	Temperature is measured most accurately by indwelling vascular or bladder thermistors, but most other sites are acceptable. Axillary measurements should not be used. Laboratory testing for the evaluation of fever should be individualized for each patient.
Blood cultures	
Level I:	For skin preparation, povidone-iodine should be allowed to dry for 2 min, or tincture of iodine for 30 s. Alcohol skin preparation, an acceptable alternative for iodine-allergic patients, need not be allowed to dry.
Level II:	Obtain a single pair of blood cultures after appropriate skin disinfection after the initial temperature elevation, and another pair within 24 h thereafter from a second peripheral site. Additional cultures should be based on high clinical suspicion of bacteremia or fungemia, and not instituted automatically for each temperature elevation. If two peripheral sites are not available, one pair of cultures may be drawn through the most recently inserted catheter, but the diagnostic accuracy is reduced. Draw at least 10–15 mL blood/culture.
Suspected intravascular catheter infection	
Level II:	Examine the catheter insertion site for purulence, and distally on the extremity for signs of vascular compromise or embolization. Any expressed purulence from an insertion site should be collected for culture and Gram stain. The catheter should be removed and cultured for evidence of a tunnel infection, embolic phenomena, vascular compromise, or sepsis. Two blood cultures should be drawn peripherally, or one may be drawn from the most proximal port (if a multilumen catheter). Both the introducer and the catheter itself should be cultured for suspected pulmonary artery catheter infection. It is not routinely necessary to culture the intravenous fluid infusate.
Suspected ICU-acquired pneumonia	
Level I:	A chest x-ray should be obtained to evaluate for suspected pneumonia. Posteroanterior and lateral films or computed tomography of the chest can offer more information.
Level II:	Lower respiratory tract secretions should be sampled for direct examination and culture. Bronchoscopy may be considered. Respiratory secretions should be transported to the laboratory within 2 h of collection. Pleural fluid should be obtained for culture and Gram stain if there is an adjacent infiltrate or another reason to suspect infection.
Evaluation of the febrile patient with diarrhea	
Level II:	If more than two diarrheal stools occur, a single stool sample should be sent for *Clostridium difficile* evaluation. A second sample should be sent if the first is negative and suspicion remains high. If illness is severe and rapid testing is unavailable or nondiagnostic, consider flexible sigmoidoscopy. If illness is severe, consider empiric therapy with metronidazole until the results of studies are available. Empiric therapy (especially with vancomycin) is not recommended if two stool evaluations have been negative for *C. difficile*, and is discouraged because of the risk of producing resistant pathogens. Stool cultures are rarely indicated for other enteric pathogens if the patient is HIV-negative or did not present to the hospital with diarrhea.

Continued

Table 38.1. *Continued*

Suspected urinary tract infection
Level II: Obtain urine for culture and to evaluate for pyuria. If the patient has an indwelling
             Foley catheter, urine should be collected from the urine port and not the drainage
             bag.
             The specimen should be transported rapidly to the laboratory, or refrigerated if
             transport will exceed 1 h.

Suspected sinusitis
Level I: Aspirate should be Gram stained and cultured.
Level II: Computed tomography of the facial sinuses is the imaging modality of choice for
             the diagnosis of sinusitis.
             Puncture and aspiration of the sinuses should be performed using sterile technique
             if mucosal thickening or an air–fluid level is present in the sinus.

Postoperative fever
Level II: Examine the surgical wound for erythema, fluctuance, tenderness, or purulent
             drainage.
             Open the wound for suspicion of infection.
             Culture and Gram stain should be obtained from purulent material if from deep
             within the wound.

Suspected central nervous system infection
Level II: Gram stain and culture of cerebrospinal fluid should be performed in cases of
             suspected infection. Other tests should be predicated on the clinical situation.
             A computed tomographic study is usually required before lumbar puncture, which
             may need to be deferred if a mass lesion is present.
             Consider lumbar puncture for new fever with unexplained alteration of
             consciousness or focal neurologic signs.
             In febrile patients with an intracranial device, cerebrospial fluid should be sent for
             culture and Gram stain.

Noninfectious causes of fever
Level II: Reevaluate all recent medications and blood products the patient has received.
             Stop all nonessential medications, or substitute medications for treatments that
             cannot be stopped.

[a] Summary of clinical recommendations, Society of Critical Care Medicine, 1998; level III guidelines excluded.
Source: Adapted from O'Grady NP, Barie PS, Bartlett JG, et al. Practice guidelines for evaluating new fever in criti-
cally ill adult patients. Task Force of the Society of Critical Care Medicine and the Infectious Diseases Society of
America. Clin Infect Dis 1998;26:1042–1059, with permission. Published by the University of Chicago. Reprinted
from Norton JA. History of Endocrine Surgery. In: Norton JA, Bollinger RR, Chang AE, et al, eds. Surgery: Basic
Science and Clinical Evidence. New York: Springer-Verlag, 2001, with permission.

The most common abnormality detected is a low urine volume, usually
less than 1 L/day, due to inadequate fluid intake. In this situation, the
patient should be encouraged to **increase fluid intake** and to maintain
a urine volume of 2 to 3 L per day. Water is the best fluid to drink, while
teas, cranberry juice, and other drinks that are high in oxalate should
be limited. Cranberry juice has been shown to be effective in reducing
the risk for recurrent urinary tract infections, but it is high in oxalate
and should be limited in patients who form stones. Patients sometimes
also are advised to **limit the intake of certain foods** that are high in
calcium and oxalate, such as cheese, spinach, and nuts; however, it is
often difficult to maintain these dietary restrictions.

Medications sometimes are necessary to prevent recurrence.
Orthophosphates decrease urinary calcium and are used to prevent
calcium stone formation. Hydrochlorothiazide prevents reabsorption
of sodium and calcium in the loop of Henle; this leads to an increase

in proximal tubular reabsorption of sodium and calcium, which decreases total urinary calcium excretion.

Acute Pyelonephritis

Acute pyelonephritis indicates infection of the kidney and renal pelvis accompanied by fever, flank pain, and infected urine. In the case presented, there is no clinical evidence for pyelonephritis. The diagnosis is made clinically. Bacterial pyelonephritis typically involves an infection of the renal interstitium and collecting system. Bacterial invasion of the kidney results in a humoral response that activates the complement cascade. The polymorphonuclear leukocytes release superoxide radicals that damage not only bacteria but also the surrounding renal tissue. **If the damage is severe, renal scar or loss can occur.**

In the United States, the majority of cases of pyelonephritis are due to the Enterobacteriaceae group of bacteria, mainly *E. coli*. *Proteus, Pseudomonas, Enterobacter, Klebsiella,* and *Staphylococcus* also can cause pyelonephritis. The urea splitting bacteria include *E. coli, Proteus,* and *Klebsiella* and are important, since they may facilitate the development of infection stones.

Patients can present with mild gram-negative bacteremia to septic shock. Renal abscess can form if treatment is delayed, with resultant renal parenchyma loss. In the pediatric population, children with vesicoureteral reflux are at risk for pylonephritis and renal scarring, since the kidney matures until approximately age 7 (**Fig. 38.1**). **The clinical onset of acute pyelonephritis can be sudden and dramatic; shaking chills with fevers of 38° to 40°C are not uncommon.** Symptoms of lower urinary tract infection, such as frequency, urgency, and dysuria, may have preceded the acute event by several days. Costovertebral angle tenderness usually is severe due to inflammation of the kidney and surrounding anatomy. Urine analysis typically demonstrates white

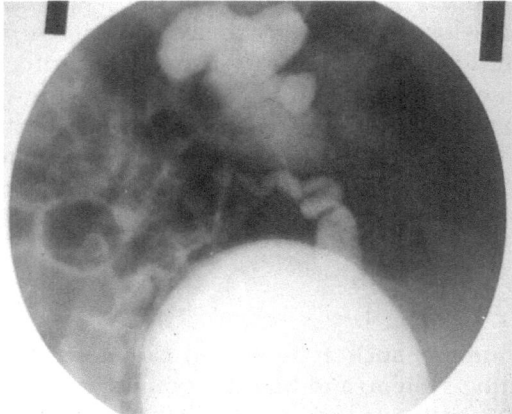

Figure 38.1. Voiding cystourethrogram demonstrating reflux. Note dilation at renal collecting system due to reflux.

blood cells (WBC), red blood cells (RBC), and bacteria. **The finding of WBC casts in the urine sample is strongly suggestive of acute pyelonephritis, and urine Gram stain can establish the diagnosis of bacteriuria.**

Risk Factors

Risk factors for acute pyelonephritis include vesicoureteral reflux, obstruction of the urinary tract, and hematogenous infection. Reflux typically occurs in children, and, since their kidneys are still maturing, acute pyelonephritis can interfere with kidney growth and development. Obstructions can be caused by several factors, including stricture, stone, or pregnancy. With pregnancy, the gravid uterus can obstruct the ureters. Obstruction leads to stasis of urine, which facilitates bacterial growth. Normally, bacteria in the urinary tract are washed out by ureteral peristalsis and proper bladder emptying; however, obstruction disables the former defense mechanism.

Other risk factors include **diabetes mellitus**, since there is increased substrate availability in the kidney. **Gas-forming organisms** could result in emphysematous pyelonephritis, which may require nephrectomy. **Patients with neurogenic bladder and the elderly** also are at increased risk, since urinary emptying may not be complete in these patients. Finally, **females** are more prone to develop acute pyelonephritis due to their shorter urethral length compared to the male urethra.

Management

Treatment of pyelonephritis consists of intravenous fluid hydration and antibiotic therapy. A standard regimen includes an aminoglycoside (gentamicin, 1.5 mg/kg IV q 8 h) plus ampicillin (2 g IV q 6 h). In mild cases, oral antibiotics can be considered; however, if a positive clinical response is not noted within 24 hours, hospitalization with intravenous antibiotics should be implemented. Following intravenous antibiotics, 75% to 80% of patients improve clinically and become afebrile within 72 hours. Once patients have been afebrile for 24 to 48 hours, they may be switched to oral antibiotics. A 14- to 21-day total course of antibiotics is recommended to ensure effective sterilization of the kidney and helps reduce the incidence of renal scarring.

Urologic intervention is necessary if pyelonephritis occurs in the presence of an obstruction, such as a ureteral calculus. In this situation, antibiotics are not effective until the purulent urine behind the obstruction is drained via nephrostomy or ureteral stent. In cases of renal abscess formation, percutaneous drainage and intravenous antibiotic therapy usually are effective.

Urinary Tract Tumors

Urinary tract tumors, such as renal cell carcinomas, tumors of the urinary collecting system, and bladder tumors, can cause flank pain when the tumor obstructs the urinary tract. These tumors also cause pain when they are large and stretch the ram capsule or when they invade surrounding structures (Fig. 38.2). Bladder and ureteral tumors

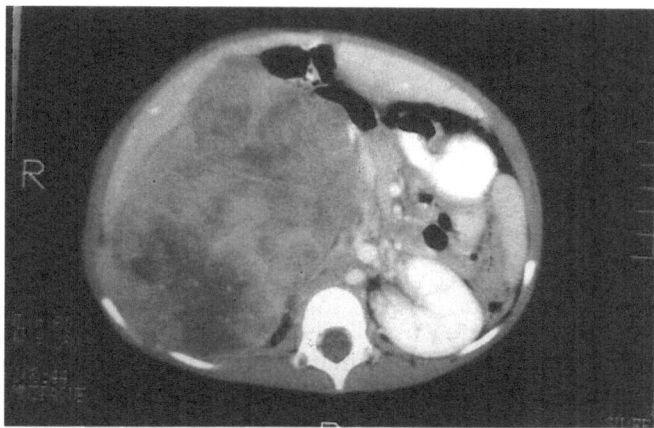

Figure 38.2. Computed tomography (CT) scan of large renal tumor. In this situation, flank pain could result from stretching of the renal capsule or direct invasion into surrounding tissues.

are seen more commonly in smokers, and gross hematuria usually is associated with the flank pain. There may be prior episodes of gross hematuria, flank pain, or weight loss in patients with urologic malignancies.

Renal cell tumors are relatively uncommon and account for 3% of adult malignancies. Most renal tumors (90%) are adenocarcinomas and originate from the cells of the proximal convoluted tubules. These tumors usually are unilateral and grow inwardly toward the medulla of the kidney. If gross hematuria is present, it indicates that the tumor has invaded the collecting system of the kidney. Only an advanced tumor would produce flank pain, since a stage 1 tumor is confined to the kidney. Tumors that penetrate the renal capsule but remain within Gerota's fascia are considered grade 2. A grade 3 tumor has spread locally and can cause flank pain, as can a grade 4 tumor, which is metastatic. **Treatment for renal tumors stage 1 to 3 is by surgical excision. Grade 4 tumors are treated with chemotherapy, but excision is sometimes necessary for relief of pain or to control bleeding.**

Tumors of the urinary collecting system, ureter, and bladder are most commonly transitional cell carcinomas. These tumors can cause flank pain when they obstruct the urinary tract, and they commonly present with gross hematuria. About 30% of patients with a renal pelvic cancer complain of flank pain, whereas only 15% of patients with a ureteral tumor experience flank pain.

Bladder tumors usually present with hematuria; however, when the tumor is located at the ureteral orifice, it can cause flank pain due to ureteral obstruction. Bladder tumors that obstruct the ureter tend to be advanced at the time of discovery, and prognosis is guarded.

Urologic tumors rarely are palpable on physical examination unless they are large; however, most renal tumors are seen during

upper tract imaging with ultrasound or CT scan (Fig. 38.2). Bladder and ureteral tumors usually require intravenous pyelogram (IVP), contrast-enhanced CT scan, cystoscopy, and sometimes retrograde urography for accurate diagnosis. For this reason, all patients with flank pain who also have gross hematuria require urologic consultation.

Traumatic Flank Pain

Flank pain due to trauma usually is obvious, given the clinical presentation. In the trauma setting, **imaging of the urinary system is necessary to exclude serious injury to the urinary tract, such as renal laceration, renal contusion, or ureteral avulsion (Table 38.2).** As seen in **Table 38.2, CT scan** is useful for evaluating the retroperitoneum in cases of blunt abdominal trauma. Renal lacerations and contusions can occur from relatively minor forces and can be diagnosed with CT (**Fig. 38.3**). **In the pediatric population, a hydronephrotic kidney, due to a congenital ureteropelvic junction obstruction, can rupture from a relatively minor traumatic event. Also, the pediatric kidney is more prone to injury since it is not well protected.** In the adult, a significant amount of fat, muscle, and bone protect the kidney from injury, but this protective barrier is not well developed in children. Therefore, **all children who present with flank pain following a traumatic event require upper tract imaging.**

If the magnitude of the injury was severe or involved a sudden deceleration injury, then **contrast imaging of the urinary tract with CT scanning** is suggested to exclude an injury to the urinary collecting system, such as ureteral injury or avulsion (**Table 38.3**). However, as seen in **Table 38.3**, the leading cause of ureteral injury in an adult is a gunshot wound. Injuries to the collecting system of the kidney usually are due to significant trauma, except in the pediatric population for the reasons mentioned above. Administration of intravenous contrast often is necessary to document these injuries, since they usually are not seen on a plain abdominal x-ray or ultrasound examination and urinalysis may be normal (**Table 38.4**). Thus, **a normal urinalysis in the trauma setting does not exclude serious urologic injury.**

Renal Artery Emboli

Renal artery emboli can result secondary to mitral valve disease, atrial fibrillation, acute myocardial infarction, endocarditis, and cardiac tumors. In addition, **atherosclerotic aortic disease and thrombi originating in renal artery aneurysms** have been known to cause renal artery emboli (**Table 38.5**).

Patients with renal artery emboli present with acute, severe flank pain. There often is a history of cardiac or atherosclerotic disease. Physical examination may demonstrate a cardiac arrhythmia or

Table 38.2. Comparison of diagnostic methods for evaluating blunt and penetrating abdominal trauma.

Test	Time required (min)	Pros	Cons	Sensitivity {specificity} and injury type	Reference	Utility: blunt vs. penetrating
Diagnostic peritoneal lavage (DPL)	5–15	Fast. Very sensitive. Minimal equipment required. Specialized training not required. May be performed in a variety of locations. Results are quantitative, objective, and operator independent.	Invasive. Not recommended if prior laparotomy. Not injury specific. May miss retroperitoneal and diaphragm injuries.	97% {99%} blunt 85–93% {67–99} penetr 99% {43%} penetr 99% {86%} penetr 100% {84%} blunt	Alyono[a] Alyono[a] Oreskovich[b] Merlotti[c] Liu[d]	Good sensitivity for both blunt and penetrating trauma. Nonspecific for both. Sensitivity and specificity highly dependent on cell count criteria used.
Abdominal CT	30–50	Very specific with good sensitivity. Good for evaluating posterior (back and flank, retroperitoneal) injuries. Allows staging of blunt organ injuries for nonoperative management. Most major injuries operator (reader) independent.	Not useful for most anterior penetrating injuries. Requires time and patient transport. Some operator (reader) dependence. May miss blunt intestinal injuries and, initially, some pancreatic injuries. Limited finding-specific or quantitative criteria mandating operation exist.	85% {100} blunt 99% {100} blunt 97% {95} blunt	Fabian[e] Peitzman[f] Liu[d]	Good sensitivity and specificity for blunt injuries and most posterior penetrating injuries. Insensitive for anterior penetrating injuries.
Abdominal ultrasonography (FAST)	5–10	Fast. Sensitive for hemoperitoneum in experienced hands. Noninvasive and no contrast required. May be performed in a variety of locations if equipment is available.	Not useful for penetrating injuries. Requires immediately accessible equipment and specialized training and experience. Nonquantitative and substantially operator dependent.	92% {95} 83% {100} 95% {95} 97% {97} 82% {99}	Liu[d] McKenney[g] Yoshii[h] Singh[i] Rozycki[j]	Good sensitivity for clinically significant blunt injuries. Poor sensitivity for penetrating injuries.

Continued

Table 38.2. *Continued*

Test	Time required (min)	Pros	Cons	Sensitivity {specificity} and injury type	Reference	Utility: blunt vs. penetrating
Diagnostic laparoscopy	20–60++	Excellent for diagnosis of diaphragmatic injuries. Good for nonquantitative dx. of hemoperitoneum. Good for determining peritoneal penetration for SW/GSW. High degree of injury specificity when visualized.	Invasive. Poor sensitivity for some injuries. Requires specialized training, experience, and equipment. Nonquantitative and substantially operator dependent. Typically requires more conscious sedation than other methods. General anesthesia may be needed in some circumstances.	88% liver/spleen 83% diaphragm 50% panc/ kidney 25% hollow viscus 100% periton penetr 18% GI injuries	Ortega[k] Ortega[k] Ortega[k] Ortega[k] Sosa[l] Ivatury[m]	Good sensitivity for peritoneal penetration, hemoperitoneum, and diaphragmatic injuries. Poor sensitivity for GI and retroperitoneal injuries.

GSW, gunshot wound; SW, stab wound.

[a] Alyono D, Morrow CE, Perry JF. Reappraisal of diagnostic peritoneal lavage criteria for operation in penetrating and blunt trauma. Surgery (St. Louis) 1982;92:751–757.

[b] Oreskovich MR, Carrico CJ. Stab wounds of the anterior abdomen: analysis of a management plan using local wound exploration and quantitative peritoneal lavage. Ann Surg 1983;198:411–418.

[c] Merlotti GJ, Marcet E, Sheaff CM, et al. Use of peritoneal lavage to evaluate abdominal penetration. J Trauma 1985;25:228–231.

[d] Liu M, Lee CH, P'eng FK. Prospective comparison of diagnostic peritoneal lavage, computed tomographic scanning, and ultrasonography for the diagnosis of blunt abdominal trauma. J Trauma 1993;35(2):267–270.

[e] Fabian TC, Mangiante EC, White TJ, et al. A prospective study of 91 patients undergoing both computed tomography and peritoneal lavage following blunt abdominal trauma. J Trauma 1986;26:602.

[f] Peitzman AB, Makaroun MS, Slasky BS, Ritter P. Prospective study of computed tomography in initial management of blunt abdominal trauma. J Trauma 1986;26:585–592.

[g] McKenney M, Lentz K, Nunez D, et al. Can ultrasound replace diagnostic peritoneal lavage in the assessment of blunt trauma? [see comments]. J Trauma 1994;37(3):439–441.

[h] Yoshii H, Sato M, Yamamoto S, et al. Usefulness and limitations of ultrasonography in the initial evaluation of blunt abdominal trauma. J Trauma 1998;45(1):45–50.

[i] Singh G, Arya N, Safaya R, et al. Role of ultrasonography in blunt abdominal trauma. Injury 1997;28(9–10):667–670.

[j] Rozycki GS, Ochsner MG, Schmidt JA, et al. A prospective study of surgeon-performed ultrasound as the primary adjuvant modality for injured patient assessment. J Trauma 1995;39(3):492–498.

[k] Ortega AE, Tang E, Froes ET, Asensio JA, Katkhouda N, Demetriades D. Laparoscopic evaluation of penetrating thoracoabdominal traumatic injuries. Surg Endosc 1996;10(1):19–22.

[l] Sosa JL, Arrillaga A, Puente I, Sleeman D, Ginzburg E, Martin L. Laparoscopy in 121 consecutive patients with abdominal gunshot wounds. J Trauma 1995;39(3):501–504, discussion 504–506.

[m] Ivatury RR, Simon RJ, Stahl WM. A critical evaluation of laparoscopy in penetrating abdominal trauma. J Trauma 1993;34(6):822–827, discussion 827–828.

Source: Reprinted from Mackersie RC. Abdominal trauma. In: Norton JA, Bollinger RR, Chang AE, et al, eds. Surgery: Basic Science and Clinical Evidence. New York: Springer-Verlag, 2001, with permission.

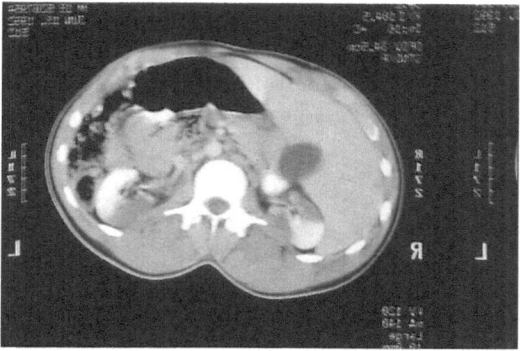

Figure 38.3. CT scan of bilateral areas of renal infarction due to trauma.

Table 38.3. Mechanism and site of ureteral injuries.

Reference	n^a	GSW[b]	SW[c]	Blunt[d]	Upper[e]	Mid[f]	Lower[g]	Data class
Peterson[h]	18	17	1	0	5	7	6	III
Liroff[i]	20	N/A	N/A	N/A	5	11	4	III
Stutzman[j]	22	22	0	0	6	3	13	III
Holden[k]	63	63	0	0	20	27	16	III
Lankford[l]	10	10	0	0	6	3	1	III
Carlton[m]	39	36	1	2	N/A	N/A	N/A	III
Eickenberg[n]	17	17	0	0	6	2	9	III
Presti[o]	18	10	6	2	15	1	2	III
Steers[p]	18	17	0	1	12	4	2	III
Rober[q]	16	16	0	0	8	4	4	III
Campbell[r]	15	12	0	3	7	4	4	III
Totals	256	219	8	8	90 (41%)	66 (30%)	61 (28%)	

N/A, not available.
[a] Number of patients in study.
[b] Gunshot wound.
[c] Stab wound.
[d] Blunt trauma.
[e] Upper one third of ureter or renal pelvis.
[f] Middle one third of ureter.
[g] Lower one third of ureter.
[h] Peterson NE, Pitts JC. Penetrating injuries of the ureter. J Urol 1981;126:587–590.
[i] Liroff SA, Pontes JES, Pierce JM Jr. Gunshot wounds of the ureter: 5 years of experience. J Urol 1977;118:551–553.
[j] Stutzman RE. Ballistics and the management of ureteral injuries from high velocity missiles. J Urol 1977;118:947–949.
[k] Holden S, Hicks CC, O'Brien DP, et al. Gunshot wounds of the ureter: a 15-year review of 63 consecutive cases. J Urol 1976;116:562–564.
[l] Lankford R, Block NL, Politano VA. Gunshot wounds of the ureter: a review of ten cases. J Trauma 1974;14:848–852.
[m] Carlton CE Jr, Scott R Jr, Guthrie AG. The initial management of ureteral injuries: a report of 78 cases. J Urol 1971;105:335–341.
[n] Eickenberg H, Amin M. Gunshot wounds to the ureter. J Trauma 1976;16:562–565.
[o] Presti JC Jr, Carroll PR, McAninch JW. Ureteral and renal pelvic injuries from external trauma: diagnosis and management. J Trauma 1989;29:370–374.
[p] Steers WD, Corriere JN Jr, Benson GS, et al. The use of indwelling ureteral stents in managing ureteral injuries due to external violence. J Trauma 1985;25:1001–1003.
[q] Rober PE, Smith JB, Pierce JM. Gunshot injuries of the ureter. J Trauma 1990;30:83–86.
[r] Campbell EW, Filderman PS, Jacobs SC. Ureteral injury due to blunt and penetrating trauma. Urology 1992;40:216–220.
Source: Reprinted from Presti JC Jr. Urology. In: Norton JA, Bollinger RR, Chang AE, et al, eds. Surgery: Basic Science and Clinical Evidence. New York: Springer-Verlag, 2001, with permission.

Table 38.4. Urinalysis and intravenous urography in the diagnosis of ureteral injuries.

Reference	n^a	Urinalysis[b]	IVU[c]	Data class
Peterson[d]	18	10/13	7/11	III
Liroff[e]	20	9/13	N/A	III
Lankford[f]	10	9/9	8/8	III
Carlton[g]	39	N/A	17/21	III
Eickenberg[h]	17	N/A	7/9	III
Presti[i]	18	11/16	3/11	III
Steers[j]	18	14/16	7/8	III
Rober[k]	16	8/11	8/8	III
Campbell[l]	15	10/13	4/12	III
Totals	171	71/91 (78%)	61/88 (69%)	

N/A, not available.
[a] Number of patients in study.
[b] Microscopic (>5 red cells/high-power field) or gross hematuria on initial urinalysis.
[c] Intravenous urography demonstrating ureteral injury.
[d] Peterson NE, Pitts JC. Penetrating injuries of the ureter. J Urol 1981;126:587–590.
[e] Liroff SA, Pontes JES, Pierce JM Jr. Gunshot wounds of the ureter: 5 years of experience. J Urol 1977;118:551–553.
[f] Lankford R, Block NL, Politano VA. Gunshot wounds of the ureter: a review of ten cases. J Trauma 1974;14:848–852.
[g] Carlton CE Jr, Scott R Jr, Guthrie AG. The initial management of ureteral injuries: a report of 78 cases. J Urol 1971;105:335–341.
[h] Eickenberg H, Amin M. Gunshot wounds to the ureter. J Trauma 1976;16:562–565.
[i] Presti JC Jr, Carroll PR, McAninch JW. Ureteral and renal pelvic injuries from external trauma: diagnosis and management. J Trauma 1989;29:370–374.
[j] Steers WD, Corriere JN Jr, Benson GS, et al. The use of indwelling ureteral stents in managing ureteral injuries due to external violence. J Trauma 1985;25:1001–1003.
[k] Rober PE, Smith JB, Pierce JM. Gunshot injuries of the ureter. J Trauma 1990;30:83–86.
[l] Campbell EW, Filderman PS, Jacobs SC. Ureteral injury due to blunt and penetrating trauma. Urology 1992;40:216–200.
Source: Reprinted from Presti JC Jr. Urology. In: Norton JA, Bollinger RR, Chang AE, et al, eds. Surgery: Basic Science and Clinical Evidence. New York: Springer-Verlag, 2001, with permission.

murmur, while urologic symptoms, such as urinary frequency, urgency, and dysuria, commonly are absent. Urine analysis may be normal, and **a study that evaluates renal function, such as an IVP, intravenous contrast-enhanced CT, or renal angiogram, is necessary to establish the diagnosis (Fig. 38.4).**

Patients who present with renal artery emboli usually are medically unstable or recently have suffered a cardiac event. In such

Table 38.5. Arteriosclerotic renovascular hypertension.

Institution	Number of patients	Operative outcome (%)			Surgical mortality (%)
		Cured	Improved	Failed	
Bowman Gray	152	15	75	10	1.3
University of Michigan	135	29	52	19	4.4
University of California, San Francisco	84	39	23	38	2.4
Cleveland Clinic	78	40	51	9	2

Source: Reprinted from Stanley JC. Surgical treatment of renovascular hypertension. Am J Surg 1997;174:102–110. Copyright © 1997 Excerpta Medica. With permission from Excerpta Medica.

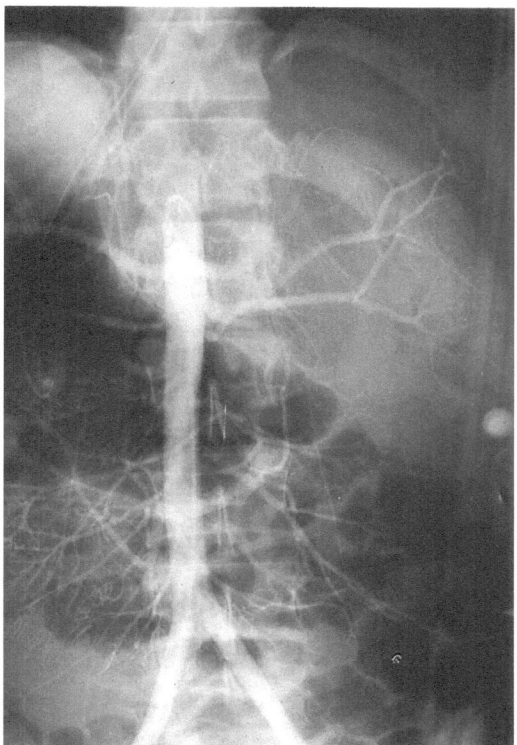

Figure 38.4. Renal artery angiogram demonstrating normal right renal vasculature and abrupt cutoff of left renal artery due to emboli.

patients who usually have unilateral renal infarction, treatment is non-operative and consists of **anticoagulation therapy**. For bilateral renal artery emboli or emboli to a solitary kidney, **streptokinase catheter embolectomy or surgical treatment may be necessary**.

Nonurologic Causes

Other problems that cause flank pain that should be considered by the clinician include *intraabdominal* **pathology** that secondarily results in flank pain. Since the kidneys are related anatomically to the colon, pancreas, spleen, ovaries, and psoas muscle, pathology involving these organs can produce flank pain. Usually, the abdominal symptoms are the primary complaint of the patient in these situations.

Musculoskeletal **causes** of flank pain are not uncommon and also need to be considered. Most patients with a musculoskeletal cause of flank pain present with pain of long-standing duration (12 weeks or more). In contrast to flank pain secondary to a urologic cause, musculoskeletal pain tends to be localized more medially, below the costal margin and above the inferior gluteal folds, with or without leg pain (sciatica).

Psychological

If the evaluation of a patient with flank pain is normal and the patient continues to complain of pain and seeks narcotic medication for relief of symptoms, consider **drug-seeking behavior or Munchausen syndrome**. These patients are well aware of the clinical presentation of stone disease and have been known to put a drop of blood from a pricked finger in the urine to simulate microscopic hematuria. Such patients may have an "allergy" to all nonnarcotic analgesics and sometimes indicate the narcotic that works best for them. Such patients also have brought in small stones that they recently have "passed" in the urine. On stone analysis, these stones usually are found to be composed of 100% quartz. Patients with drug-seeking behavior or Munchausen syndrome should not be given narcotics; however, **psychiatric evaluation is recommended**.

History and Physical Examination

History

The history is the most important component of the evaluation of the patient with flank pain. The onset and severity of the pain provide clues to the etiology of the pain. **Long-standing, dull pain is more typical of an infectious, malignant, or congenital problem. Acute, severe pain is characteristic of renal colic and most commonly results from an acute obstruction of the urinary tract due to a calculus**, as seen in the case presented. It is not uncommon for patients with renal colic to complain of prior stone episodes, since calculi tend to reoccur in up to 60% of patients.

Nausea and vomiting are common in patients who present with flank pain. These symptoms are due to irritation of the peritoneum and distention of the renal capsule. Nausea and vomiting, therefore, can occur with most causes of flank pain; however, it is most severe when the flank pain is acute and severe, such as from a renal calculi.

Associated urinary frequency and urgency are common with many causes of flank pain and are due to pain that is referred to the bladder area. The presence of **gross hematuria** is an important sign that can occur during an episode of flank pain and can be due to a renal calculi, infection, or tumor. **Gross hematuria mandates a complete urologic evaluation to rule out a malignancy of the urinary tract, such as a renal carcinoma, bladder carcinoma, or ureteral tumor.** The evaluation should include **imaging of the upper urinary tract with ultrasound or CT scan and evaluation of the bladder with cystoscopy.**

A **history of fever**, in association with flank pain, is an ominous sign that usually indicates infection (**Table 38.1**). The source of the fever typically is infected urine that remains undrained behind the source of obstruction, such as a calculi, stricture, or tumor. If no obstruction is present, yet the patient complains of flank pain in the presence of fever, it is consistent with acute pyelonephritis. In this situation, the renal tissue itself is infected, without obstruction of the urinary tract collecting system.

The **presence of comorbid conditions** must be considered when evaluating a patient with flank pain. Most healthy individuals with flank pain and no fever can be managed safely as outpatients. Problems that might predispose an individual to developing urosepsis include diabetes, immunosuppression, and pregnancy.

Tobacco use should be determined, since there is an increased risk for developing a transitional cell carcinoma in smokers. Transitional cell epithelium can be found in the bladder, ureter, and renal collecting system. Patients with transitional cell cancer typically present with gross hematuria without significant flank pain. However, if the tumor or a blood clot cause obstruction, flank pain may be identical to that produced by a renal calculi.

Patients with cardiac arrhythmias presenting with acute, severe flank pain should be evaluated for a possible thromboembolic event. In this situation, a cardiac thrombus suddenly is dislodged and obstructs the main renal artery or one of its branches. The resulting pain is identical to that produced by a renal calculi, so a history of cardiac arrhythmia is essential for establishing the diagnosis. **A functional imaging study, such as an IVP, contrast-enhanced CT, or renal angiogram, demonstrates absence of renal blood flow, indicating obstruction of the renal artery (Fig. 38.4).**

Physical Examination

A complete physical examination is indicated for patients presenting with flank pain to help determine the etiology of the pain and provide insight into the severity of the problem. It is important to perform a complete physical examination and resist the temptation to focus on the urinary tract or flank area exclusively.

Vital signs are important to determine if the flank pain might be associated with dehydration, infection, or urosepsis (**Table 38.1**). **In the patient with flank pain, urosepsis is suggested if the patient is febrile, has a rapid pulse and respiration rate, and has labile blood pressure.** If urosepsis is suspected, the patient should be hospitalized to prevent septic shock. In this situation, intravenous antibiotics, aggressive fluid replacement, and urologic relief of any hydronephrosis are indicated.

Fever from a lower urinary tract infection (bladder) may be low grade, while high spiking temperatures suggest upper tract infection (kidney). It is important to note, however, that one always cannot localize the site of the infection by the severity of the temperature. That is, a high temperature necessarily does not indicate upper urinary tract infection and vice versa; this is true especially in children.

The **carotid arteries should be auscultated** for bruits to evaluate for a possible cardiac etiology of the flank pain, such as a renal artery disease or embolus. **Heart auscultation** for rate, rhythm, and murmurs should be done for the same reason, since renal artery embolism

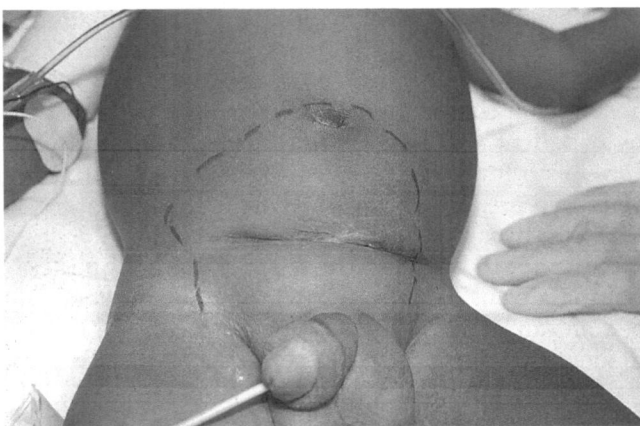

Figure 38.5. Large bladder rhabdomyosarcoma in a 2-year-old causing urinary tract obstruction. Note outline of mass and indwelling catheter.

usually occurs in patients with atrial fibrillation. The **abdomen** should be examined for bruits, tenderness, and masses. If the pain is more severe during the abdominal examination, consider intraabdominal etiologies for the flank pain. **A rectal examination**, with stool for guaiac, should be done to exclude a possible intraabdominal cause for the flank pain.

In females, it is essential to determine if the patient is pregnant with a urine or serum β-human chorionic gonadotropin (β-HCG) test. If the patient is pregnant, x-rays should be avoided, and the patient should be evaluated with ultrasound. Both males and females should have a **complete genital examination**, since referred pain is common. The bladder sometimes is able to be palpated just above the pubic symphysis. If the bladder is distended, it suggests a possible urologic etiology for the pain (**Fig. 38.5**).

The flank area should be examined for asymmetry, mass, and percussion tenderness. It is uncommon to discover a palpable flank mass, unless there is a large renal tumor present. Patients with acute pyelonephritis or obstructing renal calculi complain of severe pain when the flank is percussed, so it is important to tap lightly in order to maintain patient confidence.

To rule out a musculoskeletal etiology for the flank pain, **the lower extremities should be examined for motor and sensory function**.

Laboratory and Diagnostic Studies

Laboratory Studies

The history and physical examination help determine the *most probable* etiology of the flank pain and guide the clinician toward the selection of the most appropriate laboratory and diagnostic tests.

In almost all cases, **a urinalysis** should be performed as the initial diagnostic test. Among the most important parameters to consider on urine analysis are pH, WBCs, RBCs, bacteria, casts, and crystals. Infected urine typically has a high pH secondary to urea splitting bacteria. In contrast, patients with uric acid stones tend to have an acidic urine, since these stones do not form when the urine is alkaline. The presence of WBCs in the urine may signify infection, but it also may be due to inflammation caused by a stone. The presence of WBC casts strongly suggests urinary tract infection or acute pyelonephritis. Tumors of the urinary tract usually result in urinary RBCs, and the urine may appear grossly bloody. A stone similarly can result in RBCs in the urine, so it is important to repeat a urinalysis in patients after they have passed the stone to exclude an underlying urologic cancer. If the patient has RBCs in the urine after the stone has passed, urologic evaluation is necessary. A Gram stain should be done in the emergency room or clinic and can help determine if infection is present. In the case presented, a negative Gram stain suggests sterile urine. Finding bacteria on an unspun specimen suggests infection. Most urinary tract infections are caused by gram-negative bacteria such as *E. coli*; however, gram-positive organisms can cause urinary tract infections as well. If urinary calculi are present within the urinary tract, it is not uncommon to find crystals in the urine analysis, along with RBCs and WBCs, as seen in the illustrated case. The shape of the crystal can be used by the laboratory technician to help identify its composition. **The urinalysis may be normal if the etiology of the flank pain is due to cardiac, intraabdominal, musculoskeletal, or psychological problems.**

Limited blood tests are indicated in patients with flank pain. If infection is suspected, a complete blood count is important to determine if the serum WBC count is elevated. Anemia and a low or high platelet count might be seen in the presence of bleeding urologic tumors. An abnormally high hematocrit can be seen if the patient is dehydrated. Evaluation of serum sodium, potassium, chloride, bicarbonate, glucose, blood urea nitrogen (BUN), and creatinine are important. An elevated BUN can be due to renal disease or dehydration. In general, if the BUN is greater than 10 times the serum creatinine level, then the elevation most likely is due to dehydration. If the BUN to serum creatinine ratio is 10 or less, then renal disease is likely. The serum creatinine level directly reflects renal function. An elevated creatinine indicates impaired renal function, regardless of the BUN value. The impaired function could be due to dehydration, obstruction, tumor, infarct, or medical renal disease. Moreover, an elevated serum creatinine indicates bilateral renal disease or disease involving a solitary kidney, since only one healthy kidney is required to maintain a normal serum creatinine. In long-standing renal compromise, it is not uncommon to see a fall in serum bicarbonate along with hyperkalemia. Hyponatremia results from volume overload and can cause nausea, vomiting, and seizures. Hyperkalemia especially is dangerous, since it could result in cardiac arrhythmias. Other useful tests might include a serum uric acid level and serum calcium level, if a urinary calculus is suspected.

Diagnostic Studies

Following the history, physical exam, and laboratory analysis, a **plain film of the abdomen** can help identify urinary calculi (**Fig. 38.6**). This film is called a KUB, since it visualizes the kidney, ureter, and bladder. The entire film should be viewed for intestinal gas pattern, gallstones, bony structure, and free air, which may provide insight into the etiology of the pain. Renal cell carcinomas are osteolytic tumors, and this can be seen radiographically in metastatic disease. An abnormal intestinal gas pattern, gallstones, or free air suggest intraabdominal pathology. Aortic calcifications and aneurysms should be determined, since they might suggest renal artery disease as the etiology of the flank pain. Urinary calculi typically are seen as calcifications overlying the kidney shadow or along the course of the ureter (**Fig. 38.6**). Small stones, 1 to 2 mm in size, can cause severe flank pain if they obstruct the flow of urine into the bladder. **Stones typically become obstructive where the ureter meets the renal pelvis [ureteropelvic junction (UPJ)], where the ureter crosses over the pelvic brim, and where the ureter enters the bladder [ureterovesical junction (UVJ)].** Small stones tend to lodge at the UVJ, whereas bigger stones lodge higher in the urinary tract. **It should be noted that uric acid calculi are radiolucent and are not seen on a plain film of the abdomen, but they can be seen on ultrasound or CT scan.**

Following the history, physical examination, urinalysis, and abdominal plain film, a preliminary diagnosis is possible in most instances. However, more detailed imaging studies often are performed to confirm the diagnosis and to help plan appropriate therapy. The traditional test of choice for evaluating flank pain in detail has been the **IVP** (**Table 38.4**). The IVP is a relatively inexpensive functional study that diagnoses most urologic, infectious, and cardiac causes of flank pain. However, because it requires the administration of iodine-based

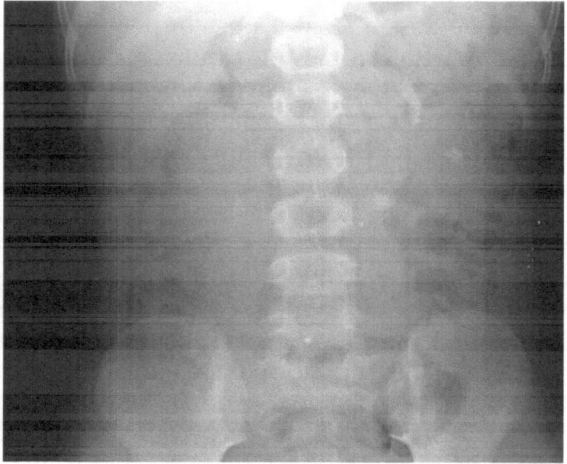

Figure 38.6. Plain film of the abdomen demonstrating multiple left renal calculi.

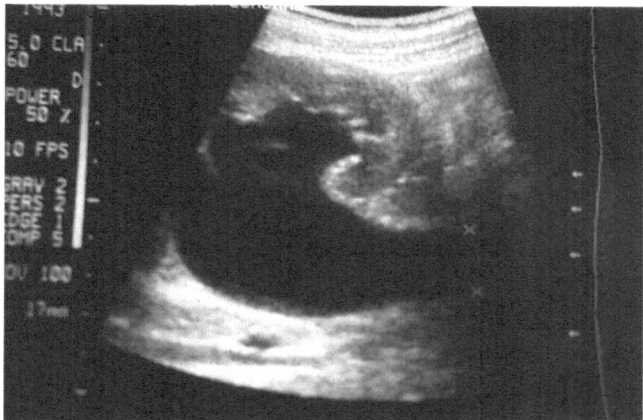

Figure 38.7. Renal ultrasound demonstrating hydronephrosis.

intravenous contrast medium, an allergic reaction to the contrast is possible. These reactions can be severe and have resulted in hemodynamic and respiratory collapse. **To avoid contrast reactions, an ultrasound or noncontrast CT can be used instead of an IVP (Fig. 38.7).** Ultrasound and noncontrast CT are noninvasive and do not require intravenous contrast administration. The disadvantage, compared to IVP, is that these studies do not provide any functional information about the kidney. These tests demonstrate anatomy, not function, and this consideration may be important in a patient's evaluation. For example, if the clinician is concerned about a possible renal infarct secondary to an arterial embolus, a renal ultrasound and noncontrast CT scan might be normal, since they do not assess renal function. In this instance, the kidney looks normal; however, it is no longer functioning due to the recent infarct. To assess function, either an IVP or intravenous contrast-enhanced CT scan could be done.

Summary

The urologist frequently evaluates patients with flank pain and diagnoses and treats conditions that may have local or systemic ramifications. Nonurologic causes for the pain always are considered during the initial evaluation. Although the history and physical examination are the most important aspect of the evaluation, laboratory and diagnostic tests help confirm the diagnosis. Since this is a commonly encountered clinical problem, all practitioners should have some familiarity with the diagnosis and management of flank pain.

Selected Readings

Ahya SN, Coyne DW. Renal disease. In: Ahya SN, Flood K, Paranjothi S, eds. The Washington Manual of Medical Therapeutics, 30th ed. Philadelphia: Lippincott Williams & Wilkins, 2001.

Dunn DL. Diagnosis and treatment of infection. In: Norton JA, Bollinger RR, Chang AE, et al, eds. Surgery: Basic Science and Clinical Evidence. New York: Springer-Verlag, 2001.

McLeod RS. Evidence-based surgery. In: Norton JA, Bollinger RR, Chang AE, et al, eds. Surgery: Basic Science and Clinical Evidence. New York: Springer-Verlag, 2001.

Presti JC Jr, Urology. In: Norton JA, Bollinger RR, Chang AE, et al, eds. Surgery: Basic Science and Clinical Evidence. New York: Springer-Verlag, 2001.

Presti JC Jr, Stoller ML, Carroll PR. Urology. In: Tierny LM Jr, McPhee SJ, Papadikis M, eds. Current Medical Diagnosis and Treatment, 39th ed. New York: Lange Medical Books/McGraw-Hill, 2000.

Stack RS. Acute pyelonephritis. In Rakel R, ed. Conn's Current Therapy, 9th ed. Philadelphia: WB Saunders, 2000.

39

Scrotal Disorders

Robert E. Weiss

Objectives

1. To discuss the diagnosis and treatment of the undescended testicle. Be sure to consider the age of the patient.
2. To generate a list of potential diagnoses for the patient who presents with pain or a mass in the scrotum. Be sure to:
   - Discuss testicular versus extratesticular origins
   - Discuss benign versus malignant causes
   - Discuss emergent versus nonemergent causes
3. To list the history and physical exam findings that help differentiate etiologies. Be sure to discuss the following issues:
   - Pain—presence, absence, onset, severity
   - Palpation—distinguish testicular from extratesticular (adnexal) mass
   - Transillumination
4. To discuss the diagnostic algorithm for scrotal swelling and/or pain.
5. To discuss the treatment of nonmalignant causes of scrotal swelling or pain.
6. To discuss the staging and treatment of testicular cancer.

Cases

Case 1

A mother brought her 15-month-old son in for evaluation because he has "only one testicle."

Case 2

A 15-year-old boy presented to the emergency department with acute testis pain and nausea.

Case 3

A 24-year-old man presented to his physician with a "lump on his testis."

Introduction

This chapter discusses the diagnosis and treatment of **cryptorchidism,** the **acute scrotum,** and **testis cancer.**

The testicle's primary responsibility is to make **sperm** and **testosterone.** Testicular development and descent are controlled intricately by the **hypothalamus-pituitary-gonad axis (Fig. 39.1).** The hypothalmus releases GNRH which stimulates the pituitary to release LH and FSH. LH and FSH stimulate the testis to grow and make testosterone. Testosterone regulates its own production by regaling feedback on the hypothalmus and pituitary. Testicular endocrine function becomes fully developed after puberty.

Descent of the testis and epididymis from the abdomen occurs only in mammals. Scrotal development in males is a result of the testis and epididymis descending, causing the skin to stretch. Sperm fertility is enhanced by being stored in a cooler region within the scrotum rather than in the abdomen. Cryptorchid or "undescended testis" results in infertility if the testis is not placed in the scrotum.

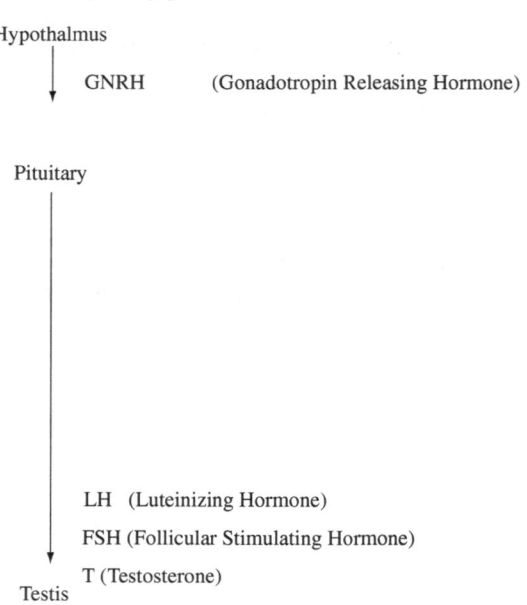

Figure 39.1. Hypothalmic-pituitary-gonadal axis.

During early development, the testes originates in the abdomen near the kidney. During early embryologic development, the processus vaginalis is an invagination at the inguinal ring. The gubernaculum attaches superiorly onto the Wolffian duct and inferiorly into the inguinal canal. As the fetus matures, the testis descends into the scrotum. This descent from abdomen to scrotum explains why the testis lymphatic drainage is to the nodes below the renal hilum and the venous drainage is to the vena cava on the right and to the renal vein on the left.

Cryptorchidism

Cryptorchidism or undescended testis is defined as an abnormal descent of the testis and can be unilateral or bilateral. The incidence is 3.4% to 5.8% in full-term boys and 1.82% at 1 year of age. The testis can be found in the upper scrotum, inguinal canal, or abdomen. Two thirds of the cases are unilateral, while one third of the cases are bilateral. It is more common in premature boys.

For the **examination**, the child should be placed in the cross-legged position. Initial visual inspection should reveal a scrotum that is developed bilaterally. The testis should be palpated between the thumb and forefinger. The testes should have equivalent size and texture. **The undescended testis may be retractile and easily manipulated into the scrotum.** Often, slight groin pressure with the forefinger brings the testis down into the scrotum. If the testis is not palpated in the scrotum or groin, **ultrasonography** may be necessary to locate it above the internal inguinal ring or within the abdomen. Most retractile testes descend by 1 year of age.

If the testis does not appear to be descending properly, **surgical orchiopexy** is the necessary treatment to place the testis in the scrotum, which allows appropriate testis maturation and eventual fertility. Most surgeons perform this procedure by the time the patient has reached 1 year of age. Cryptorchid testis is associated with inguinal hernia in 25% of patients due to a patent processus vaginalis. The hernia should be repaired when the orchiopexy is performed. Orchiopexy usually is performed through an inguinal incision, allowing the surgeon to mobilize the testis and its blood supply to reach the scrotum. Associated hernias also can be repaired. The testis is sutured to the dartos in the scrotum to keep it in place.

Case Discussion

In the child in **Case 1**, there was no history of trauma or infection, and the mother stated that she had noted this condition for several months. The child was examined in a cross-legged position. The right testis was in a normal position within the scrotum; however, the left testis was in the groin, near the external ring, and could not be manipulated into the scrotum. The mother discussed the situation with the urologist and decided that her child should have an elective orchipexy.

Scrotal Pain

Scrotal pain can be due to several etiologies that range from chronic to surgical emergency. **The differential diagnosis for a painful testis includes testis torsion, epididymitis, trauma, tumor, torsion of appendix testis or appendix epididymis, incarcerated hernia, and ureteral calculi.** See **Algorithm 39.1.** Occasionally, kidney stones that migrate to the distal ureter cause pain referred to the groin, but this pain usually is colicky in nature.

Testis Torsion

The patient who presents with acute testis pain should be treated as a surgical emergency. A patient who has a testis torsion and is not treated within 3 to 12 hours may suffer testis atrophy. Testis torsion occurs because the testis rotates or twists its blood supply, essentially strangling the testis. Vascular occlusion results in acute pain as the testis becomes edematous.

Testis torsion usually occurs in adolescent males, but it may be seen in cryptorchid testis or as a result of testis trauma. The cremasteric muscle spasms, causing the spermatic cord to rotate upon itself.

The patient's history of torsion usually is consistent with sudden onset, acute pain, nausea, and vomiting. The patient should have a urinalysis, urine culture and sensitivity, and complete blood count

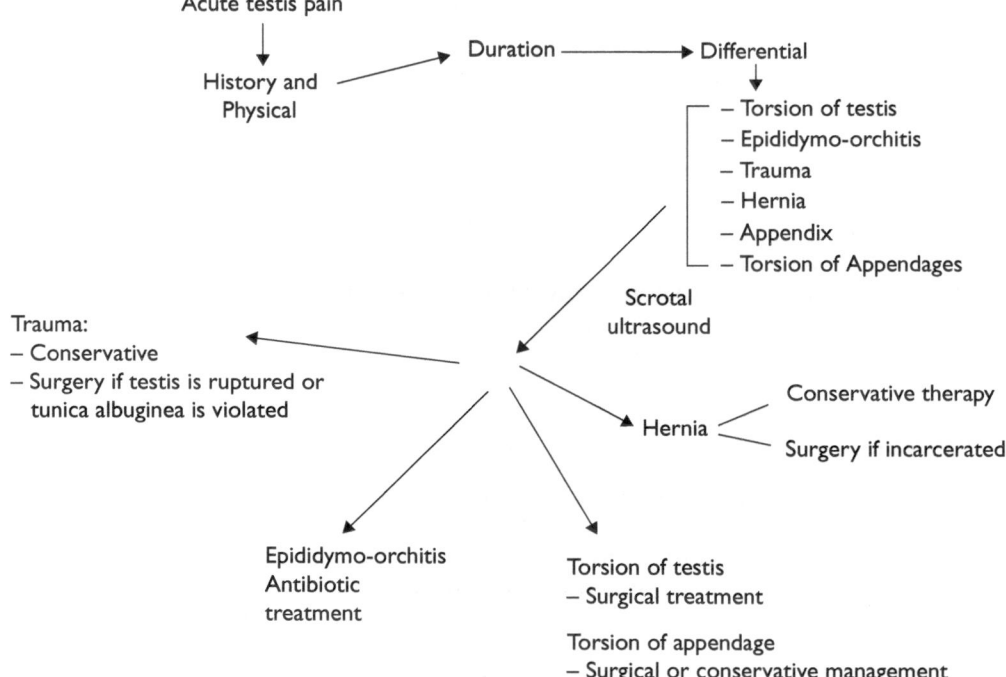

Algorithm 39.1. Algorithm for workup of acute testis pain.

(CBC) to evaluate infectious sources consistent with epididymitis. **Physical examination of the patient with torsion reveals a tender, erythematous scrotum with a high or horizontal position of the testis.** The cremasteric reflex usually is absent. Epididymitis usually presents with gradual onset, white blood cells in the urine, and increased tenderness behind the testis along the epididymis. The patient may have a history of recent sexual activity or symptoms of urinary infection or prostatitis. Differentiating the two may be difficult. Epididymitis may progress to epididymo-orchitis.

Diagnosis should be confirmed with an emergency Doppler ultrasonography. A testis torsion appears as hypovascular, while epididymitis appears as hypervascular. Since Doppler ultrasonography technology has improved, nuclear scanning rarely is necessary to confirm the diagnosis.

For **treatment**, manual detorsion may be attempted if the torsion has occurred within a few hours. This consists of infiltration of the spermatic cord near the external ring with lidocaine. The left testis is rotated counterclockwise manually, while the right testis is rotated clockwise manually. **Manual detorsion** usually is not effective because of the patient's degree of pain. **Emergent surgical scrotal exploration** should be performed under general anesthesia. A scrotal incision is made, the spermatic cord is untwisted, and the testis is inspected. If the testis appears viable, it should be sutured in place to the surrounding tissue. The contralateral testis also should undergo orchiopexy during the same procedure. Nonviable testis require orchiectomy.

Torsion of the testicular appendages may mimic testis torsion and usually occurs in boys younger than 16 years of age. The **appendix testis** (remnant of the Müllerian duct) and **appendix epididymis** (remnant of the Wolffian duct) may twist and cause venous engorgement and infarction, producing the "blue-dot sign." These cases may be managed conservatively with pain medications. If the pain persists or there is concern of testis torsion, emergent surgical exploration should be performed.

Case Discussion
The patient in **Case 2** stated that the pain occurred suddenly about 2 hours previously and continued to be unbearable. He denied trauma or sexual activity. Urinalysis was negative for white blood cells, and Doppler ultrasonography revealed decreased flow to the testis. The patient underwent emergent scrotal exploration in the operating room, where a testis torsion was found. The spermatic cord was untwisted, and the testis regained its pink color. The testis was sutured to surrounding tissue (orchipexy) to prevent future torsion and the contralateral testis also underwent orchiepexy. The patient recovered without problem.

Epididymo-orchitis

Acute epididymitis is extremely painful and may mimic the symptoms of testicular torsion. The incidence of epididymitis is much higher than that of testicular torsion. Acute epididymitis is an infectious process caused by reflux of bacteria via the vas deferens. It is caused by urinary tract pathogens, such as gram-negative organisms, and often originates from prostatitis or an indwelling urethral catheter. Acute epididymitis also can be associated with sexually transmitted diseases, such as those caused by *Chlamydia trachomatis* or *Neisseria gonorrhea*. **The patient usually presents with gradual onset of pain. Acute onset, however, may occur and mimic testis torsion. The patient complains of tenderness, scrotal erythema, and fever.**

Laboratory findings reveal white blood cells in the urine and a positive Gram stain. The CBC shows an elevated white cell count, with a shift to the left. **Ultrasonography reveals a hypervascular area** consistent with the inflammatory response of infection.

Treatment should include immediate antibiotics. If a urinary pathogen is suspected, the patient should be given a quinolone or a trimethoprim sulfate until urine and blood culture sensitivities return. If a sexually transmitted disease is suspected, the patient should be given an injection of ceftriaxone followed by oral doxycycline or tetracycline. Depending on the severity of the infection, the patient may need pain medications, ice packs to the scrotum, and bed rest.

The pain may not resolve for 2 weeks or longer. The patient should be followed closely for possible abscess. Infertility may be a long-term sequela. Some patients progress to chronic epididymitis and require long-term antibiotic coverage and nonsteroidal antiinflammatory medication.

Testis Masses

Testis masses include **benign lesions of the scrotum** and **testis tumors**. See **Algorithm 39.2**.

Benign Lesions of the Scrotum

Hydrocele
Hydroceles are a common scrotal problem. They usually are benign, but they must be differentiated from testis tumors and inguinal hernias.

Hydroceles in children usually are due to persistent patency of the processus vaginalis. The processus usually closes, and the hydrocele resolves. Persistent hydroceles after the age of 2 years usually are repaired surgically.

Hydroceles in adults usually are due to fluid collection within the tunica vaginalis. They often are due to nonspecific epididymitis or orchitis or are a result of scrotal trauma. Occasionally, they can be related to testis cancer, tubercular epididymitis, or radiotherapy.

Physical examination of the hydrocele reveals a uniformly enlarged mass in the scrotum. It usually is nontender and can be **transilluminated**. **Ultrasonography** confirms the diagnosis of hydrocele and rules out the presence of testis tumor or inguinal hernia.

Treatment of a hydrocele depends on the symptoms. If the hydrocele is small and the patient has no discomfort, the patient is managed conservatively. If the hydrocele is large, it should be explored

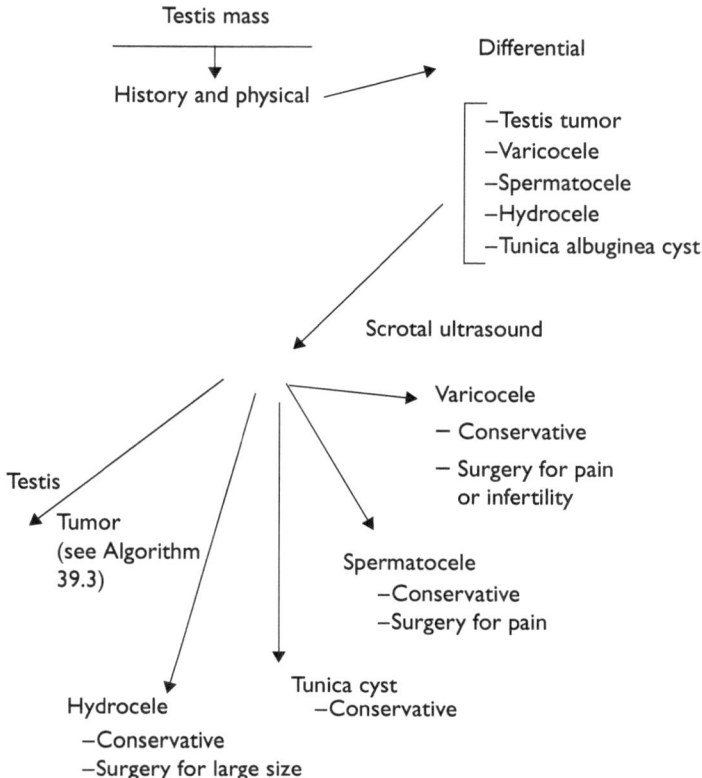

Algorithm 39.2. Algorithm for workup of testis mass.

surgically, and the tunica vaginalis should be resected. Simple aspiration of the fluid often results in recurrence or infection.

Spermatocele
Spermatocele is another common benign mass. It usually is small, with the patient complaining of a nontender, firm testis mass. The spermatocele is located in the epididymis, posterior to the testis and clearly separate. The spermatocele is caused by **obstruction of the tubules connecting the rete testis to the head of the epididymis**. The cystic nature of the spermatocele should be confirmed by **ultrasonography**. Initial **treatment** should be conservative. If the patient complains of persistent pain over a period of time, surgical excision may be performed.

Varicocele
A varicocele is the **dilation of the pampiniform venous plexus**, which drains the testis. Varicoceles probably are due to incompetence of venous valves. The higher prevalence of left varicoceles may be caused by the insertion of the left spermatic vein on the left renal vein. Approximately 20% of men have varicoceles, and they usually are benign. In a small number of men, these veins become painful, especially when standing upright for long periods of time. Rapid onset of

a varicocele in an older man may be an indication of a renal tumor obstructing the spermatic vein. Large varicoceles also have been associated with infertility. Varicoceles may affect the temperature of the testes and subsequently alter sperm count, sperm motility, and morphology.

Physical examination of men with varicoceles should be performed with the patient in the upright position. The engorged veins can be palpated superior to the testis following the path of the spermatic cord. These veins usually dilate when the patient performs the Valsalva maneuver and empty when the patient is in the reclining position. Testicular size should be compared to the contralateral side.

Most men with varicoceles do not need **treatment**. Surgery may become necessary if the patient demonstrates diminished testicular size or abnormal sperm parameters or if the patient complains of persistent pain. Surgery may be performed by **high ligation of the spermatic veins in the abdomen or ligation of the branches of inferior veins in the spermatic cord**. It is important to identify all collaterals to prevent recurrence.

Testis Tumors

Testis tumors commonly occur in young men between the ages of 20 and 40 years old. There are two to three new cases of testis cancer per 100,000 men in the United States per year. Only 1% to 2% of these cases occur bilaterally. Six percent of men with testis cancer have a history of cryptorchidism. Testis tumors tend to occur in an age group of men who often do not have routine physical examinations. **Therefore, patient awareness and self-examination are very important. Early detection is essential, as the cure rate is high.** Due to improvements of chemotherapy, the 5-year survival rate exceeds 90%. See **Algorithm 39.3.**

Testis tumors can be divided into two groups: **seminoma** and **non-seminoma**. Seminoma represents 35% of testis tumors. Nonseminomatous tumors include **embryonal carcinoma (20%), teratoma (5%), choriocarcinoma (<1%), and mixed teratocarcinoma (40%). Serum tumor markers for testis cancer are β-human chorionic gonadotropin (β-HCG), α-fetoprotein (AFP), and lactic acid dehydrogenase (LDH).** These serum markers should be drawn if testis cancer is suspected. β-Human chorionic gonadotropin is present in 5% to 10% of men with seminoma, in 40% to 60% of men with embryonal carcinoma, and in all men with choriocarcinoma. It is made by syncytiotrophoblasts and can be used to follow the tumor's response to therapy. It has a half-life of 24 hours. α-Fetoprotein is produced by the yolk sac. It is found primarily in pure embryonal carcinoma, in mixed (teratocarcinoma), and in yolk sac tumors, but it is never elevated in seminoma or pure choriocarcinoma. The half-life of AFP is 5 days. Lactic acid dehydrogenase is a less specific tumor marker that may be elevated in patients with metastatic disease.

Patients present with a palpable mass in their testis. Delay in diagnosis often occurs because young patients do not present immediately

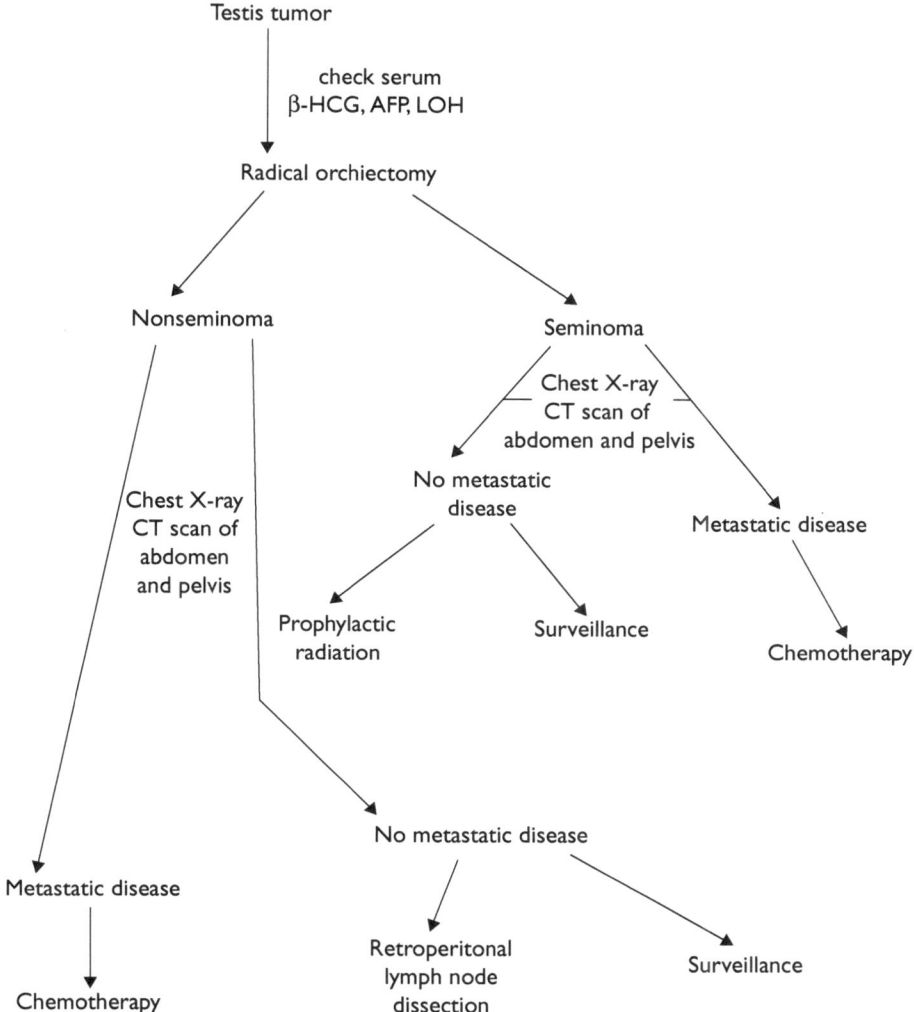

Algorithm 39.3. Algorithm for workup of testis tumor. AFP, α-fetoprotein; β-HCG, β-human chorionic gonadotropin; CT, computed tomography; CXR, chest x-ray; LDH, lactic acid dehydrogenase.

to their physicians or because they are mistakenly diagnosed as having epididymitis. **Physical examination and scrotal ultrasonography are essential in order to make the diagnosis.** For patients with indeterminate lesions, magnetic resonance imaging may assist in the evaluation.

Testis cancer is treated by radical orchiectomy. An incision is made in the groin. The spermatic artery and vein are clamped to avoid tumor spread, and the testis is removed along with the spermatic cord. Sites of metastases include the retroperitonem and the lung. Therefore, staging includes abdominal and pelvic computed tomography (CT) scan and chest x-ray. **Testis tumors on the right tend to metastasize to the interaortocaval area at the level of the renal hilum (following the drainage of the right spermatic vein) and on the left to the periaor-**

tic area at the left renal hilum (following the drainage of the left spermatic vein). Once the testis tumors metastasize to these "primary landing sites," they tend to progress in a stepwise manner to other lymph nodes in the retroperitoneum. Disease also may progress to the lung, liver, and brain. Choriocarcinoma, however, may spread initally to the lung. See **Table 39.1** for the TNM staging stystem for testis cancer.

After the orchiectomy is performed, markers should decline and eventually normalize. If they remain elevated, residual disease is present. Seminoma is very radiosensitive. Patients with no disease or minimal retroperitoneal disease are advised to have **radiation** to the retroperitoneum as prophylaxis or treatment. Patients with higher stage disease are given **chemotherapy**: etoposide and platinol (cisplatin) (EP) or bleomycin, etoposide, and cisplatin (BEP).

Patients with nonseminomatous tumors eventually should have normal serum markers after orchiectomy if there is no metastatic disease. Patients with gross mestastases or persistently positive markers are given chemotherapy (EP or BEP). Patients who have normal markers and no gross evidence of disease have an approximately 25% to 40% possibility of relapse, depending on the pathology. Because of this, they are advised to undergo a **retroperitoneal lymph node dissection**. This procedure requires an abdominal incision, and lymph nodes are removed below the renal hilum and along the vena cava or aorta, depending on the side of the testis tumor and the suspected landing site. Side effects of the surgery may include impairment of ejaculatory function (retrograde), which may result in infertility. Some patients opt not to have the surgery and require intensive surveillance with frequent CT scans in order to identify metastatic disease.

Table 39.1. TNM staging system for testis cancer.

T: Primary tumor	
Tx	Cannot be assessed
T0	No evidence of primary tumor
Tis	Intratubular cancer (CIS)
T1	Limited to testis and epididymis, no vascular invasion
T2	Limited to testis and epididymis with vascular invasion or invades into tunica vaginalis
T3	Invades spermatic cord
T4	Invades scrotum
N: Regional lymph nodes	
Nx	Cannot be assessed
N0	No regional lymph node metastasis
N1	Metastasis in a lymph node mass 2 cm or less
N2	Metastasis in a lymph node mass >2 cm and <5 cm or multiple nodes none >5 cm
N3	Metastasis in lymph node mass >5 cm
M: Distant metastasis	
Mx	Cannot be assessed
M0	No distant metastasis
M1	Distant metastasis present

Source: Reprinted from Presti JC Jr. Urology. In: Norton JA, Bollinger RR, Chang AE, et al, eds. Surgery: Basic Science and Clinical Evidence. New York: Springer-Verlag, 2001, with permission.

Patients who develop recurrence have an excellent response to BEP. **Testis tumors are one of the few tumors for which long-term cures have been achieved with chemotherapy.**

Case Discussion
The patient in **Case 3** denied trauma or pain. The physician examined the patient and found a firm nodule on the testis that did not transilluminate. The physician ordered serum β-HCG, AFP, and LDH tests and a scrotal ultrasound. The ultrasound revealed a solid left testis mass and the serum markers showed an elevated AFP level, but normal β-HCG and LDH levels. The patient underwent a left radical orchiectomy through an inguinal incision. Three weeks after the surgery, the AFP level returned to normal, and the patient's chest x-ray and abdominal CT scan showed no evidence of metastatic disease. The patient will undergo a surgical retroperitoneal lymph node dissection to determine if he has metastatic disease in the retroperitoneum.

Summary

This chapter discussed the diagnosis and management of the undescended testis, and the evaluation and management of the acute scrotum. Testis torsion must be diagnosed promptly so that the proper surgery can be performed to salvage the testis.

There are several benign etiologies for scrotal masses including hydroceles, varicoceles, and spermatoceles. Testis tumors occur in young men and must be diagnosed early for proper treatment. Ultrasonography provides the best diagnostic test to differentiate benign from malignant lesions of the testis.

Selected Readings

Albanese CT. Pediatric surgery. In: Norton JA, Bollinger RR, Chang AE, et al, eds. Surgery: Basic Science and Clinical Evidence. New York: Springer-Verlag, 2001.

Berkowitz GS, Lapinski RH, Dolgin SE, Gonzella JG, Bodian CA, Holzman IR. Prevalence and natural history of cryptorchism. Pediatrics 1993;92:44–49.

Carroll PR, Presti JC, eds. Testis cancer. Urol Clin North Am 1998;365–531.

Cuckow PM, Frank JD. Torsion of the testis. Br J Urol 2000;86(3):349–353.

Dearnaley DP, Huddart RA, Horwich A. Managing testis cancer. Br Med J 2001;322(7302):1583–1588.

Foster RS, Donahue JP. Retroperitoneal lymph node dissection for the management of clinical stage I non-seminoma. J Urol 2000;163(6):1788–1792.

Jefferson RH, Perez LM, Joseph DM. Critical analysis of the clinical presentation of the acute scrotum: 9-year experience at a single institution. J Urol 1997;158(3):1198–1200.

King LR. Undescended testis. JAMA 1996;276(11):856.

Noske HD, Kraus SW, Altinkilic BM, Weidner W. Historical milestones regarding torsion of scrotal organs. J Urol 1998;159(1):13–16.

Oliver RTD. Current opinion in germ cell cancer. Curr Opin Oncol 2000;12(3):249–254.

Presti JC Jr. Urology. In: Norton JA, Bollinger RR, Chang AE, et al, eds. Surgery: Basic Science and Clinical Evidence. New York: Springer-Verlag, 2001.

Rozanski TA, Bloom DA. The undescended testis: theory and management. Urol Clin North Am 1995;22(1):107–118.

Schmoll HJ. Treatment of testicular tumors based on risk factors. Curr Opin Urol 1999;9(5):431–438.

40

Transplantation of the Kidney

David A. Laskow

Objectives

1. To discuss the inclusion/exclusion criteria for renal transplantation.
2. To discuss the technical aspect of renal transplantation.
3. To discuss the impact of the source of the kidney donor in relationship to the outcome.
4. To discuss organ allocation.
5. To introduce the basic antirejection medications.
6. To describe the different types of rejection.
7. To discuss the management of a postoperative renal allograft recipient.

Case

A 27-year-old man presents with increasing serum creatinine 2 weeks after a renal allograft transplant. The patient is afebrile, with blood pressure at 155/85, pulse at 84, and respiration at 16. On physical exam, his wound is well healed, and the allograft is palpable and nontender in the right lower quadrant. Urinalysis, laboratory values, and ultrasound are pending.

Inclusion/Exclusion Criteria for Candidates Seeking Kidney Transplantation

Patients with **end-stage renal disease (ESRD)** have three options to replace and support their failing renal function: **hemodialysis, peritoneal dialysis, and renal transplantation**. All three are viable options in the management of a patient's renal function. These options are not mutually exclusive, and, in fact, most patients eventually are treated with all three.

Table 40.1. Causes of end-stage renal disease (ESRD): United States Renal Data System (USRDS) Annual Data Report.

Diabetes	Malignancies
Hypertension	Metabolic disorders
Glomerulonephritis	Congenital/other hereditary disease
Cystic kidney disease	Sickle cell disease
Interstitial nephritis	AIDS related
Obstructive nephropathy	Unknown
Collagen vascular disease	

Data from www.USRDS.org. Web site of United States Renal Data System.

Hemodialysis is the most common technique for the treatment of ESRD throughout the United States, although transplantation has proven to be the most effective solution to renal failure. The two most common causes of renal failure (Table 40.1), hypertension and diabetes mellitus, are significant risk factors for cardiovascular disease. The combination of underlying medical conditions leading to renal failure and dialysis itself creates an inverse relationship between time on dialysis and success with a renal transplant. Unfortunately, patients often have to wait years before receiving a transplant and have to suffer the debilitating consequences of long-term dialysis.

Prior to renal transplantation or to placement on a list for a cadaveric renal transplant, the potential recipient undergoes a thorough history and a thorough physical exam. Routinely, a complete blood count (CBC), chemistries, prothrombin time, partial thromboplastin time, chest x-ray, electrocardiogram (ECG), and blood type are obtained. In view of the significant effect the antirejection medications have on infectious agents, hepatitis B surface antigen and surface antibody (HBsAg, HBsAB), hepatitis B core antibody (HBcAB), hepatitis C antibody (HepCAb), VOR2, human immunodeficiency virus (HIV), herpes simplex virus (HSV), purified protein derivative (PPD), and cytomegalovirus (CMV) routinely are obtained. In women over 18, a Papanicolaou (Pap) smear from within the past year is required. A mammogram is required in women over 40. Last, blood routinely is sent to the tissue-typing lab for human leukocyte antigen (HLA) typing and for identification of preformed antibodies against a panel of known HLAs. This is called a panel reactive antibody test (PRA). Future workup is directed by the individual's underlying medical condition. Many patients undergo an echocardiogram, a cardiac stress test, a noninvasive vascular exam, and duplex ultrasound of the carotid arteries, since cardiovascular disease is pervasive through the renal failure population.

The contraindications to renal transplantation (Table 40.2) fall into two large categories. The first category is related to the general effect immunosuppressants have on infections and on cancer and to the patient's ability to take these drugs. The second category relates to the patient's overall medical condition, with a focus on cardiovascular status, and his or her ability to undergo a substantial operation.

Table 40.2. Contraindication to renal transplant.

Recent malignancy
Active infection
Active tuberculosis
Active AIDS
Hepatitis (with grade 2 cirrhosis or greater)
Pregnancy
Active illicit drug use
Active alcohol abuse
Noncompliance
Uncontrolled psychiatric disorders
Severe cardiovascular disease
Other end-stage organ disease (cardiac, pulmonary, hepatic)

How Organs Are Allocated Once a Patient Has Been Placed on a Cadaveric Waiting List

The goal of the **renal allocation scheme** is to **balance the benefit of matching HLA against waiting time (Table 40.3).** Patients steadily accumulate points for each year for which they wait for an organ, and therefore waiting time eventually serves as the driving force behind allocation. Patients cannot start accumulating waiting time until their glomerular filtration rate is less than 20 cc/min. Various numbers of points are given to different degrees of HLA matching, and so a patient's total points fluctuate with each potential transplant. Finally, points are given to individuals with PRAs greater than or equal to 80%. A PRA of 80% means that the recipient has antibodies against 80% of the antigens against which he/she is tested. The HLAs used are those commonly found in the local population. Patients become sensitized to HLAs and develop antibodies through exposure to human tissue through pregnancy, blood transfusions, and previous transplants of any time (except corneal). Overall, the higher the PRA becomes, the more difficult it is to find a compatible transplant. In the clinical case

Table 40.3. United System for Organ Sharing (UNOS) cadaver kidney allocation system.[a]

Kidneys allocated locally first, then regionally, then nationally to patients ranked highest, as determined by the following criteria:
Antigen mismatch (0–2 points)
Time waiting (<1 + 1 point per year)
Panel reactive antibody >80% (4 points)
Pediatric points (3–4 points)
Previous living donation (4 points)
Patients are eligible for marginal donors if specifically consented prior to listing
The individual with the highest cumulative point total is awarded the organ

[a] Individuals are placed on the waiting list only when their creatinine clearance or glomerular filtration rate (GFR) is less than or equal to 20 mL/min.

presented, it would be helpful to know what the HLA match was, as well as what the recipient PRA was prior to transplant.

The allocation scheme recognizes and rewards with points the fact that **children** on dialysis often have a difficult time maintaining good nutrition, which in turn causes poor physical and mental development, and that children derive more benefit from a transplant than adults. Special status and points are given to **patients who have donated a kidney** and who go into renal failure themselves. **As opposed to liver, heart, and lung transplant allocation schemes, with kidney transplants there are no points allocated based on medical need. Kidneys are allocated first locally, then regionally, and, last, nationally, with the exception of mandatory sharing of a zero mismatched kidney.** Usually six HLAs are identified in both the donor and the recipient. Occasionally, fewer than six HLAs are identified in the donor, making it impossible to have a perfect six antigen match. The benefit seen in these well-matched kidneys is derived from the absence of a mismatched HLA. Therefore, rather than giving special points for a six-HLA matched kidney, the United Network for Organ Sharing (UNOS) gives primacy to the zero mismatched recipient/donor combination, then a one mismatch, a two mismatch, and so on.

Kidneys donated from family members are much more likely to share common HLAs than those from a live, unrelated donor or from a cadaver donor. Among siblings, there is a 25% chance of a six-antigen match, a 50% chance of a three-antigen match, and a 25% chance of no match at all. Parent to child donations or vice versa always are at a minimum of a three-antigen match. Living, related recipient/donor match also occurs with minor HLAs that are not tested for. It is for this reason that recipients of a living, related allograft enjoy excellent long-term renal allograft function.

Who Can Serve as a Cadaveric Donor?

Cadaveric renal organ donation has come full circle. Initially, patient kidneys were harvested after **cardiac death**. After transplantation, these kidneys had a high incidence of **acute tubular necrosis**. The Harvard brain death criteria (**Table 40.4**) established in 1968 and modified by Mohandas and Chow helped set the guidelines for brain death determination.[1] Note that an electroencephalogram (EEG) is not required to make the diagnosis of **brain death**. The determination of brain death is a clinical diagnosis made after excluding agents such as hypothermia, drugs, and ethyl alcohol (ETOH), all of which can cause reversible brainstem depression. Once the diagnosis of brain death is determined, the Organ Placement Organization (OPO) is contacted, and the suitability of the various organs for donation is determined.

---

[1] Mohandas A, Chow SN. Brain death: a clinical and pathological study. J Neurosurg 1971;35:211; Report of the Ad Hoc Committee of the Harvard Medical School to examine the definition of brain death. JAMA 1968;205:337.

Table 40.4. Brain death criteria.

Absence of spontaneous movement
Absence of spontaneous respiration over a 4-minute test period
Absence of brain reflexes as evidenced by:
Fixed dilated pupils
Absent gag reflex
Absent corneal and ciliospinal reflexes
Absent doll's eye movements
Absent response to caloric stimulation
Absent tonic neck reflex
Unchanged status for at least 12 hours
Responsible pathologic process deemed irreparable
Hypothermia and the presence of CNS depressants such as barbiturates must be excluded

CNS, central nervous system.
Data from Report of the Ad Hoc Committee of the Harvard Medical School to Examine the Definition of Brain Death. JAMA 1968;205:337.

Currently, the majority of individuals are able to donate multiple organs. Individuals who have severe, nonrecoverable neurologica injuries can donate their organs as well, although this type of donation is somewhat controversial. This less common form of donation usually is determined by the family, and the organ procurement organization is contacted. Life support is withdrawn in an operating room setting, and cardiopulmonary death usually occurs within minutes. A physician other than a member of the transplant team pronounces the patient dead. This type of donation is termed a **controlled, non–heart-beating donor.** Well-functioning liver and kidney allograft can be harvested in this manner with little effect on immediate function. **Uncontrolled, non–heart-beating donations** occur when a patient is undergoing a cardiac arrest and resuscitation has failed. This often is a setting in which organ donation already has been discussed, and the patient arrests prior to brain death. Rapid infusion of preservation solution and heparinization are paramount for retrieving usable organs.

Issues that Arise with Live Donation

Since the immunosuppressive agents have become so effective at stopping acute rejection, HLA match has taken on a diminished role. ABO blood type incompatibility remains a significant obstacle to organ donation. As the need for HLA match has diminished, **the number of living, unrelated, emotionally attached donors has increased.** The focus of the live donor evaluation (**Table 40.5**) is determining the **overall health of the individual and his/her renal function.** This type of donation often is spousal, but it has occurred between distant relatives, friends, and community members. The lack of cadaveric donors has resulted in the transplant community exploring the possibility of some financial remuneration for both live and cadaveric donors.

The transplant community has an obligation to these "heroic" individuals who provide live donations to ensure that organ donation is as

Table 40.5. Live donor evaluation.

Identifying individuals who are willing to serve as live kidney donors
Discussion concerning the willingness of the individual to donate isolated from potential conflicting recipient issues
Complete history and physical
Psychosocial evaluation
Laboratory test
Urinalysis, complete blood count, complete metabolic profile, and coagulation studies
Blood type
Infectious screening for hepatitis A, B, and C, CMV, EBV, HSV, HIV, toxoplasmosis, and RPR
PSA in men over 50
Pregnancy test, Pap smear, and mammogram in women over 40
If donor and recipient are ABO compatible and there are no medical or psychological contraindications to donation then proceed with remainder of donor workup
24-hour urine collection for protein and creatinine clearance
Cardiac evaluation
ECG (if abnormal add echocardiogram)
Chest x-ray
MRI/MRA
Immunologic studies
HLA typing
Crossmatching with the recipient

CMV, cytomegalovirus; EBV, Epstein-Barr virus; ECG, electrocardiogram; HLA, human leukocyte antigen; HSV, herpes simplex virus; PSA, prostate-specific antigen; RPR, rapid plasma reagent.

safe as possible. It is important to inform the patient that, although the operation is safe, complications and rare deaths have occurred with donation. Currently, donation in this country is based solely on an altruistic basis, and paid donation is prohibited.

Surgical Techniques

The kidney transplant operation is well described in Chapter 65, "Kidney Transplantation and Dialysis Access," in Surgery: Basic Science and Clinical Evidence, edited by J.A. Norton, R.R. Bollinger, A.E. Chang, et al., published by Springer-Verlag, 2001. Here, several clinically important points will be mentioned. **An important point to note is the difference between placing a kidney obtained from a cadaver donor and placing a kidney obtained from a live donor.**

During the procurement of a kidney from a cadaveric donor, a cuff of vena cava and aorta can be left on the renal vein and artery, respectively. The renal vein anastomosis actually is sewn between the cuff of the vena cava and recipient's external iliac vein in an end-to-side fashion. This anastomosis can be done without the worry of tearing the thin wall of the right renal vein. Large hemostatic bites of the vena cava may be taken without concern for narrowing the anastomosis. Having a cuff of aorta allows for a single anastomosis even in the presence of multiple renal arteries. The cuff of aorta is sewn in an end-to-side fashion to the external iliac artery. Once again, with a large cuff, the surgeon need not be concerned with narrowing the renal artery anastomosis.

In kidneys obtained from live donors, the renal artery may be sewn to the external iliac artery in an end-to-side fashion or to the internal iliac artery in an end-to-end fashion. The left kidney often is the preferred kidney, especially from a live donor, as the left renal vein is considerably longer and thicker-walled than the right renal vein. Occasionally, the recipient's internal iliac vein is divided to enable the external iliac vein to be moved more anteriorly and out of the pelvis. If the kidney from a live donor has two arteries, they may both be sewn directly into the external iliac artery. The incidence of renal artery stenosis may be reduced by the uses of an aortic punch biopsy. More commonly, the smaller of the two arteries is sewn into the larger main renal artery in an end-to-side fashion under ice on the back table. The kidney is then placed within the recipient, and a single anastomosis between the main renal artery and the recipient iliac artery (external or internal) is performed. Vascular thrombosis of the artery and vein are rare events: arterial thrombosis occurs less than 1%, and venous thrombosis occurs less than 2%.

Posttransplant Period

The **differential of an increasing serum creatinine** is influenced significantly by the amount of time from the day of the transplant to the increase in serum creatinine (**Fig. 40.1**). Three different time periods can be created based on the most likely cause for an increasing serum creatinine post–kidney transplant: **the early period, the intermediate period, and the late period**.

Throughout the posttransplant period, **a thorough history and a thorough physical exam** help narrow the differential diagnosis of a rising serum creatinine. Drug levels, urine analysis with culture, complete blood count (CBC), and blood chemistry routinely are obtained in the workup for this problem. Duplex ultrasound identifies fluid collection around the kidney and reveals the status of blood flow through the artery and vein. A renal scan often is helpful in identifying changes in renal flow and urinary leaks, and a kidney biopsy is needed to make a definitive diagnosis of rejection. These tests are used routinely in sorting out the correct etiology for the recipient of a renal allograft who presents with a rising serum creatinine.

The following sections describe the most likely causes of deterioration in renal function, based on time from transplant to change in function, and focus the history and physical exam on the most pertinent facts (**Fig. 40.1**). **Algorithm 40.1** illustrates the **investigation into a rising serum creatinine level over time**.

The Early Period

In the **early postoperative period, day 0 to day 7**, the differential diagnosis can be broken down into **immunologic causes, technical causes**,

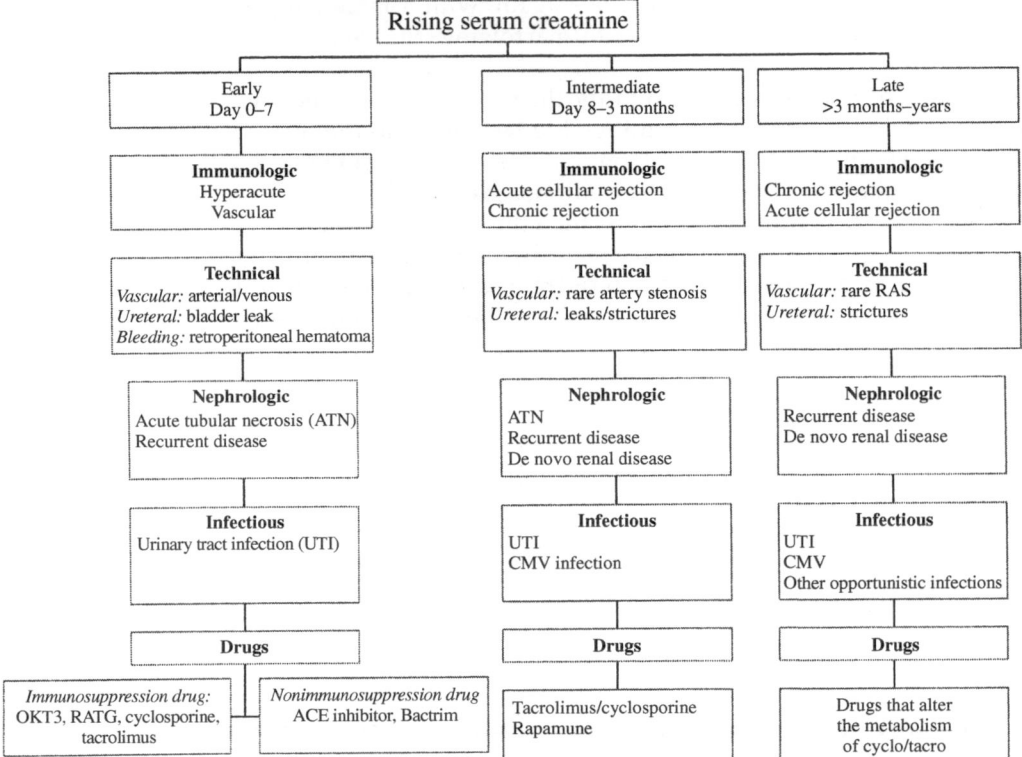

Figure 40.1. Differential for a rising serum creatinine post–renal transplant. ACE, angiotensin-converting enzyme; CMV, cytomegalovirus; RAS, renal artery stenosis; RATG, rabbit antithymocyte globulin.

nephrologic causes, infectious causes, and drug toxicity. The recipient in the case presented has passed this crucial period.

Immunologic Causes

Hyperacute rejection has become a rare event, as the ability to detect preformed antibodies prior to the transplant has improved. Hyperacute rejection derives from antibodies in the recipient's serum directed against the donor's antigens. These preformed antibodies bind to the donor tissues, activating the complement cascade, which leads to immediate graft thrombosis. The two methods for screening for donor-specific antibodies are **lymphocytic crossmatch** and **flow cytometric studies**.

A variant of hyperacute rejection is **accelerated vascular rejection.** The level of preformed antibodies is too low to be detected by the current screening test, but it quickly rises with stimulation by exposure to the new donor antigen. Clinically, the kidney often is functioning; however, urine output acutely falls off, and serum creatinine rises. Patients at risk for hyperacute rejection or early vascular rejection have been exposed previously to antigens. Patients may be exposed to human HLA through previous transplants, pregnancy, and blood transfusions. Patients, while waiting for a transplant, have their blood checked on a monthly basis for antibodies against a panel of known human antigens. Patients with a high PRA are at higher risk for immunologic complications. See **Algorithm 40.1** and **Figure 40.1**.

Technical Complications
Technical complications of the vasculature leading to vascular thrombosis of the artery or vein usually occur within the first 48 to 72 hours posttransplant. The overall incidence of vascular complications is reported to be between 0.5% and 3%. The clinical hallmark of vascular thrombosis is a rapid fall in urine output with an increase in serum creatinine and change in the color of the urine from yellow to a brick red. Thrombosis of the renal allograft often is associated with thrombocytopenia and hyperkalemia. If vascular thrombosis is suspected after a live donor, the recipient should be returned to the operating room immediately, since there is only a narrow window of time before the ischemic damage to the kidney becomes irreversible. Bleeding in the retroperitoneum space often presents with a decline in renal function and a drop in platelets. As the retroperitoneum hematoma expands, platelets are consumed, and the hematoma compresses the renal vein, resulting in a sharp drop in urine production.

Urine leaks rarely are caused by poor anastomosis. The vascular supply of a ureter in its normal anatomic position is rich in collaterals. The transplanted ureter is dependent on the blood from the renal artery traveling the length of the ureter. If the transplanted ureter has been skeletonized or is of excessive length, the distal aspect of the ureter may become necrotic, leading to a urinary leak. If the distal aspect of the ureter is ischemic, the physician needs to continue to monitor the recipient for a late developing ureteric stricture.

Nephrologic Causes
The most common cause of a rising serum creatinine in the early postoperative period is **acute tubular necrosis (ATN)**. Many factors can influence the incidence of ATN, the most important of which are the length of warm ischemic time, the length of cold ischemic time, the method of preservation, and the age of the donor; ATN also may be exacerbated by hypovolemia and dialysis.

Focal glomerulosclerosis is the only clinical entity that is seen with any frequency recurring in the immediate postoperative period. The hallmark of recurrent disease is proteinuria in the nephrotic range.

Infectious Causes
Any infection can alter the renal transplant function in the early postoperative period. The most common infections in the early postoperative period are the same that are found in the general population: **urinary tract infections, wound infections, and pulmonary infections**.

Immunosuppressive Drugs and Their Toxicities
Immunosuppression regimens often are a cocktail of multiple drugs. **Calcinurin inhibitors** are the mainstay of the majority of immunosuppressive regimens. They are known to inhibit the transcription of interleukin-2 (IL-2), a major mediation of cellular acute rejection. Calcinurin inhibitors have a profound effect on renal hemodynamics,

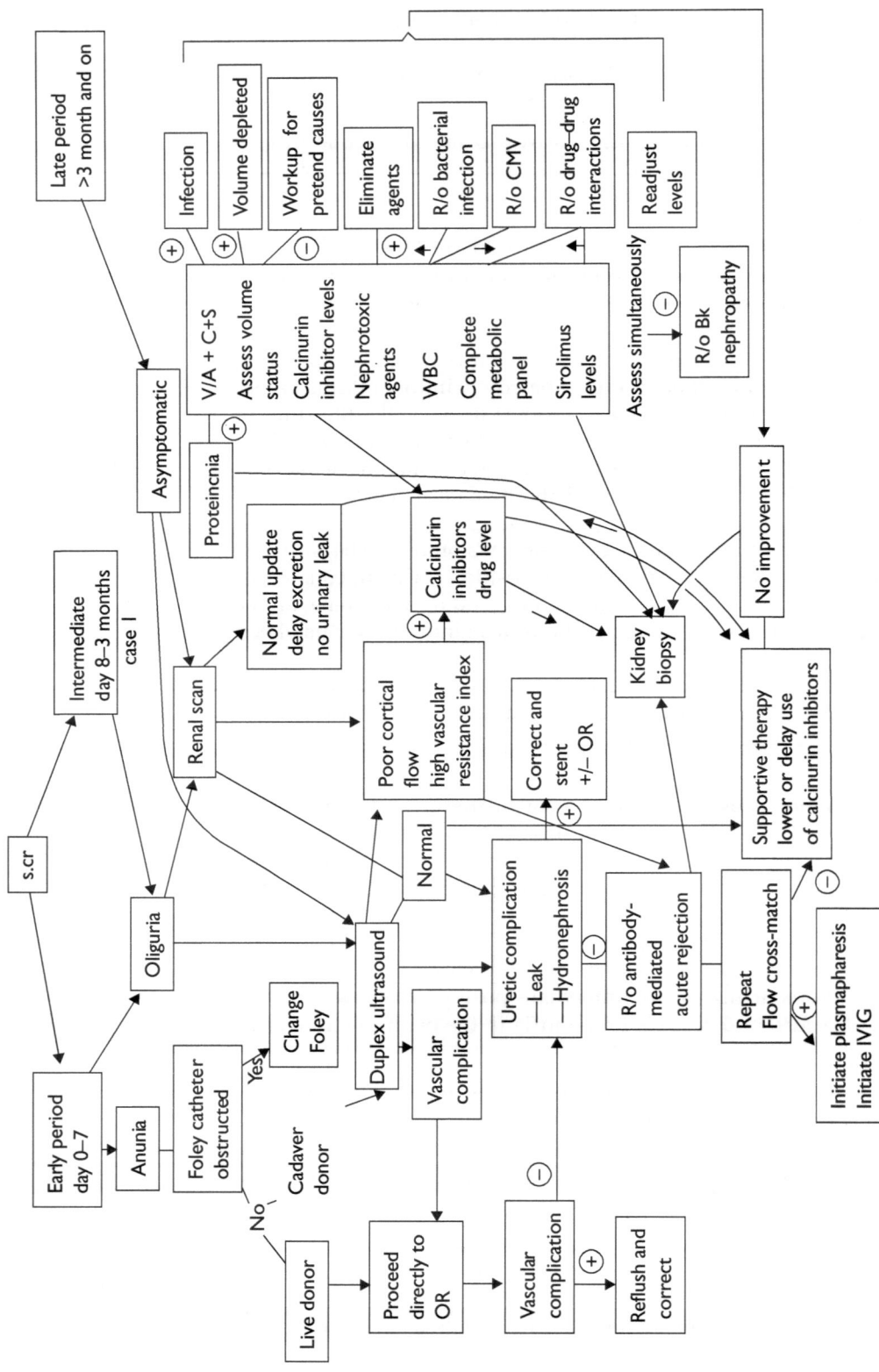

Algorithm 40.1. Investigation into a rising serum creatinine over time. BK, BK virus; C&S, culture and sensitivity; CMV, cytomegalovirus; IVIG, intravenous immunoglobulin; U/A, urinalysis.

causing afferent arterial vasoconstriction, a decrease in AFR, a decrease in renal plasma flow, and an increase in renal vascular resistance. Subsequently, the calcinurin inhibitor cyclosporine and tacrolimus are known for their nephrotoxicity. Many of the side effects of the calcinurin inhibitors parallel the nephrotoxicity. In addition, rapamycin has been shown to be nephrotoxic when combined with cyclosporine. Less appreciated is the cytokine release that occurs with OKT3 and occasionally with rabbit antithymocyte globulin (RATG) that also alters renal function. There are multiple drugs that alter the metabolism and absorption of calcinurin inhibitors; they alter the serum levels of the inhibitors, resulting in either toxicities or rejections.

Drugs that alter the renal flow, like **angiotensin-converting enzyme (ACE) inhibitors**, also may potentiate the nephrotoxic effect of the calcinurin inhibitors. Last, **drugs that usually are mildly nephrotoxic** may cause significant deterioration when given with a calcinurin inhibitor. Patients and physicians often are unaware of the significant nephrotoxicity seen when nonsteroidals are taken in combination with a calcinurin inhibitor.

The Intermediate Period

During the intermediate period, **drug toxicity in the form of calcinurin inhibitors and acute cellular rejection** are the most common causes of decrease in renal function. (See the case presented.) Acute rejection is a T-cell–mediated process that occurs most commonly between **day 8 and day 90**. The T-cell response to transplanted alloantigens is expressed either **directly on donor tissue or indirectly by professional self-antigen presenting cells** that have phagocytosed the donor alloantigens and presented them again. Once T-cell activation occurs, multiple cytokines are released, which are responsible for promoting the acute agent response. The cytokine IL-2, elaborated by T cells, plays a central role in acute rejection and has served as the focus to antirejection therapy. The details of T-cell–mediated agents are described in Chapter 62, "Immunology of Transplantation," of Surgery: Basic Science and Clinical Evidence, edited by J.A. Norton, R.R. Bollinger, A.E. Chang, et al., published by Springer-Verlag, 2001. The incidence of acute rejection has decreased steadily with changes in the immunosuppressive protocols. It is uncommon to lose a kidney immediately to acute rejection, although the presence of acute rejection, the number of acute rejections, the time to acute rejection (late rejection has a worse prognosis than early), and the severity of the rejection episode are strong predictors of late graft loss.

Calcinurin inhibitors are the most likely cause of renal dysfunction during this period. The transplanted kidney often is just recovering from ATN or is extremely susceptible to the nephrotoxic effects of these drugs. See **Algorithm 40.1** and **Figure 40.1**.

The Late Period

Last, **chronic rejection, intrinsic renal allograft disease, and drug toxicity** are predominant causes of a rise in the serum creatinine **after**

3 months. Chronic rejection is a term describing a renal allograft recipient who presents clinically with a steady rise in serum creatinine, hypertension, proteinuria, and histologically with interstitial fibrosis, subintimal thickening, and glomerular sclerosis. Chronic rejection is believed to have multiple etiologies, both immunologic and non-immunologic. Unfortunately, there are no current immunosuppression agents that stop or reverse chronic rejection. Renal dysfunction secondary to recurrent disease is most commonly caused by diabetic nephropathy, focal glomerulosclerosis, and membranoproliferative glomerulonephritis types I and II, although graft loss secondary to diabetic nephropathy is uncommon, since the deterioration of renal function is slow while the patient's risk of cardiovascular death is high. The most common cause of graft loss in all renal recipients over the age of 50 is death with a functioning allograft. See **Algorithm 40.1** and **Figure 40.1**.

Summary

It is convenient to examine the problem of deteriorating renal function over time, since the differential and focus of the workup change from the early period (days 0–7), through the intermediate period (day 8 to 3 months), and the late period (over 3 months). Throughout this time course, rejection of some kind is always a consideration; the early period is associated with antibody mediated rejection (hyperacute rejection and accelerated rejection), and the intermediate period is dominated by cellular-mediated rejection, and the late period is associated with chronic rejection. Rejection as a cause for graft loss has been minimized by the present-day armamentarium of immunosuppressive drugs. The penalty that is paid for this benefit, however, is that, as time progresses, the nephrotoxicities associated with the immunosuppressive drugs play a dominant role in allograft dysfunction. In addition, drugs that alter the metabolism of these immunosuppressive agents, as well as medications that act synergistically with them to cause nephrotoxicity, need to be monitored closely once the patient leaves the acute care setting. Finally, in the late period, the cause of renal dysfunction is further complicated by the possibility of recurrent renal disease as well as de novo renal disease. The investigation into renal allograft dysfunction often is aided by routine laboratory tests, urinalysis, complete metabolic panel, complete blood count, and immunosuppressive drug levels; ultimately, however, a renal biopsy often is required for the definitive answer.

Selected Readings

Bowen RA, Ljungman P, Carlos PV. Transplant Infections. Philadelphia: Lippincott-Raven, 1998.

Danovitch GM. Handbook of Kidney Transplantation, 3rd ed. Philadelphia: Lippincott Williams & Wilkins, 2001.

Epstein AM, Ayanian JZ, Koegh JH, et al. Racial disparities in access to renal transplantation—clinically appropriate or due to underuse or overuse? N Engl J Med 2000;343(21):1537–1544, and two pages preceding 1537.

Flye MW. Principles of Organ Transplantation. Philadelphia: WB Saunders, 2000.

Ginns LC, Cosimi AB, Morris PJ. Transplantation. Malden, MA: Blackwell Science, 1999.

Kirk AD. Immunology of transplantation. In: Norton JA, Bollinger RR, Chang AE, et al, eds. Surgery: Basic Science and Clinical Evidence. New York: Springer-Verlag, 2001.

Knechtle SJ. Kidney transplantation and dialysis access. In: Norton JA, Bollinger RR, Chang AE, et al, eds. Surgery: Basic Science and Clinical Evidence. New York: Springer-Verlag, 2001.

Levinsky NG. Quality and equity in dialysis and renal transplantation. N Engl J Med 1999;341(22):1591–1593.

Stuart FP, Abecassis MM, Kaufman DB. Organ Transplantation. Georgetown, TX: Landes BioScience, 2000.

Thistlethwaite JR, Bruce D. Rejection. In: Norton JA, Bollinger RR, Chang AE, et al, eds. Surgery: Basic Science and Clinical Evidence. New York: Springer-Verlag, 2001.

41

Transplantation of the Pancreas

James W. Lim

Objectives

1. To review diabetes mellitus (DM) in terms of prevalence, incidence, and costs to society.
2. To identify the classic complications of DM.
3. To review recipient and donor selection.
4. To discuss the three situations in which pancreas transplant is performed.
5. To describe the graft and patient survivals for pancreas transplant.
6. To describe the functions of the pancreas.
7. To describe the different surgical techniques for pancreas transplant.
8. To name the major complications of pancreas transplant.
9. To describe the impact of islet cell transplant.

Case

A 43-year-old Caucasian man with a history of type 1 diabetes mellitus (DM) since age 5 presents to the emergency room with nausea and vomiting for 72 hours. In addition, he appears to be lethargic and confused and has a fever of 39°C. The examination is significant for poor skin turgor, confusion, and right lower extremity cellulitis; he has a blood pressure (BP) of 90/50, a pulse of 125, and a respiratory rate of 35. His lab work is significant for a white blood cell count of 22,000, blood urea nitrogen (BUN)/creatinine of 55/3.4, glucose of 750, and positive serum acetone. The emergency room staff states that this is the fifth time in the past 2 years that this man has come in with similar presentations. What is the diagnosis and how should this patient be treated?

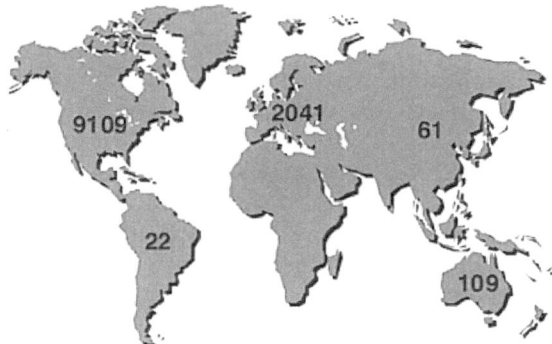

Figure 41.1. Number of pancreas transplants reported in the International Pancreas Transplant Registry (IPTR) by continent, 1987–1999. (Reprinted from Cecka JM, Terasaki PI, eds. Clinical Transplants 1999. Los Angeles: UCLA Immunogenetics Center, 2000, with permission.)

Historical Perspective

Pancreas transplant (P Tx) remains the least recognized transplant to the lay public with the exception of small-bowel transplant. Although whole-organ P Tx was first performed in 1966, it remains much of a mystery to healthcare providers at large as well as to the general public because of the paucity of news surrounding it. More kidney transplants (K Tx) have been performed in 1 year in the United States than pancreas transplants worldwide from 1987 to 1999. According to the **International Pancreas Transplant Registry (IPTR)**, 13,372 kidney transplants were performed in the United States alone in 2000, whereas the total number of pancreas transplants performed worldwide from 1966 to 1999 was 12,939.[1] Two thirds of the pancreas transplants performed are done in the United States, with one fourth in Europe (**Fig. 41.1**). With the advent of Medicare payment for pancreas transplants effective July 1, 1999, it is hoped that financial reimbursement will stimulate an increase in the total number of pancreas transplants performed. In fact, more information about islet cell transplant has emerged with the news of successful islet cell transplant in Edmonton, despite the small numbers and limited follow-up span.

Diabetes Mellitus

Overview

It is estimated that 6.3% or 18.2 million people in the United States have **diabetes mellitus (DM)**. This includes 13 million people who are diagnosed and the estimated 5.2 million people who are undiagnosed.[2]

---

[1] OPTN/SRTR 2001 Annual Report.
[2] Centers for Disease Control and Prevention. National diabetes fact sheet: general information and national estimates on diabetes in the U.S., 2002. Atlanta, GA: U.S. Department of Health and Human Services, Centers for Disease Control and Prevention, 2003.

The incidence of new cases diagnosed per year is 1.3 million people aged 20 years or older. Approximately one in every 400 to 500 children and adolescents has **type 1 DM**. Clinical reports and regional studies indicate that **type 2 DM** is becoming more common among Native American/American Indian, African American, and Hispanic/Latino children and adolescents. Diabetes was the sixth leading cause of death on U.S. death certificates in 2000. Overall, the risk for death among people with DM is about two times that of people without DM. In fact, those patients on dialysis who have DM have the highest rate of mortality on dialysis, approximating 28% per year. From a strictly economic point of view, it is estimated that direct and indirect expenditures attributable to DM in 2002 were $132 billion.[3] Per capita expenditures totaled $13,243 for people with DM and $2,560 for people without DM. Healthcare spending for patients with DM is more than double the spending for patients without DM.

Classic Complications

Diabetes mellitus is a chronic, disabling disease that affects all the major organ systems and shortens the life span by 10 years for those people in the United States who are affected by it. The **classic complications** that occur consist of **retinopathy (DM is the most common cause of blindness among adults aged 20 to 74), gastropathy/gastroparesis, nephropathy (DM is the most common cause of renal failure), neuropathy, vasculopathy (DM is the most common cause of amputations), labile control, and diabetic ketoacidosis (DKA).**[4]

Strict control clearly has been shown to delay significantly the development and slow the progression of the microvascular complications of DM. There appears to be a trend for fewer macrovascular events (strokes, myocardial infarctions, etc.) in patients who are controlled aggressively with insulin. However, this is at the cost of a 10-pound greater weight gain and a threefold higher risk of severe hypoglycemia. These results were noted with the publication of the **Diabetic Control and Complications Trial (DCCT)** in the *New England Journal of Medicine* in 1993.[5] For many patients, however, such aggressive control with its inherent problems proves to be as troublesome as the primary disease itself.

[3] Reviews/commentaries/position statements report from the American Diabetes Association. Diabetes Care 2003;26:917–932.

[4] Centers for Disease Control and Prevention. National diabetes fact sheet: general information and national estimates on diabetes in the U.S., 2002. Atlanta, GA: U.S. Department of Health and Human Services, Centers for Disease Control and Prevention, 2003.

[5] DCCT Research Group. The effect of intensive treatment of diabetes on the development and progression of long-term complications of insulin-dependent diabetes mellitus. N Engl J Med 1993;329:977–986.

Pancreas Transplant

Evaluation

With the knowledge that strict control could and did prevent some of the complications associated with DM, the need for a better alternative to insulin arose, laying the foundation for P Tx. Simply put, **any patient with DM with complications could be a considered a candidate for P Tx.** Most centers would place an **age restriction for the recipient of between 18 and 60 years of age; these recipients also would have to have no active contraindications, such as active cancer (CA), illicit drug abuse, HIV, uncorrectable cardiopulmonary disease, inability to afford the medications, and noncompliance. Relative contraindications consist of obesity [body mass index (BMI >35)], amputations (sign of severe peripheral vascular disease), severe gastroparesis (inability to tolerate oral medications postoperatively), and active smoking. Although initially patients with only type 1 DM were deemed candidates, current data from the IPTR support the use of P Tx for patients with type 2 DM as well.** The 1-year patient (95% type 1 vs. 93% type 2) and graft (84.8% type 1 vs. 85.2% type 2) survival for both types of DM were not significantly different.

As with any other transplant evaluation, **the potential patient is evaluated by a team consisting of a transplant surgeon, transplant nephrologist, transplant coordinator, social worker, and financial coordinator. Laboratory work** is done, with the most important values consisting of the serology, i.e., hepatitis (Hep) B or C, HIV, serum creatinine, and blood type. The **serology** helps to determine if patients need further clarification of their **hepatitis status** (liver biopsy if Hep B or C positive). The **serum creatinine** determines if the patient needs a K Tx with a P Tx. The **blood type** determines who the potential cadaver donor may be, since the donor must be blood type compatible. Only two programs in the country perform living donor pancreas transplants, and the numbers are small. Most donors are cadaveric. The most important workup of the possible recipient is the **cardiac imaging study**, be it a nuclear imaging study or a cardiac catheterization. The reason for this is the high rate of cardiac perioperative mortality and morbidity associated with DM.

Once the patient's testing is finished and the workup is deemed appropriate, the patient can be listed for transplant. Exactly as for a K Tx, the patient waits on a list with people of the same blood type, and those with the longest waiting time are called first. The waiting time for patients on the P Tx list tends to be shorter, since fewer people are on the P Tx list than on the K Tx list. For example, in New Jersey, approximately 200 people are on the P Tx list and 2000 are on the K Tx list.[6]

Donor Selection

The assessment of a suitable donor is more demanding objectively and subjectively. Unlike for a kidney donor in which serum creatinine

---

[6] OPS New Jersey, personal communication.

is usually the one marker used to rule a potential donor in or out, for a pancreas donor, **a number of different markers are used, such as amylase, lipase, and glucose.** However, even an elevated serum glucose does not rule out a potential donor, since studies have shown that brain-dead donors often manifest some degree of hyperglycemia, especially when high-dose steroids are given as part of any brain-swelling prevention protocol at many centers in the U.S. **Age restrictions** for donors usually range from 8 to 50 years of age, with some centers using donors up to age 60. **Weight restrictions** range from 30 to 100 kg. Donors above 90 kg often manifest increased degrees of fatty infiltration, which, when significant, rules out these donors for whole organ P Tx, but they can be used for recovery for islet cell transplant. Higher degrees of fatty infiltration have led to more successful islet cell recovery.

With respect to whole-organ recovery, the subjective findings of the amount of "fat," coupled with the texture and "feel" of the potential cadaver donor pancreas, make the procurement of the pancreas rely much more on the experience of the recovering transplant surgeon. More so than with almost any other organ, with the exception of the heart, the experience of the recovery surgeon is crucial, since the decision to accept the pancreas can be a difficult one. **The technical aspects of recovery also can be complicated.** The donor pancreas is the only organ recovered that has with it other organs attached, in this case the spleen at the tail of the pancreas and the C-loop of the duodenum that comes attached to the head of the pancreas (**Fig. 41.2**). Also removed with the donor pancreas are the donor iliac vessels. The spleen is removed either at the end of the procurement process or most commonly when the donor pancreas is prepared on the back table at the recipient hospital. The back-table work consists of cleaning up any

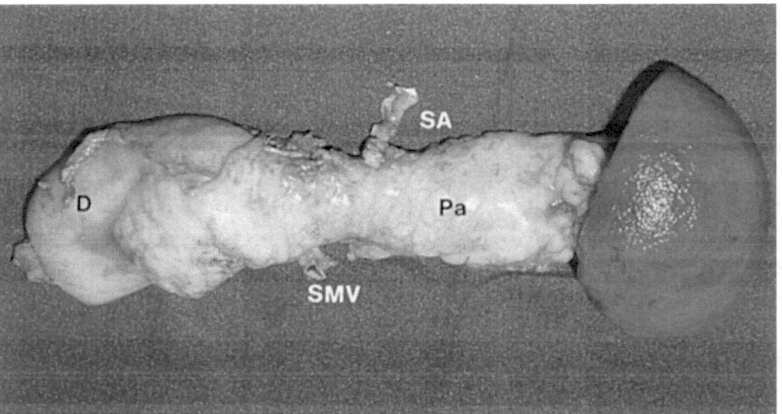

Figure 41.2. The organ is kept in ice-cold solution until transplantation. The kidneys are removed. D, duodenum; Pa, pancreas; SMV, superior mesenteric vein; SA, splenic artery. (Reprinted from Kremer B, Broelsch CE, Bruns DH. Atlas of Liver, Pancreas, and Kidney Transplantation. New York: Thieme Medical Publishers, 1994. Reprinted by permission.)

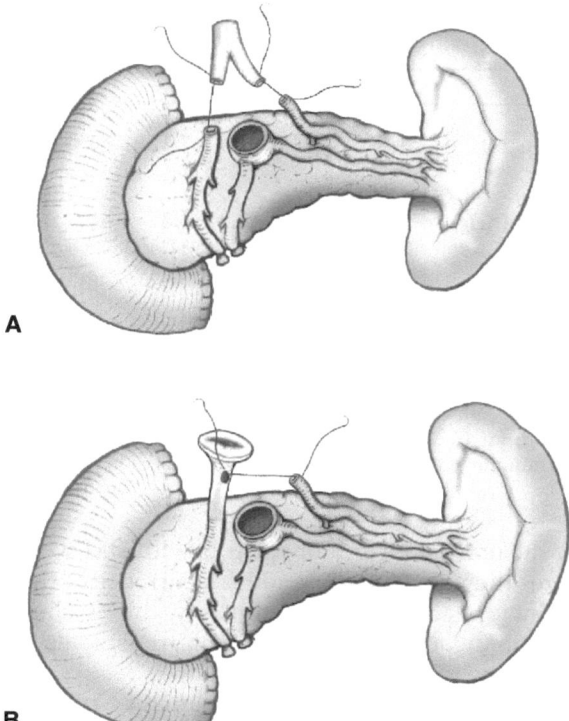

A

B

Figure 41.3. (A) Donor iliac conduit is anastomosed to the splenic artery and the superior mesenteric artery of the pancreas on the back table. (B) Alternatively, the blood supply to the donor pancreas can be reconstituted by direct anastomosis of the splenic artery to the superior mesenteric artery. (Reprinted from Harland RC. Pancreas transplantation. In: Norton JA, Bollinger RR, Chang AE, et al, eds. Surgery: Basic Science and Clinical Evidence. New York: Springer-Verlag, 2001, with permission.)

extraneous tissue and stapling off the mesenteric vessels and duodenal stumps. The donor common iliac artery with its attached external and internal iliac artery is used as a Y graft to attach to the donor pancreas superior mesenteric artery (SMA) and splenic artery (SA) so as to use the common iliac artery as a conduit for the inflow of the pancreas (**Fig. 41.3**).

Three Options for Pancreas Transplant

Renal function determines which of the three options potential P Tx candidates will undergo.

   Patients with renal failure or pending renal failure receive both a **pancreas and kidney transplant, otherwise known as simultaneous pancreas and kidney (SPK) transplant (Table 41.1).** Approximately 83% of all pancreas transplants performed in the U.S. are performed in this manner. This patient is then able to come off dialysis, much as a patient who receives a K Tx. This patient, however, would have the added benefit of no longer being a diabetic. The ramifications go

Table 41.1. Demographics: U.S. cadaver pancreas transplants, January 1996 to September 1999.

	SPK	PAK	PTA	*p* value
Frequency	3257	455	183	
Recipient age (years)	38.4 ± 7.5	39.9 ± 7.1	37.0 ± 8.6	.0001
Male recipients	58%	58%	39%	.001
Retransplants (%)	1%	28%	14%	.001
Preservation time (hr)	13.3 ± 5.8	16.3 ± 6.4	16.3 ± 6.8	.0001
Donor age (years)	27.2 ± 11.8	26.7 ± 11.3	25.8 ± 11.3	.167
No. of HLA-A,-B,-DR mismatches	4.3 ± 1.2	3.5 ± 1.4	3.4 ± 1.4	.0001
Waiting list time (days) 25–75%	92–415	48–363	48–310	.0005

HLA, human leukocyte antigen; PAK, pancreas after kidney (transplant); PTA, pancreas transplant alone; SPK, simultaneous pancreas and kidney (transplant).
Source: Reprinted from Cecka JM, Terasaki PI, eds. Clinical Transplants 1999. Los Angeles: UCLA Immunogenetics Center, 2000, with permission.

further, since the natural history of patients with DM who receive only a K Tx indicates they have nearly a 100% recurrence of their DM in the transplant kidney histologically. Fortunately, this is clinically significant only 5% of the time. As with other transplants, results have improved with time (**Table 41.2**).

A second subset of patients receives a pancreas after kidney (PAK) transplant. These patients had renal failure because of DM and already have received a K Tx. Because some of the medications that are required posttransplant can exacerbate and worsen glucose control, diabetic complications worsen to the point that these patients now become candidates for PAK. The creatinine clearance (Cr Cl) that defines these patients is >50 cc/min. Approximately 10% of all pancreas transplants are performed in this manner.

Table 41.2. Outcome of U.S. cadaveric pancreas transplants by era of transplant (level II evidence).

Type of Tx	Era	1-year patient survival (%)	1-year pancreas graft survival (%)
Simultaneous pancreas-kidney	1987–1989	90	74
	1990–1991	91	75
	1992–1993	92	79
	1994–1997	94	82
Pancreas after kidney	1987–1989	90	56
	1990–1991	96	51
	1992–1993	90	52
	1994–1997	95	71
Pancreas transplant alone	1987–1989	93	46
	1990–1991	90	51
	1992–1993	80	56
	1994–1997	93	62

Source: International Pancreas Transplant Registry (IPTR), Department of Surgery, University of Minnesota, Minneapolis, MN. With permission. Reprinted from Harland RC. Pancreas transplantation. In: Norton JA, Bollinger RR, Chang AE, et al, eds. Surgery: Basic Science and Clinical Evidence. New York: Springer-Verlag, 2001, with permission.

The third and last subset of patients to receive a P Tx has the most to benefit from this procedure and the most to lose from diabetes. This subset makes up 7% of all the pancreas transplants performed in the U.S. today. These patients have DM and some of the classic complications, most often labile sugar control or hypoglycemic unawareness. Hypoglycemic unawareness is very uncommon, but it is defined as the inability to sense when the glucose level is nearing dangerously low levels, to the point of losing consciousness. Most diabetics can sense when their glucose levels are getting low and are able to take some sort of "high sugar" tablet or juice to keep them from losing consciousness or going into seizures. Those with hypoglycemic unawareness are not able to detect this and always are fearful that they may do themselves or others harm. However, they do not have renal failure yet or, at worst, they have some early renal insufficiency. **These patients receive a pancreas transplant alone (PTA).** The Cr Cl that delineates these patients is 60 to 70 cc/min. Since nearly 35% of all patients with DM go on to suffer renal failure after 15 to 20 years, and since it has been shown that a PTA can reverse all the diabetic changes in the native kidney after 5 to 10 years, this is a very viable option.[7]

Function of the Pancreas

Before the surgical technique can be explained, the **function of the pancreas** must be understood. The pancreas has two main functions, **one endocrine and the other exocrine. The main endocrine function is insulin production.** Insulin is produced mainly in the tail of the pancreas by the beta islet cells and released into the portal vein, from which it then goes to the liver to be metabolized in what is called the **first-pass phenomenon. The exocrine function is the production and release of the protease enzymes and bicarbonate.** These are released via the pancreatic duct back into the gastrointestinal tract via the ampulla of Vater in the duodenum. The donor pancreas retains these two functions, and the surgical connections are related to these two functions. Hence, the donor portal vein is the conduit by which the insulin produced in the donor pancreas is released into the vascular system in the recipient. Likewise, the attached donor duodenum is the conduit by which the exocrine function is facilitated.

Surgical Techniques

The endocrine function can be drained into the iliac venous system of the recipient (**systemic drainage**) or into the mesenteric venous system of the recipient (**portal drainage**). The exocrine function can be drained either into the bladder (**bladder drainage**) or into the gastrointestinal tract (**enteral drainage**).

Most centers currently use systemic drainage of the endocrine function, and more and more centers are using enteral drainage of

---

[7] Fioretto P, Steffes, MW, Sutherland DE, et al. Reversal of lesions of diabetic nephropathy after pancreas transplantation. N Engl J Med 1998;339:69–75.

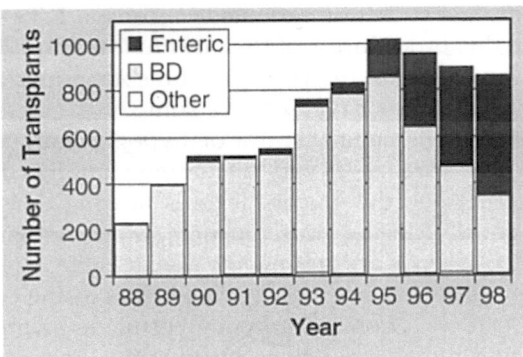

Figure 41.4. Annual number of U.S. BD, cadaver pancreas transplants for which duct management technique is known from 1988–98. (Reprinted from Cecka JM, Terasaki PI, eds. Clinical Transplants 1999. Los Angeles: UCLA Immunogenetics Center, 2000, with permission.)

the exocrine function (**Figs. 41.4 and 41.5**). The advantage of systemic drainage is more historical, in that most transplant surgeons were trained to use this method and therefore are more comfortable in its surgical technique and, even more importantly, in its results. **This is and remains the preferred technique for most centers.** The insulin production goes into the systemic system by way of the donor portal vein into the recipient iliac vein (**Fig. 41.6**). Thus, the insulin produced does not get metabolized first, since the **first-pass phenomenon** does not come into play. These patients are, in fact, hyperinsulinemic, much like a type 2 diabetic, but they do not become hypoglycemic because there is still some degree of insulin resistance present.

A few select centers are performing the portal drainage technique. The insulin production drains back into the portal system by way of the donor portal vein to the recipient's superior mesenteric vein, thereby preserving the **first-pass phenomenon (Fig. 41.7).** The advantage of

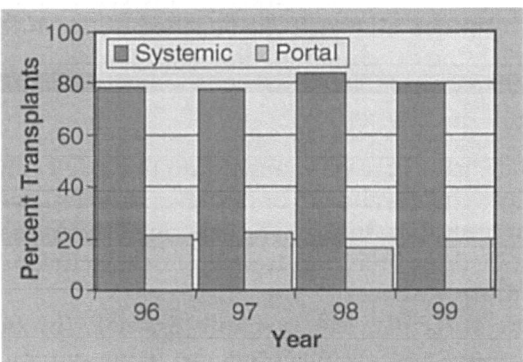

Figure 41.5. Annual percentage of U.S. cadaver ED pancreas transplants managed with systemic or portal venous drainage, 1996–98. (Reprinted from Cecka JM, Terasaki PI, eds. Clinical Transplants 1999. Los Angeles: UCLA Immunogenetics Center, 2000, with permission.)

Figure 41.6. Bladder-drained pancreas transplant. (Reprinted from Hickey DP, Bakthauatsalam R, Bannon CA, et al. Urologic complications of pancreatic transplantation. J Urol 1997;157:2042–2048. With permission from Lippincott Williams & Wilkins.)

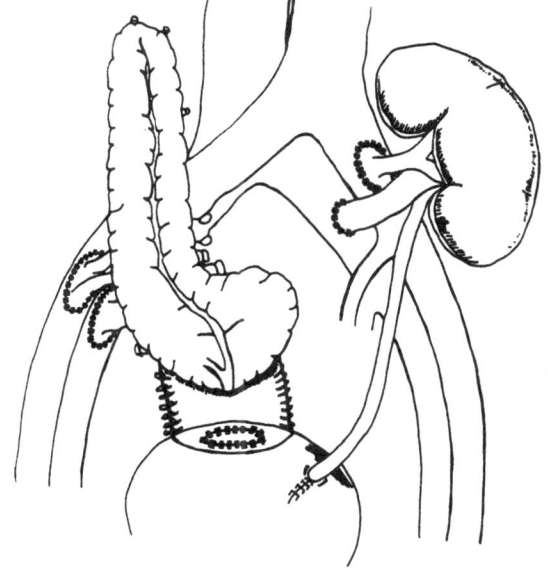

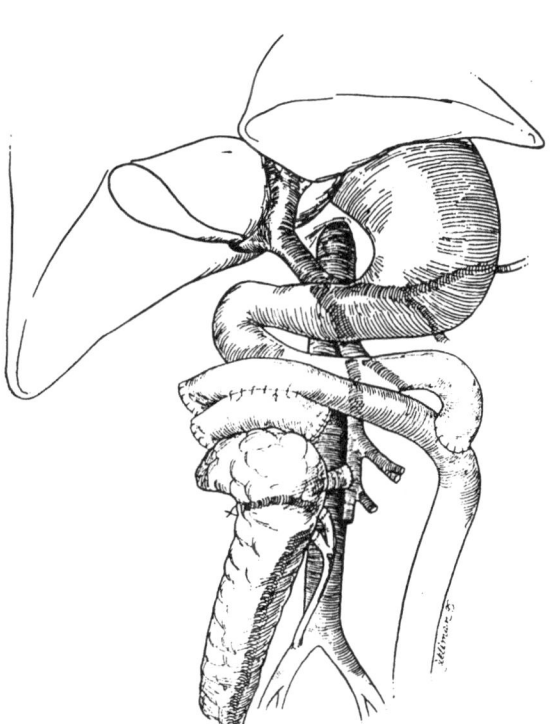

Figure 41.7. Technique for whole-organ pancreas transplantation with portal venous and enteric exocrine drainage. (Reprinted from Newall KA, Bruce DS, Cronin DC, et al. Comparison of pancreas transplantation with portal venous and enteric exocrine drainage to the standard technique utilizing bladder drainage of exocrine secretions. Transplantation: Brief Communications 1996;62(9):1353–1356. With permission from Lippincott Williams & Wilkins.)

this method is the theoretical improvement of the lipid profile of the recipient, since there is no longer any hyperinsulinemia. Other advantages consist of less rejection episodes and faster operative times.

To date, graft and patient survivals based on systemic versus portal drainage are similar. When portal drainage is used, the exocrine function drains back into the enteric system by way of the recipient loop of small bowel, be it a Roux-en-Y limb or adjacent recipient jejunum. Hence, this method preserves the physiologic nature of the pancreas by draining the endocrine function back into the portal system and the exocrine function back into the enteric system, hence, the terminology **portal/enteral drainage**. This is in distinction to **systemic/bladder drainage,** whereby the endocrine function drains into the iliac venous system and the exocrine functions drains via the bladder.

The advantages of the enteric drainage technique over the bladder drainage technique are many. First, the classic complications associated with draining active enzymes and bicarbonate with the resultant volume loss are alleviated. Therefore, the problems with hematuria, recurrent urinary tract infections (UTIs), reflux pancreatitis (reflux of the urine back into the donor pancreas), acidosis, and hypovolemia are avoided entirely by performing the enteric drainage technique. The ramifications of this cannot be understated. Approximately 12% of all patients drained via the bladder route must be corrected surgically within 2 years of the original P Tx.[8] The surgical correction consists of taking down the bladder anastomosis and reconnecting the exocrine drainage back into the enteric system (**Fig. 41.8**).

The main advantage for performing the bladder drainage technique is to measure the urinary amylase produced by the donor pancreas as a means to diagnose rejection. A decrease of 25% to 60% of the baseline urinary amylase is used by these centers to monitor for rejection. Although the ability to collect the urinary amylase is lost with the enteric drainage technique, direct biopsy of the donor pancreas is used to diagnose rejection definitively. Monitoring of the donor pancreas is performed by checking serum amylase and lipase. Any persistent increase from the baseline serum amylase and lipase is taken as being abnormal, and, if appropriate measures do not indicate infection or technical problems, then a percutaneous U.S.-guided biopsy of the donor pancreas is performed.

The other main advantage of bladder drainage over enteric drainage is that leaks at the donor duodenal anastomosis are tolerated better if urine is leaking rather than enteric contents. Most often, a placement of a Foley catheter to decompress the bladder is enough to control the urinary leak. The main advantage of performing a Roux-en-Y limb anastomosis to the donor duodenum is that, should a leak occur, the enteric contents from a defunctionalized loop of bowel usually can be better controlled than if an adjacent loop of recipient jejunum is used.

---

[8] Cecka JM, Terasaki. PI, Clinical Transplants 1999. Los Angeles: UCLA Immunogenetics Center, 2000:68.

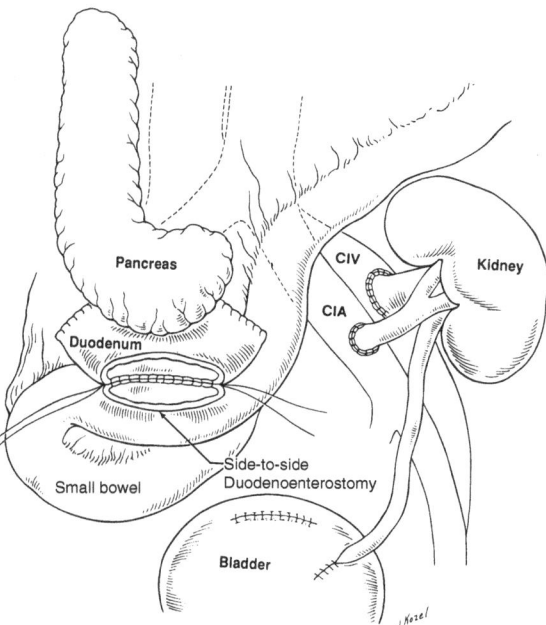

Figure 41.8. Procedure of enteric conversion after pancreas transplantation with bladder drainage. CIA, common iliac artery; CIV, common iliac vein. (Reprinted from Sollinger HW, Sasaki TM, D'Alessandro AM, et al. Indications for enteric conversion after pancreas transplantation with bladder drainage. Surgery 1992;112:842–846. Copyright © 1992 Mosby. With permission from Mosby.)

Postoperative Complications

The most urgent graft-threatening complications occurring in the perioperative period consist primarily of bleeding or thrombosis of the vascular anastomoses and leak at the duodenal anastomosis.

Bleeding enough to warrant going back to the operating room is uncommon; however, the incidence of blood transfusions either in the original operation or after the procedure approximates 5%. The incidence of **vascular thrombosis** is 12%, with 5% arterial and 7% venous.[9] Classically, thrombosis occurs immediately postoperatively and is manifested as a sharp increase in the patient's blood sugar level. Vascular thromboses can be seen as late as 1 month after the procedure. If thromboses are seen after 1 month, they usually are secondary to an immunologic issue rather than a technical one. Unfortunately, by the time this occurs, the graft already is thrombosed, with very little or no chance for salvage. The patient is taken back to the operating room, and, most often, the thrombosed graft is removed, since the incidence of graft thrombectomy to viability is exceedingly rare.

---

[9] Troppmann C, Gruessner AC, Benedetti E, et al. Vascular graft thrombosis after pancreatic transplantation: univariate and multivariate operative and nonoperative risk factor analysis. J Am Coll Surg 1996;182(4):285–316.

Duodenal anastomosis leak occurs in up to 1.4% of all cases, with the highest incidence in enteric drained PTA (**Table 41.3**). As noted above, a Roux-en-Y connection facilitates control. If undetected, the leaks may lead to deep wound infections that may cause worsening renal or pancreatic function and potential multiorgan dysfunction. Much of the cause of the leak is secondary to the attenuated donor bowel wall, which may facilitate pulling through of sutures and resultant leak. The immunocompromised state does not lend itself to faster or better healing of the duodenal anastomosis. The patient usually has a nasogastric tube to help with the perioperative ileus associated with any intraabdominal procedure.

The **usual postoperative course** consists of 7 to 10 days of hospitalization, with frequent glucose monitoring in the first 48 hours postoperation. Thereafter, the patient recovers as with any other intraabdominal procedure and proceeds to ambulate as quickly as possible. Some centers keep their patients at bed rest for at least 48 to 72 hours postoperatively so as to minimize any chance of the donor pancreas moving and potentially kinking at the vascular anastomoses. Knowledge about **immunosuppression medications** is imperative, and patients are not discharged until they have proven that they know their medications. (See Immunosuppressive Drugs and Their Toxicities in Chapter 40 for an overview of immunosuppression medications.) The same immunosuppression medications used for K Tx also are used in P Tx, i.e., **Prograf** (tacrolimus or FK506), **Neoral** (cyclosporine), **Cellcept**, and prednisone.

See **Algorithm 41.1** for postoperative monitoring.

Immunosuppression Medications

Recent immunosuppressive regimens have stressed corticosteroid sparing or elimination, with rejection-free survival rates approaching 90% at some centers. The **PIVOT Study Group** compared the conventional 5-day dose of daclizumab (DAC) versus a 2-dose DAC versus no antibody induction in SPK recipients receiving Prograf, Cellcept, and prednisone. The conclusions were that both DAC regimens significantly reduced the incidence of acuter rejection, with the 2-dose

Table 41.3. Reasons for technical failures: U.S. cadaver pancreas transplants, January 1996 to September 1999.

	SPK			PAK			PTA		
	BD	ED	p	BD	ED	p	BD	ED	p
Gft Thr	5.4%	6.6%	.215	5.4%	12.7%	.009	4.0%	15.1%	.01
Infection/pancreatitis	0.6%	1.6%	.107	1.7%	3.2%	.314	2.0%	1.4%	.76
Anastomosis leak	0.4%	1.1%	.05	0.0%	0.6%	.214	0.0%	1.4%	.238
Bleed	0.2%	0.2%	.974	0.4%	0.0%	.42	0.0%	0.0%	—

BD, bladder drained; ED, enteric drained.
Source: Reprinted from Cecka JM, Terasaki PI, eds. Clinical Transplants 1999. Los Angeles: UCLA Immunogenetics Center, 2000, with permission.

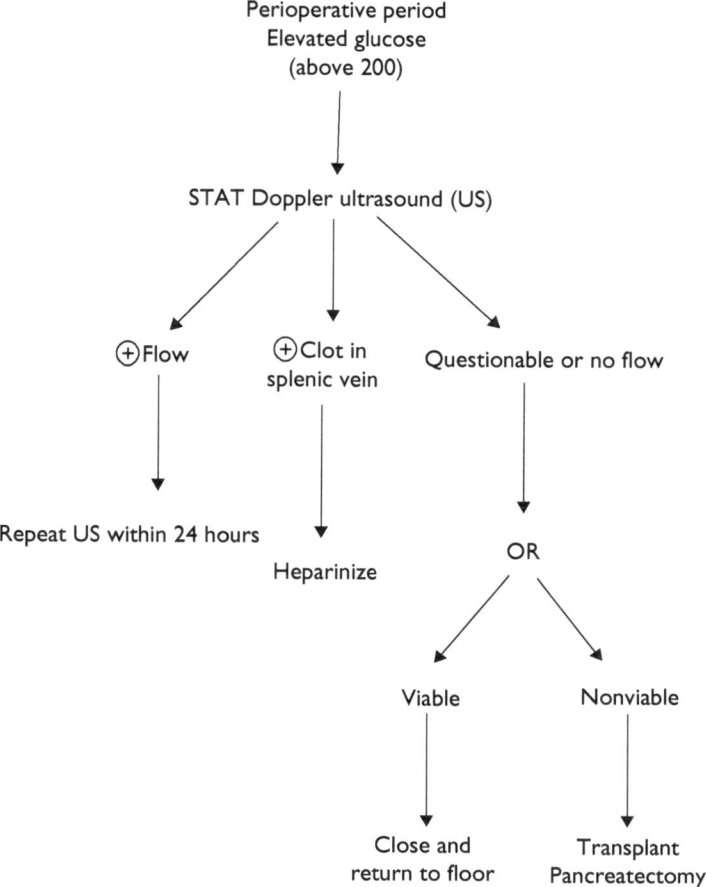

Algorithm 41.1. Algorithm for postoperative monitoring in pancreas transplant.

DAC regimen showing the highest event-free survival rate.[10] Kaufman and colleagues[11] presented their single-center, retrospective experience with a number of different protocols designed to minimize and then eventually withdraw steroids. They concluded that rapid steroid elimination can be achieved safely in SPK and PTA patients. Enough data have been reviewed to make some clear-cut recommendations on P Tx. For SPK, there appears to be very little difference with respect to graft survival using Prograf or Neoral as the first-line medication, whether

[10] Stratta RJ, Alloway RR, Hoge LA, PIVOT Investigators. One year outcomes in simultaneous kidney-pancreas transplant recipients receiving an alternative regimen of daclizumab. Program and abstracts of American Transplant Congress 2003, the fourth joint American Transplant meeting, May 30–June 4, 2003, Washington, DC. Abstract 662.
[11] Kaufman DB, Leventhal JR, Gallon LG, et al. Pancreas transplantation in the prednisone-free era. Program and abstracts of American Transplant Congress 2003, the fourth joint American Transplant meeting, May 30–June 4, 2003, Washington, DC. Abstract 665.

Table 41.4. Outcomes according to immunosuppression: U.S. pancreas transplants performed between January 1, 1994, and November 1, 1998.

Simultaneous pancreas-kidney (SPK) transplants		
	Pancreas graft function at one year	
Type of immunosuppression	%	n
Cyclosporine, azathioprine	81	1170
Cyclosporine, mycophenolate mofetil	86	850
Tacrolimus, azathioprine	80	516
Tacrolimus, mycophenolate mofetil	83	740
Pancreas after kidney (PAK) transplants		
	Pancreas graft function at one year	
Type of immunosuppression	%	n
Cyclosporine, azathioprine	58	88
Cyclosporine, mycophenolate mofetil	63	59
Tacrolimus, azathioprine	73	55
Tacrolimus, mycophenolate mofetil	79	160
Pancreas transplants alone (PTA)		
	Pancreas graft function at one year	
Type of immunosuppression	%	n
Cyclosporine, azathioprine	54	40
Cyclosporine, mycophenolate mofetil	54	14
Tacrolimus, azathioprine	63	37
Tacrolimus, mycophenolate mofetil	73	85

Source: International Pancreas Transplant Registry (IPTR), Department of Surgery, University of Minnesota, Minneapolis, MN. With permission. Reprinted from Harland RC. Pancreas Transplantation. In: Norton JA, Bollinger RR, Chang AE, et al, eds. Surgery: Basic Science and Clinical Evidence. New York: Springer-Verlag, 2001, with permission.

or not Imuran or Cellcept is used as the second-line medication (**Table 41.4**). However with respect to PAK and PTA, there does appear to be a favorable response with Prograf over Neoral. The higher incidence of potential diabetogenicity seen with Prograf does not offset its use for this subset of P Tx patients.

Islet Cell Transplant

Most recently, **a major breakthrough in pancreas islet cell transplant** was reported in the *New England Journal of Medicine*. In the past, 1-year graft survival for islet cell transplant was 8%. In this landmark report, seven of seven patients had 100% success, had no rejection, and were insulin free.[12] Although the longest follow-up was only 11 months and

[12] Shapiro J, Lakey JR, Ryan EA, et al. Islet transplantation in seven patients with type I diabetes mellitus using a glucocorticoid-free immunosuppressive regimen. N Engl J Med 2000;343:230–238.

the total number of patients reported was exceedingly small, this pre-liminary report gives hope that potentially greater and bigger things will follow. As of mid-2003, a total of 49 transplants (36 patients at nine international sites) had been performed. The immunosuppression pro-tocol included daclizumab, sirolimus, and Prograf. Median follow-up at that time was 9.4 months. The eligibility criteria are quite strict and consist of the following: presence of type 1 DM with stable require-ments, weight limit of 70 kg or less, Cr Cl greater than 80 mL/min, and no progressive diabetic complications. Of those who completed the transplant, 82.3% are insulin-free, with 52% of those who received any transplant being insulin-free. Most patients required two transplants, and some required three transplants. No deaths have been reported; however, there is a wide variation of success, with results as high as 90% at Edmonton to as low as 23% at some of the other sites.

Other centers have picked up the Edmonton protocol and, with their own variations, also have had some success. **Long-term issues that need to be addressed involve the ability to achieve success with only one transplant as opposed to the two usually required. Also, the cost of starting up an islet cell transplant program is prohibitive for many centers, and therefore certain centers may become the regional center for all the prospective patients in that area. Finally, the inability to monitor for rejection delays any therapeutic measures until it is too late.** The long-term question of potentially increasing patients' anti-body level to the extent that it makes them untransplantable should they need a K Tx in the future is another issue that can be addressed only with time.

Although solid organ P Tx still is considered to have the superior outcome for more people, the realization of successful islet cell trans-plant is closer than ever. The ability to avoid major surgery and yet undergo successful P Tx via percutaneous placement of these islet cells indeed would be a major breakthrough in the field of transplant. Although immunosuppression medications still would be required, any method that would decrease the known morbidity and mortality of an operative procedure could be considered only an advantage.

Case Discussion

The patient in the case presented exhibits the classic complications associated with someone who has DM with a severe infection. Most often, the infection is not noticed because of the lack of sensation in the lower extremities. These patients often become very ill very quickly and appear septic. Often, they are dehydrated as manifested by the elevated BUN and creatinine. In addition, as they lose their ability to control their sugars with routine subcutaneous doses of insulin, they can go into ketoacidosis, as manifested by the serum acetone. The treat-ment consists of an insulin drip and adequate intravenous hydration with empiric antibiotic coverage. The patient should be admitted and, when stable, have an imaging study to evaluate for possible osteomyelitis.

Summary

The realization of successful islet cell transplant forever has changed the face of P Tx. No longer are the prospects for islet cell transplant "just around the corner." The success of islet cell transplant after so many years of futility has spawned new interest in hepatocyte transplant for liver transplant as well as in the potential of stem cells. Not lost in this great surge of cell research are the ever improving results for solid-organ P Tx. Clearly, results have improved from era to era. Technical failure rates have improved much over the years, but they still remain the number-one reason for graft loss. Improvements in immunosuppression have helped reduce the added complication rate in the care of the immunosuppressed patient. It is hoped that, as advances continue to be made in the field of islet cell and whole-organ P Tx, more potential patients are made aware that their options are no longer restricted to insulin alone. Percutaneous insulin is not the answer for many patients, and, as more news surrounding the improved results of P Tx become known, more healthcare providers will be better able to inform their prospective patients.

Selected Readings

Cecka JM, Terasaki PI, eds. Clinical Transplants 1999. Los Angeles: UCLA Immunogenetics Center, 2000.

DCCT Research Group. The effect of intensive treatment of diabetes on the development and progression of long-term complications of insulin-dependent diabetes mellitus. N Engl J Med 1993;329:986–997.

Harland RC. Pancreas transplantation. In: Norton JA, Bollinger RR, Chang AE, et al, eds. Surgery: Basic Science and Clinical Evidence. New York: Springer-Verlag, 2001.

Nymann T, Hathaway Dr, Shokouh-Amiri MH, et al. Kidney-pancreas transplantation: the effects of portal versus systematic venous drainage of the pancreas on the lipoprotein composition. Transplantation 1995;60(12):1406–1412.

Porte D, Sherwin RS, Baron A, et al, eds. Ellenberg and Rifkin's Diabetes Mellitus: Theory and Practice, 6th ed. New York: McGraw-Hill, 2002.

Troppmann C, Gruessner AC, Benedetti E, et al. Vascular graft thrombosis after pancreatic transplantation: univariate and multivariate operative and non-operative risk factor analysis. J Am Coll Surg 1996;182(4):285–316.

Tyden G, Bolinder J, Solders G, Brattstrom C, Tibell A, Groth C-G. Improved survival in patients with insulin-dependent diabetes mellitus and end-stage diabetic nephropathy 10 years after combined pancreas and kidney transplantation. Transplantation 1999;67(5):645–648.

Transplantation of the Liver

James W. Lim

Objectives

1. To know the history behind the evolution of liver transplant.
2. To know the complications of end-stage liver disease.
3. To know the indications and contraindications for liver transplant.
4. To understand the basic technical aspects of liver transplant.
5. To know the major complications associated with liver transplant.
6. To understand the implications for a pediatric versus an adult patient.

Case

A 45-year-old Caucasian man presents with a 6-month history of increasing fatigue, itching, and abdominal distention. His past medical history is significant for blood transfusion in the 1980s and intravenous drug abuse (IVDA), but he has not used any illicit drugs for the past 20 years. His exam is significant for icteric sclera, an umbilical hernia, and abdominal ascites. His lab work is significant for an elevated total bilirubin of 4.0, prothrombin time international normalized ratio (PT INR) of 2.3, serum albumin of 2.0, and normal liver transaminases. What is the presumptive diagnosis and what is the workup for this patient?

Historical Perspective

The first liver transplant on a human model was performed in 1963. Unfortunately, this patient expired on the operating table, and it was not until 1967 that the first long-term survivor was reported. This patient was a $1\frac{1}{2}$-year-old child with hepatocellular carcinoma who survived for a little more than 1 year before succumbing to recurrent tumor. Immunosuppression medications and surgical techniques at that time still were crude by current standards, with a dismal 1-year survival rate of 15% in 1970.

As immunosuppression (mainly the discovery of cyclosporine) and surgical technique improved from the late 1970s through the early 1980s, so did the results of liver transplants. In 1983, the National Institutes of Health (NIH) established **orthotopic liver transplant (OLTX)** as definitive therapy for **end-stage liver disease (ESLD)**.[1] The pioneer in OLTX has been **Dr. Thomas E. Starzl**. It was Starzl who, after persevering through years of experimental and clinical disappointments, paved the way for and performed the world's first successful OLTX. It was his relentless quest for perfecting the OLTX process that led to **different modalities that improved the viability of the OLTX procedure**. A few of these modalities are the following[2–16]:

- The use of venovenous bypass to maintain systemic and splanchnic venous return in order to keep the patient hemodynamically stable during the anhepatic phase

[1] National Institutes of Health (NIH) consensus statement. Liver Transplant 1983; 4(7):1–15.

[2] Denmark SW, Shaw BW, Starzl TE, Griffith BP. Veno-venous bypass without systemic anticoagulation in canine and human liver transplantation. Surg Forum 1983;34:380–382.

[3] Shaw BW, Martin DS, Maequez JM, et al. Venous bypass in clinical liver transplantation. Ann Surg 1984;200:524–534.

[4] Griffith BP, Shaw BW, Hardesty RL, et al. Veno-venous bypass without systemic anticoagulation for transplantation of the human liver. Surg Gynecol Obstet 1985;160: 270–272.

[5] Starzl TE, Marchioro TL, Porter KA, et al. The use of heterologous antilymphoid agents in canine renal and liver homotransplantation and in human renal homotransplantation. Surg Gynecol Obstet 1967;124:301–318.

[6] Starzl TE, Marchioro TL, Waddell WR. The reversal of rejection in human renal homografts with subsequent development of homograft tolerance. Surg Gynecol Obstet 1963;117:385–395.

[7] Starzl TE. Experience in Renal Transplantation. Philadelphia: WB Saunders, 1964.

[8] Starzl TE. Immunosuppression in man. In: Starzl TE, ed. Experience in Hepatic Transplantation. Philadelphia: WB Saunders, 1969:242–276.

[9] Starzl TE, Todo S, Fung J, et al. FK506 for human liver, kidney, and pancreas transplantation. Lancet 1989;2:1000–1004.

[10] Jamieson NV, Sundberg R, Lindell, S, et al. Successful 24- to 30-hour preservation of the canine liver: a preliminary report. Transplant Proc 1988;20(suppl 1):945–947.

[11] Kalayoglu M, Sollinger WH, Stratta RJ, et al. Extended preservation of the liver for clinical transplantation. Lancet 1988;1:617–619.

[12] Todo S, Nery J, Yanaga K, et al. Extended preservation of human liver grafts with UW solution. JAMA 1989;261:711–714.

[13] Starzl TE, Halgrimson CG, Koep LJ, et al. Vascular homografts from cadaveric organ donors. Surg Gynecol Obstet 1979;149:737.

[14] Starzl TE, Miller C, Broznick B, Makowka L. An improved technique for multiple organ harvesting. Surg Gynecol Obstet 1987;165:343–348.

[15] Starzl TE, Demetris AJ, Van Thiel DH. Medical progress: liver transplantation, part I. N Engl J Med 1989;321:1014–1022.

[16] Starzl TE, Fung J, Tzakis A, et al. Baboon to human liver transplantation. Lancet 1993;341:65–71.

- The use of antilymphocyte globulin (ALG), azathioprine, steroids, and, most recently, FK506 (Prograf/tacrolimus) to improve outcomes
- Improvements in preservation so as to keep the donor liver viable for a longer time
- The use of systemic arterial and venous grafts for vascular reconstruction so that those patients with abnormal or occlusive diseased anatomy also can undergo OLTX safely
- Standardizing the procurement of multiple donor organs from a single cadaver donor so as to benefit as many recipients as possible
- Discovering chimerism to explain liver tolerogenicity

Starzl has been instrumental in achieving clinical success not just in OLTX but also in kidney and intestinal transplants. It has been estimated that approximately 90% of all the transplant surgeons in the United States have been trained either directly by him or indirectly by one of his fellows.

End-Stage Complications of Liver Disease

Once patients reach ESLD, they manifest **classic signs and symptoms**. Clinically, these can be divided broadly into **those associated with liver failure and those associated with portal hypertension (Table 42.1)**. These patients may have an **acute process, a chronic process, a malignant process, or an inherited metabolic process that impairs the life-sustaining daily function of the native liver (Table 42.2)**. The end result is always death if liver failure ensues and is irreversible.

Table 42.1. Liver failure and portal hypertension in cirrhosis.

Liver failure	Portal hypertension
History	History
Fatigue	Upper GI variceal bleeding
Encephalopathy	
Sleep–wake cycle reversal	
Physical exam	Physical exam
Jaundice	Ascites
Ecchymosis	Umbilical caput medusa
Tremor, liver flap	Large hemorrhoids
Gynecomastia, spider angioma	Splenomegaly
Testicular atrophy	Petechiae
Shrunken liver	
Laboratory exam	Laboratory exam
Coagulopathy	Thrombocytopenia
Hypoalbuminemia	Mild neutropenia
Elevated bilirubin	
Radiologic exam	Radiologic exam
Computed tomography: shrunken lobulated liver (a cirrhotic liver may appear normal)	Ultrasound: hepatofugal portal flow
	Portal vein thrombosis
	Splenic vein diameter >13 mm

Source: Reprinted from Ginns LC, Cosimi AB, Morris PJ. Transplantation. Malden, MA: Blackwell Science, Inc., 1999, with permission.

Table 42.2. Indications for liver transplantation.

Chronic advanced cirrhosis
  Primarily parenchymal disease
    Postnecrotic cirrhosis (viral, drug-related)
    Alcoholic cirrhosis
    Cystic fibrosis
    Autoimmune disease
  Primarily cholestatic disease
    Biliary atresia
    Primary biliary cirrhosis
    Sclerosing cholangitis
    Cryptogenic cirrhosis
  Primarily vascular disease
    Budd-Chiari syndrome
    Veno-occlusive disease
Acute fulminant hepatic failure
  Viral hepatitis
  Drug-induced (e.g., halothane, sulfonamides)
  Metabolic liver disease (e.g., Wilson's disease, Reye's syndrome)
Inborn errors of metabolism
  Glycogen storage disease
  α_1-Antitrypsin deficiency
  Wilson's disease
Primary hepatic malignancies
  Hepatoma ± cirrhosis
  Cholangiocarcinoma
  Unusual sarcomas arising within hepatic parenchyma
Retransplantation

Source: Reprinted from Ginns LC, Cosimi AB, Morris PJ. Transplantation. Malden, MA: Blackwell Science, Inc., 1999, with permission.

The complications consist of **fatigue** (the most common symptom), **refractory ascites** (associated with only a 6-month mean survival), **variceal bleeding**, **hepatorenal syndrome** (renal failure/insufficiency), **hepatic encephalopathy**, **spontaneous bacterial peritonitis (SBP)**, and **malnutrition**. Most of these complications are associated primarily with **chronic or progressive end-stage cirrhosis**, which makes up 80% of the indications at most liver transplant centers. Cirrhosis is applied to the gross pathologic appearance usually associated with ESLD. Cirrhosis in and of itself is not an absolute indication for transplant.

In the patient in the case presented above, with the complications as noted and with biochemical markers indicating chronic liver injury, cirrhosis strongly indicates the need for OLTX. Until the mid-1990s, the most common indication for OLTX was alcoholic liver disease, also called Laënnec's cirrhosis. With the advent of commercially available testing for **hepatitis C virus (HCV)** via polymerase chain reaction (PCR) in 1993, HCV has now become the most common indication for OLTX.[17] At many centers in the United States, one third of OLTXs performed are secondary to HCV. Despite major advances in the medical

---

[17] Belle SH, Beringer KC, Detre KM. Recent findings concerning liver transplantation in the United States. In: Cecka JM, Terasaki PI, eds. Clinical Transplants 1996. Los Angeles: UCLA Tissue Typing Laboratory, 1996:15–29.

treatment for HCV, including pegylated interferon and ribavirin, 20% of all patients with HCV proceed to cirrhosis. The time span to reach cirrhosis is 20 years. As cirrhosis (histopathologic diagnosis describing end-stage scarring of the liver) occurs, multiple signs and symptoms arise simultaneously, with fatigue being the most common complaint. The patient presented at the start of this chapter has some well-known risk factors for HCV; IVDA, blood transfusion, tattoos, healthcare employment, and sexual/household contact are the main risk factors. He also has classic symptoms for HCV, and his lab results are compatible with chronic HCV. A liver transplant evaluation should be part of his workup.

Transplant Evaluation

Once the patient is thought to have ESLD, ideally he/she should be **referred to a liver transplant center**. The liver transplant team is composed of **a hepatologist, a transplant surgeon, a transplant coordinator, a social worker, and a financial coordinator**. The workup focuses on identifying the cause of the ESLD and treating the symptoms and signs that have made the patient's health deteriorate. In addition to the important **history and physical, certain laboratory tests and radiologic studies** are necessary to verify the disease process (**Table 42.3**). Once the workup is finished, the transplant team meets to review the results in order to **decide if the patient is indeed a candidate and is suitable for listing**, which would then place the patient on the transplant list. In general, conditions that must be met for listing to occur are the following: **irreversible liver disease, stable cardiopulmonary status, no active illicit drug/alcohol abuse history, no active infection/cancer (CA)** (exceptions for small-sized hepatocellular carcinomas), **well-informed patient and/or family, ability to afford the medications** (via insurance), and **being a reasonable-risk candidate.**[18] Many of the acceptance criteria are similar to those for any other organ transplant candidate.

One aspect of OLTX that is very different from that of other organ transplants is that of **tissue typing**. For kidney transplant (K Tx), for example, data support the improved success rate with better matched donor kidneys. For kidney transplants performed between 1995 and 2001, matching at the human leukocyte antigen (HLA) -A, -B, -DR loci resulted in a 16% higher projected 10-year graft survival when compared with grafts mismatched for five or six HLAs (p < .001).[19] **The role of tissue typing in OLTX is minimal, and, as such, no data exist that support improved results based on matching criteria alone.** As an immunologically favored organ, no crossmatch is necessary for

---

[18] Zumeida GD, Yeo CJ. In: Turcotte JG, ed. Shackelford's Surgery of the Alimentary Tract. Philadelphia: WB Saunders, 2002:518.
[19] Ramos E, Drachenberg CB, Portocarrero M et al. BK virus nephropathy diagnosis and treatment: Experience at the University of Maryland Renal Transplant Program. In: Cecka JM, Terasaki PI, eds. Clinical Transplants 2002. Los Angeles: UCLA Immunogenetics Center, 2003:143–153.

patients who undergo OLTX, unlike for patients who undergo K Tx or pancreas transplant (P Tx), where a final crossmatch is warranted in almost all cases. However, just as in a K Tx and a P Tx, **blood typing is mandatory**, since the donor and recipient must be blood-type compatible.

Listing of Patients

The **biochemical and clinical derangements that are associated with ESLD** can be graded via the **Child-Turcotte-Pugh (CTP)** classification of hepatocellular function in cirrhosis (**Table 42.4**). Each designated group is assigned one, two, or three points depending on the severity. With five groups, the minimum and maximum number that can be achieved are five and 15 points, respectively. In this manner, patients are listed for OLTX only if they have at least seven points. Once the patient has been evaluated to have the indication for OLTX and after

Table 42.3. Routine liver transplantation studies.

Diagnostic studies
  Chest radiograph
  Colonoscopy in patients with sclerosing cholangitis, history of gastrointestinal bleeding, or other specific indications
  Duplex ultrasonography of hepatic vessels
  Electrocardiogram for those over age 40 years
  Endoscopic retrograde cholangiopancreatography in patients with sclerosing cholangitis
  Mesenteric angiography if duplex ultrasound is not definitive
  Pulmonary function testing when indicated
  Ultrasound, computed tomography, or magnetic resonance imaging of liver for cirrhotics and those at risk for cancer
  Upper gastrointestinal endoscopy
Blood studies
  ABO typing and red blood cell antibody screen
  α-Fetoprotein and carcinoembryonic antigen levels for patients with cirrhosis
  α_1-Antitrypsin and ceruloplasmin levels in patients with cirrhosis
  Arterial blood gases
  Calcium and phosphorus levels
  Cholesterol level
  Complete coagulation panel
  Creatinine and blood urea nitrogen levels; creatinine clearance determination if creatinine level elevated
  Glucose determination
  Hematology survey, including platelet count hepatitis B and C, immunodeficiency virus, cytomegalovirus, herpes virus, varicella zoster, Epstein-Barr virus, and toxoplasmosis serology
  Histocompatibility testing
  Liver function tests
  Magnesium level
  Serum electrolyte levels
  Total serum protein and albumin levels
  Uric acid determination

Source: Adapted from Zuidema GD, Yeo CJ. Shackelford's Surgery of the Alimentary Tract. Vol III: Pancreas, Biliary Tract, Liver and Portal Hypertension, Spleen. Turcotte JG, ed. Philadelphia: WB Saunders, 2002. Copyright © 2002 Elsevier Inc. With permission from Elsevier.

Table 42.4. Child-Turcotte-Pugh (CTP) score to assess hepatocellular function.

Points	1	2	3
Albumin (g/dL)	>3.5	2.8–3.5	<2.8
Bilirubin (mg/dL)	<2.0	2.0–3.0	>3.0
Prothrombin (seconds above normal)	<4	4–6	>6
(International normalized ratio)	<1.7	1.7–2.3	>2.3
Ascites	None	Mild	Moderate
Encephalopathy (grade)	0	I–II	III–IV
Score:	5–6 points	Child's A	
	7–9 points	Child's B	
	9–15 points	Child's C	

Source: Data from Sauerbruch T, Weinzierl M, Kopcke W, Baumgartner G. Prognostic value of Pugh's modification of Child-Turcotte classification in patients with cirrhosis of the liver. Panminerva Med 1992;34(2):65–68; and from Zimmerman H, Reichen J. Assessment of liver function in the surgical patient. In: Blumgart LH, ed. Surgery of the liver and biliary tract, vol 2. Edinburgh: Churchill Livingstone, 1994.

the rest of the formal evaluation (psychosocial, financial, medical clearance) has cleared the patient to receive an OLTX, then the patient is given a status to determine how urgently the liver is needed.

Status 1 indicates an acute process and warrants an emergent OLTX, since death is expected within a 7-day period. Status 2A indicates the patient is in an intensive care unit (ICU) setting and warrants urgent OLTX, since death is expected within 2 to 4 weeks. Status 2B indicates the patient is sick enough to warrant OLTX but does not require urgent transplantation and is not in an ICU setting. Status 3 indicates only that the patient has at least seven points but is able to function adequately. Most patients in the United States are either a status 1 or 2A at the time of transplant. Unfortunately, there are disparities in waiting time for a lifesaving organ in different areas of the country. Because of this disparity, a new system was implemented on February 27, 2002.[20] With the **model for end-stage liver disease (MELD)** and **pediatric end-stage liver disease (PELD)**, patients now are graded according to a formula that more objectively assesses their priority for obtaining an OLTX.

The MELD and PELD scores assess the patient's risk of dying while waiting for OLTX (**Fig. 42.1**). **These scores have replaced the previous method of listing patients based primarily on their CTP score.** The MELD score is used for adult patients (18 years of age and older) and is based on bilirubin, INR, and creatinine. The PELD score is used for patients less than 18 years of age and is based on bilirubin, INR, albumin, growth failure, and age when listed for transplant, factors that better predict mortality in children. The MELD score replaces the previous status 2A, 2B, and 3 categories; however, status 1 category remains in effect. The PELD score replaces the previous status 2B and 3 for pediatric patients (status 2A did not exist in the previous pediatric listing categories), but, again, status 1 remains in place. Waiting times are used under this current policy only to determine who comes

---

[20] Allocation of livers, amended. UNOS policy 3.6. February 2002.

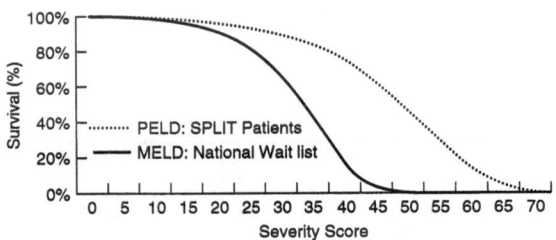

Figure 42.1. Model for end-stage liver disease (MELD) and pediatric end-stage liver disease (PELD) mortality risks at 3 months for 1230 adult and 649 pediatric patients added to the waiting list between March 1, 2001 and August 15, 2001. (Reprinted from Freeman RB Jr, Wiesner RH, Harper A, et al. The new liver allocation system: moving toward evidence-based transplantation policy. Liver Transplant 2002;8(9): 851–858. With permission from John Wiley & Sons, Inc.)

first when there are two or more patients who have the same MELD/ PELD score and blood type.

Even with the vast majority of recipients being in critical condition just prior to transplant, the 1-year graft survival is 80.2%, with the patient survival above 86.4%.[21]

Contraindications

The contraindications to OLTX can be classified as being **absolute and relative**. As is the case with most other organ transplants, **experience has led to a decreasing number of contraindications**. These are noted on **Table 42.5**. Unlike with most other organ transplants, the **psychosocial issues** more often rule out a patient for transplant. This is due to the fact that the more common reason that patients require OLTX is prior illicit behavior, such as IVDA and ethyl alcohol (ETOH) abuse. Prior to the mid-1990s, ETOH was the most common reason people required OLTX. In a landmark paper from the University of Pittsburgh, Starzl reported a recidivism rate of approximately 10% posttransplant, thus putting to rest many critics who felt that an OLTX for patients with a history of ETOH abuse was not warranted.[22] Most if not all centers implement a certain time frame for which the patient must be alcohol-free prior to being considered for transplant. Once listed, the recipient waits for a cadaver donor to be identified.

Donor Evaluation and Organ Procurement

The **evaluation of the cadaver donor** is one of the crucial steps in the success of the OLTX. Broad guidelines for acceptance criteria as a cadaver donor exist, and, as is the case for many aspects of transplant,

---

[21] 2002 OPTN/SRTR annual report, Table 9.9.

[22] Van Thiel, DH, Gavaler JS, Tarter RE, et al. Liver transplantation for alcoholic liver disease: a consideration of reasons for and against. Alcoholism Clin Exp Res 1989;13(2): 181–184.

these may differ greatly from center to center (**Table 42.6**). In general, the cadaver donors must be deemed **brain dead**, most often from a cerebrovascular accident (CVA). The definition of being brain dead also may differ from hospital to hospital, but most hospitals rely on neurologic exams by two separate physicians or tests to confirm diminished blood flow to the brain. Once the donor is determined to be brain dead, **laboratory tests** are performed to determine the patient's blood type and physiologically describe the patient's body chemistry and serology. No blood work exists to reliably predict liver function in the donor and then in the recipient. **A history of homosexuality or promiscuity, a history of heavy alcohol use, or a history of illicit drug abuse rules out many potential cadaver donors.** Once consent is obtained from the donor's family, the cadaver donor is taken to the operating room (OR) for a procurement, whereby transplant surgeons remove the organs to be transplanted.

In the operating room, the cadaver donor is placed under general anesthesia, and the entire abdomen and chest are prepped. An incision is made from the sternal notch to the pubic symphysis. The chest and abdomen are entered, and retractors are placed. Even if the heart and lungs are not procured, the chest is opened so as to optimize exposure of the intraabdominal organs, especially the liver. **The main points of the procurement process of the liver** include the following:

- Visualization of the liver, looking for sharp edges and no gross pathology

Table 42.5. Contraindications to liver transplantation.

Absolute
Advanced, uncorrectable cardiac or pulmonary disease
Severe, irreversible pulmonary hypertension
Hypotension requiring vasopressor support
Recent intracranial hemorrhage
Irreversible neurologic impairment
HIV infection
Uncontrolled sepsis
Extrahepatic malignancy[a]
Inability to comply with posttransplant regimen
Active substance abuse
Relative
Stage III or IV HCC
HBV-DNA+ and HBeAg+ hepatitis B
Cholangiocarcinoma
Age over 70 years

[a] With the exception of skin cancer and some neuroendocrine tumors. HBeAG, hepatitis B early antigen; HBV, hepatitis B virus; HCC, hepatocellular carcinoma.

Source: Reprinted from Hanto DW, Whiting JF, Valente JF. Transplantation of the liver and intestine. In: Norton JA, Bollinger RR, Chang AE, et al, eds. Surgery: Basic Science and Clinical Evidence. New York: Springer-Verlag, 2001, with permission.

- Identification of any anatomic abnormalities of the liver (replaced right or left hepatic arteries exist in up to 18% of all patients)
- Control of sites for cannulation and decompression of the blood supply of the intraabdominal organs [aorta and superior/inferior vena cava (SVC/IVC)]
- Flushing of the gallbladder
- Heparinizing the donor with approximately 20,000 to 30,000 units
- Cannulating the aorta
- Infusion of University of Wisconsin solution (preservation fluid)
- Simultaneous decompression of the organs by way of incising the SVC/IVC
- Placement of ice throughout the chest and body cavity so as to better preserve the organs

If the heart is accepted, then this is the first organ to be removed, followed by the lungs. They both have the shortest cold-ischemic times, with the heart having a desired cold-ischemic time of 4 hours. Next, the liver and pancreas usually are resected en bloc and then separated on the back table. The kidneys usually are the last organs to be removed. The liver has a desired cold-ischemic time of 12 hours.

When the donor liver has been brought back to the recipient hospital, further work is performed to clean off any extraneous tissue, muscle, or lymphatics not required for the recipient operation. This is the "back-table" work, and it may take as long as an extra hour to clean up the donor liver (**Fig. 42.2**). Usually the recipient is brought into the operating room and prepared for OLTX simultaneously with the back-table work.

Table 42.6. Guidelines of acceptability as a cadaveric liver transplant donor.[a]

Age: Neonatal to 70 years of age and older
No prolonged hypoxia or hypotension
No abdominal or serious systemic infection
No cancer except skin or primary brain cancer
Reasonable cardiac, renal, and pulmonary function while on respirator support
Negative history for chronic liver disease and intravenous substance abuse
Negative serology for human immunodeficiency virus (HIV) and syphilis
No risk factors for HIV, such as intravenous drug use or prostitution
Laboratory studies:[b]
  Total bilirubin level of less than 4.0 mg/dL
  Aspartate and alanine transaminase levels less than four times normal
  Alkaline phosphatase level less than twice normal
  Prothrombin time and partial thromboplastin time no more than twice normal
Steatosis involving less than 30% to 50% of hepatocytes

[a] Most of these guidelines are relative, and many exceptions occur. The trend is to use higher risk donors because of the severe shortage of donor livers.
[b] These guidelines are relative and vary greatly among programs.
Source: Reprinted from Zuidema GD, Yeo CJ. Shackelford's Surgery of the Alimentary Tract. Vol III: Pancreas, Biliary Tract, Liver and Portal Hypertension, Spleen. Turcotte JG, ed. Philadelphia: WB Saunders, 2002. Copyright © 2002 Elsevier Inc. With permission from Elsevier.

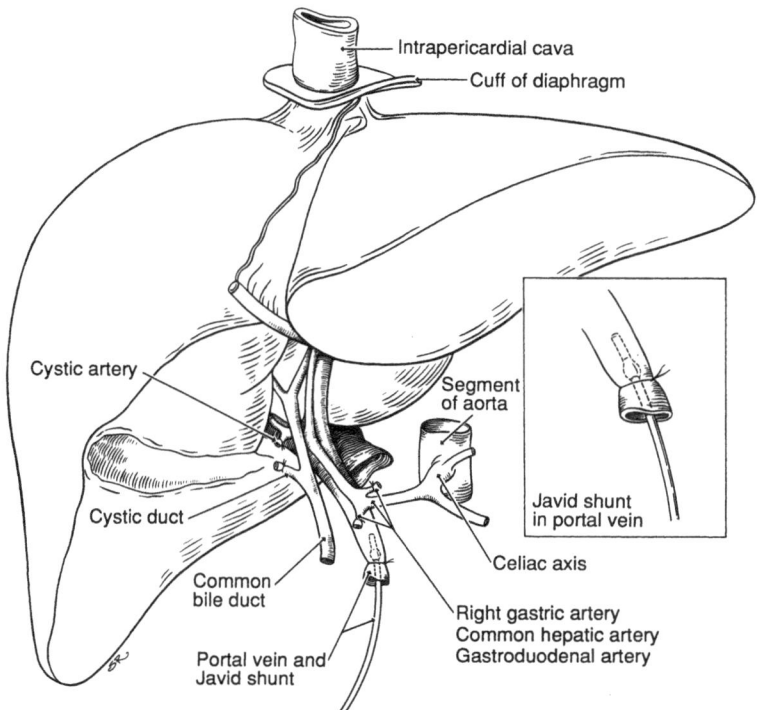

Figure 42.2. The donor liver. A thorough understanding of the details and variations of hepatic vasculature anatomy is essential for performing the donor hepatectomy expeditiously. After the donor liver has been removed, a Javid or other suitable catheter is tied into the portal vein. This is used for flushing with University of Wisconsin preservation solution on the back table and later during implantation for infusing cold lactated Ringer's solution containing albumin. (Reprinted from Zuidema GD, Yeo CJ. In: Turcotte JG, ed. Shackelford's Surgery of the Alimentary Tract, vol 3: Pancreas, Biliary Tract, Liver and Portal Hypertension, Spleen. Philadelphia: WB Saunders, 2002. Copyright © 2002 Elsevier Inc. With permission from Elsevier.)

Surgical Technical Issues

The basic technique of OLTX consists of **removing the recipient's diseased liver and replacing it with a healthy liver**. The donor liver is placed in the same position as the previously removed recipient liver, and in this manner the liver transplant is termed, appropriately, **orthotopic liver transplantation**. Removing the diseased recipient liver is fraught with technical difficulty, since large, fragile, thin-walled veins (varices) develop around the liver substance and vascular attachments. Much blood loss can be noted during this time of the operation. To alleviate this, the concept of **venovenous bypass** was introduced. In this manner, direct cannulation into the systemic venous system by way of the axillary/subclavian and femoral vein and into the portal system by cannulation of the portal vein is gained (**Fig. 42.3**). These two systems then are connected through the bypass machine. Venovenous bypass reduces the high portal pressures seen in the varices and thereby

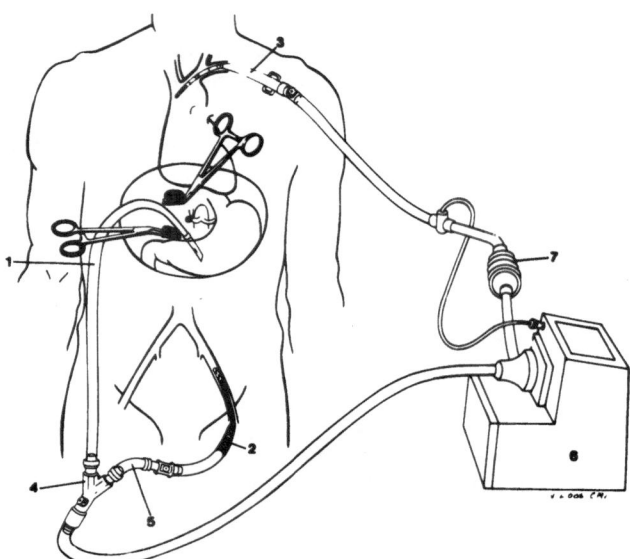

Figure 42.3. A diagrammatic representation of the venovenous bypass setup. A heparin-bonded Gott shunt is placed in the portal vein (1) and connected to a percutaneously placed femoral cannula (2) that is connected to a Bio-Medicus roller pump (6) with a flow meter (7) and heat exchanger. A return cannula is placed percutaneously into the left subclavian vein (3). (Reprinted from Johnson SR, Marterre WF, Alonso MH, Hanto DW. A percutaneous technique for venovenous bypass in orthotopic cadaver liver transplantation and comparison with the open technique. Liver Transplant Surg 1996;2:354–361. With permission from John Wiley & Sons, Inc.)

reduces the bleeding noted in the operative field. Also, because the vena cava is occluded entirely with removal of the recipient liver, the returned inferior vena caval and portal venous blood to the heart is returned via the axillary/subclavian vein cannulation. This allows placement of the donor liver and the vascular anastomoses to be performed without having to rush for fear of inhibiting inflow to the right side of the heart because of caval interruption. Once the vascular anastomoses are finished (supracaval, infracaval, portal, arterial), the biliary system is drained by way of a biliary-to-biliary or biliary-to-enteric anastomosis **(Fig. 42.4)**.

Postoperative Complications

Complications usually result from **a technical, immunologic, or infectious etiology**.

The most common complication in the perioperative period is from a **technical** source. One of the most devastating is **hepatic arterial thrombosis (HAT)**, which occurs in up to 5% of adults and in up to 20% of children. Often, there is no effective therapy, and the patient is relisted as a status 1 for emergent retransplantation. Other technical complications include **hemorrhage, thrombosis of the vena cava or portal anastomoses, and bile duct leak or narrowing**. Postoperative hemorrhage that requires reoperation for control is almost always

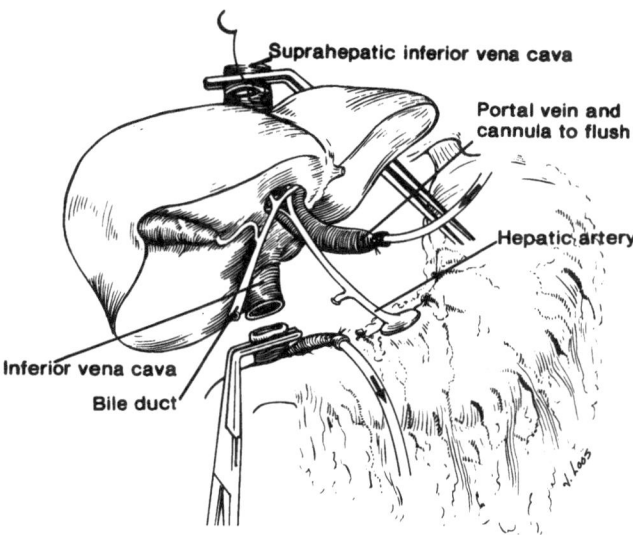

Suprahepatic inferior vena cava

Portal vein and
cannula to flush

Hepatic artery

Inferior vena cava

Bile duct

Figure 42.4. Implantation of the donor liver. The suprahepatic vena caval anastomosis is performed first, followed by the infrahepatic vena cava, portal vein, hepatic artery, and common bile duct. (Reprinted from Hanto DW, Whiting JF, Valente JF. Transplantation of the liver and intestine. In: Norton JA, Bollinger RR, Chang AE, et al, eds. Surgery: Basic Science and Clinical Evidence. New York: Springer-Verlag, 2001, with permission.)

within the first 48 hours after the initial operation. Thrombosis of the supra- or infracaval anastomosis occurs rarely, in only 1% of patients. Portal vein thrombosis has been reported to occur in as high as 10% of OLTX recipients.[23,24] Biliary tract complications occur in 15% to 20% of OLTX patients, with the vast number of them occurring within the first month after surgery.[25-32] The biliary complications include anastomotic

[23] Burke GW III, Ascher NL, Hunter D, Najarian JS. Orthotopic liver transplantation: nonoperative management of early, acute portal vein thrombosis. Surgery 1988;104:924–928.

[24] Davidson BR, Gibson M, Dick R, Burroughs A, Rolles K. Incidence, risk factors, management and outcome of portal vein abnormalities at orthotopic liver transplantation. Transplantation 1994;57:1174–1177.

[25] Colonna JO II, Shaked A, Gomes AS, et al. Biliary strictures complicating liver transplantation: incidence, pathogenesis, management, and outcome. Ann Surg 1992;216:344–352.

[26] Lebeau G, Yanaga K, Marsh JW, et al. Analysis of surgical complications after 397 hepatic transplantations. Surgery 1990;170:317–322.

[27] Stratta RJ, Wood RP, Langnas AN, et al. Diagnosis and treatment of biliary tract complications after orthotopic liver transplantation. Surgery 1989;106:675–684.

[28] Heffron JG, Emond JC, Whitington PF, et al. Biliary complications in pediatric liver transplantation: a comparison of reduced-size and whole grafts. Transplantation 1992;53:391–395.

[29] D'Alessandro AM, Kalayoglu M, Prisch JD, et al. Biliary tract complications after orthotopic liver transplantation. Transplant Proc 1991;23:1956–1990.

[30] Vallera RA, Cotton PB, Clavien P-A. Biliary reconstruction for liver transplantation and management of biliary complication: overview and survey of current practices in the United States. Liver Transplant Surg 1995;1:143–152.

[31] Egawa H, Uemoto S, Inomata Y, et al. Biliary complications in pediatric living related liver transplantation. Surgery 1998;124:901–910.

[32] Greif F, Bronsther OL, Van Thiel DH, et al. The incidence/timing, and management of biliary tract complications after orthotopic liver transplantation. Ann Surg 1994;219:40–45.

leaks and strictures, leaks after T-tube removal, leaks from T-tube exit sites, obstruction, and biliary fistula from stent migration.

Immunologic complications are more common after the initial hospitalization discharge. Rarely is any rejection seen in the immediate postoperative period (the so-called honeymoon phase), much as in a K Tx or a P Tx. However, up to 75% of patients will experience acute rejection after liver transplant.[33] Most often, the diagnosis is made after a trend of increasing liver function studies [alanine aminotransferase (ALT) and aspartate aminotransferase (AST)] necessitates a liver biopsy. Fortunately, **rejection easily is treated**, and, unlike in a K Tx in which an episode of early rejection is associated with decreased long-term graft survival, this has very little bearing on OLTX long-term survival.

Infectious complications also arise after the initial perioperative period. As the immunosuppression medications make the recipient more susceptible to a whole host of infectious agents—**bacterial, fungal, and viral**—lifelong vigilance is a priority. Infection continues to be the leading cause of death in liver transplant patients. Overall infection rates range from 60% to 80%.[34-36] Bacterial infections make up the majority of infections seen and are most common within the first month post-OLTX. Fungal infections are most commonly secondary to the *Candida* species and also most commonly occur within the first month post-OLTX. With respect to viral infections, much as with other organ transplants, cytomegalovirus (CMV) is the most common. Peak incidence is at 6 weeks. As a result of the high mortality associated with postoperative infections, all patients are placed on **preemptive antibiotics** immediately postoperatively. This often continues for many months after the initial transplant.

See **Algorithm 42.1** for an algorithm for postoperative monitoring.

Immunosuppression Protocols

Although the overwhelming majority of K Tx centers use induction immunosuppression therapy for their recipients, the opposite is true for OLTX centers, where **the overwhelming majority do not use induction therapy for their patients (Table 42.7)**. Induction therapy is defined as using polyclonal [ALG, antithymocyte globulin (ATG), thymoglobulin] or monoclonal (OKT3, Zenapax, Simulect) antibodies

[33] Wiesner RH, Demetris AJ, Belle SH, et al. Acute hepatic allograft rejection: incidence, risk factors, and impact on outcome. Hepatology 1998;28:638–645.

[34] The US Multicenter FK506 Liver Study Group. A comparison of tacrolimus (FK506) and cyclosporine for immunosuppression in liver transplantation. N Engl J Med 1994; 331:1110–1115.

[35] Whiting JF, Rossi SH, Hanto DW. Infectious complications after OKT3 induction in liver transplantation. Liver Transplant Surg 1997;3:563–570.

[36] Hadley S, Samore SH, Lewis WD, Jenkins RL, Karchmer AW, Hammer SM. Major complications after orthotopic liver transplantation and comparison of outcomes in patients receiving cyclosporine or FK506 as primary immunosuppresssion. Transplantation 1995; 59:851–859.

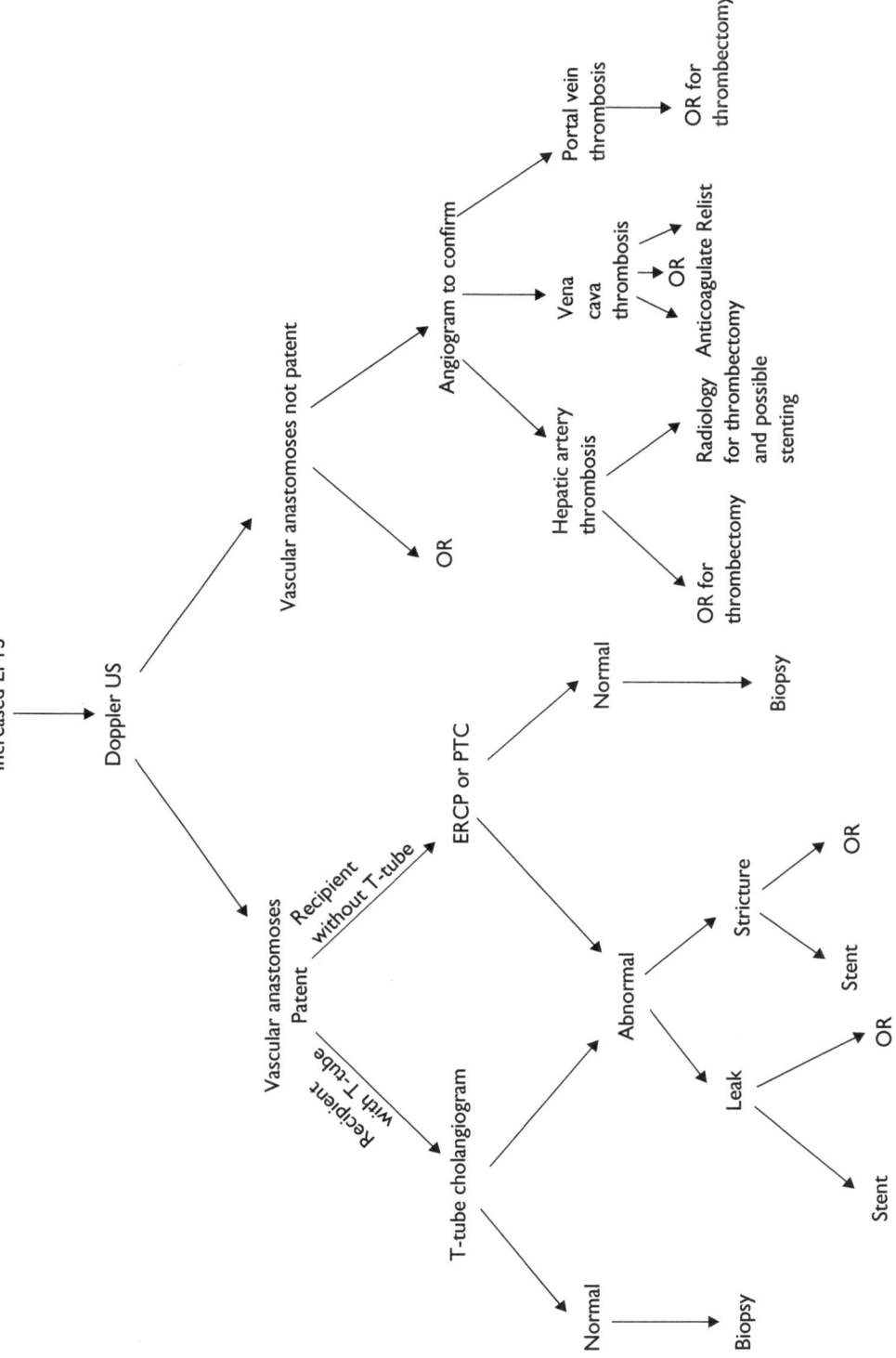

Algorithm 42.1. Algorithm for postoperative monitoring in liver transplantation. ERCP, endoscopic retrograde cholangiopancreatography; LFT, liver function test; OR, operating room; PTC, percutaneous transhepatic cholangiography; US, ultrasound.

Table 42.7. Immunosuppression use for induction, 1992 to 2001: recipients with liver transplants.

	Year of Transplant									
	1992	1993	1994	1995	1996	1997	1998	1999	2000	2001
Transplants	3064	3440	3652	3931	4077	4185	4503	4715	4962	5180
Tx with immunosuppression info	2497	2845	3093	3365	3484	3815	4083	4238	4668	4812
No induction drugs recorded	99.7%	99.3%	87.2%	86.2%	90.0%	93.0%	91.8%	87.4%	84.1%	84.8%
Drugs ALG	0.0%	0.0%	0.0%	0.0%	0.0%	—	—	—	—	—
ATG	0.2%	0.2%	4.3%	4.0%	3.6%	2.1%	1.1%	0.7%	0.6%	0.4%
NRATG/NRATS	—	—	—	—	0.0%	0.0%	0.0%	—	0.0%	—
OKT3	0.2%	0.5%	8.6%	10.0%	6.6%	4.9%	3.7%	1.5%	0.9%	0.7%
Thymoglobulin	—	—	—	—	—	—	0.1%	0.5%	1.2%	2.5%
Zenapax	—	—	—	—	—	0.0%	2.4%	6.2%	6.8%	5.9%
Simulect	0.0%	0.0%	0.0%	0.0%	0.0%	0.0%	1.0%	4.1%	6.8%	5.9%

ALG, antilymphocyte globulin; ATG, antithymocyte globulin; NRATG/NRATS, Nashville rabbit antithymocyte globulin/Nashville rabbit antithymocyte serum.
(—), drug not used anytime during the year.
Induction drugs include any reported antilymphocyte antibodies and antibodies directed against lymphocyte receptors.
Reprinted from www.transplant.org, on-line Annual Report, 2004. *Source:* OPTN/SRTR Data as of August 1, 2002.

prior to the recipient receiving the organ. As acute rejection does not appear to have any deleterious long-term impact on graft/patient survival in the OLTX patient, most liver transplant centers have not used induction therapy with its potential to decrease acute rejection, especially in the early postoperative period.

The advent of **cyclosporine (CSA)** in the late 1970s markedly increased patient and graft survival, and the later discovery of **Prograf/ tacrolimus (FK506)** added to the improved results.[37] Both drugs work to block T-cell activation primarily by inhibiting transcription of interleukin (IL)-2, IL-3, IL-4, and interferon-γ (IFN-γ). The newest form of CSA is **Neoral** and is dosed at 7 to 10 mg/kg/day in two divided doses, with a target range of 350 ng/mL. FK506 is dosed at 0.1 mg/kg/day, with a target range of 10 to 15 ng/mL.

Corticosteroids long have been part of every immunosuppression protocol for every center regardless of the organ transplanted. For many liver transplant centers, **steroids now are being phased out of the protocol** because of the deleterious long-term side effects associated with chronic steroid use and the better and stronger immunosuppression medications now available. One of the mainstay medications used in conjunction with Neoral or FK506 is **mycophenolate mofetil (MMF)**. This drug blocks proliferation of T and B lymphocytes and inhibits antibody formation and the generation of cytotoxic T cells. Usually administered as 1 g twice a day, no levels are checked. Instead, doses are lowered when toxicity occurs (usually in the form of diarrhea or nausea and vomiting).

Pediatric and Living Related Liver Transplant

The **indications for OLTX in children** differ from the indications for OLTX in adults (**Fig. 42.5**). **Biliary atresia** usually comprises 55% to 60% of the patients who receive pediatric OLTX. Unfortunately for the pediatric recipient, **finding an appropriately sized donor is more difficult**, since the pediatric cadaver donor pool is far smaller than the adult cadaver donor pool. In addition, **the percentage of cadaveric liver transplants going to pediatric patients decreased** from 15% in 1992 to 10% in 2000.[38] This is one of the reasons for the placement of the PELD score, and, in the year it was implemented, the percentage of cadaveric transplants going to pediatric recipients increased more than in any other year of the period (from 10.1% in 2000 to 10.5% in 2001).[38] Also, because of the low overall number of available organs for pediatric recipients, **living donor liver transplant (LDLT)** was a much more common procedure in the pediatric population proportionally than in the adult population. Usually this entails taking a small piece of the liver from an adult and placing it into the child. Most often, it is

---

[37] Jain B, Hamad I, Rakela J, et al. A prospective randomized trial of tacrolimus and prednisone versus tacrolimus, prednisone, and mycophenolate mofetil in primary adult liver transplant recipients. Transplantation 1998;66:1395–1398.

[38] Roberts JP, Brown RS, Edwards EB, et al. Liver and intestine transplantation. Am J Transplant 2003;3(suppl 4):78–90.

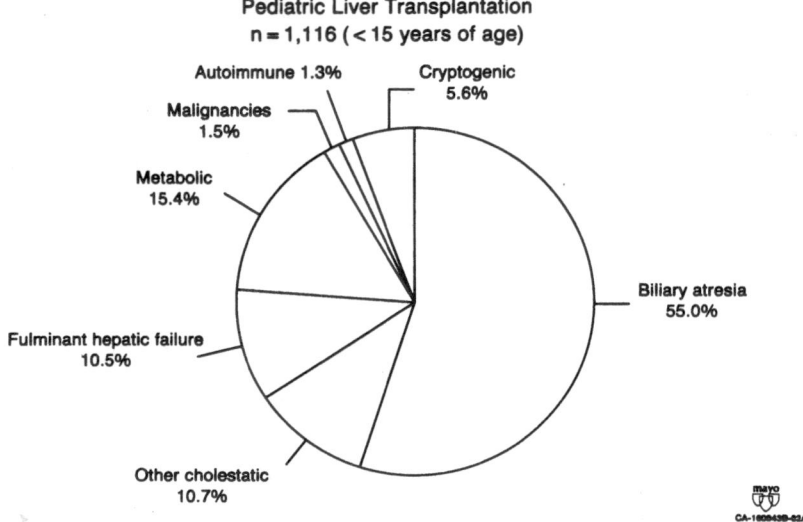

Pediatric Liver Transplantation
n = 1,116 (< 15 years of age)

Autoimmune 1.3%   Cryptogenic
                               5.6%
Malignancies
   1.5%

Metabolic
 15.4%

                                    Biliary atresia
                                       55.0%

Fulminant hepatic failure
        10.5%

Other cholestatic
     10.7%

Figure 42.5. Indications for liver transplantation in pediatric patients based on the Pitt-UNOS Liver Transplant Registry. (Reprinted from Busuttil RW, Klintmalm GB. Transplantation of the Liver. Philadelphia, W.B. Saunders Company, 1996. Copyright © Elsevier Inc. With permission from Elsevier. Data in Belle SH, Beringer KC, Murphy JB, et al. The Pitt-UNOS Liver Transplant Registry: Clinical Transplantation 1992.)

a parent-to-child donation, and, almost always, it is the left lateral segment of the left lobe of the parent that is used (**Fig. 42.6**). The 1-year graft and patient survival for pediatric OLTX are 81% and 89%, respectively, which are comparable to those for adult OLTX.[39] As is the case in kidney transplants in children, a pediatric specialist, in this case a **pediatric hepatologist,** is the key to success in the overall care of the pediatric recipient. Also, as is the case for kidney transplants in children, **a strong social situation** is crucial to the long-term success of the transplant process. The social services evaluation is vital to obtaining the pertinent information in order to help with the decision of whether or not a pediatric recipient is a suitable candidate.

The same lengthened waiting time and the mortality rate on the adult OLTX list produced a shift toward performing more LDLT in the adult recipient population as well (Fig. 42.7). This entails taking a much bigger piece of the liver, usually the whole right lobe, from the donor and anastomosing it into the recipient. As the technical difficulty of this procedure is great, the mortality and morbidity rates are noted to be as high as 0.5% and 14.5%, respectively.[40–42] Most of the compli-

[39] 2002 OPTN/SRTR Annual Report. Tables 10 and 11.

[40] Broering DC, Sterneck M, Rogiers X. Living donor liver transplantation. J Hepatol 2003;38:S119–S135.

[41] Renz JF, Roberts JP. Long-term complications of living donor liver transplantation. Liver Transplant 2000;6(6 suppl 2):S73–S76.

[42] Brown RS, Russo MW, Lai M, et al. A survey of liver transplantation from living adult donors in the United States. N Engl J Med 2003;348:818–825.

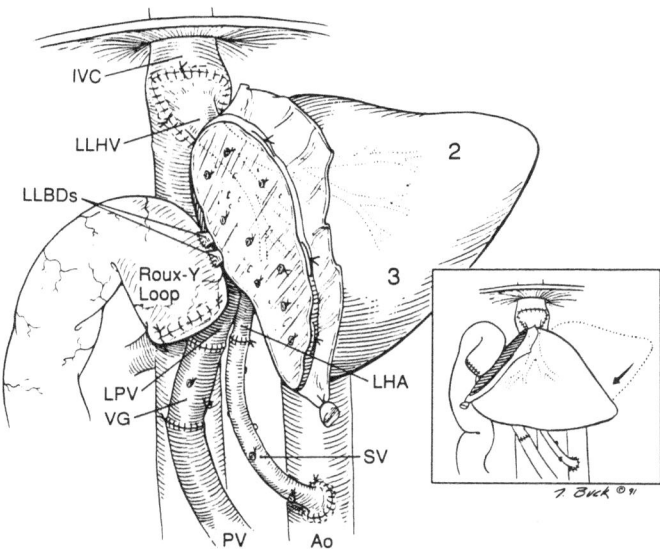

Figure 42.6. Living related donor left lateral segment after implantation. IVC, inferior vena cava; LLHV, left lateral hepatic vein; LLBDs, segment 2 and 3 bile ducts; LPV, left portal vein; VG, vein graft; LHA, left hepatic artery; SV, saphenous vein; PV, portal vein; Ao, aorta. Inset: Final position of the graft after abdominal closure. (Reprinted from Broelsch CE, Whitington PF, Emond JC, et al. Liver transplantation in children from living related donors. Surgical techniques and results. Ann Surg 1991;214:428–439. With permission from Lippincott Williams & Wilkins.)

cations are related to the donor biliary tract system. The number of LDLTs performed has doubled in the past 2 years, and this procedure now accounts for 10% of the transplants being performed.[43] Patient and graft survival for cadaver and living donor are noted in **Tables 42.8** and **42.9**. The trend in LDLT continues, and some have predicted that up to 30% of all OLTX will be using a living donor. As long as the shortage of donor liver organs exists, living donor and other ingenious methods to increase the donor pool will continue to evolve. Already at some

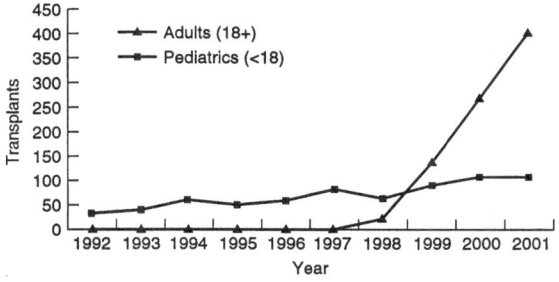

Figure 42.7. Living liver donor transplants, adults versus pediatrics, 1992–2001. (Reprinted from 2002 OPTN/SRTR annual report.)

---

[43] Roberts JP, Brown RS, Edwards EB, et al. Liver and intestine transplantation. Am J Transplant 2003;3(suppl 4):78–90.

Table 42.8. Graft survival and standard errors at 3 months, 1 year, 3 years, and 5 years; deceased donor liver transplants.

	3 Months			1 Year			3 Years			5 Years		
	n	%	Std. Err.	n	%	Std. Err.	n	%	Std. Err.	n	%	Std. Err.
Total	8735	85.8	0.4%	8735	80.2	0.4%	8191	71.4	0.5%	7630	63.5	0.6%

(+), values not determined due to insufficient follow-up; (–), values not determined since there were no transplants in the category.

Cohorts are transplants performed during 1999–2000 for 3-month and 1-year survival; 1997–1998 for 3-year survival; and 1995–1996 for 5-year survival.

Graft survival follows individual transplants until graft failure. Counts for patient and graft survival are different because a patient may have more than one transplant for a type of organ.

Center volume = Center's yearly transplants performed during the base period, based on liver transplants.

Multiorgan transplants are excluded.

Reprinted from www.transplant.org, on-line Annual Report, 2004. *Source:* OPTN/SRTR data as of August 1, 2002.

OLTX centers, single cadaver livers are being split into two so that instead of only one recipient for every one cadaver donor, there can be two recipients. The smaller left lateral segment goes into a child or into a small recipient, and the bigger, full-sized right lobe goes into an adult or into a larger recipient.

Summary

The face of liver transplant continues to evolve as human ingenuity attempts to catch up with the persistent organ shortage. Attempts at xenotransplantation and artificial livers or assist devices still are in progress. Much research has gone into growing hepatocytes to a state that they may someday save a human life, but, to date, this still is a theory and not reality. Stem cell research at this time is still that— research without any practical current use. As more and more centers start to perform LDLT, experience will accrue and benefit future patients. Currently, with the stagnant growth in the number of cadaver donors, living donation has been the lone bright spot for all of trans-

Table 42.9. Graft survival and standard errors at 3 months, 1 year, 3 years, and 5 years; living donor liver transplants.

	3 Months			1 Year			3 Years			5 Years		
	n	%	Std. Err.	n	%	Std. Err.	n	%	Std. Err.	n	%	Std. Err.
Total	605	83.0	1.6%	605	76.3	1.8%	170	72.4	3.5%	109	73.0	4.4%

(+), values not determined due to insufficient follow-up; (–), values not determined since there were no transplants in the category.

Cohorts are transplants performed during 1999–2000 for 3-month and 1-year survival; 1997–1998 for 3-year survival; and 1995–1996 for 5-year survival.

Graft survival follows individual transplants until graft failure. Counts for patient and graft survival are different because a patient may have more than one transplant for a type of organ.

Center volume = Center's yearly transplants performed during the base period, based on liver transplants.

Multiorgan transplants are excluded.

Reprinted from www.transplant.org, on-line Annual Report, 2004. *Source:* OPTN/SRTR data as of August 1, 2002.

plant, not just for OLTX. The improved results of laparoscopic donor nephrectomy have helped to increase the donor pool for the fortunate recipients with living donors. In much the same way, those patients who require OLTX and are fortunate enough to have a viable living donor now also can benefit greatly. The valuable experience of performing LDLT will only help upcoming patients. The hope is that, in the foreseeable future, LDLT will be accepted in much the same way as living donor kidney donation is accepted today.

Selected Readings

Busuttil RW, Klintmalm GB. Transplantation of the Liver. Philadelphia: WB Saunders, 1996.

Busuttil RW, Shaked A, Millis JM, et al. One thousand liver transplants: the lessons learned. Ann Surg 1994;219:490–499.

Ginns LC, Cosimi AB, Morris PJ. Transplantation. Malden, MA: Blackwell Science, 1999.

Hanto DW, Whiting JF, Valente JF. Transplantation of the liver and intestine. In: Norton JA, Bollinger RR, Chang AE, et al, eds. Surgery: Basic Science and Clinical Evidence. New York: Springer-Verlag, 2001.

Maddrey WC, Sorrell MF. Transplantation of the Liver, 2nd ed. Stamford, CT: Appleton and Lange, 1995.

Shaw BW Jr, Martin DJ, Marquez JM, et al. Venous bypass in clinical liver transplantation. Ann Surg 1984;200:524–534.

Stratta RJ, Wood RP, Langnas AN, et al. Diagnosis and treatment of biliary tract complications after orthotopic liver transplanation. Surgery 1989;106: 675–684.

Index